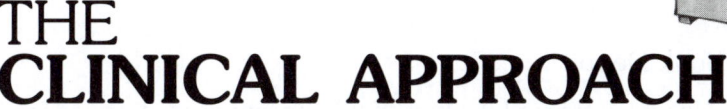

THE
CLINICAL APPROACH

A Companion for the Practising Doctor

R. D. LELE

M.B.B.S. (OSM.), DTM & H (ENG.),
MRCP (EDIN.), FRCP (LONDON),
FAMS (INDIA) HON. DSC. HON. D. LITT.

Hon. Consulting Physician & Director, Nuclear Medicine Dept.
Jaslok Hospital & Research Centre, Mumbai
Hon. Director of Nuclear Medicine & RIA Dept.
Lilavati Hospital & Research Centre (2002-2015)
Emeritus Professor of Medicine (for life) & Ex-Dean,
Grant Medical Collage & Sir J. J. Hospitals, Mumbai
Emeritus Professor of the
National Academy of Medical Sciences, India
Chairman, Research Advisory Committee,
Halfkine Institute of Research
Training & Testing, Mumbai.

Fourth Edition

www.nationalbookdepot.com

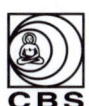

CBS Publishers & Distributors Pvt Ltd.

THE
CLINICAL APPROACH
A Companion for the Practising Doctor

Second Edition	-	2007
Third Edition	-	2015
Fourth Edition	-	2019

Published by
Vaidehi Shah Sanghavi for
The National Book Depot
Opp. Wadia Children's Hospital, Parel, Mumbai - 400 012.
Tel : (+91-22) 2416 5274 / 2413 1362 / 2413 2411 | Fax : 2413 0877
E-mail: nationalbook55@gmail.com
www.nationalbookdepot.com

and

Satish Kumar Jain
CBS Publishers & Distributors Pvt Ltd
4819/XI Prahlad Street, 24 Ansari Road, Daryaganj, New Delhi - 110 002.
Ph: 23289259 / 23266861 / 23266867 | Fax: 011-23243014
E-mail: delhi@cbspd.com; cbspubs@airtelmail.in
www.cbspd.com

ISBN : 978-93-80206-98-1

Printed by : Neel Graphics

PREFACE TO FIRST EDITION

There is growing criticism worldwide that the practice of medicine has become ädehumanizedí and highly ätechnology-orientedí, which on the one hand ignores the patient as a person and on the other makes medical care more expensive.

This book is an answer to that criticism. It emphasizes the role of history taking and physical examination, the two powerful tools available to every doctor, with which over 90 per cent of patientsí problems can be satisfactorily resolved. The WHO has determined that about 80 per cent of illness is behaviorally related. People are often harassed, worried, anxious, afraid, and seek help and reassurance. A kind and attentive doctor who is willing to spare time to listen to them and reassure them, is the most effective therapy. Thereby a lot of costly and unnecessary investigations can be avoided.

The aim of the book is to provide a core knowledge base which enables the doctor to make a proper analysis of patientsí symptoms and suggests the choice of crucial question to be asked for such an analysis. The 238 tables and 33 figures in this book make that task easy.

The book emphasizes the thoughtful and costeffective use of laboratory tests, and the right choice of tests. The ability to make optimal use of laboratory tests needs to be developed as carefully as the other clinical skills required for good practice of medicine. The entire point is how not to miss a treatable condition or a potentially serious and life-threatening condition.

An important feature of the book is the importance it gives to the role of the practising doctor as teacher-to educate patients and their families for the promotion of positive health and the prevention of sickness. The book illustrates the wide spectrum of patient care-primary prevention, secondary prevention, curative, supportive and symptomatic treatment, and rehabilitation. It describes how periodic health checks and health education can be practised very effectively by doctors as part of their professional obligations.
The book is organized in four sections.

Section I: Practice of Medicine, contains two chapters

(1) Clinical Competence

(2) Body-Mind Relationship

Section II: Emergency Medicine (chapters 3-22) contains headings arranged in alphabetical order to facilitate easy access.

Section III: General Medical Problems (chapters 23-52) contains 30 headings, again in alphabetical order.

Section IV: Special Topics (chapters 53-55) deals with Medical Oncology, Multi-System, Multi-Organ Diseases and Adverse Drug Reactions.

A list of 238 tables and 33 figures, numbered chapterwise, will allow quick access to relevant ∑nformation for the problem on hand.

It is presumed that the reader already has access to standard textbooks of medicine. I recommend that he or she uses this book as a constant companion. After reading the first and fourth sections at one stretch, the rest of the sections may be read as and when the clinical problems arise. It is the authorís hope that this companion for the practising doctor will make him or her more competent and more vigilant in the care of his patient.

R. D. LELE

PREFACE TO THE FOURTH EDITION

The tremendous popularity of the 3rd edition (2015) which is all sold out has prompted me to trying out a 4th edition. A new chapter no 62 added - prevention is better and cheaper than cure, includig a Table 1 describing the full scope of prevention including primary and secondary prevention and the scope of curative measures, supportive measures and symptomatic measures.

Table 2 describes promotive and preventive care and health education provided by the family physician.

The last chapter 63 Mobile Smart Phones Revolution in health care have an added new section initiative for mother and child healthcare.

In India 60% pregnant women are devoid of healthcare facilities. In 2014 Aditya Kulkarni, working in science for society developed a **Care Mother Kit** for estimation of Hb, urine proteins, weight, fetal heart sounds total nine parameters giving results in a few minutes. He developed an AP through which patients reports are communicated to the doctor almost instantaneously enabling timely medical care. In 2015 this was test in Aurangabad and Govandi near Mumbai with great success. This has now reached 9 states through 15 institutions, benefiting 30,000 pregnant women. It is hoped to reach 1.5 lakh pregnant women by 2020. In july 2018 Aditya Kulkarni was felicitated by Queen Elizabeth at the Buckingham Palace, for this achievement. Care nx.

R. D. LELE

CONTENT

SECTION - IV SPECIAL TOPICS

PRACTICE OF MEDICINE

1   Clinical Competence

When caring for a sick person, the doctor has to consider the following four questions:

What is wrong?	*Diagnosis*
What is going to happen?	*Prognosis*
What can be done?	*Treatment*
How did it happen?	*Aetiology, Pathophysiology*

From the viewpoint of the entire community, one more important question is:

Can it be prevented?	*Prophylaxis*

The cornerstone of the discipline of clinical medicine is the clinician's intellectual ability to conceptualize the normal and abnormal biological processes of the human body and mind, and the skills of clinical observation which lead to his ability to diagnose illness.

In the care of the patient, the clinician must continually make complex decisions, first for establishing the diagnosis and then for selecting appropriate therapy.

History taking and physical examination are the two powerful tools of the clinician. From the opening statement of the patient the clinician begins a process of conceptual thinking which leads to the formulation of hypotheses as to the nature of the problem. As data are accumulated and hypotheses become better defined, an efficient problem-solving approach leads to a reiterative, conscious matching of the information being elicited to the knowledge base stored in the clinician's memory. This matching process results in more directed data-gathering designed to confirm or refute the hypotheses. The aim of this book is to equip the doctor with a core knowledge base which enables him to formulate hypotheses, and choose key questions to pursue them. For example, when the patient presents with generalized oedema, likely initial hypotheses are that the problem is related to a cardiac, renal, hepatic or nutritional disease, or to hypothyroidism. Based on these hypotheses, a good doctor begins the diagnostic process by predicting findings that would be expected and directing his questions during his inquiry, his physical examination and his diagnostic procedures to check for the presence of the predicted findings; the outcome may support or refute the hypotheses, or may suggest a new hypothesis. This process continues till the medical problem is diagnosed. **Fig. 1.1** depicts the contribution of history, physical examination, and laboratory tests to the diagnostic process.

Analysis of Symptoms

Since symptoms call the patient's attention to his departure from health, the analysis of symptoms is the most challenging task before the clinician. Symptoms are meaningful to the extent that the doctor knows what significance to attribute to them. Since ancient times patients have been presenting to doctors with symptoms and signs as expressions of their illness. These presentations have not changed much over the centuries but our insights into what these represent have changed greatly. The clinician with the greatest insight into the pathophysiological processes of illness is best equipped to help the patient by providing a correct analysis and interpretation of symptoms and signs. While obtaining the history, the doctor tries to integrate symptoms into diagnostic hypotheses. He should recognize symptom patterns that suggest even low-frequency disease. This is where the expert does better than the general practitioner.

Generation and testing of hypotheses is constantly occurring in the doctor's mind as he is analysing symptoms. The number of hypotheses that can be generated is a function of the doctor's knowledge base. Two spectacular examples will illustrate this point.

All patients of primary hyperaldosteronism were initially labelled as 'hysterical' because their doctors could not find any apparent explanation for their weakness, flaccid paralysis and tetany. It was only in 1955 when Conn described the new syndrome that now goes by his name, that it was appreciated that the symptoms resulted from hypokalaemic alkalosis consequent on excessive potassium loss in the urine, under the influence of excessive aldosterone secretion by an adenoma from the adrenal cortex.

Before the clinical entity of acute intermittent porphyria was described by Waldenstrom and Goldberger in the 1940s, doctors misinterpreted the abdominal pain with which patients presented as perforated duodenal ulcer, appendicitis, biliary colic or renal colic, and consequently many unnecessary laparotomies resulted. This will continue to happen if the doctor's knowledge base is deficient. A doctor must have sufficient depth of knowledge that allows a thorough exploration of the symptoms relating to the patient's problem and that allows consideration of various aetiologies to explain the patient's symptoms. He must understand symptoms in terms of altered structure and function of body and mind, and must differentiate between symptoms that arise directly from a disease process and those that occur as a result of the body's response to disturbed homeostasis.

While this book emphasizes the proper analysis of symptoms, and suggests the choice of crucial questions to be asked for such an analysis, it is also necessary to appreciate the limitations of symptoms.

1. *Symptoms may be absent*
   Although it is common for disease processes to manifest themselves through symptoms, one should remember that for unexplained reasons, symptoms may be absent. Thus one encounters streptococcal tonsillitis without a sore throat, myocardial infarction without chest pain, 'silent ischaemia', 'silent thyroiditis', duodenal ulcer without peptic symptoms, viral hepatitis without jaundice, and diabetes mellitus without polyuria and polydipsia. Cirrhosis and chronic hepatitis can be totally asymptomatic during life and detected only at autopsy.

2. *Symptoms may be atypical*
   Instead of pain, the patient of ischaemic heart disease may complain of 'indigestion'; instead of epigastric pain, the duodenal ulcer patient may present with excessive watering of the mouth.

3. *Symptoms may be nonspecific*
   Anorexia, nausea and vomiting remind the doctor of possible gastrointestinal or hepatobiliary disease, but they may be the presenting symptoms of Addison's disease, chronic renal failure, hypercalcaemia or drug toxicity. Failure to remember these possibilities may lead the clinician astray. Fatigue may be a manifestation of several organic diseases as well as of mental disease.

4. *Identical symptoms*
   Hypokalaemia and hyperkalaemia both manifest the same symptoms–muscle weakness, and the same physical signs–loss of tendon reflexes and loss of muscle contraction on direct tapping. Their correct identification is made by considering the clinical setting in which they occur: vomiting, diarrhoea and diuretics provide the setting for hypokalaemia, while oliguria, anuria, crush injury and shock provide the setting for hyperkalaemia.

5. *Symptoms may remain unexplained*
   Many symptoms remain unexplained. Some people have a readiness to explain everything. Rather than adopt this self-satisfying approach, it may be better to record the fact as such– 'unexplained', or 'not understood', so that the door is still open for further inquiry.

Patient variables
Patients have different thresholds for defining themselves as sick. Symptoms which patients as well as doctors might consider as evidence of sickness are quite common in the general population. For example in a sample survey in London in a population pre-selected to be healthy, 90 per cent had headache or low backache. Social class, income, educational background and ethnic background are important determinants of whether a patient believes a symptom to represent a sickness. It may be perplexing why one patient is worried enough to seek advice while another has waited too long.

The WHO has determined that 80 per cent of problems which cause sickness are behaviourally related. Many patients seek medical care because they want to talk to someone who will hear about and sympathize with their problems. They may believe that the only 'admission ticket' to a doctor's consulting room is a physical problem, so they find one!

Other patients clearly have an illness but one which is so trivial and self-limiting that attention seems to be unnecessary from the doctor's point of view. They are harassed, worried and afraid, and seek reassurance to assuage their fears. The doctor should be sensitive to statements or symptoms which suggest psychosomatic or depressive illness. A kind and attentive doctor who is willing to spare time to listen to these patients is the most satisfactory therapy for them. Attentive listening and firm reassurance to such patients will avoid the employment of a large array of laboratory and radiological tests aimed at assuring the patient that he does not have any organic disease.

Some patients seek medical consultation not to get cured but to be defined as sick. Apart from direct financial benefits such as disability payment or compensation, 'sickness' may satisfy certain emotional needs such as dependency, or an excuse to avoid a stressful situation, or as a punishment for some guilt.

Patients may exaggerate or falsify symptoms in order to receive a particular treatment which they believe is indicated. At the other end of the spectrum is the psychological mechanism of denial which makes patients suppress their symptoms rather than seek help. The fear that their symptom may represent a serious or life-threatening disease (heart attack, HIV infection or cancer) and the fear that this will be confirmed if the doctor probes deeper into the problem, leads to a 'wishing away' attitude. Doctors themselves may show this attitude when it comes to their near relatives or themselves. Clinical detachment is not possible if the doctor is emotionally Involved in the patient's problems.

Skills in History Taking

History taking is not simply a question and answer session; it is a dialogue in which the doctor *listens with care* to what the patient is saying, *interprets* what the patient is trying to convey, *elicits* important and relevant information not volunteered by the patient and *ascertains* that the features the patient leaves unmentioned are indeed absent.

Often a symptom which has concerned the patient has little significance while a seemingly minor complaint may have considerable importance. Therefore the doctor should be constantly alert to the possibility that *any event* related to the patient and his family, however trivial or apparently remote may be the key to the solution of the medical problem.

History taking is not a one-time, circumscribed or isolated procedure. This information can be elicited during the physical examination, while reviewing laboratory test results, or later during the course of the illness. For example, finding a murmur of mitral stenosis prompts further questioning regarding previous sore throat or manifestations of rheumatic fever or paroxymal dyspnoea. Similarly, finding an apical lesion in the chest X-ray prompts re-questioning about symptoms referable to pulmonary tuberculosis.

Findings on the history and physical examination should influence each other. The history focuses the physical examination on certain organs, and findings on physical examination should encourage more detailed review of certain systems.

Clinical judgement is required to assess the reliability of the history obtained, to appropriately separate relevant from irrelevant information, and to identify information that seems incongruous with the clinical situation.

Understanding the Patient as a Person

An informative history is more than an orderly listing of symptoms; something is always gained by listening to patients and noting the way in which they talk about their symptoms. Inflections of voice, facial expression, and attitude may betray important clues to the meaning of the symptoms to the patient. They allow the doctor to evaluate the emotional status of the patient and to understand how the present problems fit into the context of the patient's social and family life. In listening to the history the physician discovers not only something about the disease but also something about the patient who has the disease. It is in obtaining the history that the physician's skill, knowledge and experience are most clearly in evidence.

The very act of taking the history provides the doctor with the opportunity to establish or enhance the unique bond that is the basis of the critically important doctor–patient relationship. Further, it helps develop an appreciation of the patient's own perception of the illness, his fears and concerns about the consequences of the illness to him and his family (fear of death, disability, loss of job etc.), the patient's expectations of the doctor and the medical care system, and the financial and social implications of the illness to the patient.

Physical and mental stress at home and at the workplace are important causes of ill-health. Stress-related disorders account for about one-third of health-care costs in developed countries. Helping to reduce stress at work (e.g. job insecurity, blocked promotion, coping with a bad boss, sexual harassment of female employees) or at home (marital problems, adolescent children) is an important area of preventive and social medicine. The family doctor can play an understanding and supportive role in helping the patient to cope with stress.

Personal and Social History

One gets immebse information by asking the patient to describe his married life, children, parents, friends, pets, association with social or charitable organizations, nature of job, hobbies, tobacco and alcohol, timmings of meal and sleep and excercise bowel habits, stress at work or at home etc.

Dieletic history is important - vegetarian or non-vagetarian, intake of fruits and vegetables.

Importance of family history

Many common and important diseases have a genetic component - such as hypertension, atherosclerotic Coronary Artery Disease, Type 2 Diabetes Mellitus, asthma many types of cancer and mental illness, thyroid disorders. These are polygenic in nature, involving interaction of multiple genes with environmental factors.

Single gene disorders (e.g. Hunlington's Disease β Thalassemia, sickle cell disease, hemophilia, muscular dystrophy, G6PD deficiency, cystic fibrosis, $\alpha 1$ antitrypsin deficiency) are also encountered especially in paediatric practice and account for upto 10 percent of paediatric admissions and childhood mortality.

Hence eliciting the family history is an important component of history taking. By questioning the patient and his relatives the clinician should ascertain the state of health of the first degree relatives- parents, siblings and off springs - since they share 50 percent of genes with the patient. If the findings suggest a genetic component the pedigree may be extended to several other family members (grand parents, maternal and paternal uncles and aunts, first cousins etc.). Family history should be recorded in the form of a pedigree, which helps to determine autosomal dominant and recessive, sex-linked dominant and recessive, and mitochondrial inheritance.

With this information the family physician can recognize the genetic components in his patients' problems and offer genetic counseling for carrier detection, early intervention and prevention of a disease in relatives of the index patient.

Importance of drug history

Eliciting a drug history from patients is extremely important, both for diagnosis and management of the patient's problem. The manifestations of drug-induced diseases frequently resemble those of other diseases, and a given set of manifestations may be produced by different and dissimilar drugs. Illness related to a drug's intended pharmacologic action is often more easily recognized (e.g. cardiac arrhythmias and digitalis, hypoglycaemia on insulin or oral sulfonylureas, and bleeding in patients on anticoagulants), than illness attributed to immune or other mechanisms, such as fever or rash which may be caused by many drugs. Many associations between particular drugs and specific reactions are described in the drug literature but there is always a "first time" for a previously undescribed association. Hence any drug should be suspect for causing an adverse reaction if the clinical setting is appropriate. (See also Chapter 55, Making Effective Therapy Safer).

Physical Examination

The findings on physical examination are less dependent on patient-generated variability than is the taking of medical history. However, the patient can still influence the conclusions of the doctor in certain instances such as eliciting tenderness over a painful region, or in sensory testing.

A doctor should be able to elicit subtle as well as obvious physical findings by inspection, palpation, percussion and auscultation, and be able to use appropriate instruments such as the ophthalmoscope, auroscope, tonometer and sigmoido-scope. When sufficient time is available, he should develop the habit of doing a complete physical examination unless inappropriate to the clinical situation. When hard-pressed for time, he should develop the skill of concentrating on *relevant* physical examination in the shortest possible time. He should undertake the physical examination with concern for the patient's comfort, privacy and sensitivity, forewarning the patient of uncomfortable or unanticipated manoeuvres. He should be able to modify physical examination procedures to adapt to particular medical situations. The pattern in a 30 minute consultation by appointment is quite different from that in a busy outpatient department where one cannot spare more than 2-3 minutes for the entire encounter. This requires more skill and efficiency than a leisurely consultation, and this skill can be developed by practice. Knowledge of anatomic relations, and knowledge of the physical and physiological mechanisms that produce normal and abnormal physical findings are essential for a proper physical examination. The doctor should understand and use physiological manoeuvres that can elicit findings that would otherwise not be apparent. He should know the range of normal variation of physical findings, and know alternative techniques capable of confirming abnormal findings. He should be able to integrate physical findings, normal or abnormal, with the diagnostic hypothesis suggested by history or other data. He should recognize patterns of findings that confirm diagnostic impressions or suggest new diagnostic possibilities.

Clinical judgement is required to be able to assess the clinical significance of physical signs. For instance, many round-faced, obese women with hairy upper lips may mimic Cushing's syndrome but their corticosteroid levels are normal. Clubbing of fingers may suggest serious diseases or it may be present in an entirely normal person.

Clinical judgement is also required to be able to determine the significance of borderline findings, and in the presence of multiple diseases, to assign findings to the appropriate disease process.

The doctor should be able to judge how often and to what extent a physical examination should be repeated on a given patient. Findings not present on the first examination may appear in a subsequent examination (e.g. pleural effusion, lymph node enlargement, skin rash, icterus etc.).

It is possible to over-interpret physical signs such as prolapsed mitral valve, café-au-lait spots, small degrees of stable scoliosis, umbilical hernia in infancy, Adie's pupil, or radiological signs like asymptomatic gallstones, colonic diverticulae, hiatus hernia, spondylosis, ptosis of a kidney etc.

Similarly, agenesis of a lobe of the thyroid, or a kidney or gallbladder may be misinterpreted as 'non-functioning' due to disease.

The imaging techniques of ultrasonography, CT and MRI have greatly enhanced the clinician's ability to detect mass lesions, but they can also create problems of 'incidentalomas' i.e. harmless lesions detected incidentally which could be misinterpreted as lesions producing the symptoms under scrutiny.

Effective Use of Laboratory Tests

The increase in the number and availability of laboratory tests has resulted in an increasing reliance by doctors on these tests for the solution of clinical problems. The impersonal quality and complexity of laboratory tests often give them an aura of authority regardless of the fallibility of the tests themselves, or of the individuals performing and interpreting the tests and of their instruments.

The clinician should understand the functions and limitations of the laboratory tests he employs. The ability to make effective use of laboratory tests should be developed as carefully as other clinical skills required for good practice of medicine. A thoughtful and cost-effective use of laboratory tests is the hallmark of clinical competence. Unintelligent use of laboratory tests is wasteful of time and money and can be harmful to the patient if the tests are invasive; hence doctors should weigh carefully the hazards and expenses in the laboratory tests they order. The question of risks versus benefits concerns medical ethics; the question of cost versus benefits concerns medical economics.

Laboratory tests can be employed for various purposes, as summarized in **Table 1.1**.

In making a choice of a diagnostic laboratory test, the doctor should consider the following:

1. How likely is the disease in question?

2. What would be the clinical consequences if (a) the diagnosis was *missed* (type I or alpha error), or (b) if the patient was mistakenly treated for a disease that was not present (type II or beta error)?

3. What is the likelihood that the test result will change the probability sufficiently to influence either the diagnosis or therapy? e.g. frozen section report determines the extent of surgery to be done–lumpectomy or radical mastectomy).

Table 1.1 CLINICAL USES OF LABORATORY TESTS

I. *Screening tests*

    A. *Healthy subjects:*

        Donors of blood: ABO Rh, hepatitis, HIV, syphilis.

        Donors of organs: tissue typing, infection screening.

        Part of periodic health check up.

    B. *Patients:* as part of initial evaluation and baseline data.

II. *Diagnostic tests*

    To confirm or to exclude diagnosis based on the hypothesis formed by history and physical examination. Here considerations of sensitivity, specificity, predictive value and efficiency of tests are important.

III. *Monitoring the response to treatment*

    ESR in rheumatic fever, tuberculosis etc.: indicator of improvement or exacerbation.

    Reticulocyte count following iron, B12, folic acid, pyridoxine therapy: predictor of beneficial response prospectively.

    Serial liver function tests during the course of viral hepatitis.

    Serial BUN/Creatinine following renal transplantation. Serial testing of glycosylated Hb in patients with diabetes mellitus.

IV. *Selection of appropriate therapy*

    Culture and sensitivity tests for antimicrobial drug therapy.

    Procalcitonin CD

    PET Fluorine-18 Deoxyglucose imagine for viable myocardium before revascularization procedures.

V. *Tests for avoiding potential harm*

    Allergy testing: penicillin, iodine contrast dyes.

    G-6-PD deficiency test: before giving certain drugs.

VI. *Monitoring drug therapy and toxicity*

    Prothrombin time: during anticoagulant therapy.

    Liver function tests: during INAH/Rifampicin therapy for tuberculosis.

    Cardiac function (EF): during adriamycin therapy. Bone marrow function: during cytotoxic drug therapy in cancer.

    Drug levels : digoxin, dilantin, cyclosporine

    Procalcitonin CD

VII. *Genetic Tests for prenatal diagnosis*

    e.g. neural tube defects, Trisomy

    1. Non-invasive   :   Serum AFP, β HCG, PAPPA

                               Ultra sonography MRI

    2. Invasive   :   Amniocentesis chorion villus biopsy foetal blood sampling fetoscopy

VIII. *Other Specific Uses :*

    Potency Test

    Legal evidence in rape, homicide, dispute paternity.

    Environmental and microbiological surveillance e.g. Hospital Infection, Water pollution, Air pollution.

4. What is the likelihood, risk and cost of obtaining *new information* from the test, weighed against the adverse consequences of delaying the test (wait and watch approach)?

An ideal test would establish the presence or absence of disease in every individual who is tested. Unfortunately such a test does not exist hence one has to consider the *sensitivity* (positivity in disease) and *specificity* (negativity in health), of every test.

If a test gives a positive result in all patients having the disease, the sensitivity of the test is described as 100 per cent.

If a test gives a negative result in all those who are free from the disease being tested for, the specificity of the test is described as 100 per cent.

Unfortunately no test has these ideal attributes; hence we have *false negatives* if sensitivity is less (α error) and *false positives* if specificity is less (β error). The *predictive value* of a test tells us how accurately a test result indicates the presence of disease if positive (positive predictive value), or the absence of disease if the test result is negative (negative predictive value).

The predictive value is determined by the complex interaction of 3 variables–*sensitivity, specificity* of the test, and *prevalence* of the disease being tested in the population.

Imagine a test with 95 per cent sensitivity and 95 per cent specificity, which may therefore be considered as a good test, yet its predictive value would vary according to the prevalence of the disease being tested for, as shown below:

Prevalence	Predictive value of positive test
0.1%	1.9%
1%	16.1%
2%	27.9%
5%	50.0%
50%	95.0%

In effect, the clinician is constantly endeavouring to *increase the prevalence* of the condition he is suspecting in the patient before deciding the choice of the diagnostic test. For instance, a history of sexual contact has 100 per cent sensitivity for venereal disease. Without sexual contact venereal disease probably cannot occur. Hence in a patient who gives a history of sexual contact, the predictive value of a positive test result for STD is 95 per cent and the predictive value of a negative test result is also high.

In contrast if an unscreened general population is subjected to the same test, the predictive value will be very low because of the low prevalence of that disease in the population.

Similarly a history of blood transfusion, intramuscular injections or IV drug abuse increases the probability of a patient having viral hepatitis or HIV.

A history of substernal pain aggravated by effort and relieved by rest/nitroglycerin increases the prevalence of ischaemic heart disease in the patient being tested; a history of substernal pain aggravated by bending forward increases the prevalence of oesophageal reflux in the patient being tested, so that the predictive value of the appropriate tests done for the two conditions would be very high, more than 95 per cent. The entire thrust of this book is to enable the clinician to make the right choice of questions to be asked to the patient and to elicit the crucial physical signs to increase the probability of the disease under consideration, so that the appropriate tests done on them will have a high predictive value. Laboratory tests should be hypothesis-directed, and not merely 'fishing nets'. This is the best approach to achieve cost containment of medical investigations, at the same time ensuring optimal care.

Right choice of test

Some general guidelines are given below for selecting tests with high sensitivity, high specificity, high predictive value, and high efficiency (highest number of true positive and true negative results).

In general, highly sensitive tests are very useful in *excluding* a diagnosis, and highly specific tests are very useful in *establishing* a diagnosis.

Highest sensitivity (preferably 100 per cent) is desired when

1. the disease is *serious* and should not be missed,
2. the disease is *treatable,*
3. false positive results do not cause serious physical, psychological or economic harm to the patient.

Examples: nutritional disorders, endocrine disorders, treatable infections.

Pheochromocytoma and insulinoma are very rare, but nearly 100 per cent curable if diagnosed, and may be fatal if missed, hence a highly sensitive test like I-123 MIBG scintigraphy is more reliable than VMA/catecholamine estimation in urine and plasma to exclude the possibility of pheochromocytoma; and insulin and C-peptide estimation during prolonged fasting (upto 72 hours) is sensitive enough to exclude insulinoma.

Highest specificity (preferably 100 per cent) is desired when

1. the disease is serious, but not treatable/curable,
2. the knowledge that the disease is absent has high psychological or public health value,
3. false positive results can cause serious physical, psychological or social damage.

Examples: HIV infection, multiple sclerosis (MS), occult cancers. One does not accept any false positives, therefore one opts for the highest possible specificity. If any case of MS is missed, there is no disaster, because the patient will return. On the other hand, false positive diagnosis can cause serious psychological harm and agony to the patient and her family. Similarly a test for lung cancer should have highest specificity possible, since no surgeon or radiotherapist wishes to treat a false positive case. Lobectomy or radiation therapy in a person without cancer can have disastrous consequences.

Highest efficiency (true positive plus true negative) is desired in the following situations:

1. The disease is *serious but treatable.*
2. False positive and false negative results are equally serious or damaging.

Example: Acute myocardial infarction and unstable angina. These conditions are potentially fatal but treatable. Equal harm can be done if the diagnosis is missed, or if a diagnosis is made wrongly and anticoagulant or thrombolytic therapy is given. Therefore one opts for tests with the maximum efficiency (e.g. coronary angiography and radionuclide tests for myocardial necrosis/viability and myocardial function.)

Importance of Time-trend Information

Review of previous data is as important as collecting new data. For instance, a patient presenting with shortness of breath and weakness has a blood pressure noted as 135/85. If a previous record of blood pressure was observed to be 190/110 and the patient has not been taking any hypotensive drugs, the clinician would wonder why, and search for further clues in the history e.g. a recent silent myocardial infarction or a gastrointestinal blood loss, or adrenal insufficiency.

Similarly, a single report of Hb 13.5 g does not tell the doctor much, but if a previous report documented the patient's Hb as 15.5 g, this may raise the question of a recent blood loss or a recent attack of malaria. A report of Hb 10 g per cent will have a different interpretation if it is known that all previous reports over a 10 year period never exceeded 10 g per cent, suggestive of a thalassaemia trait.

Recording the weight of the patient at one point of time is not as informative as weight gain or loss over a period of time.

The interpretation of a single 'coin lesion' in a recent chest X-ray would be drastically altered if a previous chest X-ray 5 years back also showed the same lesion.

Causes of Diagnostic Errors

1. Data concerning the patient's illness may be *incomplete*, that is, insufficient manifestations have been elicited to permit definition of the patient's syndrome.
2. Data may be *incorrect*, leading to the construction of an erroneous syndrome.
3. The clinician may consider various manifestations only as *isolated* phenomena rather than as parts of a syndrome (e.g. polyarteritis nodosa, SLE and other multisystem/multiorgan diseases; See also Chapter 54).
4. The doctor's medical *knowledge* may be *incomplete* that is, he may not be sufficiently familiar with the frequency of particular syndromes in a particular disease, or with the variability of syndromes in a particular disease (e.g. disseminated intravascular coagulation in septicaemia).

5. The doctor may not consider certain diseases, or may be unaware of the particular incidence of certain diseases in the population of which the patient is a sample, e.g. HIV infection, malaria, filariasis, schistosomiasis.

6. The doctor may not systematically follow the diagnostic leads obtained during the eliciting of the history of the present illness, or during the physical examination and ancillary examinations, for the purpose of eliminating possibilities, e.g. absent radial pulse.

7. The doctor may ignore the necessity of making a positive effort to reduce the probability of all other diseases as sources of the illness, that is, he is not sufficiently thorough and comprehensive in using his screening questions, general physical examination and ancillary examinations effectively for the process of eliminating possibilities.

8. Instead of using a systematic and logical approach, the doctor uses an unthinking approach that is at best inefficient and costly, and at worst ineffective. Three illustrative examples will bring home the point.

Hepatoma

A rich businessman from Indonesia came to Bombay for a holiday. After eating *bhelpuri* and *chaat* at Juhu beach he got loose motions for which he consulted a gastro-enterologist who had recently acquired modern ultrasonography equipment. The doctor did an ultrasonographic study of the patient's abdomen (for reasons which could only be guessed) and found a 'mass lesion' in the liver, for which the patient was promptly referred for a CT scan. The CT study showed an 'enhancing lesion' on contrast injection, suggesting a diagnosis of 'hepatoma'. Totally in panic, the patient came to me for a second opinion. The key elements in the history and physical examination that made the diagnosis of 'hepatoma' most unlikely were: previous and present good health; no history of viral hepatitis; good appetite; steady weight; feeling very active and energetic; no enlargement or tenderness of the liver; no stigmata of cirrhosis or alcohol abuse; system review entirely normal.

Based on the *clinical assessment* the probability of this 'highly vascular enhancing mass lesion in the liver' being a hepatoma was very low and the alternative probability of a benign haemangioma was very high. This was confirmed by a Tc-99m RBC blood pool scan of the liver (blood pool in the lesion showing rising count rate between the initial 5 minute and the 30 minute and 2 hour images). The patient was reassured that this was a benign lesion to be left entirely alone. Any attempt to biopsy this lesion 'to confirm hepatoma' could have been disastrous.

Hyponatraemia

A young lady doctor who was feeling chronically tired had an SMA/12-60 test done for further evaluation. Seeing the report of low serum sodium (120 mEq/L) she was convinced that she had Addison's disease. The key elements in the history and physical examination were: steady weight; no abdominal pain, nausea, vomiting or diarrhoea; regular periods; she could stand prolonged religious fasts without getting hypoglycaemic; no previous history of tuberculosis or auto-immune disease; she was well hydrated; blood pressure recumbent and standing both 130/80; her urine output was adequate; she was mentally alert; she was taking neither diuretics nor any drugs which could have produced inappropriate ADH secretion (dilutional hyponatraemia). Based on this assessment I suggested to her that the serum sodium report could be wrong and should be rechecked, and that she did not have Addison's disease. The repeat sodium report was normal.

Malignant Cells in Sputum

A middle aged lawyer had to cut short his visit to the USA since he developed fever and cough, followed by pericardial effusion, and he did not have insurance cover to get investigated in the USA. The patient was admitted to hospital under my care and the pericardial effusion on tapping was found to be haemorrhagic in nature. CT scan of the thorax did not show any hilar, mediastinal or retropericardial lymph nodes. Bronchoscopy did not reveal any neoplasm but bronchial aspirate showed 'abnormal cells consistent with malignancy'. Pericardial biopsy did not show any evidence of tuberculosis or malignancy. There was no clinical or laboratory evidence of Hodgkin's disease, lymphoma or SLE. His subsequent course was uneventful recovery, but what about the malignant cells in the bronchial washings? A review of the literature indicated that respiratory viral infections can occasionally cause haemorrhagic pericarditis, and can cause metaplasia in the bronchial mucosal cells leading to the appearance of malignant cells. This fact was brought to the notice of the pathologist who agreed with the alternative explanation. Follow-up of five years has confirmed that interpretation.

The moral of these three stories is that the clinician is in the driver's seat and he should do the driving. He should never blame the colleagues who carry out ancillary investigations for misleading him, because he knows the total picture which they do not.

The most common causes of errors in diagnosis are summarized in **Table 1.2**.

TABLE 1.2 MOST COMMON CAUSES OF ERROR IN DIAGNOSIS

Lack of knowledge of disease patterns
- Newly discovered diseases.
- Rare diseases.
- Rare manifestations of common diseases. Ebola, H1N1

Lack of skill in eliciting a good history
- Symptoms not identified.
- Crucial questions not asked.

Lack of skill in physical examination
- Signs not looked for.
- Signs not identified.
- Signs misinterpreted.

Lack of hypothesis-directed approach to diagnostic tests
- Not integrating test results with clinical assessment.
- Using diagnostic tests as 'fishing nets' without knowledge of sensitivity and specificity of diagnostic test and prevalence of the disease being tested for.
- Not knowing normal variations and artefacts.

Therapy

Effective patient care depends upon the quality of diagnostic work-up and the quality of therapeutic management.

After a diagnosis is reached, knowledge of the disease process must be integrated with the knowledge about the patient as a person, and his environment, in order to develop an optimal plan of treatment, taking into account the patient's psychological and socio-economic factors. As the response to therapy is observed, a need to acquire additional data, change the diagnostic hypothesis, or alter therapy may become apparent. The doctor has to constantly relate and integrate observed findings to his knowledge gained previously through education and experience. The acquisition and maintenance of the knowledge base has to be a continuing, life-long endeavour.

To know the most effective therapies available for the patient's problem, to know the correct procedure for instituting the indicated therapies, to know the inter-drug reactions and drug toxicity, to know the need to modify drug therapy in the presence of specific organ dysfunction, are all extremely demanding tasks. Considering the flood of new powerful drugs that is constantly engulfing them, many conscientious doctors might find themselves increasingly deficient in these tasks. This book provides the relevant information in a handy manner, which will hopefully inspire more confidence, as well as more vigilance in patient care.

Over-use and mis-use of antimicrobial drug.

The wide spectrum of patient care is listed in **Table 1.3**.

Rehabilitation is an integral part of medical care. It is the combined and coordinated use of medical, social, educational and vocational measures for training or retraining the individual to the highest possible level of functional activity, and enabling the disabled or handicapped to achieve social integration. Change of profession to a more suitable one or modification of lifestyle in general e.g. for the cardiac patient, may be required. Patient education is an important function of doctors. This has been emphasized in the sections on management of diabetes and stroke.

The doctor has an important role in the community as one who promotes positive health and prevents disease. This role is quite distinct from the care of the sick, but equally important in the interest of the community. **Table 1.4** gives a list of periodic health examinations of healthy people and patient education which all doctors can do very effectively as part of their professional obligations. It is worth remembering that the word 'doctor' is derived from the Latin *docere*: to teach.

TABLE 1.3 THE WIDE SPECTRUM OF PATIENT CARE

A. *Scope of primary prevention*

Advice and guidance for the following:

1. Nutrition: calories, protein, minerals (iron, iodine, calcium) vitamins A, D, essential fatty acids, green vegetables and fruits.
2. Mother and child care: family planning advice.
3. Immunization against major infectious diseases.
4. Abstinence from tobacco, alcohol and narcotic drugs.
5. Regular physical exercise and weight control.
6. Safe sex (use of condoms) for avoidance of HIY.
7. Safety measures in homes, workplaces, roads, beaches, to prevent accidents, and environmental pollution. Use of safety belts in cars; helmets for motorcyclists and scooterists.

B. *Scope of secondary prevention*

1. Penicillin prophylaxis to prevent rheumatic valvular disease.
2. Control of hypertension to prevent its complications.
3. Control of diabetes mellitus to prevent its complications.
4. Aspirin in TIA (transient ischaemic attacks to prevent strokes.
5. Anticoagulant and thrombolytic therapy in acute myocardial infarction and ischaemic strokes to prevent further damage to the myocardium and the brain.
6. Revascularization and angioplasty: heart, kidney, peripheral vessels.

C. *Scope of curative measures*

1. Infections: Antimicrobial therapy; Immunoglobulins, antivenins.
2. Replacement of deficient nutrients and hormones; correction of excess nutrients and hormones.

3. Surgical removal of tumours: removal of foreign bodies and obstructions; organ transplants; prostheses and implants, plastic and reconstructive surgery, restoration of severed limbs.
4. Desensitization of allergic patients.
5. Desensitization of phobic patients.
6. Gene therapy (futuristic).

D. *Scope of supportive measures*

1. Restoration of circulating volume: blood, plasma, plasma expanders, saline.
2. Restoration of electrolytes and acid-base equilibrium.
3. Maintenance of ventilation and circulation.
4. Measures to reduce cerebral oedema.
5. Haemodialysis and peritoneal dialysis; haemoperfusion.
6. Plasmapheresis.
7. Immuno-modulators, immunostimulants, immunosuppressors.

E. *Scope of symptomatic measures*

1. Pain relief: analgesics, antispasmodics, antacids, antianginal drugs.
2. Sedatives and hypnotics.
3. Anxiety-reducing drugs.
4. Anti-depressants.
5. Anti-convulsants.
6. Anti-tussive drugs; bronchodilators.
7. Diuretics for oedema.
8. Laxatives for constipation.
9. Anti-emetic drugs.
10. Anti-allergic and anti-inflammatory drugs.

F. *Rehabilitation*

1. Medical rehabilitation.
2. Vocational rehabilitation.
3. Social rehabilitation.
4. Psychological rehabilitation.

TABLE 1.4 RECOMMENDED PERIODIC HEALTH EXAMINATIONS AND PATIENT EDUCATION

Pregnancy

Weight, Hb, BP, urine examination for albumin and sugar.
Prenatal care.
Supplement of iron, folic acid, calcium.

Newborn

Detection and treatment of birth defects.
Neonatal hypothyroidism screen (TSH).
Neonatal jaundice (Rh, viral hepatitis, HIV).
Immunization.

Childhood

Height-weight charts to monitor growth.
Records of milestones:
Detection of mental retardation.
Dental care: caries, orthodontic conditions.
Booster dose of immunization.
Refractive errors: squint.
Hearing defects.

Adolescence

Sex education: awareness about STD and HIV.
Avoidance of teenage pregnancy.
Health-related behaviour: alcohol, drugs, smoking.
Prevention of vehicular accidents.
Emotional support: broken families.

Adult life

Training for parenthood and family planning.
Family dysfunction: marital and sexual problems.
Guidance on health-related behaviour:
    exercise, weight control
    alcohol
    tobacco smoking
Coping with stress: Relaxation techniques
Early detection of high BP, diabetes, hyper-cholesterolaemia and hyperlipidaemia.
Early detection of ischaemic heart disease in high-risk groups.

Middle age

Females:	Prevention of osteoporosis.
	Self-examination of breasts.
	Papanicolaou smears.
Males:	Rectal examination for prostate.
	Stools for occult blood.
Both sexes:	'Empty nest syndrome'.
	Joint families: closing generation gap.
	Coping with progressive incapacity of old age. Loneliness, Memory Loss, frequent falls, fractures.

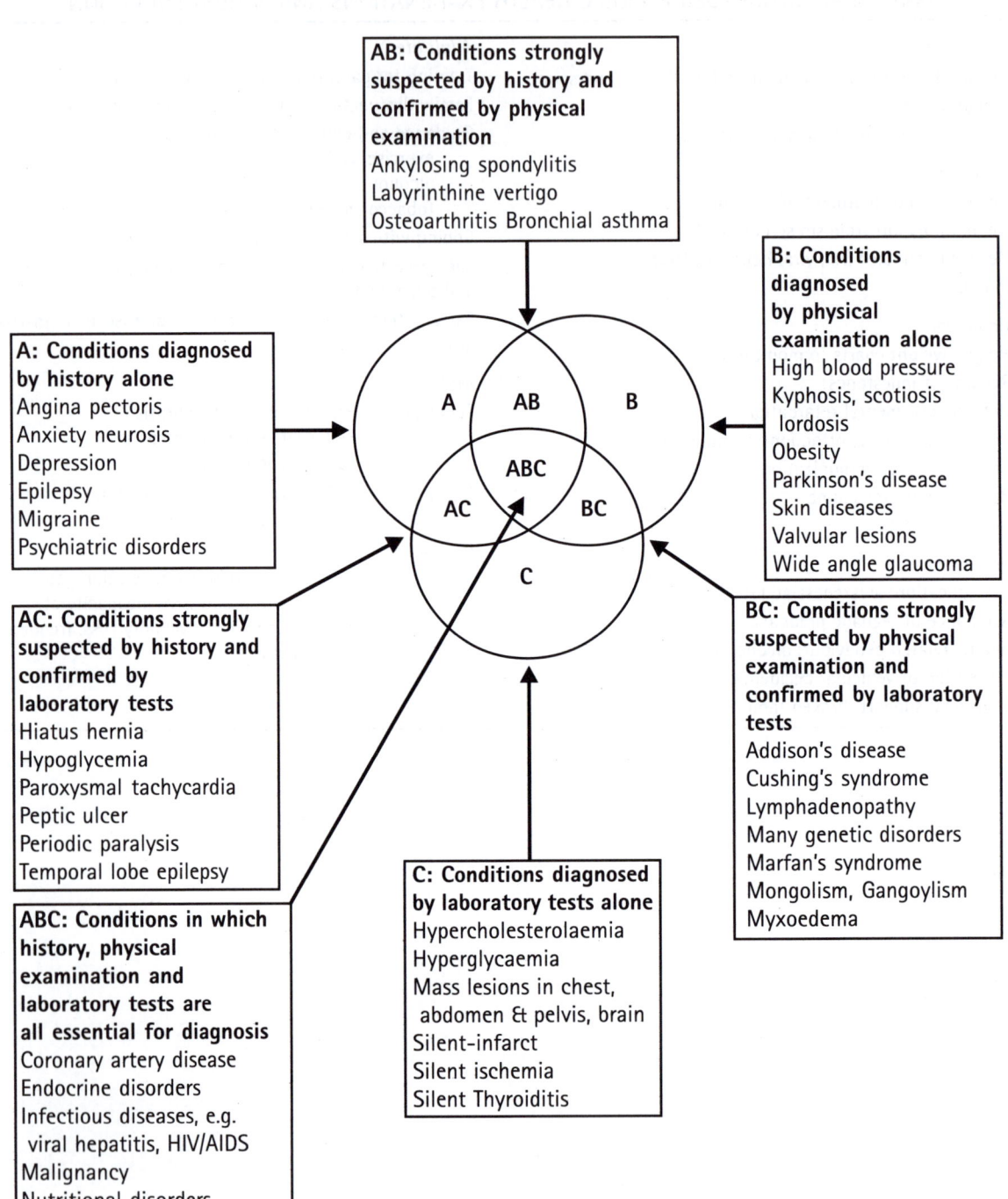

AB: Conditions strongly suspected by history and confirmed by physical examination
Ankylosing spondylitis
Labyrinthine vertigo
Osteoarthritis Bronchial asthma

B: Conditions diagnosed by physical examination alone
High blood pressure
Kyphosis, scotiosis lordosis
Obesity
Parkinson's disease
Skin diseases
Valvular lesions
Wide angle glaucoma

A: Conditions diagnosed by history alone
Angina pectoris
Anxiety neurosis
Depression
Epilepsy
Migraine
Psychiatric disorders

AC: Conditions strongly suspected by history and confirmed by laboratory tests
Hiatus hernia
Hypoglycemia
Paroxysmal tachycardia
Peptic ulcer
Periodic paralysis
Temporal lobe epilepsy

BC: Conditions strongly suspected by physical examination and confirmed by laboratory tests
Addison's disease
Cushing's syndrome
Lymphadenopathy
Many genetic disorders
Marfan's syndrome
Mongolism, Gangoylism
Myxoedema

ABC: Conditions in which history, physical examination and laboratory tests are all essential for diagnosis
Coronary artery disease
Endocrine disorders
Infectious diseases, e.g. viral hepatitis, HIV/AIDS
Malignancy
Nutritional disorders

C: Conditions diagnosed by laboratory tests alone
Hypercholesterolaemia
Hyperglycaemia
Mass lesions in chest, abdomen & pelvis, brain
Silent-infarct
Silent ischemia
Silent Thyroiditis

Fig. 1.1: The contribution of history, physical examination and laboratory tests to the diagnostic process (illustrative examples)

2   Body–Mind Relationship

The World Health Organization (WHO) has defined health as 'a state of complete physical, mental and social well-being and not merely the absence of disease or infirmity'. Further, mental health has been defined as 'the full and harmonious functioning of the whole personality'. In the words of Rene Dubos, 'Whatever its precipitating cause and its manifestation almost every disease involves both body and mind, and these two aspects are so inter-related that they cannot be separated one from the other'.

Folklore language is full of expressions that show the appreciation of the connection between the body and the mind. We 'see red', become 'blind with rage', or are struck 'dumb with horror'. One suffers from 'heartache' or 'heartbreak'. Fear makes one's 'heart come up into one's mouth' or 'sink into one's boots'; or it may 'make one's flesh creep', or make one 'limp as a rag' or 'go weak at the knees', or cause the teeth to chatter, or make the mouth dry. One cannot 'stomach' or 'swallow' a situation, disgust 'makes one sick', grief produces a 'lump in the throat', anxiety produces a 'load on the chest' or makes one feel 'knotted up' inside. Relief is expressed as 'getting something off one's chest'. Certainly there is nothing new in the recognition of body–mind unity in medicine. John Hunter said two hundred years ago that his life was in the hands of any rascal who chose to provoke him.

Psychosomatic Medicine

Dunbar in 1934 coined the adjective 'psychosomatic' to describe the mind-body relationship. His book *Emotions and Bodily Changes* published in 1935, contained 2385 references; this figure was doubled to 4717 in the 4th edition published in 1954.

The American journal, Psychosomatic Medicine, was first published in 1937. The 14th edition of Osler's *Principles and Practice of Medicine* edited by Christian in 1942, had the opening chapter on psychosomatic medicine. Weiss and English in 1943 published the first text book on *Psychosomatic Medicine*, with a wealth of evidence to illustrate the psychosomatic concept as seen in clinical practice. Balint in 1957 wrote a book entitled *The Doctor, His Patient and The Illness*, in which he emphasized the need for a more comprehensive and deeper diagnosis of each patient than is normally thought necessary: an overall diagnosis which includes everything that the doctor knows and understands about the patient as a person. The emphasis which had shifted (from the time of the Renaissance in Medicine) to *illness-centred medicine* had to be brought back to *patient-centred medicine*. This approach was also emphasized in a book edited in 1972 by Hopkins, entitled Patient-centred Medicine.

Norman Cousins, former editor of the US literary journal, *Saturday Review*, wrote an article in the *New England Journal of Medicine* describing how he cured himself of ankylosing spondylitis with a combination of laughter, vitamin C and an understanding physician. He stressed the importance of people mobilizing their innate self-healing powers. Patients have the responsibility and capacity to become and remain well; the doctor acts only as a teacher and facilitator.

An interesting study was reported in *Science* (USA) in 1984 on patients who underwent gallbladder surgery in a hospital. Twenty-three patients assigned to rooms with windows looking out on natural scenery had shorter post-operative hospital stay, needed fewer potent analgesics and gave less calls to nurses than 23 matched patients in rooms with windows facing a brick wall. Apparently pleasant surroundings elicit positive feelings, hold interest, reduce fear in stressed subjects, and reduce anxiety.

Sending flowers to a sick person is thus not merely a social ritual.

Just as the negative emotions of fear, hate, anger, greed, jealousy, and frustration are injurious to health, the positive emotions of love, hope, confidence, faith, creativity and the will to live and help others to live, could contribute to health and well-being.

In 1989 David Spiegel and his colleagues from Stanford University published a paper in the *Lancet*: 86 women with metastatic breast cancer were divided into two groups; both groups received standard medical care, but one group also participated in group therapy. The latter group lived an average of almost twice as long (36.6 months) compared to the former group (18.9 months). This observation has important implications. Perhaps positive emotions enhance the immunological surveillance function in some way.

A new concept is linking the brain, the endocrine and the immune system: psycho-neuro-endocrinology and psycho-neuro-immunology. The nervous system and the immune system communicate with each other probably massively, extensively and continuously through chemical signals. Felton from Rochester University, New York has demonstrated nor-adrenergic nerve endings deep into the parenchyma of lymphoid organs; the implications are that the mind may be controlling the immune system which may be amenable to behavioural treatment.

The Brain and the Mind

The human brain weighs only 1.5 kg but contains about 100 billion neurones (contrast the liver which weighs the same, with probably 100 million cells). The brain contains a diversity of nerve cells which Santiago Ramon y Cajal, the father of modern brain science, described as 'the mysterious butterflies of the soul the beating of whose wings may some day–who knows–clarify the secrets of mental life'. With the advent of PET (positron emission tomography) and SPECT (single photon emission computed tomography) it has indeed become possible to study the physiological and biochemical changes associated with mental processes in the living human brain. With the help of radio-labelled tracers the distribution of several neurotransmitters and their receptors can be mapped and changes occurring in their activity along with changes in regional blood flow and metabolism can be imaged. Characteristic changes are seen in anxiety, depression, obsessive-compulsive neurosis, schizophrenia and manic depressive psychosis.

Three series of brain SPECT studies are illustrated in **Fig. 2.1**.

SPECT brain perfusion studies have indicated that disruption of circuits linking frontal cortex, temporal cortex, cingulate cortex and striatum, whether structural or functional, may underlie depression, independent of the cause.

One PET study during a panic attack has shown decreased perfusion of the left parahippocampal region. PET and SPECT studies have shown abnormalities in the frontal lobes and caudate nucleus (either increased or decreased activity) in obsessive compulsive disease (OCD), which normalizes with drugs like fluoxetine which relieve the symptoms of OCD.

The complaint of 'always feeling tired' is seen in at least 10-20 per cent of patients in general practice, more so in women patients. These patients do not have any organic disease or depressive illness to account for their physical and mental fatigue. An epidemic form of this disease 'The Royal Free Disease' was described in 1955 in the student nurses of the Royal Free Hospital in London. The illness was characterized by extreme fatiguability of muscles, associated with profound alteration of mood and behaviour, lasting for a few weeks, with no neurological or biochemical abnormal findings and ultimately leading to full recovery. New light has been thrown on this enigmatic 'benign myalgic encephalomyelitis' or chronic fatigue syndrome (CFS) by brain perfusion studies with HMPAO-Hexamethylene Propylene Amine Oxime) SPECT. The pattern of blood flow is abnormal in the fronto-parietal and temporal areas-changes similar to those seen in depression and in HIV infection of the brain, causing dementia.

These new developments renew the emphasis on the body-mind unity and the need for the doctor to consider the totality of the patient's problem.

Enigma of chronic Fatigue syndrome

The pathogenesis of Chronic Fatigue Syndrome (CFS) is still not clear. Many studies in the 1980's and

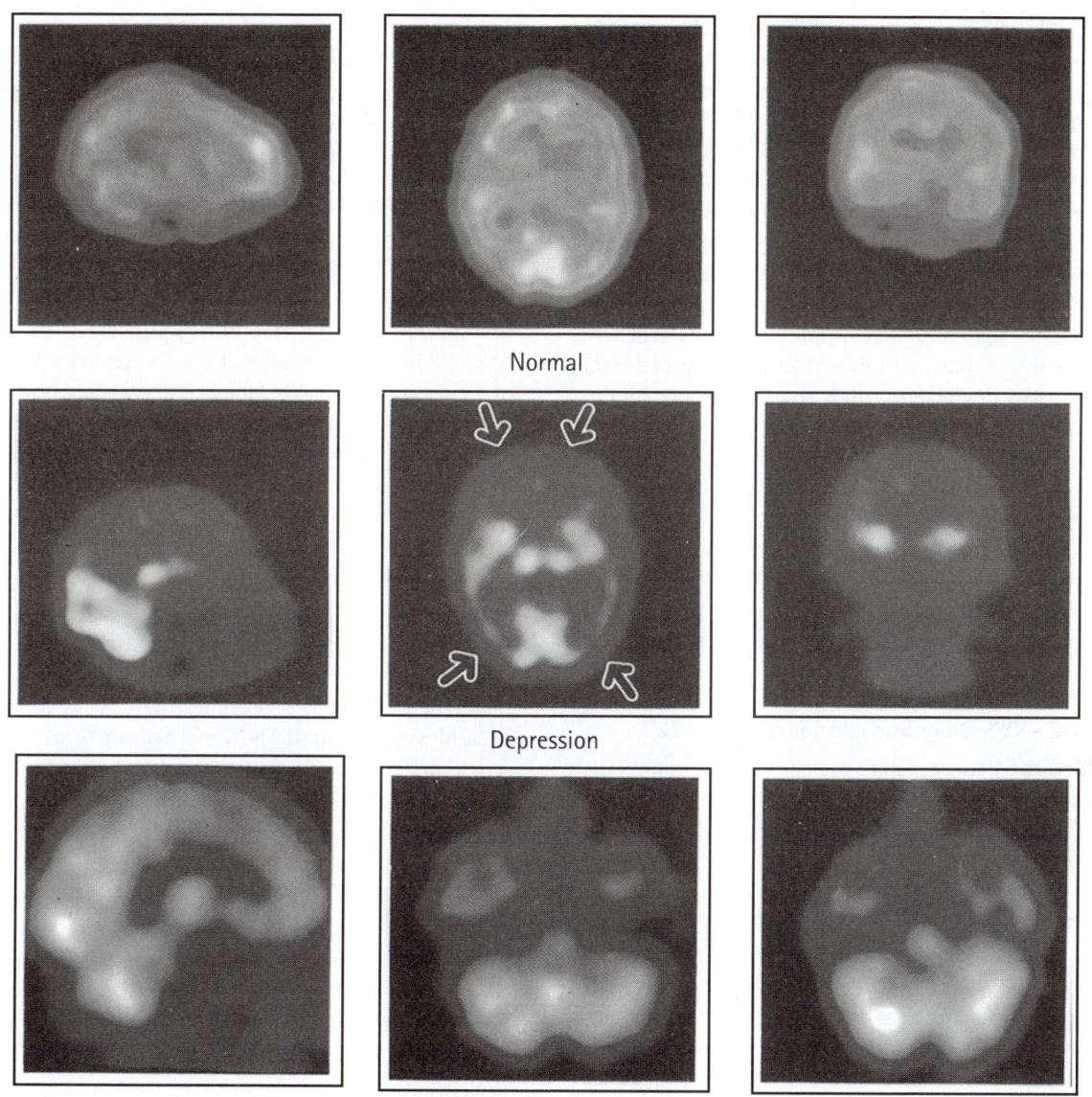

Normal

Depression

Chronic fatigue syndrome

Fig. 2.1: Brain SPECT

1990's attempted to link CFS with EBV or other viruses, yet a direct viral pathogenesis is unproved. Careful comparisons of affected and unaffected monozygotic twins showed no substantive immunlogical differences eg. IL-1, TNFα. Disturbance in the hypothalamic – pituitary adrenal function have been identified in several controlled studies of CFS. Mild to moderate depression is present in half to two-third of the patients. Most patients remain capable of meeting family, work or community obligations despite their continued symptoms such as headache, sore throat, muscle and joint aches, disturbed sleep, difficulty in concentrations and depression. Patients may be come annoyed at doctors for failing to acknowledge or resolve their problem, but no laboratory test can diagnose this condition or measure its severity. But patients are relieved when the doctor takes their complaints seriously, and offers symptomatic relief, with advice regarding life style. CFS exemplifies the need for a comprehensive approach to physical, psychological and social aspects of well-being.

CDC – CFS Diagnosis cdc.gov 2012, 7–22

Medication plays a minor role (anti-depressants such as fluoxeline, buprion). Cognitive behavioral thereby (CBT) and graded exercise therapy (GET) is found useful.

Behavioural and Emotional Disturbances

In a recent study of consecutive patients attending hospital with complaints of recurrent or persistent abdominal pain, organic disease could be found in only 15 out of 96 patients. Of the rest, 31 were depressed; 21 had chronic anxiety state; 17 had symptoms arising out of hysterical mechanism; and 12 resulted from unrecognized alcoholism.

The dilemma before the general practitioner is that while he does not wish to overlook emotional disorders, he should also not diagnose them too readily. To make matters complicated for him:

1. The patient may have *both* physical and emotional problems. To react, to worry or to be upset when faced with a physical illness is a universal phenomenon.

2. The depressed person may complain more of *physical* than mental symptoms of depression.

3. Depression can reduce tolerance for an established physical condition.

4. Depression may lead to changes in behaviour which bring about physical illness, for instance excessive drinking of alcohol or overeating.

Increased complaints about pre-existing conditions such as low back pain, osteoarthritis, constipation, chronic bronchitis and menstrual disorders should suggest depression when there is no evidence that the physical condition has worsened.

Asking a few questions about the cardinal symptoms of depression will help to 'unmask' depression: Is there a low mood, loss of interest in work or hobbies, poor sleep or early morning waking? Morning exacerbation of symptoms is a useful clue that distinguishes depression from anaemia and other physical causes. The full symptomatology of major depression is listed in **Table 2.1** anxiety in **Table 2.2**, panic attacks in **Table 2.3** and hysteria in **Table 2.4**.

Depression is very common after bereavement. Common symptoms which accompany depression are: anorexia, indigestion, headache, dizziness, tiredness, breathlessness, palpitations, and skin rashes.

Sympathetic listening, discussion and explanation of the problem, and reassurance are therapeutic measures in themselves.

Depressed persons who mainly complain of physical symptoms often complain of side-effects of anti-depressant medication. Therefore, if these are prescribed, it is important to give a full explanation of their purpose and side-effects. It is wise to start with a small dose and gradually go up to the full therapeutic dose. Weight loss during anti-depressant drug treatment is an important warning sign since these drugs usually lead to some weight gain. Another hint for a review of the physical state is the persistence of the physical symptoms as the depressed mood improves.

Anxiety, like depression, is a normal reaction to physical illness. There can be real difficulty in distinguishing physical symptoms due to anxiety from those due to physical illness (e.g. migraine, hypoglycaemia, paroxysmal tachycardia, pheochromocytoma).

TABLE 2.1 DIAGNOSTIC CRITERIA FOR MAJOR DEPRESSION

A. At least five of the following. Symptoms occur during the same 2-week period and represent a change from previous function.

At least one of the symptoms is either 1 or 2.

1. Depressed mood
2. Loss of interest or pleasure
3. Poor appetite
4. Weight loss
5. Insomnia or hypersomnia nearly everyday
6. Fatigue or loss of energy nearly everyday
7. Feeling of worthlessness or guilt
8. Inability to concentrate
9. Recurrent thoughts of death (not just fear of dying)

B. It cannot be established that an organic factor initiated or maintained the disturbance, nor is the disturbance a normal reaction to the death of a loved one.

C. No delusions or hallucinations.

D. Not superimposed on schizophrenia or psychotic disorders.

Dysthymia is a chronic milder form of depression. It is twice as frequent in adult females as in males.

Atypical major depression: Overeating and hypersomnia. A significant amount of concurrent anxiety.

TABLE 2.2 DIAGNOSTIC CRITERIA FOR ANXIETY DISORDERS

Motor
1. Tremors, twitching or feeling shaky
2. Muscle tension, aches or soreness
3. Restlessness
4. Easy fatiguability

Autonomic
5. Shortness of breath or smothering sensation
6. Palpitations along with tachycardia
7. Sweating, cold clammy hands
8. Dry mouth
9. Dizziness, lightheadedness
10. Nausea, abdominal distress, diarrhoea
11. Flushes or chills
12. Frequent urination
13. Trouble in swallowing, or 'lump in throat'

Vigilance and scanning
14. Feeling eyed upon, on edge
15. Exaggerated startled response
16. Difficulty in concentration due to anxiety
17. Trouble falling or staying asleep
18. Irritability

Exclusin of organic disease is essential

Thyrotoxicosis; Caffeine overuse

A patient with long-standing tension headache or chest pain may seek urgent advice when he hears that a colleague or friend with a similar complaint died suddenly of a brain tumour or a heart attack.

Burn Out Syndrome

Herbert Freudenberger, a New York psychoanalyst coined the term "burnout syndrome" in the early 1970's to describe a state of mental and physical exhaustion caused by one's professional life and its chronic stresses. In response to mounting task loads, the wretch piles on the hours at work, pulling late nights at the office, ignoring exercise, skipping meals or eating unhealthful fast foods on the run, cancells personal commitments to family and friends. Sooner or later the work efficiency declines, with poor concentration, fewer creative ideas, self dis-satisfaction and flagging self-esteem and anxiety about failure, and depression. Some may seek solace in alcohol or pills. Some even attempt suicide.

The anti-stress measures that are required are as simple as they are effective. They include eating wholesome food at regular meal time, exercising regularly and getting enough sleep, spending time with family and friends and developing a hobby or a pleasurable activity like listening to music or relaxation techniques including Yoga and meditation ("Yoga" literally means equilibrium).

Psychogenic Pain

Psychogenic pain can be experienced in any part of the body, but the head, neck and lower back are common sites. Abdominal pain occurs especially in the irritable bowel syndrome. Chest pain is a feature of anxiety states. Diagnosis is based on a careful analysis of the site of pain, radiation and timing which allows it to be compared with the features or pain due to organic causes. These details are given in the appropriate sections In subsequent chapters of this book.

TABLE 2.3 DIAGNOSTIC CRITERIA FOR PANIC DISORDERS

During the attack of panic:

1. Shortness of breath or smothering sensation
2. Dizziness, unsteadiness, faintness
3. Tachycardia and palpitation
4. Trembling and shaking
5. Sweating
6. Choking
7. Nausea and abdominal distress
8. Tingling, numbness (paraesthesia)
9. Depersonalization and derealization
10. Flushes (hot flushes) or chills
11. Chest pain or discomfort
12. Fear of dying
13. Fear of going crazy or doing something uncontrolled

Differential diagnosis of panic attacks:

Pheochromocytoma

Hypoglycaemia

Complex partial seizures (temporal lobe)

Hyper and hypothyroidism

Beta agonist and alpha adrenergic receptor antagonist drugs

Psychogenic Pain

Psychogenic pain can be experienced in any part of the body, but the head, neck and lower back are common sites. Abdominal pain occurs especially in the irritable bowel syndrome. Chest pain is a feature of anxiety states. Diagnosis is based on a careful analysis of the site of pain, radiation and timing which allows it to be compared with the features or pain due to organic causes. These details are given in the appropriate sections In subsequent chapters of this book.

There seems to be no explanation as to why some emotionally disturbed patients complain of pain whereas others do not. Suggestions that pent-up anger or guilt provoke pain are not convincing as general explanations though they have some truth in particular cases.

Treatment consists of reassurance, though hypochondriac patients cannot easily be reassured and often demand long interview and repeated testing. Like drugs, doses of reassurance may also be needed three times daily!

Diagnostic Problems

Even though depression and anxiety are distinct clinical entities, anxiety is one of the most common and most severe features of depression. Treatment of depression often alleviates anxiety.

Symptoms of depression and anxiety such as fatigue, insomnia and poor concentration can be caused by a large variety of physical illness or drugs (**Tables 2.5, 2.6 and 2.7**).

The whole thrust of this chapter is to bring home the intimate and inseparable relationship of the mind (psyche) and body (soma) and the need to look at the person who has the disease, and not just at the disease which the person has. It has been well said, 'There are no diseases. There are only sick persons'. Some psychiatric disorders are so common that the primary physicians (general practitioners) see them frequently and see more of them than do psychiatrists. The practitioner should remember that many depressed and anxious patients do not present with any psychologic symptoms but focus on somatic complaints only. Frequently these patients may initially deny subjective feelings of depression and may even appear superficially cheerful. A clinician who is not alert to this possibility may miss the diagnosis and may pursue futile diagnostic tests. It is usually true if, after a well taken history, the doctor has no reasonable idea of the diagnosis, it is unlikely that he will be much wiser after various investigations.

A good general practitioner should become familiar with the use of anxiolytic and antidepressant drugs and learn to use them intelligently, since it is not possible for him to send all his patients to psychiatrists. These drugs are described in **Tables 2.8 and 2.9.**

Table 2.4 DIAGNOSTIC FEATURES OF HYSTERIA (CONVERSION SYMPTOMS)

	Diagnostic features
Motor Symptoms	
Rigidity	Proportional to the force used to overcome it, on passive movement. Associated contraction of antagonistic muscles can be palpated when the patient attempts voluntary movement.
Flaccid paralysis	No wasting of muscles. Tendon ret1exes and cutaneous ret1exes are normal. Normal reaction of muscles to electrical stimulation.
Tremors and tics	Increased by attention. Blepharospasm fairly common.
Aphonia	Patient whispers while talking but phonates normally on coughing.
Sensory symptoms	
Sensory loss	Affects only cutaneous sensibility and is usually complete. Sense of position normal.
Analgesia	Upper level is horizontal; varies from time to time on successive examinations. Transition from analgesic area to normal is abrupt without any area of hypo or hyperaesthesia.
Hemianaesthesia	Corneal ret1exes remain intact. Sensory loss abruptly ceases in midline in front (of organic disease; continues for a short distance across the midline).
Blindness	Often sudden in onset. Patient commonly avoids obstacles placed in his path. Pupils and optic disc are normal. Perimeter chart: unequal constriction of visual fields.
Deafness	Patient can be awakened from sleep by calling his name, but when awake cannot hear.
Anosmia	Patient shows loss of sensation to ammonia vapour (which is a function of 5th cranial nerve, not the 1st).
Visceral symptoms	
Globus hysteticus	Difficulty in swallowing but no weight loss.
Aerophagy	May lead to enormous abdominal distension, simulating pregnancy or ovarian cyst.
Vomiting	No nausea; no weight loss.
Abdominal pain	Often leads to futile laparotomy for 'adhesions', 'fixation' etc.
Hysterical convulsions	Take place in the presence of an audience. No incontinence or tongue biting. Patient never injures herself.
Hysterical gait	Patient walks with bent knees or trunk. Bizarre gait which does not conform to any of the known gaits encountered in organic disease.

Management of chronic pain

Tricyclic antidepressants (TCAs) are extremely useful for management of patients with chronic pain. Although developed for the treatment of depression, the TCAs have a spectrum of dose-related biological activities including producing analgesia by an unknown mechanism in a variety of clinical conditions. The onset of analgesic effect is more rapid and occurs at a lower dose than is typically required for treatment of depression. TCAs can be used for chronic pain relief in patients who are not depressed. TCAs potentiate the opioid analgesia hence they are useful adjuncts for treatment of severe persistent pain e.g. malignant tumours. Painful conditions that respond to TCAs include post-herpetic neuralgia, diabetic neuropathy, central post-stroke pain, chronic low back pain, migraine and tension headache, rheumatoid arthritis and cancer.

Side-effects of TCAs such as orthostatic hypotension, cardiac conduction delay, memory impairment, constipation and urinary retention are particularly problematic in the elderly patients Venlafaxine (Effexor), a non TCA that blocks both serotonin and norepinephrine uptake, retains most of the analgesic effects of TCAs without the side effects of TCAs.

Acupuncture and acupressure: encephalins/endorphins, cannabinoids

These procedures release endogenous encephalins and endorphins and cannabinoids which relieve pain. One in three members of the general population can produce enough endorphins even to undergo major Surgery without conventional anesthetics. This approach is used in Traditional Chinese medicine.

Special cutaneous areas on skin surface in hands and feet and external ear, are exploited for relief of pain in low back and elsewhere - concept of meridians.

Laser acupuncture induces significant brain activation within the thalamus, nucleus subthalamicus, nucleus rubber, brain stem specific cerebral cortical and subcortical activation Broadman areas 40 and 42 in humans [Siedentopf E et al Lasers in Medical Science 2005, 20(2), 68-73].

Reflexology is based on the assumption that particular body surface areas are interconnected to internal body parts- for example areas on fact related to lumbar vertebrae.

Krishna Dalal et al, Department of Biophysics at AIIMS have used swept source optical coherence tomography (SS-OCT) in subjects with or without low back pain. The skin SS-OCT images of lumbar reflexology areas could determine grade 0 (normal) grade 1 (early degeneration), grade 2 (moderate degeneration), grade 3 (severe degeneration) (I Dougans: The new reflexology - a unique blend of Traditional Chinese Medicine and Western Reflexology Practice for better health and healing).

TABLE 2.5 ORGANIC DISEASES CAUSING DEPRESSION

Endocrine	Cushing's syndrome
	Hyper and Hypothyroidism
	Hyper & Hypoparathyroidism
	T2DM
Neurologic	Stroke
	Parkinsonism
	Alzheimer's disease
	Multiple sclerosis
	Brain tumours: frontal lobe, temporal lobe
Viral infections	Influenza
	Hepatitis
Vitamin deficiency	Vitamin B12
	Thiamine
	Niacin
Collagen vascular diseases	SLE, Temporal arteritis
	alphamethylodopa
Drugs (chronic administration)	anti-cancer drugs
	benzodiazepines
	cimetidine
	cycloserine
	gluco-corticosteroids
	indomethacin
	levodopa
	neuroleptic drugs
	propranolol
	reserpine

TABLE 2.6 ORGANIC DISEASES MIMICKED BY ANXIETY

Angina pectoris	Paroxysmal tachycardia
Carcinoid tumour	Pheochromocytoma
Complex partial seizures	Post-prandial dumping syndrome
Cerebral atherosclerosis	Post-viral syndromes
Hypoglycaemia, Insulinoma	Pulmonary embolism
Hypoxic states	Thyrotoxicosis
Migraine	Withdrawal of CNS depressant drugs: alcohol,
Myocardial infarction	cocaine, benzodiazepines, meprobamate
Mitral valve prolapse	

TABLE 2.7 DRUGS CAUSING ANXIETY SYMPTOMS

Caffeine: excessive use.
Sympathomimetic amines.
Bronchodilaters, e.g. theophylline overdose.
Excessive thyroid medication.

Hysteria: Somatoform Disorders

The essential concept of hysteria is that physical symptoms and signs arise when there is no organic pathology to cause them, and that these symptoms and signs result from unconscious mental processes; they are not deliberately produced as in malingering, but there is some advantage which the symptoms confer on the patient.

How sure can one be, on the basis of history and physical examination, about the absence of physical or mental disease (depression, schizophrenia)? Since one can never be certain, hysteria is at first a provisional diagnosis to be confirmed with adequate follow-up during which new evidence of disease does not appear.

The patient's age is important, for hysteria seldom appears for the first time after the age of 35-40. A careful history of previous attacks, however mild, which suggest hysteria, is a useful clue.

Hysterical symptoms begin at times of stress, and if no stress can be found, the diagnosis should seldom be made though it is important to question informants as well as the patient, because the latter may have repressed memories of the stressful event.

Physical symptoms related to the nervous system are common e.g. headache, paralysis, fits, aphonia, gait disorders, paraesthesia, anaesthesia, blindness and deafness.

The acute cases often encountered in the emergency departments which arise in relation to definite stress, usually improve quickly. Chronic cases of the kind admitted to psychiatric wards have a worse prognosis.

Munchausen's syndrome is a rare disorder in which patients present repeatedly with dramatic symptoms suggesting severe physical illness, of a kind which suggests the need for urgent surgical treatment or the administration of powerful analgesics. Patients are more often men and the commonest symptoms include acute abdominal or loin pain, haematemesis and haemoptysis. The symptoms and signs are produced deliberately and there is other evidence that the patient is trying to deceive the doctor; for instance his account of previous hospital admissions, and even his name and address are often incorrect. However, the extreme lengths to which these patients go to imitate illness and undergo multiple operations suggest a profound disorder of personality.

Compensation neurosis: Such cases are seen most often after accidents or injuries for which disability payment is due. The symptoms are more frequent after accidents at work or on the road than in injuries during sporting events or in the house. The symptoms usually persist despite treatment until the claim for compensation is settled. It is difficult to decide if this is a hysterical phenomenon or malingering.

TABLE 2.8 SELECTED ANXIOLYTIC DRUGS

	Drug	Dose	Half-life	Comments
A.	Benzodiazepines			
	Alprazolam	0.25 mg tid max. 4 mg/day	11–45 hr	Useful for anxiety with depression.
	Chlordiazepoxide (Librium)	15–30 mg tid max. l00 mg	6–30 hr	Caution: drug dependence. taper off slowly.
	Diazepam	2–5 mg tid max. 40 mg/day	20–50 hr	Commonest drug in use currently. Caution: drug dependence.
B.	Buspirone	5 mg tid max. 30 mg/day		Lacks sedative, hypnotic and muscle relaxant effects. Suitable for chronic anxiolytic therapy.
C.	Barbiturates Phenobarbitone	15–30 mg PO/bid		Suitable drug for daytime sedation, e.g. in case of nervous diarrhoea.

TABLE 2.9 SELECTED ANTIDEPRESSANT DRUGS

Drug	Dose	Sedative	Anti-cholinergic
Amiytriptyline	25 mg bid max. 300 mg/day	+++	+++
Nortriptyline	10 mg bid max. 100 mg/day	++	+
Imipramine	25 mg bid max. 300 mg/day	++	++
Desipramine	25 mg bid max. 300 mg/day	+	+
Fluoxetine	10 mg bid max. 80 mg/day	±	±

Dermatitis artefacta: In this condition the lesions are produced knowingly by the patient who conceals this from his doctor. It is usually one episode in a long history of emotional disorder which indicates a disorder of personality.

Other examples of patient-induced illness are: (i) self-induced infection, (ii) simulated fever, bleeding, anaemia, (iii) chronic 'non-healing' wounds, (iv) surreptitious self-medication, e.g. eltroxine, cathartics and diuretics.

Schizophrenia, mania and obsessive compulsive disorders, alcohol and drug addiction are not discussed here since they fall entirely in the domain of the psychiatrist.

EMERGENCY MEDICINE

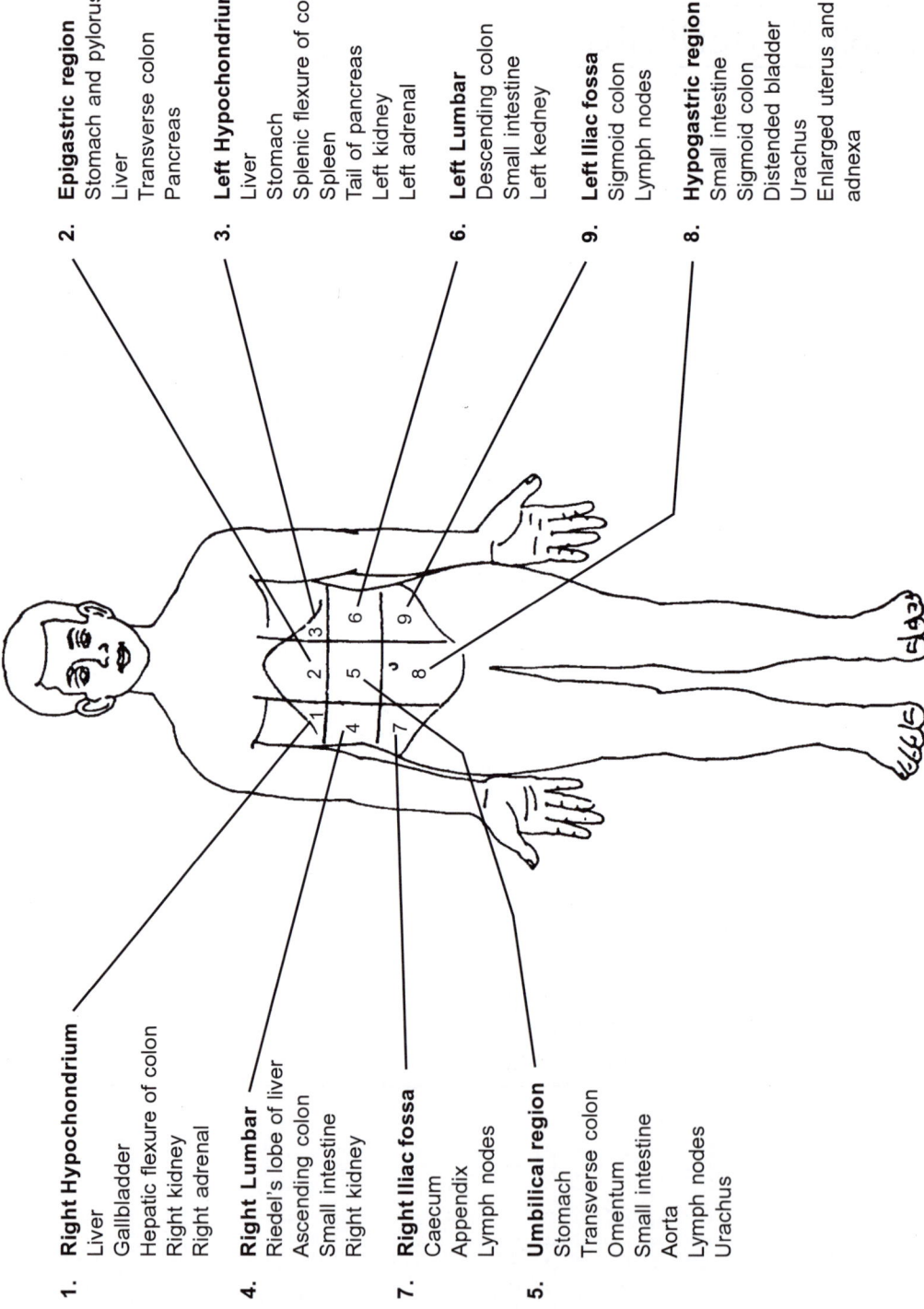

2. Epigastric region
Stomach and pylorus
Liver
Transverse colon
Pancreas

3. Left Hypochondrium
Liver
Stomach
Splenic flexure of colon
Spleen
Tail of pancreas
Left kidney
Left adrenal

6. Left Lumbar
Descending colon
Small intestine
Left kedney

9. Left Iliac fossa
Sigmoid colon
Lymph nodes

8. Hypogastric region
Small intestine
Sigmoid colon
Distended bladder
Urachus
Enlarged uterus and
adnexa

1. Right Hypochondrium
Liver
Gallbladder
Hepatic flexure of colon
Right kidney
Right adrenal

4. Right Lumbar
Riedel's lobe of liver
Ascending colon
Small intestine
Right kidney

7. Right Iliac fossa
Caecum
Appendix
Lymph nodes

5. Umbilical region
Stomach
Transverse colon
Omentum
Small intestine
Aorta
Lymph nodes
Urachus

Fig. 3.1: Sites of abdominal pain

Acute abdominal pain is a frequent and often baffling symptom with which the doctor must deal. There are few situations in clinical medicine that demand decisive action as frequently as acute abdominal pain does; The doctor who knows the crucial clinical features of the several diseases which cause acute abdominal pain (as described in **Table 3.1**), can utilize this knowledge, and by careful analysis of the age and sex of the patient (**Table 3.2**), the onset and subsequent course of the pain, the character of the pain, its location and radiation (**Table 3.3 and Fig. 3.1**), he can arrive at the most probable diagnosis, or at least narrow down the possibilities to two or three conditions.

Acute abdomen has been described by de Dombal as 'the last bastion of clinical acumen, where investigation is a thief of time'. There are problems and pitfalls in the investigation of acute abdomen. The success of clinical approach is to detect early

1. Those conditions in which surgery is rewarding (**Table 3.4**)
2. Those conditions in which surgery is futile (**Table 3.5**)
3. Those conditions III which surgery is dangerous (**Table 3.6**)

Clinical Approach to a Case of Acute Abdominal Pain

The immediate concern is to assess the gravity of the situation.

A. *General examination:*
   Is the patient restless? (colic)
   Is the patient immobile? (peritonitis)
   Is the patient vomiting? (inflammation, obstruction)
   Is there evidence of impending shock or vascular collapse?

   Rapid weak pulse
   Low blood pressure
   Cold moist skin
   Restlessness
   Are there signs of generalized peritonitis?
   Diffuse pain and tenderness
   Muscle guarding
   Absent bowel sounds

If these signs are present, immediately start an IV drip of glucose saline, stop everything by mouth, and insert a nasogastric tube for continuous suction. Since the whole picture is suggestive of perforation of a viscus (including ruptured ectopic pregnancy), this is a surgical emergency for which surgical consultation should be promptly obtained.

B. If there are no definitive findings in the abdomen, the crucial question should be asked:
   Is the cause of trouble elsewhere?

It is a sobering reminder to all clinicians that in a large series of over 6,000 cases of acute abdomen fully studied by the World Federation of Gastro-enterologists, where the initial diagnosis was acute appendicitis, perforated peptic ulcer, cholecystitis, pancreatitis, small bowel obstruction, renal colic etc, the final diagnosis was one of the following in many cases:

   Acute myocardial infarction
   Pneumonia
   Congestive heart failure
   Diabetic ketosis
   Diabetic neuropathy
   Asthma
   Intercostal herpes zoster (pre-eruptive)

These conditions, along with those listed in **Tables 3.5** and **3.6** should keep the clinician on the alert. Lack of awareness of rare diseases like acute intermittent porphyria has led many unfortunate

---

patients to futile laparotomies on the presumed diagnosis of acute appendicitis, cholecystitis, peptic ulcer perforation etc.

Specific symptoms to check

There are common situations in clinical practice where a decision has to be made on clinical grounds between two most likely possibilities; the following will be found useful.

Appendicitis vs non-specific abdominal pain

Points favouring appendicitis are:

>Symmetric pain moving to RLQ
>Pain aggravated by movement or coughing
>Anorexia, nausea, vomiting
>Flushing of the face
>Focal tenderness RLQ and rebound tenderness

Appendicitis vs cholecystitis

>Cholecystitis is more common in patients over 25 years
>History of previous dyspepsia
>Pain and tenderness worse over RUQ
>Pale stools and dark urine, jaundice

Appendicitis vs renal problems

>Renal colic is common in middle-aged men
>UTI is common in young adult females
>Loin pain and tenderness implies renal origin
>Pallor favours stone
>Flushing of face favours UTI or appendicitis
>Frequency of urine/dysuria favours renal colic
>Rebound tenderness and guarding favour appendicitis
>Pain moving downwards to thigh and drawing up of legs favour renal colic

Appendicitis vs gynaec problems

>Pain which moves favours appendicitis
>The following favour gynaec problems:
>>Radiation of pain outside abdomen
>>Short history plus shock
>>Careful obstetric history–amenorrhoea
>>GI symptoms may occur
>>Tenderness outside RLQ
>>PV: pain on moving cervix

Renal vs gynaec problems

>Loin pain/tenderness favour renal problems
>Frequency/dysuria favour renal problems

>A detailed gynaec history is mandatory
>Guarding/rebound tenderness favour gynaec problems
>PV-pain on moving cervix favours gynaec problems

Beware rushing to X-ray. It may show no UTI but may harm an early pregnancy.

Pancreatitis vs perforated DU

>Dramatic onset of pain favours perforated DU
>Profuse vomiting favours pancreatitis
>Limited pain/tenderness favours pancreatitis
>Early distension favours pancreatitis
>Presence of bowel sounds favours pancreatitis

X-ray abdomen and chest; erect and supine positions.

Lateral decubitus films and serum amylase will help.

Appendicitis vs Crohn's disease

>Age over 30 years favours Crohn's
>Pain site focal favours appendicitis
>Pain duration more than 48 hours favours Crohn's
>Abnormal bowel movement favours Crohn's
>Previous surgery favours Crohn's
>Pallor favours Crohn's while flushing favours appendicitis
>Rebound/guarding favours appendicitis

Cancer vs non-specific abdominal pain

The following should raise suspicion of cancer:

>Patient's age over 50 years
>Pain lasting 48 hours or more
>Constipation/altered bowel habit
>Bloating or distension
>Intra-abdominal mass

Perforated DU vs perforated colon

>Perforated colon common in the elderly
>Site of onset of pain below umbilicus favours colon perforation

Abdominal pain in elderly patients
Cancer:

>10 per cent of all unexplained acute abdominal pain in patients over age 50 turn out to be cancer, mostly of the large bowel. Hence never send an elderly patient away without making sure that someone else will follow up the case urgently.

TABLE 3.1 CRUCIAL CLINICAL FEATURES FOR ACUTE ABDOMEN DIAGNOSIS

Acute appendicitis
  Pain RLQ
  Pain aggravated by movement/coughing
  Nausea, vomiting, anorexia
  Focal RLQ tenderness
  Rebound tenderness and guarding
  PR: tender right side

Acute diverticulitis
  Pain LLQ
  Tenderness LLQ
  Constipation/diarrhoea
  Rectal bleeding/mucus
  Abdominal distension
  Abdominal mass

Perforated peptic ulcer
  Known history of ulcer
  Sudden pain
  General pain
  Abdominal tenderness
  Abdominal rigidity
  Bowel sounds quiet

Acute cholecystitis
  Patient usually over 40
  RUQ pain and tenderness
  History of gallstone/jaundice, patient jaundiced
  Pain radiation right shoulder
  Murphy's sign positive

Acute pancreatitis
  History of gallstone/pancreatitis
  Onset sudden
  Pain/tenderness mostly upper abdomen
  Jaundice
  Alcohol history
  Serum amylase raised

Intestinal obstruction
  Patient has vomited
  Constipation
  Distension
  History of previous abdominal surgery
  Scars
  Bowel sounds abnormally increased

Intussusception
  Child under age 2 years

Severe central pain
Anorexia, vomiting
Blood in stools
Distension of abdomen
Diffuse tenderness
Abnormal bowel sounds
Palpable mass (confirmed by ultrasound)

Aneurysm
  Usually male, elderly
  Pulsating mass in abdomen
  Local tenderness
  Gastrointestinal symptoms absent
  Femoral pulse weak, delayed
    (compare wrist and groin pulse
    simultaneously)
  Plain X-ray may show calcification in aneurysm
  wall
    (especially in lateral decubitus film)

Mesenteric ischaemia
  Elderly patient, both sexes
  Pain often severe, diffuse
  Short history of continuous pain
  Patient pale and restless
  No abdominal findings early
  50% have distended abdomen later on
  75% have quiet/absent bowel sounds later on

Colonic perforation
  Pain often for 24 hours, even days
  Pain begins in lower abdomen
  Bowel habit often abnormal before pain
  Examination may show distension and mass

Acute renal colic
  Loin pain and tenderness
  Radiation of pain to groin
  Pain comes and goes
  Dysuria, frequency, haematuria

Non-specific abdominal pain
  Pain only moderate in severity
  Not aggravated by cough/movements
  No rebound tenderness
  No muscle guarding
  Bowel sounds normal
  Movement pain free

Table 3.2 CAUSES OF ACUTE ABDOMEN ACCORDING TO AGE AND SEX OF PATIENT

Child	**Young female adult**
Intussusception	Urinary tract infection
Urinary tract infection	Salpingitis (PID)
Renal colic	Ovarian cyst: torsion of pedicle
Hernia	Ectopic pregnancy
Torsion of testis	Incomplete abortion
Chest infection	Ruptured Graafian follicle
Acute tonsillitis	Endometriosis (has mimicked appendicitis)
Young male adult	**Patients above age 50**
Peptic ulcer	Cancer, esp. large bowel
Trauma	Vascular episodes:
Alcoholic gastritis	Myocardial infarction
Crohn's disease	Aortic aneurysm
	Mesenteric ischaemia
	Hernia: inguinal, femoral
	Colonic perforation

The duration of pain, often moderate, may be for days.
The site is often vague, diffuse.
The bowel habit is often abnormal before the onset of pain.
Abdominal examination may reveal distension and a mass.
Rectal examination may reveal blood, or a mass may be felt.

Vascular:
Over 10 per cent of all acute abdominal pain in patients over 70 have a vascular cause.

Table 3.3 CAUSES OF ACUTE ABDOMEN SUGGESTED BY ONSET, CHARACTER AND LOCATION OF PAIN

Sudden onset	1. Perforation of a viscus: peptic ulcer; ruptured ectopic pregnancy
	2. Ischaemia of the gut or organ; strangulated hernia; mesenteric vascular occlusion; torsion of pedicle of ovarian cyst; torsion of the testicle
	3. Sometimes acute pancreatitis may have sudden onset although more commonly it is gradual
Gradual onset	1. Inflammation: appendicitis; cholecystitis; salpingitis
	2. Obstruction: intestinal obstruction; intussusception
Character of pain	Colicky
	Obstruction to a hollow viscus: gallbladder; appendix; intestine; ureter
Location of pain	
Mid-epigastric	Stomach, duodenum; liver, biliary tract, pancreas; spinal nerve roots T6–T8 Acute myocardial infarct
Peri-umbilical	Small intestine, appendix; upper ureters; testes, ovaries; spinal roots T9–T10
Hypogastric	Colon; lower ureters, bladder; uterus; spinal roots T11 and T12
Right upper quadrant	Liver, gallbladder; right lower lobe pneumonia, referred pain from parietal pleura; acute myocardial infarct in congestive hepatomegaly
Left upper quadrant	Pancreas; spleen; left lower lobe pneumonia
Left lower quadrant	Diverticulitis
Loin	Kidney, ureters

TTable 3.4 ABDOMINAL PAIN WHERE SURGERY IS REWARDING

I. Inflammatory lesions involving wall of viscus which, without prompt surgery, may perforate:
   Acute appendicitis
   Acute cholecystitis

II. Compromise of blood supply-danger of gangrene
   Strangulated hernia
   Intussusception
   Volvulus
   Torsion of pedicle of a cyst
   Mesenteric vascular occlusion

Table 3.5 ABDOMINAL PAIN WHERE SURGERY IS DANGEROUS

Condition	Diagnostic clues
Acute pancreatitis	High serum amylase; CT scan.
Paralytic ileus	Absent bowel sounds; abdominal distension.
Acute hepatitis	High SGOT, SGPT, bilirubin.
Myocardial infarct	ECG, CPK-MB in serum high.
Pneumonia (esp. basal)	Chest X-ray.

Table 3.6 ABDOMINAL PAIN WHERE SURGERY IS FUTILE

Condition	Diagnostic clues
Acute intermittent porphyria	Red coloured urine on exposure to air: urine for porphobilinogen.
Lead colic	Gray lines in gums; Basophilic stippling of RBCs
Haemolytic crisis	Pallor, icterus; Sickle cells, spherocytes in peripheral blood smear.
Uraemia (pseudo-obstruction)	BUN and creatinine high.
Diabetic ketosis	Urine for acetone and sugar.
Diabetic neuropathy and radiculopathy	Other features of neuropathy; urine for sugar.
Tabes dorsalis with crisis	Absent ankle jerks; Argyll Robertson pupil.
Henoch-Schonlein purpura	Knee pain and swelling; skin purpura.
Mesenteric adenitis	Children with tonsillitis; filariasis–lymphangitis, lymphadenitis.

Table 3.7 CONDITIONS IN WHICH SERUM AMYLASE IS HIGH

1. Pancreas: acute pancreatitis; pancreatic pseudocyst; pancreatic abscess; pancreatic trauma
2. Perforated peptic ulcer: peritonitis
3. Strangulated bowel; intestinal obstruction
4. Mesenteric vascular occlusion: intestinal
5. Ruptured ectopic pregnancy
6. Renal insufficiency
7. Morphine administration
8. Chronic liver disease
9. Post-operative hyperamylasaemia
10. Aortic aneurysm
11. Salivary gland: mumps, radiation sial adenitis infarction
12. Carcinoma of lung, oesophagus, breast and ovary

Note: Amylase is found in many organs-pancreas, salivary glands, small intestine, liver, kidney, fallopian tube; ectopic production of the enzyme is found in some cancers.

Pancreatic isoamylase (P) is different from non-pancreatic isoamylase(s). Measurement of isoamylases is clinically important.

Striking elevations of amylase more than 500 are due to acute pancreatitis if mumps, gut perforation and infarction are excluded.

Pain for more than 24 hours favours colon perforation
Abnormal bowel habit favours colon perforation
Mass favours colon perforation

Gallstone pancreatitis vs no-stone pancreatitis
General pain and tenderness favour non-stone pain Focal/maximal pain and tenderness RuQ favour gallstone.

History of alcoholism favours no-stone pancreatitis
Positive Murphy's sign favours stone

The Role of Laboratory Investigations

Hb and Hct
Low Hb suggests ruptured ectopic, ruptured spleen, or mesenteric vascular occlusion High Hb suggests polycythaemia vera (prone to vascular occlusion)

WBC count
> 13,000 favours appendicitis
< 8,000 does not favour appendicitis
Counts in between do not influence decision

Plain X-ray abdomen and chest
Gas under diaphragm: perforation
Fluid levels in intestine: obstruction
Lateral decubitus film

Urine
For: Albumin, pus cells, RBCs
Sugar and acetone
Amylase

Serum amylase (Table 3.7)

Therapeutic Plan

It is extremely dangerous to treat acute abdominal pain without knowledge of its source. Analgesics may only confuse the examiner; however in certain situations in which the patient has little pain tolerance and is severely agitated, analgesics or sedatives may have to be used to obtain the history and perform an examination.

Individual treatment for abdominal disorders will be determined by the definitive diagnosis. The diagnosis of appendicitis should be sufficiently precise to keep the finding of normal appendix on surgical exploration at or below 10 per cent. At the same time, the incidence of perforation should also be at or below 15 per cent.

In diverticulitis, the presence of free perforation is an indication for surgery with diverting colostomy and/or resection.

The treatment of acute pancreatitis is conservative and largely supportive. Surgical therapy may be required for severe haemorrhagic or necrotizing pancreatitis, abscess, persistent pseudocyst, and rarely, common bile duct or duodenal obstruction.

In acute cholecystitis, if the diagnosis is certain and the patient is a good surgical risk, early cholecystectomy is the procedure of choice. In older patients who are not good surgical risks at the time of the acute episode, initial antibiotic therapy (ampicillin + gentamicin) is followed by surgery 4–6 weeks later. Empyema of the gallbladder and perforation need early surgery. If the patient is diabetic, early surgery is preferable since the signs and symptoms may not be as obvious in these patients.

Acute occlusion of the superior mesenteric artery or vein is a surgical problem. The absence of abdominal findings early in the course of illness may delay the diagnosis. The absence of visceral findings in an elderly person complaining of severe abdominal pain should strongly suggest mesenteric occlusion.

There are patients who do not fall into any category. They generally have a long or intermittent history of protracted pain, have seen several consultants or have required surgical exploration for poorly defined reasons. Cancerphobia often localizes in the abdomen, hence a close surveillance and follow-up is worthwhile in patients above age 50.

One important condition which should be remembered is retroperitoneal fibrosis which can occur at any age but most commonly in middle age. The symptoms include abdominal pain, fever, anorexia, fatigue, malaise, weight loss and occasionally oedema of the feet. IVP shows medial displacement of the ureter. Surgical relief of the ureter dramatically abolishes the pain and fever.

4   Acute Gastrointestinal Bleeding

Haematemesis is vomiting of blood. Freshly vomited blood may be bright red in colour. Blood that remains in the stomach for a while is altered by gastric acid to haematin (coffee ground colour).

Melaena is the passage of black tarry stools (due to passage of more than 100 ml blood), occurring anywhere from the mouth to the small intestine. Fresh blood in the stools indicates the colon as the source, usually the recto-sigmoid. Bright red blood in the stool without change in vital signs indicates an anorectal source (e.g. piles, fissure, tumour). However, brisk upper GI tract bleeding with rapid intestinal transit may present with passage of bright red blood in the stools. In such cases vital signs are always affected.

The first indication of GI bleeding may be dizziness and fainting while getting up from the toilet seat (symptoms of blood loss); only later to be followed by melaena.

Assessment of Blood Loss

The first step in the examination of a patient with haematemesis and melaena is to ascertain the severity of blood loss.

1. Appearance of the patient: Signs of distress (including confusion), cold and sweating skin, pulse is rapid and thready; the patient is in shock due to severe blood loss.

2. Count the heart rate and take the BP with patient supine and sitting upright. Postural hypotension (supine to upright fall in systolic pressure more than 10 mm Hg) or rise in heart rate of more than 20 beats per minute indicate moderate blood loss (10-20 per cent of circulatory volume).

Supine hypotension suggests more severe blood loss (usually more than 20 per cent of circulatory volume).

Shock is evidenced by hypotension (systolic BP below 90 mm Hg), tachycardia, peripheral vasoconstriction, sweating, confusion (indicating reduced cerebral blood flow), and decreased urine output (indicating poor renal blood flow). Rapid restoration of circulatory volume is essential in this setting. Emergency therapy should be instituted as soon as a haemodynamically compromised patient is identified. The immediate step is to take blood for typing and cross-matching, and do a complete blood count (CBC), platelet count, prothrombin time (PT) and partial thromboplastin time (PTT), and blood chemistry (electrolytes, SGOT, SGPT, alkaline phosphatase, serum albumin and globulin).

Emergency Therapy

1. Two large-bore IV lines should be established with No. 14 to 18 gauge catheters in large peripheral veins. The blood bank must be notified of the potential demand for blood products, and at least 3-6 units of whole blood or packed RBCs should be held available at all times until the patient has stabilized.

2. Volume infusion: Till blood is available, rapid restoration of circulatory volume with isotonic saline, Ringer lactate solution or 5 per cent hetastarch (Hespan) may be achieved. The rate of infusion should be guided by the patient's condition. Patients in shock may require fluids or blood to be pumped or hand-infused using large syringes and stopcocks.

3. Packed RBCs and fresh frozen plasma (FFP) can be used when large volume transfusions are needed. Transfusion should be continued until the patient is haemodynamically stable and the haematocrit (Hct) remains at 30 per cent or higher.

Early consultation with a gastro-enterologist, surgeon and radiologist is essential. Timely involvement of such specialists will expedite optimal management in these cases.

Evaluation of the Stabilized Patient

In the haemodynamically stable patient, further evaluation is indicated to identify the source of bleeding and detect risk factors for further bleeding.

Localization of the bleeding site can often be accurately predicted from the history and physical examination. The crucial clinical features of various causes are given in **Tables 4.1** and **4.2**. **Table 4.3** lists the possible sources of bleeding indicated by inspection of stools.

History

Symptoms at presentation may be helpful in differentiating upper from lower 01 bleeding and may also suggest a particular diagnosis.

For example:

Haematemesis virtually means upper 01 source, mostly due to peptic ulcer or varices.

Forceful vomiting followed by haematemesis suggests Mallory-Weiss syndrome (mucosal tear at gastro-oesophageal junction).

TABLE 4.1 CRUCIAL CLINICAL FEATURES OF CAUSES OF HAEMATEMESIS

Disease	Clues in the history	Physical examination
Peptic ulcer (gastric, duodenal)	May be the first symptom; usually typical ulcer pain relation to food; night pains relieved by antacids; previous indigestion	Nil, or tenderness over epigastrium
Acute gastric erosion	Ingestion of aspirin; NSAIDs; corticosteroids	Nil
Acute intestinal erosion	Enteric-coated KCl tablets; reserpine	Nil
Stress ulcers	Head injury; Burns; Trauma; CNS disease	Nil
Portal hypertension (cirrhosis)	Previous episodes of jaundice, ascites or GI bleed; chronic alcoholism	Jaundice Hepatomegaly Splenomegaly Ascites, pedal oedema Abdominal wall dilated veins, Flapping tremors
Hiatus hernia (reflux oesphagitis)	Lower chest (retrosternal) and upper abdominal distress worse on lying down or bending forwards; relief on sitting up	Nil
Mallory-Weiss syndrome	Severe bout of vomiting followed by haematemesis; alcohol intake	Nil
Gastric cancer	Epigastric pain; anorexia; weight loss	Palpable mass in epigastrium and supraclavicular lymph node
Bleeding disorders	Previous bleeding episodes; bleeding from skin, nose, urinary tract, lungs	Bruises, purpuric spots on the skin, splenomegaly, pallor
Hereditary haemorrhagic telangiectasis	Previous episodes of nose bleed; family history	Red spots on tongue, lips, nose, fingertips

TABLE 4.2 CRUCIAL FEATURES OF LOWER GI BLEEDING

Haemorrhoids; anal fissure	Common with small recurrent bleeds Proctoscopy
Polyps	Small but frequent bleeds Sigmoidoscopic detection-single/multiple
Meckel's diverticulum	Abdominal pain with melaena
Solitary ulcer rectum	Possibly tuberculous
Inflammatory bowel disease (IBD), e.g. ulcerative colitis, Crohn's disease, amoebic colitis	Diarrhoea, blood and mucus Previous similar episodes Fever, anaemia, tachycardia
Diverticulosis	Age 60 and above; LLQ pain; short history LLQ tenderness; Previous similar episodes
Cancer colon	Age 60 and above; No pain at onset Rectal bleeding; PR: mass felt
Angiodysplasia of colon	Chronic renal failure patients; Commonly seen in ascending colon
Ischaemic colitis	Acute onset of abdominal pain; Bright red blood in stools; Sigmoidoscopy: no mucoid lesion

TABLE 4.3 INSPECTION OF STOOLS AND POSSIBLE SOURCE OF GI BLEEDING

- Blood coating the well-formed stool = source distal to sigmoid colon.
- Red blood mixed with stool = source proximal to sigmoid colon.
- Melaena–black tarry stool = source proximal to the caecum.
- Maroon stool = site distal to small bowel or right colon.
- Bright red blood without change in vital signs = anorectal source.
- Blood only on toilet paper = perianal lesions.

NOTE: Brisk upper GI bleeding with rapid intestinal transit may present with bright red blood in stools, but vital signs are always affected in that case.

Laboratory testing

Hct to assess the response to blood transfusion.

Hct should rise approximately 3 per cent for each unit of packed RBCs transfused.

Hct is also useful to assess the end point of transfusion.

Platelet count should be done in all bleeding patients. A patient with active bleeding and a platelet count of less than 50,000/µml should receive platelet transfusion or other therapy to increase the count. Hypersplenism secondary to portal hypertension is a common cause of thrombocytopenia.

PT and PTT should be measured in all patients but especially in those with suspected liver disease. Patients with active bleeding and prolonged PT or PTT should receive FFP to correct the defect. In the stable patient, correction of a prolonged PT may be attempted with inj. Vit. K 10 mg IV qid.

Nasogastric (NG) tube

In patients with haematemesis an NG tube should be inserted into the stomach as a means of detecting fresh or old blood. A positive gastric aspirate is in over 90 per cent of cases associated with an identifiable upper GI tract bleeding site.

Diagnosis confirmation

Confirmation of diagnosis of upper GI bleeding is by oesophagogastroduodenoscopy; it offers high diagnostic accuracy (85-95 per cent), low morbidity, the ability to recognize potential bleeding sites even when active bleeding is not occuring, and the potential for rapid therapeutic intervention. The procedure can be completed at the patient's bedside.

Endoscopy may be most helpful in determining which of the several potential lesions are actually bleeding and which patients have lesions with an increased risk of recurrent bleeding. Stigmata of recent haemorrhage (e.g. a visible bleeding vessel or adherent fresh blood clot found at the base of an ulcer) are associated with a recurrent bleed in 25-69 per cent of patients. Endoscopy also helps in precise identification of the site of bleeding prior to the introduction of oesophageal balloon tamponade with a Sangstaken tube.

Risk factors for increased morbidity and mortality
1. Age greater than 65 years.
2. More than one co-morbid illness.
3. Severe blood loss (more than 5 units).
4. Recurrent bleeding (within 72 hours).
5. 'Visible' bleeding or fresh clot on endoscopy.

Therapy of Specific Lesions

It is worth remembering that 85 per cent of bleeding episodes will resolve with supportive treatment alone.

Peptic ulcers
These are the most common cause of upper GI bleeding.
1. *Therapeutic endoscopy* with electro-coagulation or laser coagulation of actively bleeding ulcers offers the advantage of decreasing the blood transfusion requirements, length of hospital stay and the need for surgical intervention. Therapeutic endoscopy should not delay appropriate resuscitative measures outlined earlier.

   In patients with high risk ulcers (active bleeding, non-bleeding visible vessel, adherent clot), along with appropriate endoscopic therapy high dose constant IV infusion of omeprazol (80 mg bolus and 8 mg/ hour) raises the intragastric pH to between 6 and 7 helps to enhance clot stability and decrease further bleeding.

   Prevention of recurrent bleeding focuses on the 3 main factor in ulcer pathogenisis H. Pylori, NSAIDS and acid. Eradication of H. Pylori in patients with bleeding reduced the risk of the re-bleeding to less than 5 percent.

Endoscopic therapy is indicated for actively bleeding Mallory-Weiss tears.

2. *Surgery* is required for intractable or recurrent bleeding for peptic ulcer. Surgical consultation should be obtained early in the management of a patient with active GI bleeding. The indications are:
- Severe haemorrhage especially in patients over age 50 (needing more than 5 units of blood in 24 hours).
- Recurrent bleeding requiring additional blood transfusion during the same hospitalization.
- Ulcers with 'visible vessels'.
- Complicating medical conditions that would make elective surgery preferable to emergency surgery.

3. *Interventional radiography* with selective arterial catheterization. (a) *Intra-arterial vasopressin* infusion produces cessation of bleeding in 50-85 per cent of gastric ulcers and 12-60 per cent of duodenal ulcers. Patients with known coronary artery disease are at increased risk for ischaemia due to systemic effects of vasopressin. (b) *Arterial embolization* with absorbable gelfoam particles or metal coilsprings to produce immediate clotting. Ideally recanalization will occur after bleeding has been controlled, allowing healing of the ulcer. The success rate is variable and may be related to the location and type of lesion. Most complications occur in patients with previous gastric surgery or mesenteric vascular disease.

Oesophageal varices
In portal hypertension oesophageal or gastric varices cause bleeding with a high morbidity and mortality (35 per cent) despite modern resuscitative and therapeutic techniques.

1. *Endoscopic sclerotherapy* can be done at the bedside and is effective in controlling the primary bleeding (7-96 per cent). Results of serial sclerotherapy for the obliteration of varices after the initial bleeding episodes are comparable to other therapeutic options. Sclerotherapy is associated with a 10-15 per cent rate of significant complications, and recurrent bleeding is common.

Band ligation physically inhibits blood flow leading subsequently to thrombosis and obliteration of the varices. It is more effective than sclerotherapy and has fewer complications.

2. *Intravenous vasopressin* 100 units in 250 ml of 5 per cent dextrose in water (0.4 units/ml) is delivered by a microdrip infusion pump into a peripheral vein, on the following schedule: 0.3 units/minute every 30 minutes until haemostasis is achieved, side effects develop, or the maximum dose of 0.9 units/minute is reached.

   The infusion should be given in the ICU under cardiac monitoring. The infusion should be reduced or stopped if the patient develops angina pectoris, abdominal angina or arrhythmias. Concomitant IV nitroglycerin (NG) infusion has been shown to reduce side-effects and may improve the efficacy of vasopressin therapy. NG is administered only if the systolic BP is greater than 100 mm Hg. The dose is 10 µg/minute, increased by 10 µg/minute every 10-15 minutes until systolic BP falls to 100 mm Hg or a maximum dose of 400 µg/minute is reached.

   Control of variceal bleeding can be achieved by I. V. infusion of Octreotide (50 µg bolus and 50 µg/hour) for 2-5 days, and this has replaced vasopressin as the medical therapy of choice for acute variceal bleeding in USA.

3. *Balloon tamponade* with a Sangstaken-Blakemore tube (both a gastric + oesophageal balloon) or Linton tube (large volume gastric balloon only) or the Minnesota tube (large volume gastric balloon plus an oesophageal balloon) is effective in immediately stopping bleeding from varices, but there is a high incidence of major complications and significant mortality rate due to tube displacement. The use of the tubes should be undertaken only by experienced persons in ICU conditions.

4. *Shunt Surgery* (porta caval or distal splenorenal shunt) provides definitive therapy for patients with recurrent variceal bleeding; for patients with failed sclerotherapy; or for those who live away from a medical centre, or who live in places where it is difficult to obtain blood transfusions.

TIPS (transjugular intrahepatic portocaval shunt) has become available as an alternative approach in cases of failed sclerotherapy and re-bleeding which cannot be stopped. It can be performed under local anaesthesia. TIPS decreases rebleeding more effectively than endoscopic therapy, although hepatic encephalopathy is more common and the mortality rates are comparable. Most patients with TIPS have shunt restenosis within 1-2 years and require reinstrumentation hence TIPS is most appropriate for patients with more severe liver disease and those in whom liver transplant is anticipated.

Stress ulcers
These are a common cause of GI bleeding in the hospitalized patient. Prophylactic therapy should be provided to all patients at risk (head injury, burns, shock, sepsis, major trauma, prolonged mechanical ventilation, and CNS disease) requiring intensive care. Histamine H2 blockers are as effective as antacids and Sucralfate (in a slurry form) is given.

Angiodysplasia
Arteriovenous malformation (like telangiectasia) of the stomach or small intestines is an uncommon cause of GI bleed in the general population (7 per cent) but represents the most frequent source of upper GI bleeding in patients of chronic renal failure. These very small mucosal lesions (2 to 10 mm in diameter) can be single or multiple; some are most commonly diagnosed by endoscopy. These lesions bleed recurrently requiring a large number of transfusions over time. Oestrogen-progesterone therapy may decrease bleeding episodes in patients with renal failure.

Therapy for patients with lower GI bleeding in whom arteriography detects the source of bleeding: selective intra-arterial vasopressin stops the bleeding in upto 90 per cent of cases.

Ulcerative colitis
A short course of corticosteroids: maintenance therapy with Salazopyrine. If no response to medical management is seen then surgery is indicated.

GI Bleeding of obscure origin

In a significant proportion of recurrent acute and chronic GI Bleeding (7-25%) no source can be identified by routine endoscopic and angiographic studies. Push enteroscopy (specially designed to inspect the entire duodenum and part of the jejunum) may identify 20-40% bleeding sites. Video capsule endoscopy allows access to the entire small intestine and identifies 30-65% lesions. Tc-99m labeled RBCs is highly sensitive to detect active bleeding and provides the basis for super selective coeliac angiography both for detection and embolization of the bleeding site.

When all tests are unrevealing, intra-operative endoscopy is indicated in patients with severe recurrent or persistent bleeding requiring repeated transfusions.

5   Acute Myocardial Infarct

Acute Coronary Syndromes

Patients with atherosclerotic coronary artery disease fall into 2 large groups (1) stable angina going on for years; and (2) acute coronary syndromes (ACS) due to rupture or erosion of a vulnerable plaque with superimposed non-occlusive thrombus causing reduction in flow resulting in chest pain at rest or with slighest excretion. When the flow reduction is caused by a completely occlusive thrombus, it leads to acute myocardial infarction with ST segment elevation on presenting ECG (STEMI), the majority of whom ultimately develop a Q wave (QWMI). Patients with subtotally occlusive thrombus do not show ST elevation when they present with chest pain. They may remain as unstable angina (UA) but the majority will develop non-ST segmental elevation myocardial infarction, (UA/NSTEMI) as evidenced by rise in CK-MB or cardiac troponin in the blood. They will develop a non-Q wave MI.

Acute myocardial infarct (AMI) is a medical emergency requiring prompt hospitalization in an intensive care setting and careful medical management.

More than 50 per cent of the deaths associated with acute myocardial infarct occur within the first two hours after the onset of symptoms and are attributed to ventricular arrhythmias, usually ventricular fibrillation. The problem is how to arrange expeditious transport to the hospital ICU and what to do in the absence of these facilities, or in the time interval pending hospitalization.

The clinical diagnosis of AMI is based on the following features:

1. Chest pain resembling angina pectoris but of greater severity and duration (more than 20 minutes) and not relieved by nitroglycerin or nifedipine.

2. Chest pain may occur at rest or during sleep; only a minority of patients are engaged in strenuous activity at the time of infarction. Emotional factors are more likely to have precipitated the attack in the waking patient.

3. Accompanying symptoms: dyspnoea, vomiting, sweating, fatigue and palpitations.

Atypical presentations are equally important to remember.

1. Isolated dyspnoea
2. Isolated sweating and vomiting
3. Acute confusion

Silent infarct can occur especially in middle-aged post-operative patients, elderly patients, diabetics and hypertensive patients.

Physical examination may reveal an anxious patient with cold extremities. Elevation of jugular venous pressure (JVP) indicates congestive heart failure or right ventricular dysfunction. Auscultation of the lungs may reveal coarse rales and wheezing of pulmonary oedema. Palpation of the precordium may reveal a dyskinetic apex suggestive of regional wall motion abnormality. Auscultation of the heart may reveal an S_3 or S_4 gallop, systolic murmur (suggesting mitral incompetence or a ruptured interventricular septum).

The differential diagnosis of AMI includes other medical emergencies such as aortic dissection, pericarditis, myocarditis, pulmonary embolism, pneumothorax, perforated peptic ulcer, pancreatitis, cholecystitis and rupture of the oesophagus (See **Table 28.2**). Various spinal and musculoskeletal disorders can simulate AMI.

ECG, taken serially, plays an essential role in the diagnosis of AMI. An ECG should be obtained

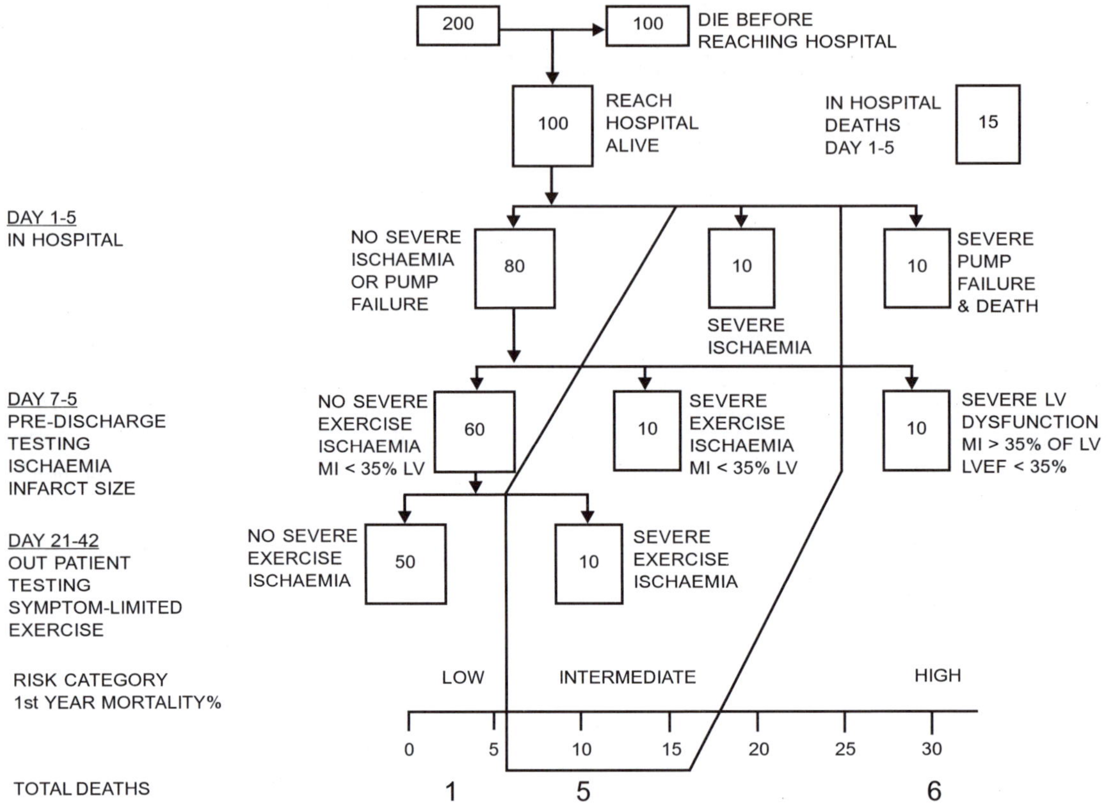

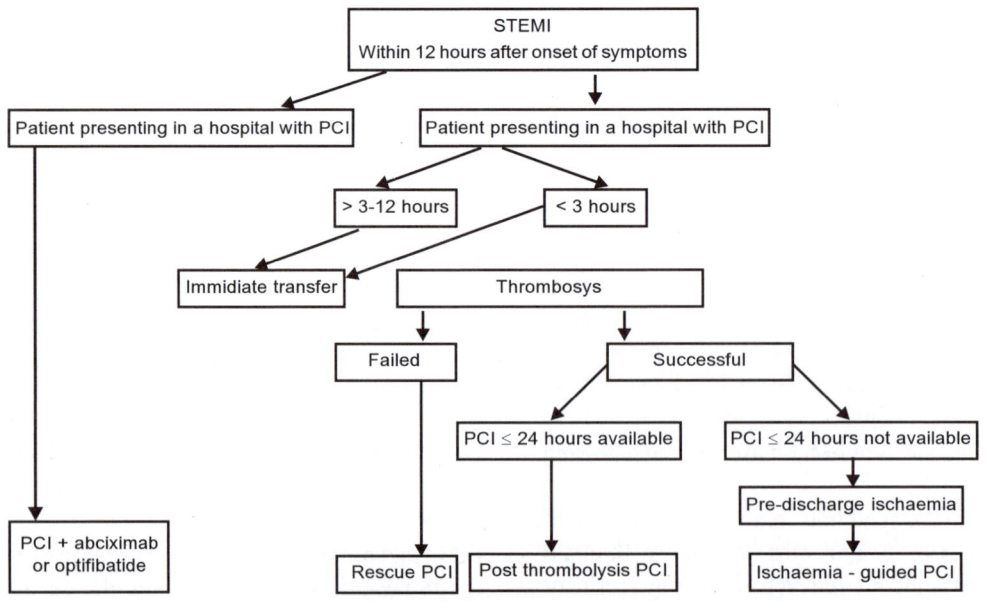

Fig. 5.1: Natural course of acute myocardial infarct

Fig. 5.2: Guidelines for management of STEMI from the Association of Physicians of India

Acute Myocardial Infarct

immediately on admission and daily during hospitalization, as well as for evaluation of recurrent chest pain or arrhythmias. It must be appreciated that initially the ECG may be *normal* and changes may evolve slowly over several hours, or upto 72 hours. Since the ECG is neither sensitive nor specific for the differentiation of transmural from non-transmural infarcts, the terms Q wave and non-Q wave infarction are preferable. Generally Q wave infarcts are associated with total thrombotic coronary artery occlusion and a greater area of necrosis than non-Q wave infarcts which are seen with partial coronary occlusion. Non-Q wave MIs have a higher prevalence of infarct extension than do Q wave infarcts. But the long-term prognosis is similar in both types.

The diagnostic ECG changes of AMI may be masked in the presence of left bundle branch block or ventricular arrhythmias. Changes in the ST segments and T waves on serial tracings may be the only clues present.

Cardiac enzymes and *proteins*, released into the circulation by myocardial injury and necrosis are useful in the definitive diagnosis of AMI. The earliest serum indicator of infarction is myoglobin (within 1-2 hours), followed by CPK-MB (rise within 4-6 hours, peak in 12-20 hours, return to baseline in 36-48 hours). LDH (lactic dehydrogenese) is elevated within 12 hours, peaks in 24-48 hours and remains elevated for 10-14 days after AMI. The measurement of plasma LDH isoenzymes LDH1 and LDH2 (ratio greater than one is considered evidence of AMI) is a valuable adjunct to CPK determination in patients presenting 1-2 days after the onset of symptoms.

Cardiac-specific troponin T (cTnT) and cardiac specific Troponin I (cTnI) have amino acid sequences different from those of skeletal muscle. They are not normally detectable in the blood of healthy individuals, but increase after STEMI to high levels and remain elevated for 7-10 days after STEMI hence they are more specific and more reliable than CK and CKMB.

Table 5.1 lists the complications of AMI.

Fig. 5.1 gives the natural course of AMI. Mortality results both from arrhythmias and pump failure. Myocardial infarct size is the primary determinant of in-hospital and post-discharge mortality. When 40 per cent or more of the LV myocardium is infarcted, prognosis is extremely poor. Since MI evolves over a period of several hours, restoration of myocardial perfusion through early thrombolytic therapy or other interventional therapy is worth attempting.

Fig. 5.2 API guidelines for management of ST elevation myocardial unfarct.

Management in ICU

1. *Analgesia:* Control of pain with *morphine sulphate* 1-4 mg slow IV, repeated after 5-10 minutes until pain is controlled or side-effects emerge. Nausea and vomiting can be avoided by concomitant use of an anti-emetic agent e.g. Cyc1izine 50 mg IV.

   Nitroglycerin 0.15 to 0.6 mg sublingually or 25-50 µg IV, followed by a 10 µg/minute infusion is useful to relieve ischaemic pain and also to reduce myocardial oxygen consumption.

2. *Sedation:* low doses of a benzodiazepine.

3. *Oxygen therapy:* 2-4 litres/minute via nasal cannula.

4. *Beta-adrenergic antagonists:* to reduce sympathetic overactivity (tachycardia, hypertension, continued pain).

   Propranolol 0.1 mg/kg IV given in 3 doses at intervals of 5-10 minutes followed by 20-40 mg PO every 6-8 hours.

   Esmolol hydrochloride, ultra-short active B blocker initial 250-500 µg/kg IV bolus over a minute and titrated to a heart rate of 55-60 p.m., has the added advantage of rapid withdrawal if adverse effects develop.

Caution: Beta blockers are contraindicated if:

1. Resting heart rate is below 50-55 p.m.

2. Systolic BP is less than 95 mm Hg.

3. PR interval is more than 0.24 seconds (significant first degree heart block), or 2nd or 3rd degree heart block.

4. Obstructive lung disease by history or wheezing on physical examination.

5. Evidence of heart failure by physical examination or chest X-ray.

TABLE 5.1 Thrombolytics use in PE

Sr. No.	Thromolytic	Dosage/Special Point	Remarks
1	Alteplase	A 15mg bolus, followed by 85mg administered over 2 hours	USFDA approved
2	Urokinase	4400 U/kg as a loading dose over 10 minutes, then continuous infusion of 4400 U/kg/h for 12-24 hours	USFDA approved
3	Streptokinase	250,000 U loading dose over 30 minutes, then 100,000 U/h over 12-24 hours	USFDA approved
4	Reteplase/ Tenecteplase	Same doses as AMI	Not USFDA approved

Thrombolytic therapy (**Table 5.1**)

This is suitable in the following settings:

- patient younger than 75 years of age.
- angina persisting 30 minutes or more associated with new ST segment elevation of at least 0.1 mV in at least two leads in the inferior, anterior or lateral location.
- admitted within 1-2 hours of onset of chest pain.

Fibronolysis should ideally be initiated within 30 minutes of presentation (door to needle time) to promptly restore the full coronary artery patency. TPA, streptokinase, tenecteplase (TNK) and retaplase (g PA) all act by promoting the conversion of plasminogen to plasmin which subsequently lyses fibrin thrombi. When administered within the first hour of the onset of symptoms of STEMI, fibrinolysis can reduce the relative risk of in-hospital death by upto 50%.

Contraindications

1. Bleeding disorder, or history of GI or GU bleed.
2. Patient is already on anticoagulants.
3. Uncontrolled hypertension.
4. History of cerebrovascular accident.
5. Surgery or prolonged CPR in the last two weeks.
6. Concurrent serious illness.

Specific agents

Urokinase 6000 IU/minute intracoronary infusion for upto 1-2 hours, or IV 1-2 million units infused over 1 hour.

Streptokinase 20,000 IU bolus followed by 2000 IU/minute intracoronary, or IV 1-5 million units infused over one hour.

Recombinant tissue plasminogen activator (RTPA).
100 mg IV over a total period of 3 hours:
10 mg: as initial bolus followed by continuous infusion for a total of 60 mg over first hour.
20 mg over each of the next 2 hours.

Reperfusion arrhythmia (VT, VF) may be prevented by prophylactic lidocaine 1 mg/kg IV bolus followed in 10 minutes by 0.75 mg/kg IV bolus and then a 2 mg per minute continuous infusion. Heparin 100 units/kg (IV bolus followed by 1000 units/hour infusion should be given at the time of thrombolytic therapy to prevent reocclusion.

Primary Percutaneous Coronary Intervention (PCI) (angioplasty and stenting without preceding fibronolysis) is effective in restoring perfusion in STEMI when carried out on an emergency basis in the first few hours of AMI. It is more effective than fibronolysis in opening occluded coronary arteries, when performed by experienced operators with "door to balloon time < 2 hours". Compared to fibronolysis, PCI is generally prefered when cardiogenic shock is present, bleeding risk is increased or symptoms have been present for at least 2-3 hours when the clot is less easily lysed by fibrinolytic drugs.

Alternative pharmacological regimens for reperfusion combine IV GpIIb/IIIa inhibitor, Aspirin and clopidogrel. These have reduced the risk of death with recurrent ischemia events.

TABLE 5.2 Recommendations of antiplatelet agents in ACS

Recommendeations	Class	Level
Aspirin should be given to all patients without contraindications at an initial loading dose of 150-300 mg. and at a maintenance dose of 75-1 00 mg daily long-term regardless of treatment strategy and continued indefinitely in patients who tolerate it.	1	A
A P2Y$_{12}$ inhibitor should be added to aspirin as soon as possible and maintained over 12 months, unless there are contraindications such as excessive risk of bleeding.	1	A
A proton pump inhibitor (preferably not omeprazole) in combination with DAPT is recommended in patients with a history of gastrointestinal hemorrhage or peptic ulcer, and appropriate for patients with multiple other risk factors (H, elicobacter pylori infection, age $\geq$ 65 years, concurrent use of anticoauglants or steroids).	1	A
Prolonged or permanent withdrawal of P2Y$_{12}$ inhibitors within 12 months after the index event is discouraged unless clinically indicated. In patients with DES a longer duration can be considered.	1	C
Ticagrelor (180 mg loading dose, 90 mg twice daily) is recommended for all patients at moderate-to-high risk of ischaemic events (e.g. elevated troponins), regardless of initial treatment strategy and including those pre-treated with clopidogrel (which should be discontinued when ticagrelor is commenced).	1	B
Prasugrel (60 mg loading dose, 10 mg daily dose) is recommended for P2Y$_{12}$ inhibitor naive patients (especially diabetics) in whom coronary anatomy is known and who are proceeding to PCI unless there is a high risk of life threatening bleeding or other contraindications. Prasugrel is used only in cath lab for planned PCI. It is not to be used in emergency department or in medically treated patient.	1	B
Clopidogrel (300 mg loading dose, 75 mg daily dose) is recommended for patients who cannot receive ticagrelor or prasugrel.	I	A
A 600 mg loading dose of c1opidogrel (or a supplementary 300 mg dose at PCI following an initial 300 mg loading dose) is recommended for patients scheduled for an invasive strategy when ticagrelor or prasugrel is not an option.	I	B
A higher maintenance dose of clopidogrel 150 mg daily should be considered for the first 7 days in patients managed with PCI and without increased risk of bleeding.	IIa	B
Icreasing the maintenance dose of c1opidogrel based on platelet function testing is not advised as routine but may be considered in selected cases.	IIb	B
Genotyping and/or platelet function testing may be considered in selected cases when c1opdiogrel is used.	IIb	B
In patients pre-treated with P2Y$_{12}$ inhibitors who need to undergo non-emergent major surgery (including CABG), postponing surgery at least for 5 days after cessation of ticagrelor or c1opidogrel and 7 days for prasugrel, if clinically feasible and unless the patients is at high risk of ischemic events should be considered.	IIa	C
Ticagrelor or c1opidogrel should be considered to be restarted after CABG surgery as soon as considered safe.	IIa	B
The combination of aspirin with an NSAID (selective COX-2 inhibitors and non-selective NSAID) is not recommended.	III	C

Complications of AMI

Heart Failure (HF)

This is a common complication of AMI and is associated with increased mortality in comparison to uncomplicated AMI, and prompt diagnosis and therapy are essential. Haemodynamic monitoring with a balloon-tipped pulmonary artery catheter should be considered in all patients of AMI complicated by HF, and should definitely be carried out in patients who do not promptly respond to appropriate treatment.

1. The balloon flotation catheter measures the pulmonary artery pressure (PA); pulmonary artery occlusive pressure (PAOP) which reflects left atrial pressure; right atrial pressure (RA); and cardiac output by thermodilution.

2. The femoral arterial catheter allows frequent determination of systemic blood pressure, when cuff pressure is unreliable or difficult to obtain (as in cardiogenic shock).

3. Hourly urine output is measured, with an Indwelling bladder catheter if necessary.

TABLE 5.3 COMPLICATIONS OF AMI

Complications	Consequences
A. Arrhythmias	VF and complete heart block can be dangerous.
B. Pump failure	Cardiogenic shock– major cause of death.
C. Infarction of mitral papillary muscle	Mitral incompetence and pulmonary oedema.
D. Rupture of inter- ventricular septum	Severe hypotension.
E. Rupture of ventricle into pericardium	Tamponade.
F. Mural thrombus in LV	Cerebral embolism.
G. Venous thrombosis –leg veins	Pulmonary embolism.
H. Ventricular aneurysm	Cerebral embolism, decreased left ventricular ejection fraction (LVEF).
I. Pericarditis	Marker of extensive infarction.
J. Post myocardial infarction syndrome (Dressler's).	Self-limiting but course may be lengthy. Rarely constrictive pericarditis.

Haemodynamic monitoring is indicated for:

i.   Moderate or severe left ventricular failure.

ii. Hypotension unresponsive to simple measures (e.g. IV fluids).

iii. Severe cyanosis, hypoxaemia, tachypnoea, sweating and acidosis.

iv. Unexplained or refractory tachycardia or other tachyarrhythmias.

v.   Clinical signs suggestive of mitral regurgitation, ruptured interventricular septum or haemodynamically significant pericardial effusion.

vi. Use of inotropic agents or vasodilators in the context of AMI.

TABLE 5.4 UNFAVOURABLE PROGNOSTIC SIGNS IN AMI

Persistent angina

Cardiomegaly

Persistent tachycardia and signs of heart failure

$S_3 S_4$ gallop

Chest-x-ray

2D echocardiography-low LVEF

Persistent ST-depression

Non-Q wave infarction is associated with a higher risk of infarct extension or recurrence (35-40%) than Q wave infarction (10-15% risk)

Most extensions occur within 7-10 days of Infarction Diltiazem 90 mg qid as preventive in non-QAMI

Diuretics are the first line of treatment for mild to moderate HF (i.e. S_3 gallop, pulmonary basal rales).

Dobutamine, a synthetic beta-adrenergic agonist is the preferred parenteral inotropic agent if the HF does not improve with diuretics, or if symptoms worsen. Continuous infusion is started with 1-2 µg/kg/minute and is gradually increased until haemodynamic improvement occurs or a dose of 10 µg/kg/minute is reached. Cardiac output is increased and LV end-diastolic pressure is decreased at this dosage.

Amrinone, a bipyridine derivative, produces both positive inotropic and vasodilator effect. A slow IV infusion (0.75 mg/kg) over several minutes, followed by a continuous infusion at 5-10 µg/kg/minute titrated to the haemodynamic response, decreases the pulmonary wedge pressure (PWP) and systemic vascular resistance (SVR).

Vasodilator therapy with nitroglycerin given as a continuous infusion beginning with 10 µg/minute is useful to reduce hypertension and pulmonary congestion.

Combination therapy with dobutamine and nitroglycerin is beneficial for patients with moderate to severe CHF.

Cardiogenic shock is indicated by systolic BP below 80, or mean BP less than 60 mm Hg, urine output less than 500 ml in 24 hours, elevated filling pressure with PAOP greater than 18 mm Hg (normal 5-6 mm Hg), cold clammy skin and mental confusion. It signifies 35-40 per cent loss of functioning myocardium, leading to a high (80 per cent) mortality despite aggressive intervention.

When inotropic measures fail, intra-aortic balloon counter-pulsation (IABC) can reduce oxygen demand through reduction in both preload and afterload and additionally increases coronary perfusion pressure and collateral flow, especially when a surgically treatable complication such as mitral regurgitation or ruptured interventricular septum is present.

Arrhythmias in AMI
Nearly all patients with acute myocardial infarction (AMI) have some form of arrhythmia, but in most cases it is mild and of no haemodynamic or prognostic significance.

25 illustrative ECG trainings are shown as under:

1. *Sinus tachycardia:* This is the commonest arrhythmia; anxiety may contribute to it. Persistence of sinus tachycardia may be a warning of incipient cardiac failure.
2. *Sinus bradycardia:* This is more common after inferior AMI.
    Usually it does not need treatment unless it is associated with hypotension.
    Severe bradycardia may lead to ventricular escape and the development of more dangerous rhythms.
3. *Atrial tachycardia or fibrillation:* This occurs in about 15 per cent of patients. These arrhythmias may exacerbate hypotension or cardiac failure

and require prompt treatment if the ventricular rate is excessively fast.

4. *Ventricular ectopic beats:* These are almost invariably present, and are frequently numerous. They can cause concern under the following conditions:
    1) Multifocal instead of unifocal.
    2) More than 6-8 per minute.
    3) 'R on T' i.e. the ectopic falls on the T wave of the preceding beat.
5. *Ventricular tachycardia:* This is also common. If it persists at a fast rate for more than 30 seconds it may have serious haemodynamic effects.

Differential diagnosis
All that looks like VT (ventricular tachycardia) may not be so. Two other common conditions should be remembered: (1) Supraventricular tachycardia (SVT) with aberrant conduction, and (2) SVT with conduction over accessory pathways.

QRS interval less than 140 msec, with RBBB morphology of QRS in lead V1 is more in favour of SVT.

Presence of AV dissociation, fusion beats, ventricular capture beats, V-A conduction are the most useful diagnostic criteria which confirm VT.

6. *Accelerated idioventricular rhythm* (AIVR): This is commonly seen after AMI especially after reperfusion. AIVR is slower ventricular tachycardia with the rate limit of 55-108 beats per minute. The rate is usually slightly faster than sinus rate and there is gradual take over from one rhythm to another. Due to this, fusion beats are common.
7. *Ventricular fibrillation:* This occurs in about 5-10 per cent of hospitalized patients. The highest risk is in the first hour after infarction, and may kill the patient before he has a chance of reaching the hospital. Hence the doctor who sees him at home should give a lidocaine bolus, if the blood pressure is above 100 mm Hg.

    Ventricular fibrillation is uncommon with AIVR and hence usually does not require treatment.
8. *Heart block:* Myocardial infarct is the most frequent cause of heart block which develops suddenly.

ECGs for practice

ECG 1

II

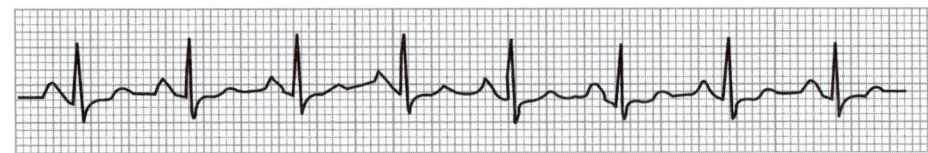

ECG 2

VI

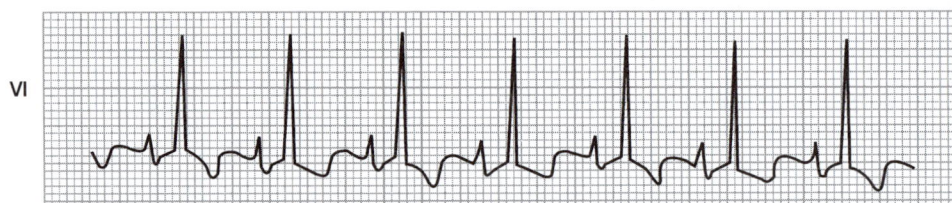

ECG 3

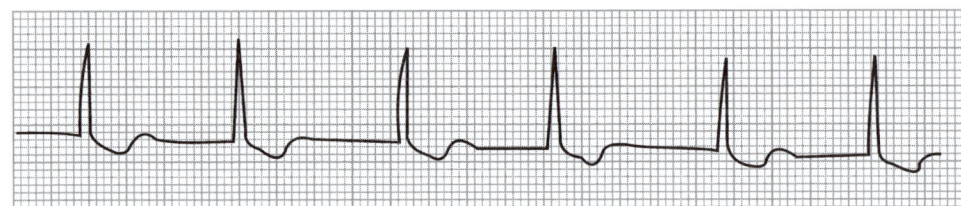

ECG 4

II

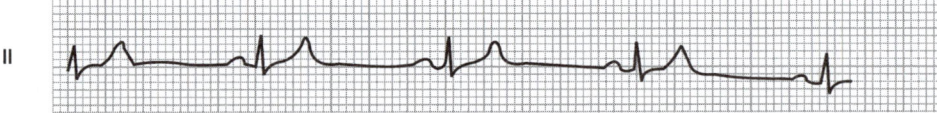

ECG 5

II

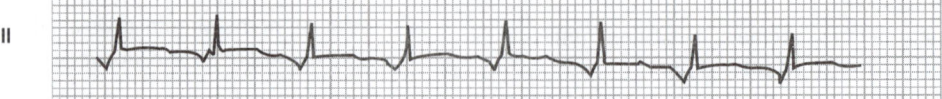

ECG 6

V1

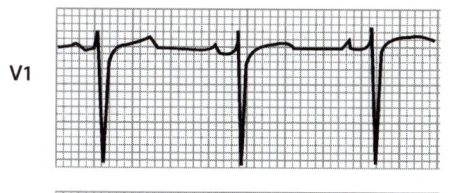

V6

ECG 9

V1

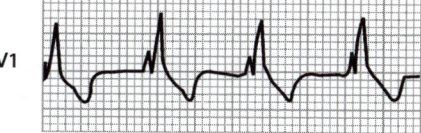

V6

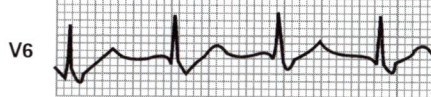

ECG 7

V1

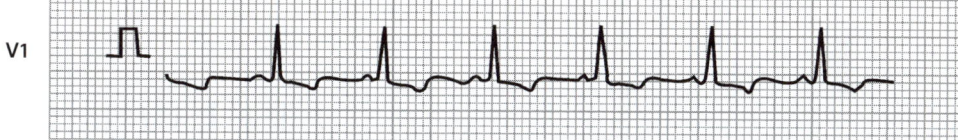

ECG 8

I

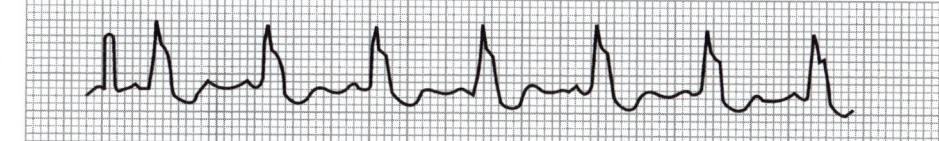

ECG 10

II

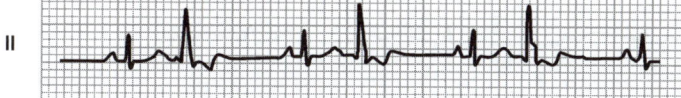

ECG 11

II

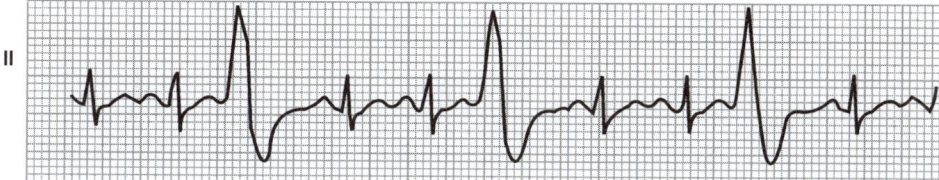

ECG 12

V1

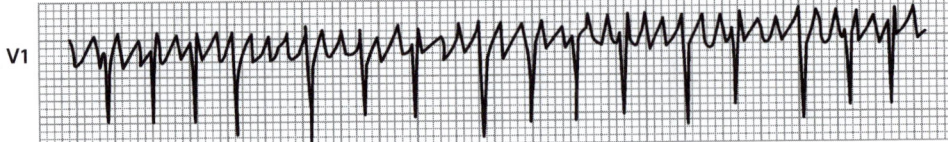

ECG 13

II

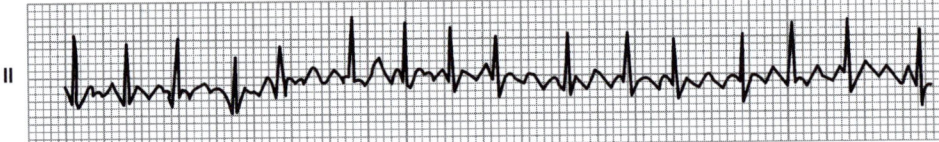

ECG 14

II

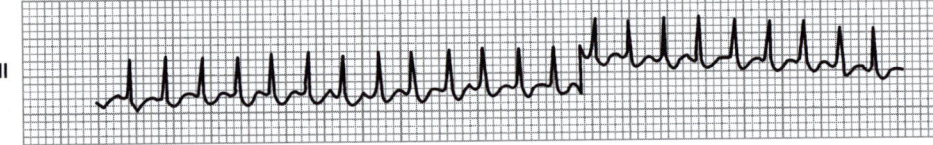

ECG 15

I

II

III

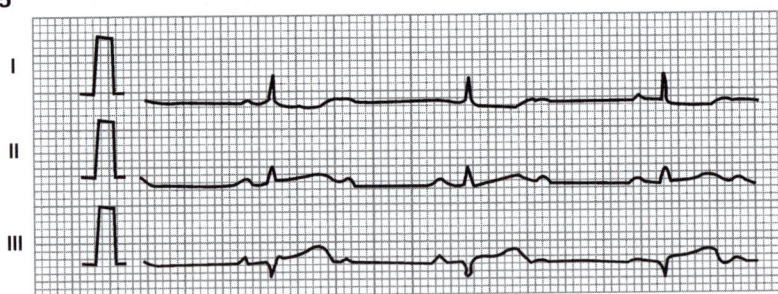

ECG 16

III

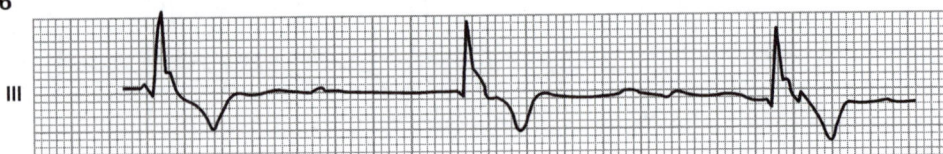

ECG 17

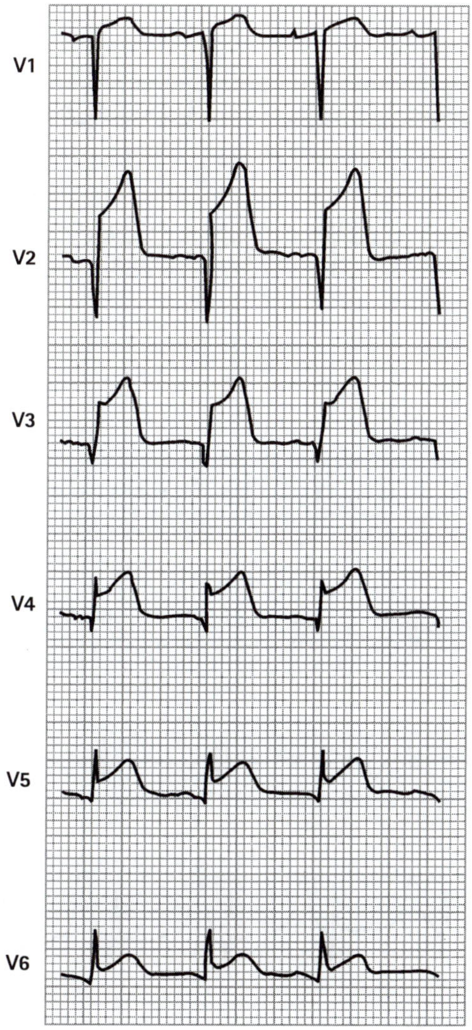

V1

V2

V3

V4

V5

V6

ECG 19

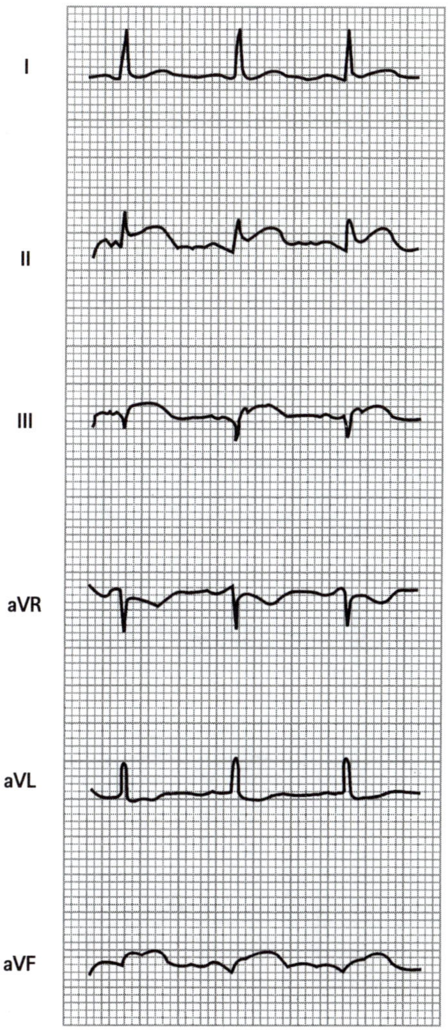

I

II

III

aVR

aVL

aVF

ECG 22

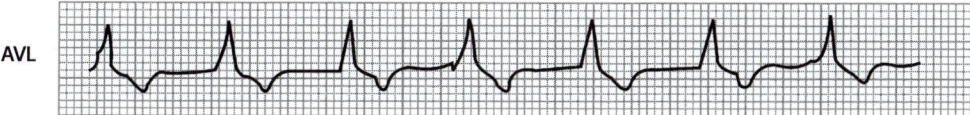

AVL

ECG 20

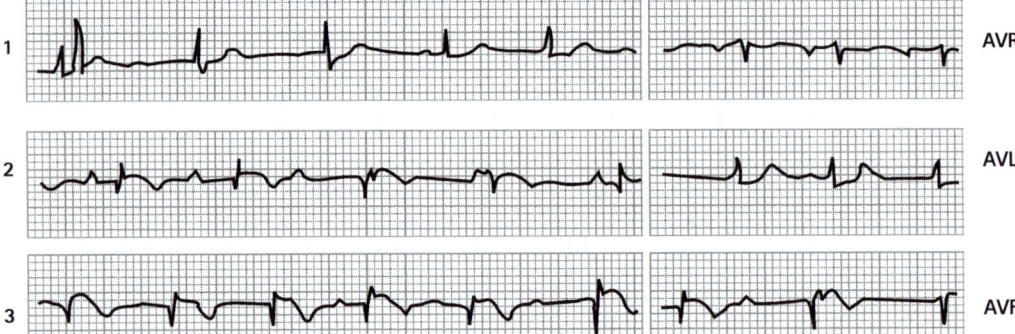

1	AVR
2	AVL
3	AVF

ECG 21

1	AVR
2	AVL
3	AVF

V1   V2   V3

V4   V5   V6

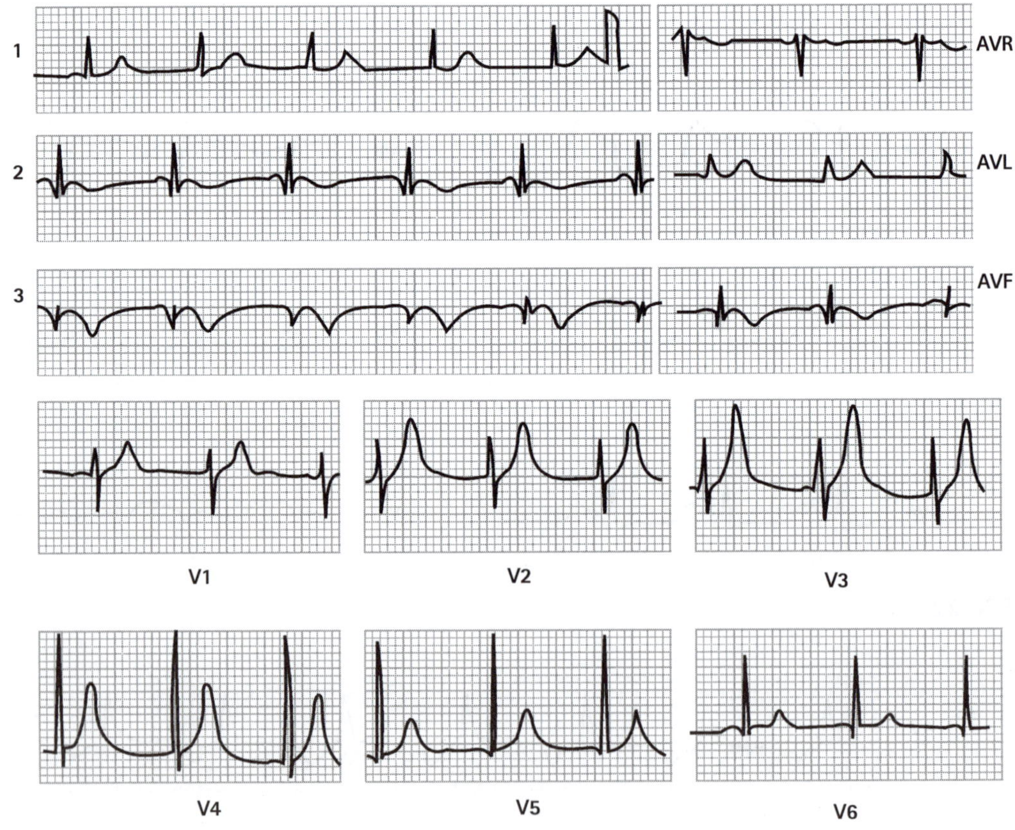

ECG 18

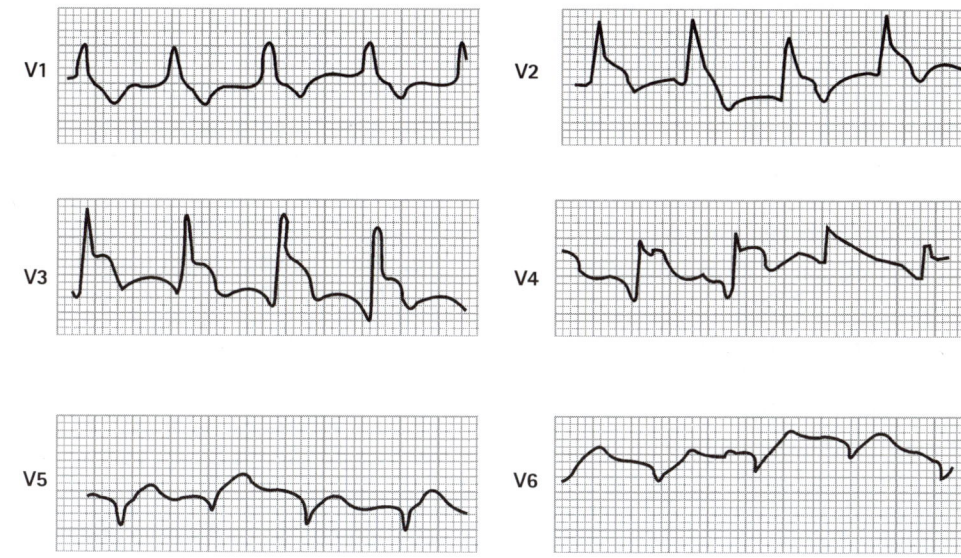

ECG22

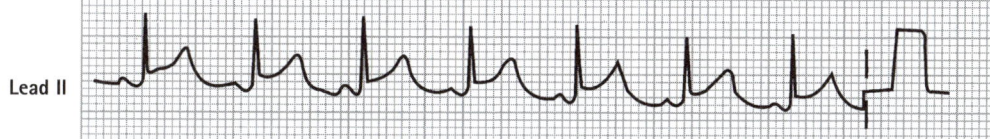

ECG24

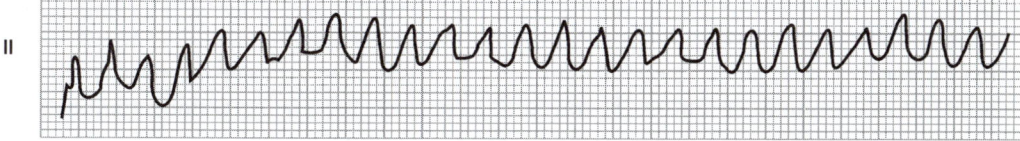

ECG25

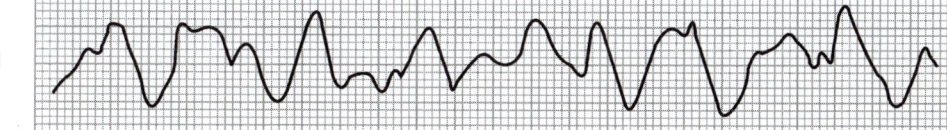

Answers to ECGs

1. **P mitrale** - Note wide notched P wave of greater than 0.10 seconds in duration.

2. **Biatrial hypertrophy with RVH with strain** – Biphasic P wave in VI, initial peaked P wave (P pulmonale) followed by negative deflection (P mitrale) and tall R wave with T wave inversion seen in VI (RVH with strain).

3. **Digitalis effect (hockey stick T wave)** - The ST segment with T wave appears like the mirror image of the correction mark.

4. **Sinus bradycardia** - Rate less than SO/minute; otherwise normal P-QRST

5. **Idiojunctional (nodal) rhythm** - Note P is inverted and PR interval is short; QRS complex is normal (like sinus beat).

6. **Left ventricular hypertrophy with strain** - The sum of S in VI and R in V6 is greater than 35 mm (LVH by voltage criteria) with ST-T depression in V6, suggesting strain.

7. **Right ventricular hypertrophy with strain** - In lead VI, tall R is greater than S mm along with ST - T depression, which indicates RVH with strain.

8. **Left bundle branch block** - Note wide and notched R waves in lead I.

9. **Right bundle branch block** - Note wide rSRI pattern in VI and slurred S waves in V6.

10. **Bigeminy** - Note SB and VPB followed by compensatory pause (pulsus bigeminus) coming in cycles.

11. **Trigeminy** - Note VPBs coming after every two SBs giving pulsus trigeminus rhythm.

12. **Atrial flutter (2:1, 3:1) block** - Note sawtooth appearance of two or three flutter (F) waves followed by QRS complex.

13. **Flutter fibrillation with fast ventricular response** - Note flutter fibrillatory waves followed by fast QRS complexes coming at irregular interval.

14. **Paroxysmal atrial tachycardia** - Note fast regular (greater than I60/minute) atrial tachycardia.

15. **2:1 AV block** - Note slow regular ventricular rate (less than SO/pm) preceded by two P waves with constant PR interval in every cycle confirming 2:1 AV block.

16. **Complete heart block** - Note very slow (less than 3D/minute), regular ventricular heart rate (idioventricular rhythm) with AV dissociation.

17. **Acute anterior wall MI** - Note Q waves and ST elevation in leads V2, V3, V4, VS (hyperacute phase of AMI) and also a small Q wave in lead V6 with ST elevation.

18. **Right bundle branch block with anterior wall MI** - Wide R waves in lead VI (RBBB); note coved up ST segment elevation in leads V2, V3 and V4; Q waves in leads V2-V6 suggestive of anterior wall MI.

19. **Acute inferior wall MI** - Note Q waves and coved up ST segment elevation in leads II, 1II and aVF suggestive of acute inferior wall MI.

20. **Inferior wall MI in evolution** - Note Q waves, elevated ST with coving downwards and T wave inversion in leads II, III and aVF; opposite changes (ST depression) in leads I and aVL.

21. **Inferior wall infarction with true posterior wall MI** - Note Q waves, coved up ST segment elevation and T wave inversion in leads II, III and aVF (inferior wall MI). Also note tall R waves and peaked tall T wave in leads VI, V2, V3 and V 4, diagnostic of true posterior wall MI.

22. **Acute pericarditis** - Note ST elevation with concavity upwards, suggestive of acute pericarditis.

23. **Wolff–Parkinson**-White syndrome - Note a very tiny P wave with very short PR interval, delta wave and wide QRS complex with ST depression and T wave inversion, diagnostic of WPW syndrome.

24. **Ventricular tachycardia** - Note wide notched QRS complexes at fast and regular intervals.

25. **Ventricular fibrillation** - Note chaotic irregular ventricular complexes without any recognizable wave pattern.

First degree heart block: delayed AV conduction. This can be diagnosed only by ECG (PR interval more than 0.20 sec.).

Second degree heart block: or partial heart block. Some atrial impulses fail to get through to the ventricles. When the atrial and ventricular contractions bear a simple ratio to one another such as in 2:1 and 3:1 block, the pulse is slow and regular.

Changes in the degree of partial heart block may give rise to sudden changes in the pulse rate.

More complex ratios such as 3:2 or 4:3 block give rise to dropped beats.

Partial heart block following AMI is usually transient.

Complete heart block: This is suspected when the pulse rate is very slow (30 to 40 per minute) and does not vary with change of posture or exertion.

Intermittent complete heart block may produce Stokes-Adams syndrome. First degree and asymptomatic second degree heart block do not need treatment. Symptomatic second degree block following inferior AMI usually responds to atropine (0.3 mg IV, repeated to a maximum of 1.2 mg). If it does not, a temporary pacemaker may be needed.

Complete heart block complicating inferior AMI is often accompanied by an escape rhythm at a satisfactory rate. It may need no treatment or it may respond to atropine; if that is unsuccessful a temporary pacemaker is needed.

Complete heart block following anterior AMI requires a temporary pacemaker. If the patient presents with asystole, atropine and isoprenoline (1-5 mg in 500 ml glucose) infused intravenously at the minimum rate needed to produce a satisfactory heart rhythm, may help to maintain the circulation until a temporary pacing electrode can be inserted.

SAECG (Signal-averaged ECG)

SAECG is a new diagnostic tool which allows the detection of late potentials (LPs)-low amplitude signals which prolong the terminal portion of the QRS complex, not picked up by conventional ECG. LPs indicate high risk for arrhythmic events and sudden cardiac death following AMI. It is known that even patients with uncomplicated AMI with an uneventful course in the ICU without arrhythmias

may have arrhythmic events in the subsequent 1-2 years. Hence it is desirable to do a pre-discharge SAECG on every patient to identify the subgroup with LPs. Thrombolysis in the early hours following AMI diminishes the incidence of LPs.

Subsequent Management of AMI

Unfavourable prognostic signs are listed in **Table 5.4**. Timetable for rehabilitation is given in **Table 5.5**.

If uncomplicated, the patient may sit out of bed on day 2, walk to the toilet on day 5 (when the heparin subcutaneous injection should be discontinued), go home on day 7-10, and return to work after 4-12 weeks depending upon the degree of physical labour.

TABLE 5.5 TIME TABLE FOR REHABILITATION ON AN UNCOMPLICATED COURSE OF AMI

1. Move toes/feet actively while in bed to prevent venous thrombosis
2. Sit in a chair within 24 hours-help himself for shaving, feeding and bed-side toilet
3. Walk in the room on 3rd day. Fully ambulatory by day 5-7. Visit toilet.
4. Sub maximal treadmill ECG test prior to discharge from hospital (better still if radionuclide tests are available) to identify patients at low and high risk for subsequent cardiac events.
5. Normal sexual activity after 6 weeks.
6. Return to work within 2 months at which time supervised exercise rehabilitation may be started.
7. Cessation of tobacco use permanently.
8. Aspirin 300 mg/d and beta blocker long-term use.

Under supervision, the level of physical exercise can be increased slowly. The patient should be encouraged to join a planned fitness training programme. He and his spouse should be specifically told that it is safe to resume normal sexual activity.

A pre-discharge radio nuclide ventriculography (which has a better sensitivity and specificity than ECG stress testing), is the most cost-effective test for assessing future risk. If the LVEF at rest is more than 40 per cent and shows no fall on exercise, if the LV size is normal and there are no exercise-induced regional wall motion abnormalities outside the infarct region, the patient can be considered to be at low risk for future coronary events or sudden death.

On the other hand LVEF at rest less than 40 per cent or a fall in exercise EF to less than 40 per cent with wall motion abnormality outside the area of infarct indicate high risk for future events and the need for further evaluation by coronary angiography. The aim is to seek the opportunity for revascularization and save the jeopardized myocardium from future insult.

TABLE 5.6 RISK FACTORS FOR ISCHAEMIC HEART DISEASE

Male Sex.

Age over 40 (although infarcts are now occurring at a young age).

Family history: death due to IHD under age 50, in father, uncle or brothers.

Smoking tobacco.

Hypertension.

Diabetes mellitus with insulin resistance.

Cholesterol HDL ratio more than 4.5 (HDL less than 30). LD (a) > 30

Waist-hip ratio (WHR) 1+.

Type A behaviour; unsuccessful aggression.

ACE gene (DD) genotype.

Risk factors should be controlled (**Table 5.6**). Aspirin 75 mg PO/once daily and beta blocker (atenolol 50 mg PO/once daily may be given as prophylactic against future coronary occlusion and ventricular fibrillation.

NOTE: Hyperinsulinaemia with insulin resistance is gaining increasing consideration as an initiating event in IHD, hypertension, obesity and diabetes.

The capability of localizing arrhythmogenic foci with cardiac catheterization has led to the possibility of cure of certain dangerous arrhythmias through the delivery of ablative radio frequency (RF) or chemicals via the catheter.

A subgroup of patents in whom RF ablative surgery has been particularly gratifying are those patients with recurrent VT early after AMI.

Antiplatelets

1. Phosphodiesterase inhibitors
   a) Dipyridamole
   b) Cilostazol

2. P2Y12 receptor antagonists
   a) First generation (Irreversible)
      i) Ticlopidine
      ii) Clopidogrel
      iii) Prasugrel
   b) Second generation (Reversible and non-competitive)
      i) Ticagrelor
      ii) Cangrelor
   c) Third generation (Reversible and competitive)
      i) Elinogrel

3. PAR-1 antagonists
   a) Vorapaxar
   b) Atopaxar

4. GPIIb/IIIa receptor antagonists
   a) Abciximan
   b) Trofiban

6 Cardiac Arrest

Cardiac arrest is sudden and complete loss of cardiac function, usually due to ventricular fibrillation, less often due to asystole. **Table 6.1** gives the mechanisms of cardiac arrest, and **Table 6.2** gives the various settings in which cardiac arrest occurs.

When the physician is faced with a patient whose pulsations cannot be felt (carotid, femoral, brachial) and whose heart sounds cannot be heard, a life-threatening emergency has arisen where instantaneous action will make all the difference between life and death. Since cessation of effective cardiac action has occurred and the brain is not receiving blood supply, urgent measures have to be adopted by the man-on-the-spot to restore blood flow to the brain. Every second counts. Most attempts at resuscitation have to be commenced before an ECG is available.

Every doctor, nurse, paramedical staff, ambulance driver, in fact every citizen especially family members of cardiac patients should be fully trained in carrying out the following cardiopulmonary resuscitation (CPR) drill effectively (**Fig 6.1**).

A. Positioning the Patient

1. Place the patient on a hard flat surface. A wooden board may be slipped under him on the cot. If that is not available he can be placed on the floor.

2. Elevate the legs, and keep them raised (resting on a table-top or chair) so as to facilitate venous return from the lower limbs by gravity.

3. Lower the patient's head and extend it as far as possible to ensure a clear airway.

4. Give one or two sharp thumps or blows with the closed fist over the middle of the sternum. This

may restore the heart beat in a fair percentage of cases. If this does not happen, then start external cardiac massage.

TABLE 6.1 MECHANISMS OF CARDIAC ARREST

Common result:	No audible heart sounds. No palpable pulsations.
Clinical distinction NOT possible	*ECG alone can decide it*
I. Ventricular fibrillation	ECG shows abnormal pattern.
II. Cardiac asystole	ECG shows flat line.
III. Extremely feeble heart beats	ECG shows normal QRS configuration.

B. External Cardiac Massage

1. Place yourself in a kneeling position by the side of the patient and with the heel of one hand placed on the lower end of the sternum and the heel of the other hand placed over it for reinforcement.

2. Exert sufficient downward pressure to depress the sternum 4-5 cm (1½ to 2 inches). Release the pressure suddenly to allow the sternum to recoil and repeat this process rhythmically 60-70 times a minute.

3. Gauge the effectiveness of cardiac massage by noting
   i.   production of a palpable carotid pulse; and
   ii. pupil reaction.

   The pupil which was dilated and fixed, will now become small, and reactive to light.

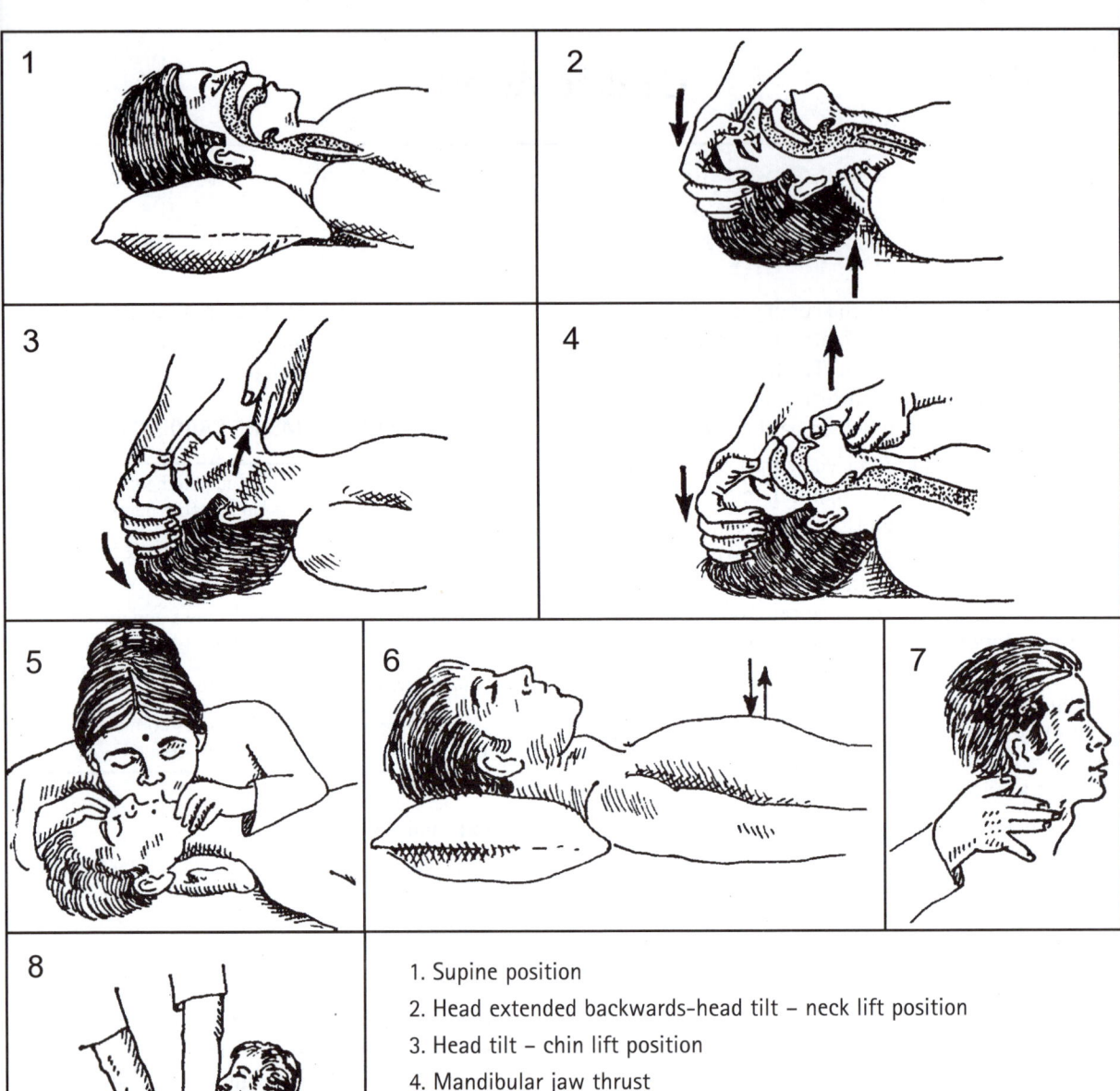

1. Supine position
2. Head extended backwards-head tilt – neck lift position
3. Head tilt – chin lift position
4. Mandibular jaw thrust
5. Mouth-to-mouth breathing
6. Observe rise and fall of chest (chest expansion)
7. Check carotid pulse
8. External cardiac massage

Fig. 6.1: Cardiopulmonary resuscitation

Table 6.2 CAUSES OF CARDIAC ARREST

	Setting	Examples	Remarks
A.	Diseases of the heart	Myocardial infarction Pulmonary embolism Cardiac tamponade Acute viral myocarditis	History of pain Sweating Shock
B.	Surgical Predisposing causes: asphyxia, excessive blood loss hypotension	During major abdominal operations, chest operations, ENT operations	Monitor ECG Always keep defibrillator and pacemaker ready Avoid excessive blood loss, hypotension, asphyxia
C.	Drug toxicity	Quinidine Procaine amide Digitalis Adrenaline Fluothiane	Always monitor ECG
D.	Electrolyte disturbances	Excess of Ca, Mg Excess of K+ Deficit of K+	Renal failure Vomiting
E.	Investigatory procedures	Paracentesis: pleural, pericardial, peritoneal, IVP Angiocardiography Cerebral angiography Percutaneous cholangiography	Prophylactic: inj. atropine to avoid vagal over-action
F.	Miscellaneous causes	Drowning Electrocution Severe trauma	

C. Mouth-to-mouth Breathing

This has to be started simultaneously with the external cardiac massage.

1. Clear the oropharynx of all contents (dentures, food, vomitus).

2. Pinch the nostrils of the patient firmly together with the thumb and index finger of one hand, which remains firmly placed on the patient's forehead. Take a deep inspiration and blow into his mouth.

3. If you are the only person on the spot, after every 15 cardiac compressions do the breathing 3 times. If you have an assistant, ask him to do it rhythmically 16 times a minute.

4. The effectiveness of mouth-to-mouth respiration is assessed by finding expansion of the chest.

If an S-shaped airway (**Fig. 6.2**) is available, this is much more effective and cleaner. Every doctor should carry one in his pocket and every household with a cardiac patient should have this handy.

By the above manoeuvres, the patient can be kept alive for more than an hour, by which time arrangements to shift him to a hospital would have become possible. On no account should the patient be left alone.

The brain suffers irreversible damage unless some circulation of oxygenated blood can be achieved within 2-3 minutes.

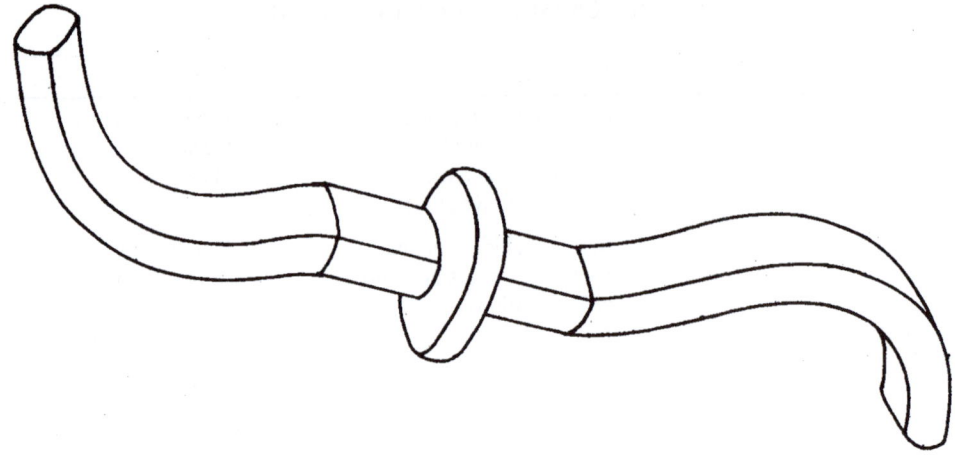

Fig. 6.2: S-shaped airway

D. Drug Therapy

1. If normal effective beating of the heart has not been restored, try the effect of 0.5 ml adrenaline 1:1000 solution. Use a long .22 gauge needle and insert it in the left 4th intercostal space parasternally. Aspirate blood into the syringe and then inject.

2. 10 ml of 10 per cent calcium gluconate may be injected in the heart if the cardiac arrest recurs after revival.

3. Lidocaine (Xylocaine) 5 ml of 1 per cent solution may be injected into the heart if ventricular fibrillation recurs after defibrillation.

4. Noradrenaline drip can help to maintain adequate blood pressure. Hypotension facilitates fibrillation.

5. Sodium bicarbonate 100 ml of 7.5 per cent solution by slow IV drip combats acidosis (which again facilitates fibrillation).

> If the pupil remains fixed and dilated and if more than 4-5 minutes of cardiac arrest have occurred before you have started resuscitation, the effort is futile.

Inappropriate CPR

The indications for CPR are clearest when the cardiac arrest has occurred as a result of an accident such as electrocution or drowning, or when it occurs during an investigation such as cardiac catheterization or from myocardial infarction without severe heart failure. In cases of cardiac rupture, cardiac tamponade and massive pulmonary embolism, CPR will nearly always be unsuccessful. One of the problems in hospital practice is to determine when it is inappropriate to attempt resuscitation because the nature of the patient's illness precludes even any remote possibility of recovery. Inevitably the hospital staff initiates CPR till someone who is familiar with the patient can make the decision as to whether the attempt should be given up (as in terminal cancer) to let the patient die in dignity.

Definition and Terminology

The pump function of the heart muscle consists of systolic shortening (inotropic function) and diastolic lengthening (lusitropic function). Inotropic and lusitropic function, along with heart rate and rhythm, preload and afterload determine the overall cardiac function.

Cardiac failure or congestive heart failure (CHF), is defined as a condition in which the heart is unable to pump blood at a rate commensurate with the metabolic requirements of the tissues. This may result from (i) a primary abnormality in the heart muscle, as in myocarditis and cardiomyopathy; (ii) loss in the quantity of normally contracting muscle, as in ischaemic heart disease and myocardial infarction; (iii) excessive pressure overload, as in hypertension and aortic stenosis; (iv) excessive volume overload, as in aortic regurgitation and left-to-right cardiac shunts; (v) severe prolonged anaemia, such as sickle cell disease and thalassaemia; (vi) disturbance of myocardial energy production as in beriberi.

It is important to distinguish cardiac failure from (1) circulatory insufficiency due to hypovolaemic or haemorrhagic shock or cardiac tamponade in which there is no primary impairment in myocardial function; (2) circulatory overload because of abnormal salt and water retention imposed on a normally functioning heart; (3) conditions in which a normally contracting myocardium is suddenly presented with a load which exceeds its capacity, e.g. rupture of a valve cusp in infective endocarditis, massive pulmonary embolism, or hypertensive crisis.

The descriptive clinical terminologies such as 'forward failure' (syncope, fatigue) and 'backward failure' (Pulmonary and systemic venous congestion), acute or chronic failure, left-sided or right-sided failure, high output or low output failure, do not signify a fundamentally different pathophysiology.

Diastolic Dysfunction and Diastolic Heart failure (DHF)

In heart failure, commonly both systolic and diastolic dysfunction are present. In most heart disease diastolic dysfunction precedes systolic dysfunction. It is noteworthy that 40–50 per cent patients with heart failure have a normal systolic function (LVEF $\geq$ 50%) with only diastolic dysfunction hence they are called diastolic heart failure (DHF). Patients with DHF tend to be older, more of them are females and 75 percent of them are hypertensive (40 per cent of whom have LV Hypertrophy – LV mass > 125 g/m^2). All have a normal end-diastolic volume (EDV) as shown by radionuclide ventriculogrphy or 2D echocardiography and Doppler. Grading of the severity of diastolic dysfunction (Grade I–IV) is now possible based on Doppler velocities.

Many signaling molecules such as endothelin, TNFα, TGFβ, and angiotensin cause proliferation of collagen, fibrosis and apoptosis especially under conditions of left ventricular pressure overload. Increase in passive stiffness along with decrease in active relaxation explains diastolic heart failure. Major goal in management of DHF is to reduced ischemia, hypertrophy and fibrosis (which caused the dysfunction) and to reduced pulmonary and/or systemic venous congestion, a major consequence of DHF. Dietary Sodium restriction and diuretics are useful for this purpose. Slowing the heart rate provides more time for diastolic filling, for which purpose beta blockers or non-dihydropyridine calcium antagonists are useful. ACE inhibitors and angiotensin 1 receptor blockers (such as condensartan 32 mg/once daily) help to reduce the number of hospital deaths. Statin therapy may reduce mortality in DHF. Digitalis is not indicated in DHF.

ANP, BNP pro BNP

1) Atrial Natriuretic peptide (ANP) is a 28 amino acid peptide with a 17 amino acid ring in the middle of the molecule. It is produced, stored and released from cardiac myocytes in the atria of the heart. It is secreted in response to stretch (atrial distension), sympathetic stimulation via B-adrenoreceptors, hypernatremia (raised serum concentration), angiotensin II and endothelin. ANP counters the increase in blood volume and blood pressure caused by renin-angiotensin system - actions opposite to those of aldosterone. Synthesis of ANP also takes place in the ventricles, brain, kidneys, supraenals, and placenta.

2) Brain Natriuretic Peptide (BNP) is a 32 amino acid polypeptide secreted in response to excessive stretching of cardiomyocytes. It was originally named because it was originally identified from extracts of porcine brains, although in humans it is produced mainly in cardiac ventricles. BNP is secreted along with a 76 amino acid N-terminal fragment -NJ pro BNP that is biologically inactive. Since its biological half-life is much longer (1-2hrs) than BNP (20 minutes) and ANP (5 minutes) it is more suitable for diagnostic testing. Normal levels (< 100 pg/ml) rules out acute heart failure with 90% sensitivity and 76% specificity. BNP < 50 pg/ml has 97% sensitivity and 62% specificity. In septic shock, values > 650 pg/ml is associated with high mortality. Values between 100-400 pg/ml are seen in heart failure.

Treatment of Cardiac Failure

The three cardinal components of treatment are:

1. Removal of the precipitating cause (**Table 7.1**)

2. Correction of the underlying aetiology wherever possible.

3. Control of the congestive heart failure state (**Table 7.2**).

ACE Inhibitors

The rationale for ACE inhibitors is given in **Table 7.3**. The usual dose of captopril ranges from 25-150 mg/day. Enalapril (2.5-40 mg/day) and lisinopril (2.5-20 mg/day) have a greater affinity for ACE receptors and a longer duration of action (upto 36 hours) than captopril, resulting in prolonged and more complete suppression of angiotensin II formation. This translates into a prolonged decrease in systemic vascular resistance and blood pressure. Hence there is an increased risk of adverse reactions especially in elderly patients (low-flow cerebral infarction, renal failure). Thus the longer-acting enalapril and lisinopril have little advantage over the short-acting captopril and should not be used in large fixed doses.

Overall, the ACE inhibitors are safe and well-tolerated. The associated adverse effects (dizziness, headache, fatigue) are mild and reversible with stoppage of therapy. Monitoring for hypotension and renal hypoperfusion (BUN, creatinine) are desirable. A leucocyte count every 2 weeks will guard against neutropenia which may develop within the first 3 months of therapy especially in patients with evidence of renal or collagen vascular disease.

Vasodilator Therapy

Since several neural and humoral influences which constrict the peripheral vascular bed increase the afterload, which impairs cardiac function, the

TABLE 7.1 PRECIPITATING CAUSES OF CHF

1. Physical over-exertion and emotional stress.
2. Excessive sodium intake.
3. Systemic hypertension.
4. Myocardial infarction.
5. Infection-pulmonary or elsewhere.
6. Pulmonary embolism.
7. Infective endocarditis.
8. Rheumatic/other myocarditis.
9. Anaemia.
10. Pregnancy
11. Thyrotoxicosis.
12. Arrhythmias.

pharmacologic reduction of afterload with vasodilator drugs (of which captopril is one category) is an important adjunct in the management of cardiac failure. Currently available vasodilator drugs are listed in **Table 7.4**. Vasodilator therapy is useful in the treatment of all forms of congestive failure. It is effective in acutely improving the deranged haemodynamics of heart failure and has also shown beneficial long-term effects.

TABLE **7.2 CONTROL OF CONGESTIVE HEART FAILURE**

A. Reduction of cardiac workload: systolic and diastolic
   i. Reducing physical activity.
   ii. Emotional rest.
   iii. Restricted caloric intake and weight reduction in overweight patients.
   iv. Reducing afterload-vasodilator, ACE (angiotensin converting enzyme) inhibitors.

B. Control of excessive salt and water retention
   i. Reduction of dietary intake of sodium.
   ii. Diuretics to increase urinary sodium loss.
   iii. Mechanical removal of excessive fluid: thoracocentesis, paracentesis, dialysis.

C. Enhancement of myocardial contracility
   i. Digitalis glycosides.
   ii. Sympathomimetic amines.
   iii. Phosphodiesterase inhibitors.
   iv. Co-enzyme Q-10 to augment intracellular myocardial energy supply.

The ideal vasodilator for the treatment of acute heart failure should have a rapid onset and a brief duration of action when given intravenously. Sodium nitroprusside qualifies as such a drug but its use requires careful monitoring of intra-arterial and pulmonary artery wedge pressure, and ECG monitoring in an intensive care unit.

For the treatment of chronic CHF, the agent should be effective orally and its action should last for at least six hours. ACE inhibitors satisfy these requirements and are widely used currently.

Nitroglycerin can be given by the IV route, or as a skin ointment for prolonged use, while isosorbide dinitrate is most effective via the sublingual route. A combination of hydralazine and isosorbide dinitrate orally is beneficial in chronic CHF and has been shown to prolong survival of patients with CHF. Prolonged use can lead to tolerance to nitrates.

Calcium channel blockers such as nifedepine reduce afterload thereby benefiting patients with left ventricular failure in hypertensive, ischaemic and valvular heart disease and cardiomyopathy.

Vasodilators should not be used in patients with hypotension.

Diuretics in CHF

The most common prescription for CHF is a low sodium diet and a diuretic, the dose of which should be tailored closely to suit the patient's need. A small gain in weight, particularly if accompanied by a sensation of congestion should prompt diuretic therapy. Excessive use of potent diuretics promotes hypokalaemia; and azotaemia and further aggravates the RAAS (renin angiotensin aldosterone system) over-compensation. The list of currently used diuretics in CHF is given in **Table 7.5**. All these drugs can be given orally. The loop diuretics are more potent than the thiazides and can act in the face of low glomerular filtration.

Sympathomimetic Amines

The adrenergic nervous system is vital for normal cardiac function. The adrenergic receptors in the heart, lung and blood vessels are listed in **Table 7.6**. Both beta-l and beta-2 receptors are present in the myocardium: their stimulation activates the enzyme adenylate cyclase (AC) which converts ATP to cyclic AMP, 'the second messenger'. AC may also be activated by H_2 and glucagon receptors. The positive inotropic response of alpha receptors is not coupled to AC activation but is probably linked to calcium influx. Beta 1 receptors are present on coronary vessels while beta 2 receptors are present on all vascular smooth muscle and bronchioles; on stimulation they cause dilatation. Alpha receptors are present on arteries, veins and bronchi and cause constriction. In the normal myocardium maximum beta adrenergic stimulation (as in physical exercise) causes an increase in contractility which exceeds that by other mechanisms. In congestive heart failure there is increased adrenergic activity as shown by elevated circulating catecholamine levels even at rest, and the prognosis varies inversely with their concentration. However, persistent sympathetic stimulation leads to a change in the beta receptors either as a reduction in the number or in sensitivity to stimulation ('down regulation'). This in turn results in diminished capability to activate AC. Depletion of beta neurones in CHF has been shown by cardiac imaging with radiolabelled tracer I-123 MIBG (Meta-iodo-benzyl guanidine), an analogue of guanethidine. Depletion of beta neurones has been shown in cardiomyopathy and in myocardial infarction. This depletion as well as reduced content of non-epinephrine in CHF

provides the rationale for the use of beta agonists as therapeutic agents to improve myocardial contractility. But this is achieved at a price-excessive energy depletion, mitochondrial damage and even cell necrosis. Long-term therapy with beta agonists may, therefore, have adverse effects on the myocardium and cause arrhythmias by their direct oxygen-washing effect on the ischaemic myocardium as well as mobilization of free fatty acids.

The currently available sympathomimetic amines with their activity on B_1, B_2, alpha and dopamine receptors are listed in **Table 7.7**.

TABLE 7.3 EFFECTS OF ACE INHIBITORS IN CHF

Haemodynamic benefits	Neurohumoral changes
Decreased systemic vascular resistance.	Decreased angiotensin II.
Decreased pulmonary capillary wedge pressure.	Decreased argenin-vasopressin.
Decreased right atrial pressure.	Decreased nor-epinephrine (NE).
Decreased ventricular ED and ES dimensions.	Decreased or no change in aldosterone.
Increased cardiac output, stroke volume and cardiac index.	Increased synthesis of vasodilator prostaglandins and nitric oxide.

TABLE 7.4 VASODILATOR THERAPY IN CHF

Site of action	The effect	The drug and dosage per day
Arterial bed	Primarily increase in stroke volume	Hydralazine 25 mg-200 mg per oral route (PO) bid Minoxodil 2.5 mg-20 mg PO bid nifedipine 10-40 mg tid PO
Venous bed	Primarily reduce ventricular filling pressure	Nitroglycerin IV 10 mg/min. or skin ointment 0.5-1 inch Isosorbide dinitrate 10 mg-60 mg PO
Both vascular beds	Reduce ventricular filling pressure in all patients. Increase cardiac output in CHF	Sodium nitroprusside IV 10 mg/min. Prazosin 1-10 mg PO Captopril 12.5-25 mg PO Combination of hydralazine plus isosorbide

Table 7.5 DIURETIC AGENTS USED IN CHF

Agent	Site of action	Onset of action	Duration of action	Average daily dose
Thiazides				
Chlorothiazide	Distal tubule	2 hr	6-12 hr	250-500 mg
Hydrochlorothiazide	Distal tubule	2 hr	12 hr	25-100 mg
Chlorthalidone	Distal tubule	2 hr	48 hr	25-100 mg
Metolazone	Proximal and distal tubule	1 hr	24-48 hr	2.5-20 mg
Indapamide	Distal tubule	2 hr	24 hr	2.5-5 mg
Loop diuretics				
Frusemide	Loop of Henle	1 hr (IV/IM 5 min.)	6-8 hr 2-4 hr	20-80 mg 10-80 mg
Ethacrynic acid	Loop of Henle	30 min. (IV 5 min.)	6-8 hr 3 hr	25-80 mg 50 mg
Bumetanide	Loop of Henle	30 min. (IV/IM 5 min.)	2 hr 30 min.	0.5-2 mg 0.5-2 mg max. 10 mg
Potassium-sparers				
Spironolactone	Distal tubule and collecting ducts	1-2 days	2-3 days	50-200 mg
Triamterine	Distal tubule and collecting ducts	2-4 days	7-9 days	100-200 mg
Amiloride	Distal tubule and collecting ducts	2 hr	24 hr	5-10 mg

Comparisons between Dopamine, Dobutamine and Other Drugs

There have been several reports comparing dopamine and dobutamine in patients with various types of CHF: dilated cardiomyopathy, acute MI and septic shock. Dobutamine progressively increases cardiac output in doses of 2.5 to 10 µg/kg/minute, decreases systemic and pulmonary vascular ectopics. Dopamine increases cardiac output upto 4 µg/kg/min following which there is no further increase. In contrast, there is an increase in pulmonary wedge pressure and the number of ventricular ectopics. Renal and hepatic blood flow are not altered by either drug. It may be concluded that dobutamine has a place in patients with chronic CHF with severely impaired pump function with low cardiac output and elevated LV filling pressures. It should be avoided in the presence of extreme hypotension, in which situation dopamine is to be preferred, because of its additional alpha adrenergic effect causing vasoconstriction.

Dopexamine
A new substance derived from dopamine which stimulates beta 2 and dopamine receptors and has been shown to have beneficial effects on cardiac work without adverse effects.

Table 7.6 EFFECTS OF ADRENERGIC RECEPTORS

	Receptor affinity	Physiological result
Heart	Beta 1 > Beta 2	Increased contractility
		Increased automaticity
	Beta 1	Increased conduction velocity (chronotropic response)
Blood vessels	Alpha	Constriction of arteries and veins
	Beta 1	Dilatation of coronary arteries
	Beta 2	Dilatation of arteries
Lungs	Alpha	Bronchoconstriction
	Beta 1 > Beta 2	Bronchodilatation

Ibopamine
An orally active analogue of dopamine which has been shown to have beneficial effects on LV work but its long-term effects have been questioned.

Xamoterol
A partial beta 1 agonist. Because of its dual action as an agonist and antagonist, the drug will increase cardiac response at low levels of sympathetic stimulation, whereas at high levels it exerts a beta-blocking effect. It seems a promising new approach to the treatment of mild to moderate heart failure regardless of the cause.

Amrinone
A non-catecholamine, non-glycoside bipyridine compound which exerts positive inotropic and vasodilator action by inhibiting a specific phosphodiesterase, thereby increasing the availability of cyclic AMP. It can only be given intravenously (5-10 µg/kg/min.). By simultaneously simulating cardiac contractility and dilating the peripheral vascular bed, it reverses the major haemodynamic abnormalities associated with CHF.

Digitalis glycosides By stimulating myocardial contractility in the failing heart, digitalis improves ventricular emptying, augments ejection fraction, reduces diastolic pressure and volume and end-systolic volume of the failing ventricle, with consequent reduction in pulmonary congestion and lowering of the systemic venous pressure.

Table 7.7 SYMPATHOMIMETIC AMINES WITH SITE OF ACTION AND APPLICATION

Name	Type of receptor				Clinical use
	β1	β2	Alpha	Dopamine	
Adrenaline	+	+	+	0	Only in anaphylactic shock
Noradrenaline	+	+	+	0	Only in hypotensive shock
Isoprenaline	+	+	0	0	For chronotropic support in patients
Orciprenaline	+	+	0	0	recovering from cardiopulmonary bypass
Dopamine	+	0	+	+	IV in acute CHF
Dobutamine	+	+	0	0	IV in acute CHF and chronic CHF
Dopexamine	+	+	0	+	IV in acute CHF
Ibopamine	+	0	+	+	Oral use in CHF
Prenalterol	±	+	0	0	Available for oral use in CHF, antidote to beta blockers
Xamoterol	±	0	0	0	IV or oral use in CHF
Pirbuterol	+	+	0	0	Oral use in CHF
Salbutamol	+	+	0	0	IV or oral use in CHF
Terbutaline	+	+	0	0	IV or oral use in CHF

In the absence of heart failure, however, when cardiac output is not limited by cardiac contractility, the drug does not increase cardiac index. Digitalis exerts a clinically significant negative chronotropic action (slowing the heart rate by prolonging the refractory period of the AV node) only in the setting of ventricular failure. In the non-failing heart the slowing effect is negligible.

The use of digitalis for the control of sinus tachycardia is irrational unless heart failure is present. The greatest benefit of slowing of ventricular rate is seen in patients with atrial fibrillation or flutter with rapid ventricular rate. It is also beneficial in CHF with sinus rhythm and impaired systolic function. Recent awareness that *diastolic function abnormality* may be the main pathophysiology in some patients of congestive heart failure leads to the conclusion that digitalis therapy should not be given to such patients. The appropriate therapy for such patients is calcium channel blockers like nifedepine.

Digitalis is a double-edged weapon, especially dangerous when used with vigorous diuretic therapy causing hypokalaemia. Old age, renal dysfunction, ischaemic heart disease and AMI, hypoxaemia, hypercalcaemia, electrical cardioversion, hypothyroidism, may all reduce tolerance to the drug and increase toxicity.

Chronic digitalis toxicity may be insidious in onset and manifest as worsening of heart failure, weight loss, cachexia, neuralgia, gynaecomastia, yellow vision and delirium. Toxic cardiac arrhythmias may *precede* the usual gastrointestinal manifestations of toxicity (anorexia, nausea, vomiting) in about 50 per cent of cases, hence the need for constant vigilance to watch out for premature ventricular contractions (which may take the form of bigeminy because of increased myocardial irritability and facilitation of re-entry), AV junctional and multifocal ventricular tachycardia.

When tachyarrhythmias result from digitalis toxicity, withdrawal of the drug and replacement of potassium are needed, along with phenytoin (for control of supraventricular tachycardia), lidocaine (for control of digitalis-included ventricular tachycardia in the absence of pre-existing AV block). A cardiac pacemaker may be required in digitalis-induced AV block. Fab fragments of purified intact digitalis antibodies represent a lifesaving approach to the management of severe digitalis toxicity. Each 40 mg vial of Fab neutralizes 0.6 mg digoxin. 4 ml should be given IV over a 30 minute period. The dosage should be repeated if toxicity is not adequately reversed with the initial dose.

Monitoring drug levels by RIA and maintaining a safe blood level (1–1.5 mg/ml digoxin) is a safeguard against toxicity. When signs of toxicity are present the serum levels are often more than 2.5 mg/ml digoxin. It must be remembered that many factors other than serum levels of the drug, determine digitalis toxicity, hence drug levels should not be the sole guide.

With the availability of alternative therapy such as diuretics plus ACEIs, these are safer alternatives for patients of CHF with sinus rhythm than digitalis. Especially in AMI, the continued administration of digitalis may increase mortality.

Refractory Heart Failure

When response to standard treatment is not forthcoming, heart failure is considered to be refractory. Before concluding that this represents an advanced pre-terminal myocardial depression, one should carefully consider if one or more underlying precipitating factors are being overlooked (**Table 7.1**). Over zealous treatment with diuretics, compounded by digitalis toxicity is a common situation to guard against. Temporary easing of salt restriction and diuretic administration and correction of depletional hyponatraemia may Improve the condition for a while. Hyponatraemia, if not due to vigorous diuretic therapy, is a late manifestation of refractory heart failure. The combination of an IV vasodilator such as sodium nitroprusside along with a potent sympathomimetic amine such as dopamine or dobutamine, often results in an additive effect, raising cardiac output and lowering filling pressure. Intravenous amrinone, along with an ACE inhibitor may also be useful in refractory heart failure.

When patients with heart failure become unresponsive to a combination of all the abovementioned measures, are in class IV category of CHF, and are unlikely to survive one year, they are candidates for cardiac transplantation. The technique has now been practised successfully over 24 years, and with the advent of cyclosporine, 1500 cardiac transplants are done annually with a 1-year survival rate of 90 per cent and a 5-year survival rate of 70 per cent.

8 Coma

Approach to a Case of Coma

The standard clinical approach consists of history taking and physical examination to arrive at a provisional diagnosis, to confirm it by appropriate laboratory or other tests, and then to start appropriate therapy.

When a patient is brought in an unconscious state, the usual process has to be altered, in that certain therapeutic procedures have to take precedence over anything else.

1. Ensure that the airway is clear.
2. Ensure that the patient is not in shock, as assessed by pulse rate and volume, blood pressure and skin temperature.
3. Ensure that the patient is not bleeding actively from a wound, if trauma has occurred.
4. In case of a head injury, be cautious about moving the head and neck, lest the spinal cord be inadvertently injured.
5. If the patient is sweating, suspect hypoglycaemia. After drawing a sample of blood for subsequent laboratory test, give in the same vein 50 per cent 50 ml hypertonic glucose.

Having ensured stability of the breathing and circulation, the next step is to interrogate the persons who have brought the patient:

1. Circumstances in which the patient was found.
2. Was the onset sudden or gradual?
3. Was there a head injury?
4. Was there a convulsion?
5. Was there fever?
6. What was the patient's previous state of health?

Up to this point some idea can be formed about the probable causes to be considered.

1. Sudden onset in a previously healthy person: poisoning; head injury and subdural haematoma: subarachnoid haemorrhage.
2. Rapid onset following fever: cerebral malaria; acute infection-meningitis, encephalitis; heatstroke.
3. Onset with convulsions: status epilepticus; cerebrovascular accidents; Stokes-Adams syndrome; encephalitis; cortical thrombophlebitis.
4. Previously ill person-sudden or gradual worsening: diabetic coma; uraemia; hepatic failure; respiratory insufficiency (CO_2 narcosis).

Note the temperature:

Fever would indicate an acute infection such as meningitis, pneumonia, malaria, or a pontine lesion (embolism, haemorrhage).

High fever 107-110°F would suggest heatstroke, especially when the skin is dry.

Lower than normal temperature would suggest:
- narcotic poisoning
- dehydration
- peripheral circulatory failure
- myxoedema

Note the respirations:

1. Slow (6-9 per minute): morphine poisoning; barbiturate poisoning.
2. Rapid and deep:
   a. acidosis; diabetic ketosis; uraemia; methyl alcohol poisoning; salicylate poisoning.
   b. Midbrain damage or dysfunction: well-marked active contraction of lower chest wall during expiration.
3. Rate and depth irregular: meningitis; medullary dysfunction.

4. Cheyne Stokes breathing: lesions in the brainstem.

Note the pulse rate:
Slow – 30-40 per minute: Stokes-Adams syndrome.
Slow and irregular: raised intracranial pressure.
Rapid – 140 per minute: shock.
      – 180-200 per minute: paroxysmal tachycardia.
Rapid and irregular: atrial fibrillation.

Note the blood pressure:
High: Hypertensive encephalopathy; toxaemia of pregnancy; cerebral haemorrhage.
Low: Dehydration; myocardial infarction; diabetic coma; gram-negative septicaemia; internal bleeding; Addisonian crisis; narcotic poisoning.

Inspect the skin:
Moist and sweating: Hypoglycaemia.
Dry skin: diabetic coma; uraemia; heatstroke.
Cyanosis of lips and nail beds: CO_2 narcosis.
Cherry red colour: carbon monoxide poisoning.
Multiple bruises: hepatic failure.
Pallor: internal bleeding; chronic renal failure.
Haemorrhagic rash: meningococcal septicaemia.
Icterus: hepatic coma; haemolytic crisis.
Marks of needle puncture: insulin; narcotic addiction.

Note the odour of the breath:
Alcohol, kerosine, turpentine, diazone insecticide.
Cyanide poisoning: (smell of bitter almonds).
Acetone: diabetic ketosis (sweet smell).
Foetor hepaticus: liver cell failure (smell of rotting apples).
Uraemia: (Ammoniacal smell).

Assess the responsiveness of the patient:
(First evaluation; hour-by-hour evaluation.)
Does he answer when his name is called?
Does he obey simple commands ('show your tongue')?
Does he respond to painful stimuli?
Supra-orbital notch-deep pressure on both sides.
Corneal reflex, gag reflex, cough reflex.

Note posture of patient:
Flexion of arms and extension of legs: decorticate posture.
Extension of arms and legs: decerebrate posture-midbrain damage.

Total flaccidity: lower pontine or medullary damage.
Now make a systematic survey, region by region, of the whole body.

Skull: Bruises; bogginess; swellings; depressed fracture; in babies: fontanelles.

Ears: discharge-pus, blood, CSF.

Nose: Blood, CSF.

Eyes: Conjugate deviation of head and eyes to one side (towards the lesion).
    Doll's eye movements–absent in midbrain lesions.
    Irrigation of external ear with 30-60 ml ice water for 20-30 seconds: absence of slow movement of eyes to same side–midbrain damage or depression.

Pupils:
1. Pinpoint-opium/diazinon poisoning, pontine lesions.
2. Very small (2 mm) reacting to light–compression of brainstem at thalamic level.
3. 3-5 mm pupil not reacting to light–compression at midbrain level.
4. Inequality-space-occupying lesion, haematoma, abscess.

Fundus oculi: Papilloedema, choroid tubercles. subhyaloid haemorrhages.

Tongue: Bone dry-uraemia; dehydration.
Marks of being bitten-epileptic fits.

Neck: Rigidity on flexion only:
      Meningitis;
      Subarachnoid haemorrhage;
      Posterior fossa tumours;
      Decerebrate rigidity (brainstem lesions).
    Rigidity in all directions:
      Disease of cervical spine.

Carotid pulse: inequality-bruit.

Heart: Triple rhythm, murmur, pericardial rub.

Lungs: Tuberculosis-(miliary TB and meningitis).
    Bronchiectasis-lung abscess; empyema (septic cerebral emboli, cerebral abscess).
    Malignancy-(metastases in brain).
    Emphysema-chronic bronchitis (CO_2 narcosis).

Abdomen: Liver; spleen; ascites.

In physical examination, two important questions to decide are

1. Are signs of meningeal irritation present?
   i. Neck stiffness on flexion.
   ii. Kernig's sign.
2. Are lateralizing signs present?
   i. One side more flaccid that the other.
   ii. Absence of spontaneous or pain-induced movements on one side.
   iii. Flattening of nasolabial furrow on one side.
   iv. Greater flapping of the paralysed cheek during expiration.
   v. One pupil wider in size than the other.
   vi. Extensor plantar on one side.

These are suggestive of: abscess; tumour; haematoma; cerebral infarction and haemorrhage (confirmed by CT scan).

Coma without focal, lateralizing or meningeal signs is suggestive of: poisoning; intoxication; metabolic causes (diabetic ketosis, uraemia, hepatic failure, CO_2 narcosis); systemic infections; shock; heat hyperpyrexia.

Remember, our main concern is not to miss a treatable condition.

Conditions which are treatable:
   Poisoning - barbiturates, diazenon.
   Infections - meningitis, cerebral malaria.
   Diabetic coma.
   Hypoglycaemia.
   Cerebral abscess (neurosurgical).
   Subdural or extradural haematoma (neurosurgical).

To this end, certain laboratory investigations are directed:

1. Urine for sugar and acetone.
2. Peripheral blood smear for malarial parasites.
3. CSF examination.

In cases of coma following fever, one is perfectly justified in suspecting cerebral malaria and after preparing a blood smear for subsequent examination, give IM inj. Chloroquine 250 mg or IV inj. Quinine sulph 600 mg repeated after 6 hours. This can be life-saving, and the effects really dramatic. No harm is done by giving these drugs to non-malarial cases of coma, provided hypotension is guarded against.

For conditions apart from hypoglycaemia and cerebral malaria, the attending physician will do well to refer the patient at once to an institution, where CT and MRI are available.

Management of an Unconscious Patient

1. Maintain ventilation; keep airway patent.
   Prevent hypoxia.
   Suction of secretions in throat.
   Intubation (cuffed endotracheal tube).
   Mechanical ventilators.

2. Maintain circulation: Restore blood, plasma or fluids to maintain systolic blood pressure around 100 mg Hg.

3. Apply a condom catheter for draining urine into a bottle to avoid soiling the bed. In the case of retention of urine, put in an in-dwelling Foley's catheter with a coverage of nitrofurantoin 100 mg tid to prevent urinary infection.

4. Insert a Ryle's tube for feeding. If the patient is vomiting, a cuffed tracheostomy tube will prevent aspiration pneumonia. Give 1600 cal + 70 g protein per day.

5. Maintain an intake/output chart: aim at a urine output of at least 1 litre in 24 hours. This will generally be achieved by intake of 2500 ml fluid.

6. Change the position of the patient every 2 hours (unless contraindicated), to avoid pressure sores on skin and hypostatic congestion of lungs.

7. Keep the skin clean and dry: use a liberal amount of talcum powder; use spirit to harden the skin; use air cushions to protect pressure points.

8. Move the legs passively 3 times daily to avoid leg vein thrombosis and embolic complications.

9. Move the arms passively 3 times daily to avoid 'frozen shoulder'.

TABLE 8.1 GLASGOW COMA SCALE FOR PROGNOSIS

Eye opening (E)	Spontaneous	4
	To loud voice	3
	To pain	2
	Nil	1
Best Motor Response (M)	Obeys	6
	Localises	5
	Withdraws (flexion)	4
	Abnormal felxion posturing	3
	External posturing	2
	Nil	1
Verbal Response (V)	Oriented	5
	Disoriented, confused	4
	Inappropriate words	3
	Incomprehensive sounds	2
	Nil	1

NOTE : Coma Score = E + M + V

Patients with head trauma scoring 3 or 4 have 85% chance of dying or remaining in vegetative state.

Score above 11 indicates 5-10% likelihood of death or remaining vegetative.

Diagnosing Brain Death

With the advent of organ transplants and legislation regarding 'beating heart brain death', the criteria for diagnosing brain death have assumed great importance. These are presented in the 'box' below. The purpose of diagnosing brain death is twofold:

1. Withdrawal of life-support measures, with the concurrence of the next of kin.

2. Removal of organs for donation while the heart is still beating, which avoids hypoxic damage to the organs to be donated.

CRITERIA FOR BRAIN DEATH

A. Clinical: Evidence of absence of brainstem reflexes
- Fixed, unreacting pupils; absence of corneal reflexes, oculocephalic reflex (doll's eye).
- Absence of vestibulo-ocular reflex (no eye movement during or after slow injection of 20 ml ice-cold water into each ear). Visualize tympanic membrane first to avoid false negative test.
- Absence of gag reflex; no response to bronchial stimulation.
- Apnoea for atleast 4 minutes.

B. EEG: Flat; absence of electrical activity on two occasions. (Required only if A is inconclusive)

C. Radionuclide cerebral angiography: Absence of cerebral circulation (useful in cases of coma due to intoxication where observations from A and B are doubtful).

The brain-stem criteria of death have been accepted in India by the Transplantation of Human Organs Act 1994. The performance of EEG and angiography are not required if there is conclusive evidence of brain stem death, as dtermined by two expert neurologists (who have no interest or benefit in any way from cadaver transplantation) do two sets of tests six hours apart.

Confusional States and Delirium

The cardinal feature of a confusional state or delirium is clouding of consciousness manifested by impaired alertness, awareness and attention.

Every medical practitioner should be able to perform a simple examination called the Mini-mental status examination, that provides an objective evaluation of the patient's mental state. The numerical score gives both an estimate of the severity of mental impairment, and a reference point for later comparison. The examination of cognitive function is an important bedside clinical skill to be acquired and practised.

MINI-MENTAL STATUS EXAMINATION

	Score	Maximum
Orientation		
What is the (year) (season), (date), (day) & (month)?	( )	5
Where are we (state) (district) (town), (hospital), (floor)?	( )	5
Registration		
Name 3 unrelated objects, taking one second for each, e.g. pen, watch, chair.		
Ask patient to repeat them.	( )	3
Attention and Calculation		
Ask patient to subtract 7 from 100; stop after 5 subtractions (93, 86, 79, 72, 65)	( )	5
Recall		
Ask for the 3 objects repeated above.	( )	3
Language		
NAMING: Show two objects, e.g. wrist watch & pencil; & ask patient to name them.	( )	2
REPETITION: 'No ifs, ands, or buts'.	( )	1
THREE STAGE COMMAND: Take a paper in your right hand; fold it in half; put it on the floor.	( )	3
READ AND OBEY: Close your eyes.	( )	1
WRITE A SENTENCE: Must contain a subject & verb & make sense.	( )	1
COPY DESIGN.	( )	1
Total Score	( )	30

Assess level of consciousness along a continuum

Alert	Drowsy	Stupor	Coma
(30)			(0)

Clinical Approach

When confronted with a patient who is in an acute confusional state, the four questions to be asked are:

- Is it due to a neurological disorder? (Focal neurologic signs mayor may not be present) **Table 9.1**.
- Is it due to a systemic illness? (Focal neurologic signs uncommon) **Table 9.2**.
- Is it due to an acute psychiatric illness? **Table 9.3**.
- Is it due to drugs? **Table 9.4**.

Investigations and Treatment

Investigation and treatment of the underlying disease should be undertaken. All current drug therapy should be reviewed and, where possible, stopped. The patient should be carefully nursed and rehydrated. If high fever is present, it should be brought down by fans, ice-packs and antipyretic drugs. Hypoglycaemia and hypoxia should be corrected.

Management of Disturbed or Violent Patients

Psychotic, organically impaired or intoxicated patients may be frightened, aggressive, confused, hallucinated, and difficult to manage. A well-lighted, tranquil environment is most conducive to their management. It is important that those involved in their acute management refrain from threatening behaviour, appear in control and avoid being drawn into a confrontation.

TABLE 9.1 NEUROLOGICAL CAUSES OF ACUTE CONFUSIONAL STATE

Cause	Clinical Clues	Confirmation
Trauma		
Concussion	History of trauma.	CT scan
Intracranial haematoma	Headache, vomiting.	
Subdural haematoma	Unequal pupils.	
Vascular disorders		
Multiple cerebral infarcts	Middle-aged pr elderly patient,	CT scan
Right hemisphere/posterior circulation infarcts	Known hypertensive or diabetic.	
Hypertensive encephalopathy		
Vasculitis: SLE, PAN, giant cell arteritis	Other systemic features of collagen diseases.	
Air and fat embolism	Clinical picture	
Subarachnoid haemorrhage	Clinical picture	CT scan
Neoplasia		
Multiple parenchymal metastases	Middle aged smoker.	X-ray chest
Meningeal carcinomatosis	Other features of lung cancer	CT scan skull
Mid-line brain tumours	or other cancers.	
Paraneoplastic		
Infection		
Encephalitis and meningitis	Onset with fever, headache, vomiting.	Blood smear for malaria parasites
Cerebral malaria, typhoid, typhus, plague		Blood culture
		Lumbar puncture
Epilepsy		
Temporal lobe seizures	History of similar previous episodes.	EEG, MRI

Table 9.2 SYSTEMIC ILLNESS CAUSING ACUTE CONFUSIONAL STATE

Causes	Clinical Clues	Confirmation
Hypoglycaemia	In elderly, focal signs may be seen	Blood sugar < 60 mg
Hypoxia-cardiac, pulmonary, CO poisoning	Clinical setting	Blood gases
Metabolic encephalopathy		
Diabetic ketoacidosis	Acidotic hyperventilation	Blood sugar and acetone
Renal failure and uraemia	High BUN and creatinine	
Hepatic failure	Flapping tremors, jaundice	High SGOT, SGPT
Electrolyte, fluid and acid-base imbalance	Other features of ECF volume depletion	Blood electrolyte pH
Nutritional deficiency		
Thiamine (Wernicke's encephalopathy)	} Especially in alcoholics	
Nicotinic acid (pellagra)	Features of deficiency	
B_{12} deficiency		
Endocrine overactivity or underactivity		Serum B_{12} < 200
Thyroid, parathyroid, adrenal	Features of the respective diseases	Serum calcium, PTH,
Heat hyperpyrexia	Rectal temperature above 107°F	T_3T_4TSH, ACTH + Cortisol
Septicaemia	Hypotension, shock	Blood culture
Hyperviscosity syndromes	Skin bruises or purpura	Coagulation profile

Table 9.3 PSYCHIATRIC ILLNESSES CAUSING ACUTE CONFUSIONAL STATE

Causes	Comments
Acute mania	Orientation for person and
Depression or extreme anxiety	place is preserved.
Schizophrenia	Orientation and attention, sleep-wake cycle and consciousness preserved.
Hysterical fugue states	Psychogenic amnesia. Focal nature of amnesia: only some things are forgotten.

Close observation of the patient is necessary. Some organic disorders initially showing signs and symptoms of psychosis, such as meningitis and encephalitis, hypoxia and poisoning, may be life-threatening. Sedatives can aggravate the symptoms.

Table 9.4 DRUGS CAUSING CONFUSIONAL STATE

Anticonvulsants
Anticholinergics
Anxiolytic/hypnotic opiates
Chronic barbiturate withdrawal
Alcohol withdrawal
Industrial poisons e.g. DDT, trichloroethylene
Heavy metals: organic mercurials, manganese
Carbon monoxide poisoning

Benzodiazepine is suitable for management of mild restlessness. In severe delirium, haloperidol (2-10 mg IM inj.) followed by 10-60 mg orally per day may be more effective.

Parenteral thiamine 100 mg (IM inj. qid for 3 days) is given to all patients suspected of Wernicke's encephalopathy (commonly seen in alcoholics).

Alcohol Withdrawal

Alcohol withdrawal carries a significant risk of death and requires a high index of suspicion for diagnosis.

Delirium tremens is manifested by tremulousness, hallucinations, agitation, confusion, disorientation and autonomic overactivity, including fever, tachycardia and profuse perspiration. It usually occurs 72-96 hours after cessation of drinking. Physical restraints should be avoided if possible, but injury should be prevented.

Chlordiazepoxide is an effective sedative in this situation. An initial dose of 100 mg IV or PO is repeated if needed every 2-6 hrs with a maximum dose of 500 mg in the first 24 hours. One half of the initial 24-hour dose may be administered over the next 24 hours; with dose reduction by 25-50 mg/day each day thereafter.

Thiamine 100 mg qid should be given IM for 3 days and subsequently given orally at the same dosage.

Alcohol withdrawal seizures (which usually occur 12-48 hours after cessation of drinking) can be controlled with phenytoin or paraldehyde (5-15 ml PO every 24 hrs).

Approach to a Case of Convulsions

An attack of convulsions followed by loss of consciousness is a frightening episode for a patient to experience, and for his relatives to witness, and is a sure occasion to call a doctor. By the time the doctor arrives on the scene, the convulsion is most probably over, and the patient may appear dazed, confused and incoherent, or may be fast asleep. He may have hurt himself in the fall, bitten his tongue, or passed urine into his clothes. The first thing for the doctor to do is to see that no fracture or severe injury has occurred, and then to allay the alarm and anxiety of the attendants and relatives, especially if this is the first episode they have witnessed. If a convulsion occurs in the presence of the doctor, he can demonstrate to the relatives how to (1) prevent the tongue from being bitten by putting a rolled up cloth or a piece of rubber between the patient's teeth; (2) loosen the patient's collar and turn the patient's head to one side to prevent the tongue from falling back and choking the patient. He will stop the relatives from forcefully attempting to smother the convulsion, which is not only futile but also harmful.

The doctor should then proceed to find out if this was the first episode or there were similar episodes before. The patient may have a record of previous examinations and prescriptions.

Sometimes the situation is not so clear-cut, and the doctor would like to ascertain if the episode of unconsciousness was a fit or a faint. The causes, significance, prognosis and management being quite different in the two conditions, the distinction is important to make (**Table 10.1**). Sometimes, especially in dealing with a young female, the problem is to decide between an epileptic fit and a hysterical fit (**Table 10.2**).

Main Questions on First Encounter

1. Is it due to idiopathic epilepsy (an excessive abnormal electrical discharge)? Ask the relatives for a history of previous fits.
2. Is it due to Stokes-Adams attack? Count the pulse rate.
3. Is it hypertensive encephalopathy? Take the blood pressure.

Examination of the Patient

1. *Pulse rate:* This is important so as not to miss Stokes-Adams attack (due to complete heart block) as a cause of convulsions (see also pp. 41 and 64).
2. *Blood pressure:* Acute glomerulonephritis and toxaemia of pregnancy (pre-eclampsia) can cause hypertensive encephalopathy as a complication of the transient hypertension. Apart from convulsions there will be a history of headache, drowsiness, oedema of the face and feet, and albumin in the urine.
3. The fit may have been due to subarachnoid haemorrhage or a vascular stroke. Hence after the convulsion is over, do a thorough neurological examination for evidence of meningeal irritation (neck stiffness, Kernig's sign) or focal deficit such as weakness of face or limb on one side, difference in deep reflexes, or extensor plantar response on one side.

The causes of convulsions according to age group are listed in **Table 10.3**.

The classification of idiopathic epilepsy and the preferred drugs for each type are given in **Table 10.4**.

TABLE 10.1 POINTS OF DIFFERENCE BETWEEN EPILEPSY AND SYNCOPE

Feature	Epilepsy	Syncope
Description of attack	Loss of consciousness with absolute suddenness; cannot be averted.	Rapid but never absolutely sudden; may be averted by lying down promptly.
Position at the beginning of attack	Any position.	Patient nearly always in upright position at onset of attack, either sitting or standing or voiding urine in standing position. Exception: Stokes-Adams attack in any position.
Warning signals	Usually no warning: aura may be present for a few seconds, which is really the first part of the seizure.	Usually gets enough warning: giddiness, tinnitus, blurred vision, nausea, vomiting.
Appearance of face	Cyanosed and suffused face during attack.	Striking pallor or ashen grey colour of face during attack; drenched in cold sweat.
Attitude of limbs	Tonic and clonic convulsions.	Flaccid: falls like a log; convulsions very rare.
Accompaniment	May fall and hurt himself; may bite the tongue; sphincter control may be lost.	Hurtful fall exceptional; no tongue biting; sphincter control is usually maintained.
Duration of attack	About a minute.	Variable-seconds to minutes.
Sequelae	Headache, confusion, drowsiness, often deep sleep.	No sequelae after recovery from attack.
EEG	Normal or abnormal.	Normal.

TABLE 10.2 POINTS OF DIFFERENTIATION BETWEEN A CONVULSION AND A HYSTERICAL ATTACK

Feature	True convulsion	Hysterical attack
Setting	Anywhere, any time, also during sleep.	Attacks often in public, and a repeat performance may be given for the newly arrived doctor. Never during sleep.
Attacks	Tonic & clonic movements.	Movements of a thrashing nature or bizarre nature.
Accompaniments	No moans and groans except stridor due to laryngeal spasm.	Moans and groans may be very marked, with sudden recurrence of thrashing.
Duration	Rarely goes beyond a minute.	Attack lasts much longer than a minute.
Sequelae	Patient may fall and hurt himself or bite his tongue; incontinence of urine and faeces.	Patient never falls, never hurts herself, never bites her tongue; NOT incontinent.
Plantars	Extensor, bilateral.	Remain flexor.
Eyelids	Eyelids opened easily, passively.	Patient screws up the eyelids when an attempt is made to open them.
EEG	Normal or abnormal.	Normal.

Table 10.3 IMPORTANT CAUSES OF CONVULSIONS ACCORDING TO AGE GROUP

Age at onset	Probable causes	Remarks
Infancy (0-2 yrs)	Congenital maldevelopment.	Take careful obstetric history.
	Birth injury.	
	Hypocalcaemia.	Evidence of tetany and rickets. Therapeutic response to calcium and Vit. D.
	Hypoglycaemia.	Response to glucose.
	Pyridoxine deficiency.	Response to pyridoxine
	Phenyl ketonuria.	Urine test.
	Febrile convulsions: coming on first day of fever likely to be due to pyrexia; but convulsions after some days likely to be due to infections like pyogenic meningitis.	Commonest cause in infancy. Later potentiality for epilepsy.
Childhood (2-10 yrs)	Birth injury.	Take careful obstetric history.
	Trauma.	Inquire about past injury,
	Infections.	encephalitis, meningitis.
	Thrombosis of cerebral arteries and veins.	In the setting of dehydration and infection.
	Neurotuberculosis.	Focal and generalized convulsions occur in 10-15% of children and young adults with neurotuberculosis.
	Beginning of idiopathic epilepsy.	
Adolescence (10-18 yrs)	Idiopathic epilepsy.	
	Trauma.	
	Congenital defects.	
	Neurotuberculosis.	
	Neurocystilcercosis.	Focal and generalized convulsions occur in 25-95% of patients of neurocysticercosis. Look for subcutaneous or tongue nodules and pseudohypertrophy of calves.
Early adulthood (18-35 yrs)	Trauma.	
	Neoplasm.	
	Idiopathic epilepsy.	
	Drug addiction and alcohol.	
	Cysticercosis.	
Pregnant women	Eclampsia.	High BP, albuminuria.
Puerperium	Cerebral venous thrombosis.	MRI for confirmation.
Middle age (35-60 yrs)	Neoplasm.	
	Trauma.	
	Vascular disease.	
	Alcohol.	
	Stokes-Adams syndrome.	
Old age (over 60 yrs)	Vascular disease.	
	Degeneration tumour.	
	Presenile/senile dementia.	
Any age	Cerebral malaria.	Most of these conditions are treatable with prompt diagnosis.
	Cerebral abscess.	
	Encephalitis.	
	Meningitis.	
	Angiomatous malformations.	
	Trauma.	
	Subdural haematoma.	
	Hypoglycaemia.	

TABLE 10.4 CLASSIFICATION OF EPILEPSY

Generalized seizures	Preferred drug
1. Tonic-clonic seizures (grand mal, major epilepsy)	Valproate Carbamazepine Phenobarbitone Phenytoin
2. Tonic seizures	- do -
3. Myoclonic seizures	Valproate Clonazepam
4. Akinetic seizures	
5. Absence of seizures (a) typical petit mal: spike and wave EEG (b) atypical: other EEG changes	Ethosuximide Valiproate
Partial Seizures	
1. Simple partial: no loss of consciousness e.g. Jacksonian epilepsy	Carbamazepine Phenytoin
2. Complex partial: with impaired consciousness	Carbamazepine Phenytoin
3. Partial seizures evolving to tonic-clonic seizures (secondary generalization)	Valproate
4. Apparent generalized tonic-clonic with EEG (but not clinical) evidence of focal onset	Carbamazepine Valproate Phenytoin

Akinetic seizure may be confused with syncope. Temporal lobe seizure may present as an acute psychotic episode.

From the clinical point of view the important question to decide is between idiopathic epilepsy and symptomatic (or secondary) epilepsy. This is particularly important if the seizure begins after the age of 20.

Symptomatic epilepsy should also be suspected in (1) all cases with headache and neurological signs; (2) where general examination of other systems reveals a possible cause for the fits; (3) focal (Jacksonian) fits especially if the fits are followed by increasing weakness of a limb; and (4) patients showing cutaneous naevi, or pigmented moles or skin lesion of epiloia (adenoma sebaceum), or subcutaneous or tongue nodules (cysticercosis).

A solitary fit (once in a lifetime) is not an uncommon occurrence especially in the background of infection, emotional stress, alcoholic excess and dehydration. It is wise not to label the person as epileptic nor put him on anticonvulsant drugs at once, but to wait for a further attack to occur before diagnosing epilepsy.

Investigations in a case of epilepsy
Blood and CSF for VDRL.

Chest X-ray (tuberculosis lung-tuberculoma of brain; malignancy lung-metastasis).

Plain X-ray skull: calcification.

EEG: Resting record is normal in about one-third of patients of epilepsy. A normal record renders unlikely any gross focal cause for the attack.

Brain scan/CT scan/MRI for cysticercosis, tuberculoma or mass lesions.

If these investigations are negative, follow-up examinations for the appearance of new evidence are essential.

Hypoxia

Hypoglycaemia of hyperglycaemia

Hyponatraemia or hypernatraemia

Hypocalcaemia or hypercalcaemia

Hypokalaemia

Hypomagnesaemia

Acidosis or alkalosis

Hypothyroidism or hyperthyroidism

Addison's disease

Dehydration

Uraemia

Management of Status Epilepticus

Recurrent grand mal convulsions without the patient regaining consciousness in between two fits, is a serious situation, needing prompt referral for hospitalization.

Sudden stoppage of drugs, especially in a longstanding epileptic patient, may precipitate status epilepticus; hence the treating physician must particularly emphasize this point to the patient and ask him to ensure that his stock of drugs does not get suddenly exhausted.

Occasionally, a non-specific fever, alcohol or excessive fatigue may be the cause of status epilepticus.

Metabolic conditions that may cause or contribute to status epilepticus are listed in **Table 10.5**. Anticonvulsant drugs are listed in **Table 10.6**.

1. The practising physician should always keep ampoules of diazepam (valium) in his emergency kit. A dose of 10 mg IV may be sufficient to terminate the convulsions promptly and safely. If it only partially abates the attack, then it has to be repeated by IM or IV injection at five minute intervals; thereafter, an IV drip may be given (2 mg/min) depending upon the patient's response.

Table **10.6 ANTICONVULSANT DRUGS**

Drug	Daily dose range		Toxic effects
	Oral	Blood level µg/ml	
Phenobarbitone	0-1 yr 30-60 mg 1-5 yr 90 mg 6-12 yr 120 mg Adult 1.5 mg/kg	10-30	Drowsiness, nystagmus, ataxia, fever, rash.
Diphenylhydantoin	1-5 yr 30-60 mg 6-12 yr 90 mg Adult 300-500 mg	10-20	Gum hyperplasia, hirsutism, rash, blood dyscrasia, megaloblastic anaemia, erythema multiforme.
Primidone	Child 5-20 mg/kg Adult 125-1000 mg		Nystagmus, ataxia, drowsiness, gastric upset, depression, rash.
Trimethadione	Child 10-15 mg/kg Adult 600-2100 mg		Blood dyscrasia, rash, lupoid reaction, lymphadenopathy, nephrotic syndrome.
Carbamazepine	Child 5-25 mg/day Adult 5-10 mg/kg upto 1600	5-12	Bone marrow suppression, hepatotoxicity, GI irritation, ataxia, dizziness, diplopia, vertigo: blood level decreased by phenytoin, barbiturate.
Sodium Valproate	Child 30 mg/kg Adult 750-1250 mg/day (upto 60 mg/kg)	50-150	Bone marrow suppression, hepatotoxicity, GI irritation, ataxia, dizziness, diplopia, vertigo: blood level decreased by phenytoin, barbiturate.

Along with diazepam, the patient should be started on regular anticonvulsant drugs, phenobarbitone 25 mg and diphenylhydantoin 100 mg which can be given via Ryle's tube every 6 hours.

Diazepam can then be withdrawn once the status epilepticus is under control. It is not useful for routine control of fits as an oral drug.

2. If diazepam is not available, paraldehyde 10 ml IM inj. in adults (1 ml/year age of child) is a useful drug. The injection can be repeated 4 hourly if convulsions persist; upto 30 ml paraldehyde daily.

3. IV or IM phenobarbitone 200 mg can be given but the main disadvantage is respiratory depression by a dose which is necessary to control the fits. Up to 300 mg can be given safely.

4. IV or IM phenytoin sodium 100-200 mg may be given (upto 500 mg in saline in 24 hours). Overmedication results in deep drug coma and respiratory depression. The infusion rate should not exceed 50 mg/minute. A loading dose is 20 mg/kg. Close monitoring of cardiac rhythm and BP is necessary.

The intractable case has to be managed by an expert anaesthesiologist by an intravenous thiopentone drip (I g in 550 ml of Ringer lactate solution at the rate of 15 drops per minute) or clonazepam IV. The anaesthesiologist can manage respiratory complications by positive pressure respiration.

Medical management of neurotuberculosis
INAH, rifampicin and pyrazinamide, and streptomycin (or ethambutol): 4 drugs regime for short-term therapy of 6 months has been effective for tuberculosis. Surgery is indicated for hydrocephalus.

Medical management of neurocysticercosis
Praziquantel (PZQ) 50 mg/kg/day for 15 days.

Oral prednisolone is started 2 days prior to starting PZQ (to avoid reactive cerebral oedema following death of larvae), and is tapered off after conclusion of PZQ treatment.

Cysts located in the pathway of CSF drainage (foramen of Monroe, aqueduct of Sylvius and outlet of 4th ventricle) are contraindications for larvicidal therapy (this can be ascertained by CT/MRI).

Albendazole 400 mg bid for 30 days is also a promising drug. 75 per cent of cases show satisfactory clinical and CT response. The drug acts slowly hence side effects are not florid (in contrast, with PZQ 20-40 per cent cases experience marked aggravation of ICT and recurrent seizures during therapy.

Patient Education

The patient, especially a child or adolescent, should not ride a bicycle, or swim unattended. All open fires in the house should be screened. Till the fits are well controlled, an adolescent or adult should not drive a car (i.e. no fits during waking hours for 2 years).

An adult patient should be guided into an occupation in which neither the patient himself nor the community is put to risk by a propensity to fits. Exposure to moving machinery and work at heights should be avoided.

Note should be made of factors which precipitate attacks, such as deprivation of sleep, fever, hot water baths, flickering lights, watching television, or emotional disturbances.

All anti-epileptic drugs (**Table 10.6**) may cause drowsiness, osteomalacia and folate deficiency resulting in megaloblastic anaemia. Phenytoin also gives rise to gingival hyperplasia in children and coarsening of features in adults. All of these drugs have some teratogenic effect, which is probably most marked with phenytoin, hence it is prudent to give carbamazepine or sodium valproate for the treatment of epilepsy in women in the reproductive years.

After the patient has been free from epilepsy for at least two years, antiepileptic drugs can be gradually withdrawn in many cases.

Five per cent of epilepsy patients have intractable seizures not responding to 3 or more drugs. Patients of partial complex seizures have a temporal lobe focus which can be surgically ablated to cure the patient. Modern PET and SPECT tests help to identify such foci.

11 Cyanosis

Cyanosis refers to a bluish colour of the skin and mucous membranes resulting from an increase in the amount of reduced haemoglobin (or of non-functional haemoglobin derivatives-methaemoglobin or sulfhaemoglobin) in the small blood vessels of those areas. It is particularly marked in the lips, ears, nail beds and malar eminences. The 'red cyanosis' of polycythaemia vera must be distinguished from true cyanosis.

The degree of cyanosis is modified by the quality of cutaneous pigment, the thickness of the skin, and the colour of the blood flowing in the cutaneous capillaries.

The accurate clinical detection of the presence and degree of cyanosis is difficult, as proved by oximetry. In some instances, central cyanosis can be reliably detected when the arterial oxygen saturation has fallen to 85 per cent. In others it may not be detected until the saturation has declined to 75 per cent.

In general, cyanosis appears when the mean capillary concentration of reduced haemoglobin exceeds 5 g/dl. As little as 1.5 g/dl methaemoglobin and 0.5 g/dl sulfhaemoglobin can produce cyanosis. It is the absolute rather than the relative quantity of reduced haemoglobin which is important in producing cyanosis. Hence in patients with severe anaemia (Hb less than 5 g/dl), even marked oxygen desaturation will not produce cyanosis. Conversely, patients with polycythaemia vera will display cyanosis at higher levels of arterial oxygen saturation than patients with normal haemoglobin. Similarly local passive congestion, resulting in an increase in the total amount of reduced haemoglobin in the vessels in a given area, may cause cyanosis.

Clinically cyanosis can be subdivided into *central* and *peripheral* types.

In central cyanosis there is arterial blood unsaturation (or an abnormal haemoglobin derivative), and the mucous membranes and skin are both affected.

In peripheral cyanosis, arterial oxygen saturation is normal, but there is an abnormally greater extraction of oxygen due to slowing of blood flow to an area. It results from vasoconstriction and diminished peripheral blood flow such as exposure to cold, shock, congestive heart failure and peripheral vascular disease. In those conditions the mucous membranes of the oral cavity and the tongue may be spared.

In cardiogenic shock with pulmonary oedema there may be a mixture of central and peripheral cyanosis.

Table 11.1 lists the causes of generalized cyanosis, and **Table 11.2** lists the causes of regional cyanosis.

Approach to the Patient with Cyanosis

Certain features should be elicited in order to recognize the cause of cyanosis.

1. *History:* How long is the cyanosis present? Cyanosis since birth: usually due to congenital heart disease with right to left shunt.
   Acquired in later life: Reversal of left to right shunt; chronic obstructive pulmonary disease (COPD), interstitial lung disease.

2. *Exposure to oxidizing chemicals* (nitrates, chlorates, aniline dyes) and drugs (phenacetin, sulfonamides).

3. *Clinical distinction between central and peripheral cyanosis:* Massage or gentle warming of a cyanotic extremity will increase peripheral blood flow and abolish peripheral but not central cyanosis.

TABLE 11.1 GENERALIZED CYANOSIS

I. *Central cyanosis*

A. Decreased arterial oxygen saturation

1. Decreased atmospheric pressure: High altitude over 5000 metres (16,000 feet)

2. Impaired lung function
   (a) alveolar hypoventilation
   (b) mis-match between ventilation/perfusion, (perfusion of hypoventilated alveoli), e.g. bronchial carcinoma, tuberculous bronchial stenosis
   (c) impaired oxygen diffusion, e.g. fibrosing alveolitis, pulmonary oedema

3. Anatomic shunts-admixture of venous and arterial blood
   (a) congenital heart disease e.g. Fallot's tetralogy
   (b) pulmonary arterio-venous fistulas
   (c) multiple small intrapulmonary shunts (e.g. cirrhosis of liver)

4. Mutant haemoglobin with low affinity for oxygen (Kansas Hb) - Detected by Hb electrophoresis

B. Haemoglobin abnormalities: arterial oxygen saturation normal

1. Methaemoglobinaemia
   hereditary
   acquired due to drugs
   (phenacetin, sulfonamides)

2. Sulfhaemoglobinaemia
   acquired due to drugs

II. *Peripheral cyanosis:* arterial oxygen saturation normal

A. Exposure to cold air or water

B. Reduced cardiac output-shock, acute left ventricular failure, severe mitral stenosis

C. Arterial obstruction, e.g. embolus, vasospasm, Raynaud's phenomenon, hyperviscosity syndromes

D. Venous obstruction/hypertension, tricuspid valve disease, constrictive pericarditis.

An important point in the differentiation of cyanosis due to a central veno-arterial shunt from that due to primary lung disease is the *response to oxigen.*

TABLE 11.2 REGIONAL CYANOSIS

I. *Face and upper limbs only*
Superior vena cava obstruction: oedema plus cyanosis: distended non-pulsatile veins

II. *One extremity only*
Phlebothrombosis of a large vein with few collateral channels Arterial embolism in an extremity

III. *Lower extremities only*–not in upper extremities (Differential cyanosis) Patent ductus arteriosus with pulmonary hypertension and right-to-left shunt

IV. *Acrocyanosis*
Hands and fingers only

V. *Erythrocyanosis*
Lower part of the legs on exposure to cold: in young women with short skirts and thin stockings

In the latter a considerable reduction in cyanosis results from a rise in the alveolar PO_2. In congenital cyanotic heart disease oxygen administration produces virtually no change in the oxygen saturation since veno-arterial mixing occurs downstream from the pulmonary vascular bed.

The cyanosis due to methaemoglobinaemia is also unrelieved by oxygen therapy. However the PO_2 is normal in this condition.

4. *Presence or absence of clubbing of fingers and toes:* clubbing is marked in Fallot's tetralogy, interstitial pulmonary fibrosis, or pulmonary arteriovenous shunts. Peripheral cyanosis or acutely developing central cyanosis is not associated with finger clubbing.

5. *Detection of functionally abnormal haemoglobin derivatives: Methaemoglobin:* This is done by spectroscopic analysis of a 1:100 dilution of blood; in the presence of methaemoglobin a band is seen at 630 μ which disappears on the addition of a reducing agent.

Management of Cyanosis

Obstruction of the upper airways causing cyanosis (e.g. occlusion of the larynx by a foreign body, acute laryngeal oedema, diphtheritic laryngitis) need urgent tracheostomy.

Obstructive lesions of the main bronchi, such as bronchial carcinoma, adenoma, or tuberculous stenosis, may produce cyanosis if perfusion of the unventilated areas of the lung continues. These lesions can be corrected surgically.

In COPD with varying degrees of bronchitis and emphysema the severity of cyanosis depends to a considerable extent on the sensitivity of the respiratory centre to the raised arterial PCO_2. In the so-called 'pink puffers' the respiratory centre retains its normal behaviour and responds to the hypercapnia by hyperventilation which maintains near-normal oxygenation at the expense of severe dyspnoea. In the 'blue bloaters' on the other hand, the respiratory centre has lost its ability to respond to a rising PCO_2. Dyspnoea is less severe but hypoxaemia and cyanosis are marked.

Fallot's tetralogy is the most common congenital cardiac lesion which causes cyanosis. The four classic features are: infundibular pulmonary stenosis, VSD, overriding aorta, and right ventricular hypertrophy. Corrective surgery is advisable at some point in almost all patients with this anomaly. Successful correction avoids progressive infundibular obstruction, delayed growth and complications due to hypoxaemia and polycythaemia.

Raynaud's phenomenon occurs in 80–90 per cent of patients with scleroderma and is the presenting symptom in 30 per cent. It may be the only symptom of scleroderma for several years.

Atherosclerosis of the extremities is a frequent cause in men over age 50. Drugs that are useful include reserpine (adrenergic blockade), phenoxybenzamine, methyldopa, calcium channel blockers especially nifedepine (10–30 mg tid).

Occasionally, surgical sympathectomy is helpful in patients unresponsive to medical therapy but the benefits are often transient.

Methaemoglobinaemia
Blood levels greater than 50 per cent are indicative of severe toxicity, and levels greater than 70 per cent are often fatal. Treatment includes supplemental oxygen and methylene blue 1–2 mg/kg IV over 5 minutes if there are signs of hypoxia, or if the methaemoglobin level is over 30 per cent. The dose may be repeated once after 1 hour if there are persistent signs of hypoxia.

12 Dyspnoea

Breathing is the only involuntary act which is carried out by voluntary muscles, and normally this is so. Dyspnoea is a subjective sensation in which there is an abnormally uncomfortable awareness of breathing. The perception of the sensation and the person's reaction to that perception are both important. For instance, during vigorous physical exercise or sporting activity the volume of ventilation is markedly increased–*hyperpnoea*; and the rate of respiration is also markedly increased–*tachypnoea*, but the person though aware of this, is not abnormally uncomfortable about it. This is in contrast to the anxious and fearful patient who uses a large number of verbal expressions to describe his abnormally uncomfortable awareness of his breathing, such as: 'cannot get enough air', or 'air does not go all the way down', or 'smothering feeling in the chest', 'tightness in the chest', 'choking in the chest', or 'fatigue in the chest'.

Dyspnoea occurs as a symptom in a wide variety of diseases. The critical questions that the doctor should raise are:

Is it due to cardiac dysfunction?
Is it due to pulmonary dysfunction?
Is it due to renal dysfunction? (volume overload)
Is it due to severe anaemia?
Is it due to psychogenic problems?

The causes of dyspnoea are listed in **Table 12.1**. Dyspnoea due to mechanical embarrassment to breathing such as extreme obesity, massive ascites or advanced pregnancy, does not pose a diagnostic problem. Causes of dyspnoea according to onset are given in **Table 12.2**.

By analysis of the history, as regards onset, circumstances in which it occurred–at rest (orthopnoea) or during exertion, or during emotional stress; and the position the patient adopts during the episode, some idea can be formed about the cause.

Breathlessness on exertion is frequently the first symptom of heart failure. From the history alone it is usually hard to distinguish this from the dyspnoea due to lung disease but the differentiation is often possible if the patient is observed at the time. Typically patients with cardiac failure take rapid shallow breaths; wheezing and the excessive use of accessory muscles of respiration (seen in bronchial asthma), are uncommon. However, occasionally, in the presence of pulmonary oedema, a cardiac patient will wheeze. The clinical points of difference between cardiac asthma and bronchial asthma are given in **Table 12.3**.

Paroxysmal nocturnal dyspnoea is characteristic of mitral stenosis and left ventricular failure. A patient with respiratory disease may also have nocturnal worsening of symptoms but, unlike the cardiac patient who stops coughing and goes to sleep, the bronchitic patient continues to have disturbed sleep due to cough, and brings out a lot of sputum, throughout the night.

Orthopnoea is characteristic of congestive heart failure, bronchial asthma and COPD, and in bilateral diaphragmatic paralysis.

A sudden and unexpected episode of *dyspnoea at rest* suggests an inhaled foreign body, pulmonary embolism, spontaneous pneumothorax, or anxiety and panic reaction.

The dyspnoea of chronic bronchitis and emphysema (COPD) tends to develop more gradually than that of heart disease. However, episodes of superadded respiratory infection (e.g. pneumonitis, pneumothorax or exacerbation of asthma) may present as acute episodes of dyspnoea.

TABLE 12.1 CAUSES OF DYSPNOEA

A. *Cardiac diseases*
1. Coronary artery disease, leading to left ventricular failure.
2. Hypertensive heart disease, leading to left ventricular failure.
3. Valvular heart disease, e.g. mitral stenosis.
4. Hypertrophic cardiomyopathy.
5. Dilated cardiomyopathy.
6. Restrictive cardiomyopathy: amyloidosis; sarcoidosis; haemochromatosis.
7. Constrictive pericarditis.
8. High output heart failure:
   severe chronic anaemia;
   thyrotoxicosis;
   beriberi;
   intracardiac shunts.

B. Respiratory diseases
1. Bronchial asthma.
2. COPD.
3. Interstitial fibrosis various causes).
4. Massive pleural effusion.

C. Acute glomerulonephritis
   Volume overload.

D. Severe Anaemia (irrespective of the cause)

E. Mechanical embarrassment to breathing
   Pregnancy-later months.
   Ascites.
   Extreme obesity.

F. Psychogenic
   Anxiety, panic attacks.

In patients in whom the etiology of dyspnoea is not clear, pulmonary function testing is helpful in determining whether dyspnoea is produced by heart disease, lung disease, abnormalities of the chest wall or anxiety. It is possible to identify

Obstructive (asthma, COPD), brochiectasis, brochiolitis, cystic fibrosis).

Restrictive (parenchymal) – sarcoidosis, pneumoconiosis, idiopathic pulmonary fibrosis, drug/ radiation induced interstitial lung disease.

Restrictive (extraparenchymal) – Neuromusclar weakness or chest wall (kyphoscoliosis, ankylosing spondylitis obesity.

The coexistence of both cardiac and pulmonary disease in the same patient makes matters difficult.

TABLE 12.2 CAUSES OF DYSPNOEA ACCORDING TO ONSET

1. Dramatic onset (over minutes):
   Pneumothorax
   Pulmonary embolism
   Pulmonary oedema

2. Acute onset (over hours):
   Pneumonia
   Allergic alveolitis
   Asthma
   Left ventricular failure

3. Subacute onset (over days):
   Pleural effusion
   Bronchogenic carcinoma
   Sarcoidosis
   PCP in AIDS
   mycobacterial, fungal pneumonia

4. Chronic onset (over months):
   COPD
   Diffuse fibrosing conditions
   Anaemia
   Hyperthyroidism

5. Intermittent (episodic):
   Asthma
   Left ventricular failure

Examples are coronary artery disease in a heavy smoker with chronic bronchitis; mitral stenosis with tropical eosinophilia.

Echocardiography with dobutamine stress or radionuclide ventriculography at rest and during symptom-limited exercise are useful techniques by which left ventricular ejection fraction (LVEF) and right ventricular ejection fraction (RVEF) can be compared between rest and exercise. Normal response is a rise in EF of at least 5 per cent over the rest value. The LVEF falls on exercise in left ventricular disease at an early stage when RV response is normal. A normal LV response and abnormal RV response (fall on exercise) is indicative of dyspnoea due to lung disease. In isolated right coronary artery lesions, the RV response to exercise is abnormal, while LVEF response to exercise may be normal; additionally there will be wall motion abnormality in the inferior wall. The RV response may improve markedly with sublingual nitroglycerin.

TABLE 12.3 DIFFERENTATION BETWEEN CARDIAC AND BRONCHIAL ASTHMA

Points	Cardiac Asthma	Bronchial Asthma	Remarks
Age	Usually older age group	Any age; common in young and under 45	
Past history	Coronary artery disease; hypertension; valvular disease	Previous attacks of asthma; other allergic manifestations	Two conditions can coexist e.g. mitral stenosis with tropical eosinophilia; hypertension with chronic bronchitis.
Family history	Usually non-contributing	Bronchial asthma; atopy; allergy	
Precipitating factors	May be none, or exertion; infarction	No relation to exertion; allergens	Allergen may not always be obvious.
Symptoms	Wheezing not marked; cough with pink frothy sputum	Wheezing marked; cough with thick sticky sputum	Occasionally symptoms may be identical.
Blood pressure	May be high (HT), normal, or low (myocardial infarction; tight stenotic lesion)	Normal	Look particularly for pulsus alternans while taking blood pressure.
Pulse	Rapid; pulsus alternans may be present	Rapid (may be feeble in prolonged asthma); no pulsus alternans	This is valuable evidence of left ventricular failure; not seen in bronchial asthma.
Chest	Shape normal	May be barrel-shaped	Not reliable.
Apex beat	May be heaving (hypertension, myocardial infarction, aortic valvular disease); or tapping (mitral stenosis)	Normal; may be difficult to palpate due to emphysema	In obese persons difficulty in assessing cardiac enlargement by palpation.
Heart size	There may be evidence of cardiac enlargement	No cardiac enlargement	Assessment may be difficult clinically, needs X-ray chest for confirmation.
Auscultation of heart	Triple rhythm; murmurs	Normal heart sounds	Wheezing may drown cardiac sounds especially 3rd sound.
Breath sounds	Expiration not prolonged; Wheezing not marked; earlier, basal crepitations, gradually involves whole lung	Expiration markedly prolonged; wheezing marked all over the chest; not confined to bases	Occasionally cardiac asthma may totally mimic signs of bronchial asthma.
Circulation time using decholin or calcium gluconate	Arm-to-tongue time prolonged	Arm-to-tongue time normal	Valuable bedside test in a difficult case where clinical differentiation is not sure.
Therapeutic dilemma	Morphine is the drug of choice; adrenaline is contraindicated	Morphine is dangerous; adrenaline very useful especially early in attack	When in doubt avoid morphine and adrenaline, and give IV aminophylline 0.25 g slowly.

Both ventricular responses to exercise are normal in dyspnoea due to anxiety or malingering, or that due to obesity.

Severe anaemia can cause dyspnoea on exertion but the patient prefers to lie flat rather than sit up (unlike cardiac patients with pulmonary congestion).

Management of an acute attack of bronchial asthma

I. *Assessment of severity*

History: Patients with a long history of asthma can often reliably compare the present attack with previous ones. Past or present use of corticosteroids, frequent hospitalization, previous need for mechanical ventilation and recent emergency room visits should raise the suspicion of a severe and unresponsive attack necessitating hospitalization.

Physical examination: Dyspnoea at rest, orthopnoea, sweating, difficulty speaking in sentences, and use of accessory muscles of respiration indicate severe bronchospasm. Respiration rate over 30 p.m., pulse rate over 120 p.m. and pulsus paradoxus greater than 18 mm Hg indicate a dangerously severe episode. The intensity of wheezing is unreliable because breath sounds decrease with severe obstruction. Somnolence and agitation suggest impending respiratory failure. Subcutaneous emphysema should raise suspicion of associated pneumothorax.

If the initial FEV 1 is less than 30 per cent of the predicted value or does not increase to at least 40 per cent of the predicted value after one hour of vigorous therapy, hospitalization is recommended.

A chest X-ray is useful to exclude complications such as pneumothorax or pneumomediastinum, to suggest or confirm a diagnosis of pneumonia, and to reveal evidence of other conditions that mimic asthma.

II. *Treatment of acute attack*

1. *Oxygen:* should be given bilaterally at low flow rates (2-3 litres per minute) by nasal cannula. Most asthmatics hyperventilate hence $PaCO_2$ is usually low.

   A 'normal' or increased $PaCO_2$ > 40 mm Hg with mental confusion may require mechanical ventilation, with very high pressures (> 80 cm H_2O).

2. *Beta adrenergic agonist bronchodilators:* are given as a metered dose inhaler (MDI) with a spacer device or reservoir. Albuterol, terbutalin and metaproterenol are equally effective. Large doses and frequent administration may be required in seriously ill patients. 2-4 initial puffs followed by 1-2 puffs every 10-20 minutes are given until improvement occurs, or until tremors or cardiac arrhythmia develop.

   In the absence of MDI or nebulizer facilities, epinephrine 0.3 mg SC 15-20 minutes for upto 3 doses may be used.

3. *Aminophylline drip:* IV loading dose 6 mg/kg body weight is infused slowly over 20 minutes (This should be reduced or omitted if the patient has recently taken aminophylline). Maintenance dose by constant IV infusion (0.5 mg/kg/hour). In the elderly or in patients with heart or liver failure, lower infusion rate (0.2 mg/kg/hour).

   Serum levels should be monitored and kept below 40 mg /litre to avoid toxicity (seizures, ventricular arrhythmias).

4. *Systemic steroids:* Methyl prednisolone 0.5-1 mg/kg IV 6 hourly is given for its anti-inflammatory effects. The beneficial effect is evident only after 4-6 hours.

III. *Maintenance therapy*

   MDI with beta adrenergic agonist should be used regularly even when asymptomatic, after the acute attack is over.

   Precipitating factors such as allergens, cold weather, chemical irritants, exercise, medication such as aspirin and NSAIDs, beta adrenergic antagonists and cholinergic drugs (including eye drops) should be avoided.

   Inhaled corticosteroids by MDI may reduce or eliminate the need for systemic steroids. The usual dose is 2 puffs 4 times daily, 5-10 minutes after inhaled bronchodilators.

   Cromolyn sodium 2 puffs 4 times daily and MDI improves baseline pulmonary function, reduces frequency and severity of the attacks, and reduces the requirement for other medication including steroids. Cromolyn has no role in the treatment of acute attacks.

The body of a normal man of 65 kg contains about 40 litres of water of which 28 L is intracellular and 12 L extracellular. The latter is composed of 10 L interstitial fluid and 2-3 L plasma.

Sodium, potassium, calcium, magnesium and phosphorus are important electrolytes which, along with hydrogen ions, are maintained within narrow limits in the tissue cells and in the extracellular fluid which bathes them. The kidneys play an important part in maintaining the 'constancy of the internal environment of the body' which is a pre-condition of life.

Derangement of water and electrolyte balance and disturbances in hydrogen ion concentration occur in a wide variety of clinical conditions.

These derangements (depletion or excess of water, sodium, potassium, calcium and magnesium) can present considerable diagnostic difficulties. Furthermore, it is not uncommon for multiple electrolyte deficits to develop simultaneously.

1. When both sodium and water are lost (as is the case in most clinical situations listed in **Table 13.1**) estimation of serum sodium is *not* going to give any indication of the volume depletion. Clinical assessment of dehydration and the laboratory tests of raised haematocrit, BUN and creatinine are helpful while the serum sodium may be within the *normal range* in spite of severe depletion.

2. On the other hand, a *low serum sodium* by itself does not indicate what should be the management of the patient. It is the *clinical setting* which indicates if the hyponatraemia is *depletional* (which needs replacement of sodium) or *dilutional* (which does not need replacement of sodium but needs restriction of water to 500 ml per day). Hyponatraemia associated with oedema is more complex. Its management is again determined by the clinical setting, assisted by estimation of urinary concentration of electrolytes.

3. Potassium and magnesium are mainly intracellular ions and severe deficits may occur without significant alterations in their plasma concentrations. Clinical setting and the ECG are helpful in assessment of their deficiency or excess.

4. The measurement of electrolytes in the urine is useful only in the clinical context (**Figs. 13.1, 13.2**). A very simple and cheap test for the presence of sodium in the urine is the *Fantus test*, which is based on the fact that urine (which contains sodium chloride) will give a white precipitate of silver chloride-sodium nitrate when added to a solution of silver nitrate. In a cholera patient with hypovolaemia the urine will *not* show a white precipitate; whereas in a patient with Addison's disease in crisis with hypovolaemia, the urine will show a white precipitate indicating continued loss of sodium in the urine. Doctors in the developed world stopped using this test about 50 years ago. However, there is no reason why this simple test should be discarded. There is no simple test for urinary potassium.

In patients who are found unexpectedly to have hypokalaemia, the finding of urinary K^+ of more than 20 mmol per day indicates excessive renal loss of potassium. On the other hand urinary K^+ of less than 10 mmol/day in the presence of hypokalaemia indicates an extra-renal source of loss (usually gastrointestinal).

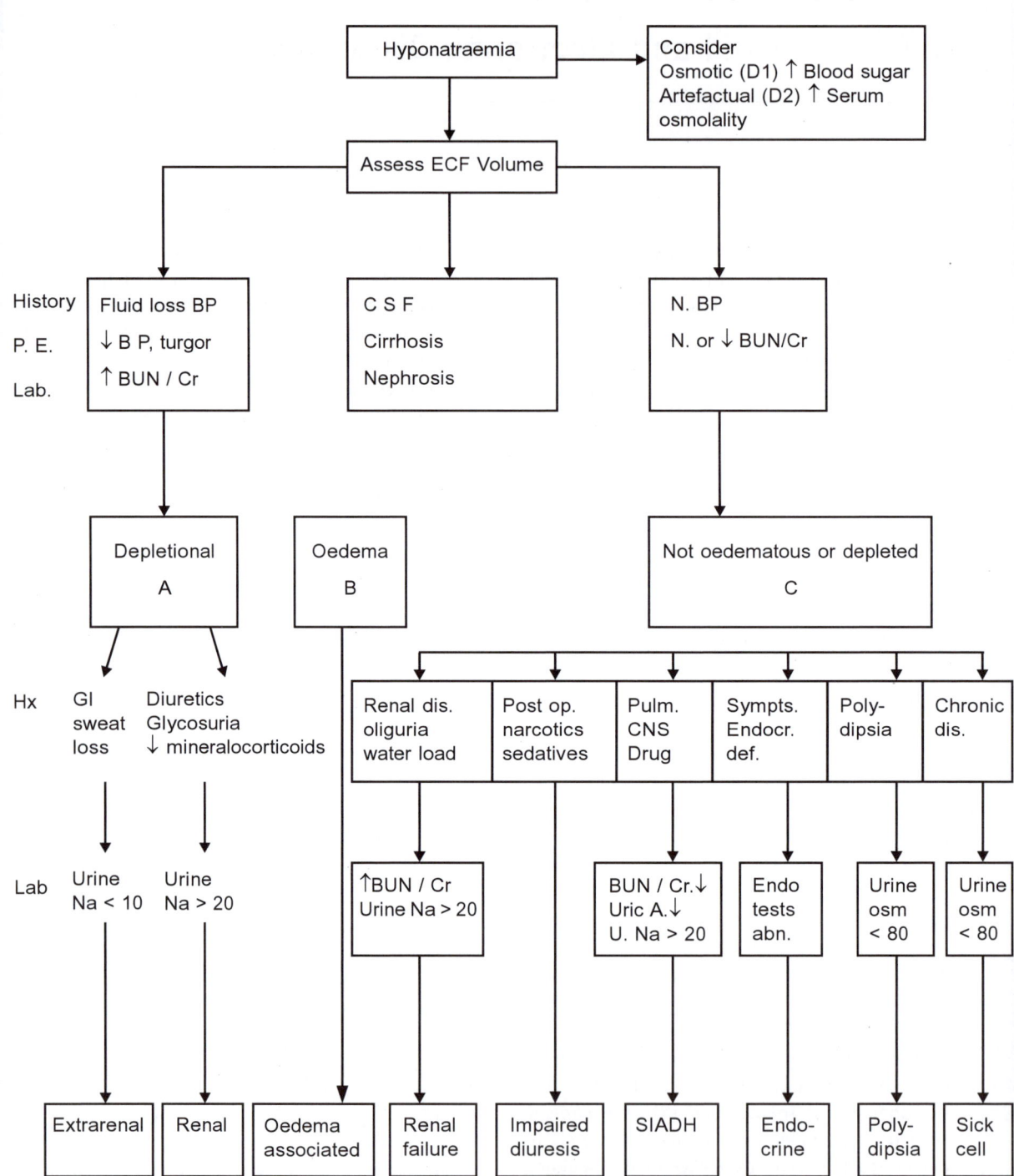

Fig. 13.1: Clinical approach to hyponatraemia

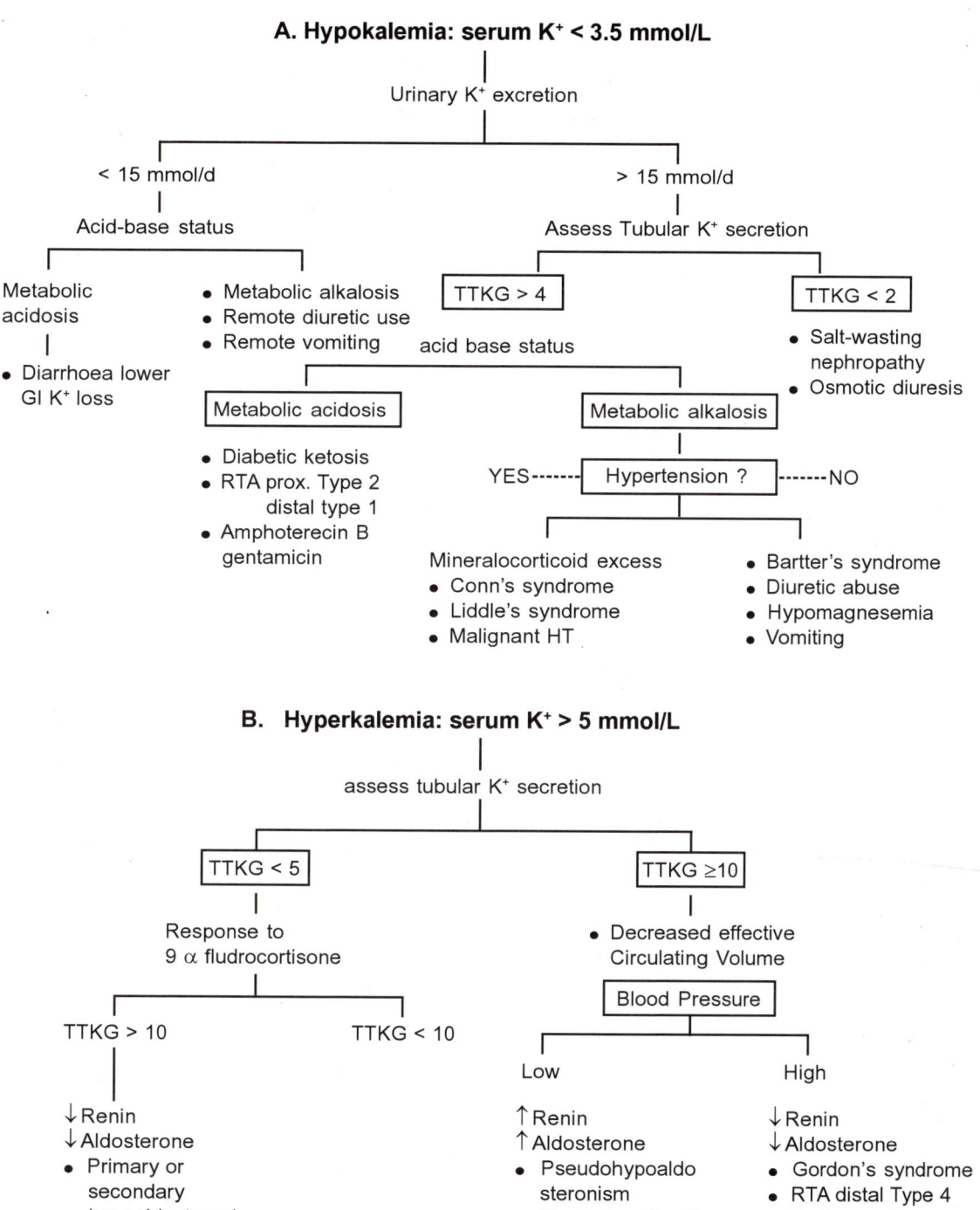

A. Hypokalemia: serum K⁺ < 3.5 mmol/L

Urinary K⁺ excretion

< 15 mmol/d

Acid-base status

Metabolic acidosis

• Diarrhoea lower GI K⁺ loss

• Metabolic alkalosis
• Remote diuretic use
• Remote vomiting

> 15 mmol/d

Assess Tubular K⁺ secretion

TTKG > 4

acid base status

Metabolic acidosis

• Diabetic ketosis
• RTA prox. Type 2 distal type 1
• Amphoterecin B gentamicin

Metabolic alkalosis

YES------- Hypertension ? -------NO

Mineralocorticoid excess
• Conn's syndrome
• Liddle's syndrome
• Malignant HT

• Bartter's syndrome
• Diuretic abuse
• Hypomagnesemia
• Vomiting

TTKG < 2

• Salt-wasting nephropathy
• Osmotic diuresis

B. Hyperkalemia: serum K⁺ > 5 mmol/L

assess tubular K⁺ secretion

TTKG < 5

Response to 9 α fludrocortisone

TTKG > 10

TTKG < 10

↓Renin
↓Aldosterone
• Primary or secondary hypoaldosteronism

TTKG ≥10

• Decreased effective Circulating Volume

Blood Pressure

Low

High

↑Renin
↑Aldosterone
• Pseudohypoaldo steronism
• K⁺ sparing diuretics

↓Renin
↓Aldosterone
• Gordon's syndrome
• RTA distal Type 4
• Cyclocsporine

Fig. 13.2 Hypokalaemia and Hyperkalaemia

Table 13.1 ECF VOLUME DEPLETION

Clinical conditions	Common manifestations
A. *Gastrointestinal loss* (Urine Na less than 10 mmol/L)	Anorexia Nausea
1. External loss:	Vomiting
Vomiting, diarrhoea	Apathy
Nasogastric suction	Lethargy
Fistula drainage	Weakness
2. Internal loss:	Orthostatic
Intestinal obstruction	dizziness
Paralytic ileus	Syncope
Peritonitis, ascites	
B. *Skin loss* (Urine Na less than 10 mmol/L)	Hypotension Weight loss
Excessive sweating	Poor skin turgor
Burns	Sunken eyes
Pemphigus	Tachycardia Oliguria
C. *Renal loss* (urine Na more than 20 mmol/L	
1. Renal disease	
Acute tubular necrosis	Polyuria
recovery phase	Dry tongue
Relief of prolonged obstruction	
Chronic renal failure	
2. Prolonged diuretic therapy esp. in cirrhosis and ascites	
3. Osmotic diuresis:	
Uncontrolled diabetes	Urine: sugar
mellitus	+++
4. Deficiency of mineralocorticoids:	Pigmentation,
Addison's disease	asthenia
Hypoaldosteronism	

Sodium and Water

Both physiologically and clinically sodium and water metabolism are closely inter-related.

Primary sodium deficits are nearly always accompanied by water deficit, leading to the clinical syndrome of extracellular fluid (ECF) volume depletion. The causes and clinical manifestations of ECF volume depletion are given in **Table 13.1** and those of ECF volume excess are given in **Table 13.2**.

Table 13.2 ECF VOLUME EXCESS

Conditions	Manifestations
Congestive heart failure	Weight gain Dyspnoea Raised JVP Pulmonary basal creps
Nephrotic syndrome	Generalized oedema
Renal failure	Volume overload
Cirrhosis liver	Ascites Lower limb oedema

The normal serum sodium is 140 mEq/L. A lower level of serum sodium (less than 135 mEq/L) is hyponatraemia. It can occur clinically in three sets of conditions:

  A. Depletional.

  B. Associated with oedema.

  C. Not associated with depletion or oedema.

The clinical approach to hyponatraemia is depicted in **Fig. 13.1**.

The causes of hypernatraemia (serum sodium more than 150 mEq/L) are listed in **Table 13.3**.

The syndrome of inappropriate ADH secretion (SIADH) is described along with its causes in **Table 13.4**.

Cholera represents the most striking example of the rapid loss of fluids and electrolytes from the gastrointestinal tract resulting in hypovolaemic shock, metabolic acidosis and, if untreated, death. *Addison's disease* represents the most striking example of loss of sodium from the kidneys in the absence of mineralocorticoids. Addisonian crisis is a life-threatening situation. The treatment of cholera and Addison's disease are therefore given in detail below.

Treatment of Cholera

Successful therapy demands only prompt replacement of gastrointestinal losses of fluids and electrolytes.

A 'diarrhoea treatment solution' recommended by WHO may be prepared by adding 4 g sodium chloride, 6.5 g sodium acetate and 1 g potassium chloride to a litre of sterile, pyrogen-free distilled water.

TABLE 13.3 CAUSES OF HYPERNATRAEMIA

1. *Inability to take in water* (hypothalamic dysfunction)
   Encephalopathy
   Strokes
   Delirium
   Overwhelming infection
   Surgery
   Drugs causing delirium or impaired thirst

2. *Volume contraction* (with inadequate water replacement)
   Diarrhoea
   Osmotic
     diuresis
     mannitol
     glucose
     urea

3. *Sodium overload*
   Exogenous: hypertonic saline
   Endogenous: Conn's syndrome
                 Cushing's syndrome

Alternatively, lactated Ringer's solution may be administered. Either of these solutions should be infused intravenously and rapidly, at the rate of 50-100 ml per minute in adults, until a strong radial pulse has been restored. The same fluid should later on be infused in quantities equal to the gastrointestinal losses (if they can be measured accurately) or at a rate sufficient to maintain a normal pulse volume and normal skin turgor. Enormous volumes of fluid may be required to be replaced, which in extreme cases may exceed twice the weight of the patient. Observation of the jugular venous pulse and auscultation of the lung bases will avoid over hydration. Since adult patients can lose as much as one litre of isotonic fluid per hour during the first 24 hours of the disease, close observation of the urine output is mandatory during this critical period.

Delayed or inadequate restoration of electrolyte and fluid losses results in a very high incidence of acute renal shutdown and death.

In children complications are both more frequent and more severe. The most serious include stupor, oedema and cardiac arrhythmias due to potassium depletion. The diarrhoea treatment solution recommended by WHO is useful to correct acidosis, hypokalaemia and hypoglycaemia without provoking hypernatraemia.

TABLE 13.4 SYNDROME OF INAPPROPRIATE ADH SECRETION (SIADH)

1. Urine osmolality exceeds plasma osmolality.

2. Plasma BUN and creatinine and uric acid are *normal* or *low* (these are high in hyponatraemia due to volume depletion).

Causes:
1. Neoplasms.
2. CNS disorders: meningitis, encephalitis, trauma, tumour, stroke.
3. Pulmonary: wide variety of infections including tuberculosis, asthma, COPD.
4. Drugs: chlorpropamide and tolbutamide;
          cyclophosphamide and vincristine;
          psychoactive drugs: haloperidol.

In patients who are alert (both children and adults) oral rehydration therapy (ORT) is also remarkably effective. The ORT solution is prepared by adding 20 g glucose (or 40 g of cane sugar), 3.5 g sodium chloride, 2.5 g sodium bicarbonate and 1.5 g potassium chloride to one litre of drinking water. This solution can be given to mild cases of cholera throughout the course of illness, and it is also satisfactory in more severe cases once the hypovolaemic shock has been corrected by the initial rapid intravenous fluid therapy.

Although fluid and electrolyte treatment alone leads to rapid recovery in virtually all cholera patients, adjunctive antimicrobial therapy dramatically reduces the duration and volume of diarrhoea and eradicates the vibrio from the stools. Tetracycline (50 mg/kg body weight) daily in 4 divided doses for 2 days is the drug of choice.

Treatment of Adrenal Crisis

I. *Emergency measures*
   1. Establish intravenous access with a large gauge needle.

   2. Draw blood for immediate serum electrolyte and glucose assay, plasma ACTH and cortisol. Do not wait for results.

   3. Infuse 2-3 litres of 0.9 per cent saline (154 mmol/L NaCl) or 50g/L (5 per cent) dextrose in 0.9 per cent saline as quickly as possible.

Monitor for signs of fluid overload by following central or peripheral venous pressure and listening for pulmonary rates. Reduce the infusion rate if indicated.

4. Inject 4 mg dexamethasone sodium phosphate intravenously. 100 mg hydrocortisone can also be given IV immediately and every 6 hours thereafter (but it will interfere with measurement of plasma cortisol during the short ACTH stimulation test).

5. Use supportive measures as needed.

II. *Subacute measures after stabilization of the patient*
1. Continue IV 0.9 per cent saline at a lower rate for the next 24-48 hours.
2. Search for and treat possible infections precipitating the crisis.
3. Perform a short ACTH stimulation test to confirm the diagnosis of adrenal crisis if the patient is not known to have had adrenal insufficiency previously.
4. Determine the type of adrenal insufficiency and its cause if not already known.
5. Taper glucocorticoid to maintain dosage over 1-3 days if precipitating or complicating illness permits.
6. Begin mineralocorticoid replacement with fludrocortisone 0.1 mg by mouth daily (when saline infusion is stopped).

III. *Treatment of chronic primary adrenal insufficiency*

Maintenance therapy

Glucocorticoid replacement
Dexamethasone 0.5 (0.25-0.75) or prednisolone 5 mg orally (2.5-7.5) at bedtime.

Supplement with hydrocortisone 5-10 mg orally in midafternoon if indicated.

Alternative therapy with hydrocortisone 15-20 mg on awakening and 5-10 mg in early afternoon.

Monitor clinical symptoms and plasma ACTH levels.

Mineralocorticoid replacement
Liberal salt intake.
Fludrocortisone 0.1 mg (0.15-0.2) mg orally.

Monitor BP and pulse rate in lying down and standing position, oedema, serum potassium and plasma ACTH levels.

Educate patient about the disease, how to manage minor illness and major stress and how to inject IM dexamethasone.

Provide the patient with a medical alert bracelet and emergency information card.

IV. *Treatment of minor illness or stress*
Increase glucocorticoid dose by 2-3 times for the few days of illness. Do not change mineralocorticoid dose.

General anaesthesia or IV sedation should not be used in office practice.

V. *Steroid coverage for illness or surgery in hospital*
For moderate illness give hydrocortisone 50 mg orally twice daily;

For severe illness give hydrocortisone 100 mg IV every 8 hours; taper dose to maintenance level by decreasing by half everyday. Adjust dose according to course of illness.

For minor procedures under local anaesthesia no extra supplement is needed.

For moderately stressful procedures e.g. barium enema, endoscopy or arteriography, give single 100 mg IV dose of hydrocortisone just before the procedure.

For minor surgery, give hydrocortisone 100 mg IV just before induction of anaesthesia and continue every 8 hours for the first 24 hours; taper dose rapidly, decreasing by half per day to maintenance level.

Potassium

Hypokalaemia (Serum K < 3.5 mEq/L)
Clinically significant depletion can occur without alteration in plasma potassium concentration (since potassium is mainly an intracellular ion and there is as yet no method available to measure it). Potassium lack may be suggested by an associated elevation of the plasma bicarbonate level.

Clinical features of potassium depletion are: apathy, muscular weakness, mental confusion and abdominal distension (due to paralytic ileus). It is worth emphasizing that these features are identical with those seen in hyperkalaemia, but the clinical setting in which hypo- and hyperkalaemia occur are entirely different (**Fig. 13.2**); hence the importance of history and ECG.

ECG changes in hypokalaemia:
ST depression and small T wave.

ECG changes in hyperkalaemia:
Tall T waves; A-V conduction defects; irregular rhythm; ventricular fibrillation and asystole.

The clinical setting in which hypokalaemia occurs can be anticipated and the condition prevented by giving potassium supplement orally 3-4 g/day.

The danger of hypokalaemia is death from cardiac arrest or respiratory muscle paralysis. A hypokalaemic patient is more susceptible to digitalis intoxication.

Treatment of hypokalaemia
Oral: potassium chloride 2-3 g/day In divided doses.
IV: 1.5 g KCl in sterile ampoule added to 500 ml of normal saline or 5 per cent glucose solution. The solution then contains 40 mmol/L of potassium. This should be given at a *slow rate* over 2 hours (not more than 20 mmol per hour). This is especially important in oliguric or anuric patients to avoid the danger of hyperkalaemia.

Hyperkalaemia (Serum K > 5.5 mEq/L)
This occurs most often in the setting of severe oliguria or anuria. Common causes are circulatory failure from blood loss or injury (especially crush injury causing muscle damage), and in severe cases of adrenal insufficiency. It may occur in diabetic ketosis prior to adequate treatment with insulin and intravenous solutions. Potassium-conserving diuretics (e.g. spironolactone) especially when given with potassium supplement can lead to hyperkalaemia in patients with poor renal function.

Cardiac disturbances are often the first and only manifestation of hyperkalaemia. The pulse becomes irregular and heart block of varying degrees occurs. The danger of cardiac arrest is imminent with concentrations of plasma potassium above 7.5 mmol/L.

Treatment of established case of hyperkalaemia

1. Migration of potassium into the cells is encouraged by glucose 50 ml of 50 per cent solution plus 5-10 units of crystalline insulin. This can be repeated if increased K+ returns. Alternatively, 20 per cent glucose solution containing 6-12 units of soluble insulin is infused slowly over 6-12 hours.

2. Provided there is no evidence of circulatory overload, isotonic sodium bicarbonate solution should be infused slowly until the plasma bicarbonate is in the upper reference range.

3. When severe ECG changes are present, 10 ml of 10 per cent calcium gluconate should be given intravenously to reduce the cardiotoxic effects of the potassium ions. The ECG is monitored throughout the procedure.

4. Any deficit of sodium or water should be replaced in order to restore normal circulation. Metabolic and respiratory acidosis should be corrected.

Prevention of hyperkalaemia can be achieved by:

1. Dietary restriction of foods rich in potassium (bananas, fruit juice, coconut water).

2. Administration of sodium- or calcium-loaded resins which, in the intestine, absorb potassium from the blood and intestinal secretions and contents.

3. If the above measures fail, or if the rise of potassium is rapid, removal of potassium by peritoneal or haemodialysis is indicated.

Calcium

Precise control of the extracellular calcium level is essential for many important biological functions such as neuromuscular excitation and transmission of nerve impulses.

In normal serum, 45 per cent of calcium is protein-bound (mainly to albumin), 5 per cent is complexed to ions, and 50 per cent is a solution in an ionized state (Ca^{2+}). The concentration of (Ca^{2+}) is controlled by the action of parathyroid hormone (PTH) and Vit. D.

PTH is secreted in response to a decrease in the extracellular Ca^{2+} concentration, and acts rapidly to restore Ca^{2+} level to normal by (a) increasing bone resorption by osteoclastic activity; (b) promoting renal tubular reabsorption of filtered calcium, and (c) stimulating intestinal absorption of minerals indirectly through increased production of 1-25 dihydroxy vitamin D3 (1, 25 $(OH)_2$ D). PTH also promotes urinary phosphorus excretion through decreased availability of this ion to form calcium complexes.

1, 25 $(OH)_2$ D3 enhances intestinal absorption of calcium, magnesium and phosphorus from the diet; it also facilitates, bone resorption, in concert with PTH.

The normal range of serum calcium is 9-11 mg per cent.

Hypocalcaemia (Serum Ca < 8.4 mg/dl)

When a clinician sees a laboratory report of a low serum calcium, it represents a reduction in the protein-bound calcium and *not* a change in the ionized calcium (Ca^{2+}). Hence he should at once check the serum albumin. Total serum calcium decreases approximately 0.8 mg/dl for each 1 g/dl decrease in albumin. This commonly occurs in malnutrition, cirrhosis and nephrotic syndrome and does not need any treatment with calcium. Clinically significant hypocalcaemia results from a decrease in Ca^{2+} and may be caused by hypoparathyroidism, vitamin D deficiency or malabsorption, magnesium deficiency, acute pancreatitis, and renal failure and distal renal tubular acidosis.

Drugs e.g. gentamicin, cisplatin, phenobarbitol, diphenylhydantoin, loop diuretics and phosphate salts may also cause significant hypocalcaemia through a variety of mechanisms.

Alkalosis can depress Ca^{2+} levels. Therefore hyperventilation may produce or exacerbate symptoms of hypocalcaemia.

Clinical manifestations

These vary greatly among patients, and depend on severity, duration and rate of development. Additional hypokalaemia and hypomagnesaemia can potentiate the cardiac and neurologic abnormality of hypocalcaemia.

Tetany is a manifestation of neuromuscular irritability. Latent tetany can be detected by tapping on the jaw over the facial nerve, resulting in contraction of the facial muscle (Chvostek's sign), or by occluding the arterial blood supply to the arm with a blood pressure cuff for 3 minutes, producing carpopedal spasm (Trousseau's sign).

Other neurological signs include circumoral paraesthesia, muscle cramps, memory impairment, confusion, delusions, hallucinations, paranoia and seizures.

ECG manifestations of hypocalcaemia include prolongation of the QT interval and non-specific T wave changes (identical changes are also produced by hypomagnesaemia).

I.   *Acute management*
     Symptomatic hypocalcaemia is a medical emergency. Prompt administration of IV calcium gluconate, 20 ml of a 10 per cent solution (available as 90 mg elemental calcium per 10 ml ampoule) intravenously over 10-15 minutes reverses tetany. This should be followed by a slow IV infusion of calcium gluconate 60-80 ml of a 10 per cent solution (540-720 mg of elemental calcium) in 1 litre of 5 per cent D/W. An infusion rate of 0.5-2 mg/kg/hour is usually adequate to relieve symptoms.

Calcium should not be mixed with bicarbonate because precipitation of calcium carbonate may occur.

ECG monitoring of calcium infusion is prudent in patients receiving digitalis as calcium potentiates the effects of this drug.

II. *Chronic management*
     Patients of hypoparathyroidism, pseudo-hypoparathyroidism (end-organ insensitivity to PTH), and chronic vitamin D deficiency states need life-long supplementation of dietary calcium and Vit. D to maintain total serum calcium between 8.5 and 9 mg/dl to allow a margin of safety for the calcium to fluctuate upward to levels that are not dangerous. Measurement of 24-hour urinary calcium is essential in monitoring therapy.

Normal range of urine Ca is 50-150 mg/day.

Hypercalciuria (4 mg/kg/day or 250 mg calcium/ g creatinine) may occur, with a consequent risk of nephrolithiasis and nephrocalcinosis.

Patients with hypercalciuria may benefit from thiazide diuretics and dietary salt restriction, to facilitate increased renal reabsorption of calcium.
Oral calcium supplement: 1g elemental Ca/day, in the form of 1 g $CaCO_3$, tid.
Vit. D calcitriol 0.25 μg PO qid.
DHT (dihydrotachysterol) 0.2-0.4 mg PO qid.

Hypercalcaemia (Serum Ca > 10.4 mg/dl)

Only elevation of *ionized* Calcium (Ca^{2+}) is clinically significant and it is good to measure this with a calcium electrode to evaluate a hypercalcaemic patient.

Hypercalcaemia may arise from several different pathophysiological mechanisms, including
(1) Increased calcium mobilization from bone (e.g. malignant metastases, primary hyperpara-thyroidism, hyperthyroidism, immobilization, Vit. D intoxication).
(2) Increased calcium absorption from the GI tract (e.g. sarcoidosis and other granulomatous disease, Vit. D intoxication, milk-alkali syndrome).
(3) Decreased urinary calcium excretion (e.g. thiazide diuretics, familial hypocalciuric hypercalcaemia).

Clinical manifestations
These are variable and depend upon the level and the rate of rise. The most common symptoms are: nausea, vomiting, polyuria, polydipsia, fatigue, lack of concentration, somnolence, obtundation and coma.

The cornerstone of treatment of hypercalcaemia is treatment of the underlying cause.

Hypercalcaemia of malignancy is described in Chapter 53 on Medical Oncology, and the treatment is also described in the same chapter.

Magnesium

Magnesium is an essential co-factor for a variety of enzymes and has important effects on neuromuscular function. Of the body store of magnesium, 60 per cent is in bone, 20 per cent in muscle and the remainder in other tissues. In contrast to calcium, only 20 per cent of Mg is protein-bound, hence it is less affected by changes in serum protein concentration and pH.

Disorders of magnesium metabolism are occasionally responsible for otherwise puzzling clinical features. These are susceptible to therapeutic control, hence the need to know them.

Magnesium Deficiency

The most frequent cause of magnesium deficiency is prolonged diarrhoea or vomiting, which has been treated with parenteral fluids without magnesium supplement. It also occurs in protein energy malnutrition and malabsorption syndrome, and chronic alcoholism. Excessive urinary losses can occur due to diuretics.

Clinical features are predominantly neuromuscular with anorexia, vomiting, tremors, choreiform movements and aimless plucking of the bedclothes. Mental depression, confusion, vertigo, ataxia, agitation, epileptiform convulsions and hallucinations also occur. ECG changes include prolongation of QT and non-specific T wave changes. Severe hypomagnesaemia may precipitate ventricular arrhythmia.

The diagnosis is confirmed by finding the concentration of magnesium in the plasma to be less than 0.75 mmol/L (Normal range 1.5-2.1 mmol/L or 1.8-2.2 mg/dl).

Acute management

For patients requiring immediate control of seizures or tetany, 1-2 g of $MgSO_4$ (2-4 ml of a 50 per cent solution containing 8-16 mmol of Mg) may be given IV over 15 minutes. Further parenteral therapy should be given as 1 g $MgSO4$ (2 ml) IM inj. every 4-6 hours, depending on the serum Mg level and the clinical status. Serum magnesium level should be monitored during replacement therapy, when repeated doses are to be given parenterally. The deep tendon reflexes should be tested before each dose. If they are absent, magnesium should be withheld.

Treatment consists of parenteral magnesium chloride 30-50 mmol added to 1 litre of 5 per cent glucose or other isotonic solutions, given over a period of 12-24 hours. The infusion should be repeated daily until the plasma concentration remains within the normal range.

Magnesium excess

This occurs in acute and chronic renal failure due to impaired urinary excretion of magnesium. Mild hypermagnesaemia is usually asymptomatic but with serum magnesium levels of 5-6 mg/dl there may be a decrease in deep tendon reflexes and some degree of mental confusion. With serum magnesium levels of 7-9 mg/dl, the respiratory rate slows, PR, QT and QRS duration are prolonged, and hypotension occurs. Further increase can result in profound hypotension, respiratory failure, complete heart block and asystole.

Treatment
Volume expansion with saline, and diuresis with frusemide in a manner similar to that for hypercalcaemia. However, care is required since this regimen will also increase the excretion of calcium in the urine, potentiating the toxic effect of hypermagnesaemia. Hence calcium gluconate (1-3 ampoules per litre of saline) should be added to the infusate.

In patients with poor renal function, dialysis using magnesium-free dialysate should be started.

Phosphorus

In the adult human body there are 700-800 g of phosphate. Phosphorus is the main component of bone along with calcium. About 85 per cent of the total body phosphorus is in bone in the form of hydroxyapatite. Of the non-osseus 15 per cent, 99 per cent is intracellular in organic compounds or is a component of phospholipids in cell membranes. It is the body's major intracellular ion.

Phosphorus influences the rate of ammoniagenesis, glycolysis, and gluconeogenesis, and can affect the oxygen dissociation of haemoglobin through the regulation of 2.3 diphosphoglycerate.

In serum 85 per cent of the phosphorus exists as HPO_4^{2-} or H_2PO_4 (orthophosphate ions) whereas only 15 per cent is protein-bound. The ratio of the two species of orthophosphate ions changes with pH. Therefore the serum concentration of inorganic phosphate (Pi) is most conveniently expressed as elemental phosphorus in mg/dl or mmol/dl. The normal range is 2.5 to 4.5 mg/dl (0.8-1.45 mmol/L.)

Serum phosphate level is influenced by pH, PTH and Vit. D levels, renal function and dietary phosphorus intake, and does not always reflect total body stores. Phosphorus is ubiquitous in food, and improved nutrition generally ensures adequate phosphate stores.

Hypophosphataemia

Hypophosphataemia may occur due to four mechanisms:

(1) *Increased excretion of phosphorus in the urine* e.g. hyperparathyroidism, renal tubular defects, diuretic phase of acute tubular necrosis, postobstructive diuresis, after renal transplants, extracellular fluid volume expansion.

(2) *Decreased intestinal absorption of phosphorus* e.g. malabsorption, malnutrition/starvation, administration of phosphate-binding minerals.

(3) *Abnormality of Vit. D metabolism* e.g. Vit. D deficient rickets, familial hypophosphataemic rickets, Vit. D dependent rickets, tumour-associated hypophosphataemia.

(4) *Shifts in the intracellular space* e.g. treatment of diabetic ketoacidosis, severe respiratory alkalosis, chronic alcoholism, alcohol withdrawal, recovery phase of starvation, initiation of hyperalimentation.

Clinical effects
Severe hypophosphataemia (serum Pi < 1 mg/dl) may cause muscular weakness, rhabdomyolysis, neurologic abnormalities ranging from paraesthesias to coma, haemolysis, platelet dysfunction and myocardial depression.

Treatment of hypophosphataemia depends upon the severity and chronicity of the process and on its associated symptomatology.

Mild hypophosphataemia (serum Pi 1-2.5 mg/dl) Improved nutrition is generally a equate.

Severe hypophosphataemia (serum Pi 1 mg/dl) Supplement of Neutra-phos 2 capsules/day.

Hyperphosphataemia

Hyperphosphataemia (serum P > 5 mg/dl) is seen in adults in severe renal insufficiency, hypoparathyroidism, pseudohypoparathyroidism, acromegaly and treatment with diphosphonates e.g. for Paget's disease. Ectopic calcification and metabolic bone disease are the most important consequences.

The clinical manifestations of hyperphosphataemia are related to secondary changes in calcium metabolism.

Treatment

1. Dietary restriction of phosphorus intake (0.7-1 g/day).

2. Phosphate binders: aluminium hydroxide and aluminium carbonate gel (5-10 ml lid) (1-2 tab tid) before meals to effectively bind ingested phosphate.

   Aluminium compounds should not be given in patients of renal insufficiency for fear of development of aluminium toxicity.

   Calcium carbonate can be given in those patients, but the Ca x P product should be kept below 70 to minimize the risk of soft tissue calcification.

14   H⁺ Ion Concentration Disturbances

Life is possible only if blood is kept within a narrow range of alkalinity. In health, physiological hydrogen ion concentration of 36-44 nmol/L corresponding to a pH between 7.37 and 7.45 is maintained by two widely different mechanisms which are closely integrated. Some understanding of these mechanisms is necessary to appreciate the clinical implications of acidosis and alkalosis.

The blood is alkaline because it contains bicarbonates, phosphates and proteins which are quite strong bases. The blood also contains carbonic acid as its main acid component.

The $[H^+]$ of the blood depends upon the ratio of carbonic acid and bicarbonate. The bicarbonate buffer acts in the following way:

$$H^+ + HCO_3^- \Rightarrow H_2CO_3 \Rightarrow CO_2 + H_2O$$

The CO_2 is ultimately eliminated by the lungs. The concentration of carbonic acid in the plasma is determined by the partial pressure of carbon dioxide (PCO_2) in the alveoli. On the other hand, the concentration of bicarbonate is regulated by renal tubules, which are responsible for elimination of fixed acids.

A great many metabolic processes result in the production of acids which must re eliminated to maintain the pH in the normal mild, alkaline range. The effective blood buffer mechanism minimizes the increase in H⁺ concentration. In health, on a normal diet, 40-80 mmol of non-volatile acid are excreted in the urine. The renal tubules form carbonic acid and much of the H⁺ is excreted in the form of ammonium ions along with the acid anion. The bicarbonate ion generated in this process in the renal tubules is returned to the blood and reconstitutes the depleted buffer.

Abnormalities in the reaction of body fluids are reflected in changes in the concentration of carbonic acid (i.e. $PaCO_2$) and bicarbonate (which ranges between 22 and 25 mmol/L at a standard value of $PaCO_2$ of 5.3 KPa or 35-45 mm Hg.

The two mechanisms (respiratory and renal) of elimination of acid are closely integrated. Disturbance in one mechanism leads to compensatory adjustments in the other, as shown by **Table 14.1**.

Most acid-base disturbances can be diagnosed with a careful history, arterial blood gases (ABG) analysis and serum electrolytes. Urinary pH and electrolytes may also be helpful. Unfortunately facilities for ABG are denied to most clinicians in developing countries hence they have to rely on the clinical setting in which these disturbances occur and act accordingly. Mixed acid-base disturbances are common in the acutely ill patient and can often be predicted from the clinical situation. Careful evaluation of the expected compensatory responses of the pH, PCO_2 and HCO_3 is necessary **(Table 14.1)**. Measurements of electrolytes and calculation of the anion gap must also be performed. The treatment of mixed acid-base disorders must be directed at the underlying abnormalities.

TABLE 14.1 COMPENSATORY MECHANISMS IN ACID-BASE DISTURBANCES

	Primary change	pH	Compensatory response
Metabolic acidosis	↓ HCO_3^-	↓	↓ PCO_2
Metabolic alkalosis	↑ HCO_3^-	↑	↑ PCO_2
Respiratory acidosis	↑ PCO_2	↓	↑ HCO
Respiratory alkalosis	↓ PCO_2	↑	↓ HCO_3^-

TABLE 14.2 CAUSES OF METABOLIC ACIDOSIS

Increased lactic acid production	Shock and circulatory failure Cardiac arrest Severe myocardial infarction Severe liver failure Acute alcoholic intoxication Biguanides (oral antidiabetics in the elderly)
Other acids produced in excess	Diabetic ketosis: β-hydroxy butyric acetoacetic acid Salicylate intoxication: salicylic acid Methyl alcohol poisoning: formic acid
Decreased bicarbonate production	Renal tubular acidosis Acute and chronic renal failure
Loss of bicarbonate from the body	Acute & chronic diarrhoea Fistulae Continuous aspiration of intestinal contents

Gradations of metabolic acidosis
Normal range of plasma bicarbonate: 22-26 mmol/L
Moderate acidosis: bicarbonate 15 mmol/L
Severe acidosis: bicarbonate below 10 mmol/L

Metabolic Acidosis

This may result from either (a) accumulation of excess acid; or (b) loss of bicarbonate from the body (**Table 14.2**).

Causes of metabolic acidosis can be categorized using the anion gap

Anion gap (AG) = $[Na^+] - [Cl^-] + [HCO_3^-]$ = 12 + 4

An increased AG is due to increases in: anionic proteins, phosphates, sulphates, organic ions, drug intoxications.

Normal AG indicates loss of bicarbonate, decreased renal ammonia production or addition of hydrochloric acid.

The clinician should anticipate the occurrence of metabolic acidosis in any conditions that would result in hypoxia of the tissues and the resultant accumulation of organic acids, particularly lactic acid. Shock and circulatory failure, severe myocardial infarction and cardiac arrest are important clinical situations in which metabolic acidosis is seen.

Acute alcohol intoxication and severe liver failure also lead to lactic acidosis. Biguanides (e.g.

phenformin) used in the treatment of diabetes mellitus may cause lactic acidosis, especially in the elderly.

In uncontrolled diabetes, β-hydroxybutyric acid and acetoacetic acid are produced in abnormally large amounts and at a rate which is greater than the capacity of the body to oxidize them.

Salicylate intoxication produces metabolic acidosis as well as respiratory alkalosis. Intoxication with methyl alcohol (methanol consumed as illicit liquor) results in the oxidation product formic acid, and that with ethyleneglycol results in the production of oxalic acid.

Depletion of body bicarbonate occurs from direct loss of sodium bicarbonate in the stools in chronic or severe acute diarrhoea, or from the loss of intestinal contents from fistulae or by intestinal aspiration.

In patients with acute or chronic renal failure and renal tubular acidosis, the ability of the kidneys to conserve and generate bicarbonate ions and to produce and secrete hydrogen and ammonium ions is impaired.

The clinical picture in the individual case is largely determined by the underlying condition, and by the presence of other concomitant disturbances of water and salt balance. The diagnosis is facilitated by an awareness of those conditions in which it is likely to arise. The diagnosis is confirmed by the determination of blood pH (concentration of H^+ ions) and of bicarbonate in the blood. The normal range of plasma bicarbonate is 22-26 mmol/L.

In acidosis, a bicarbonate level of 15 mmol/L indicates a moderate degree, and a level below 10 mmol/L indicates a severe degree of acidosis.
BUN and creatinine along with Na and K should also be routinely estimated in all cases.

Treatment of metabolic acidosis
1. IV infusion of 0.9 per cent NaCl to correct sodium and water depletion which is almost invariably present. Provided the kidneys are not primarily diseased, and provided the sodium and water depletion is not so severe as to impair renal function seriously (urine output more than 30 ml per hour), this measure alone is enough to correct metabolic acidosis of moderate severity.

2. Acidosis with pH below 7.2 should always be treated with parenteral bicarbonate, since acidosis of this degree can result in severe myocardial depression, hypotension and resistance to vasopressor administration. An approximation of the amount of bicarborate needed to replete serum concentration to normal can be found by the following formula:

HCO_3 deficit = (kg body wt) (0.4) x
(desired HCO_3^- - measured HCO_3^-).

Usually 2-3 ampoules of 7.5% $NaHCO_3$ (44.6 mEq per ampoule) are added to 1000 ml of 5% D/W. One-half of the calculated deficit may be replaced in 3-4 hours if severe heart failure is not present. No further bicarbonate therapy should be given when the pH reaches 7.2. Over-alkalinization can cause tetany, seizures, cardiac arrhythmias and increased lactate production.

Correction of acidosis without correction of potassium deficit may lead to life-threatening hypokalaemia (due to intracellular shift of potassium). Potassium supplementation should be undertaken when the acidosis is partially corrected and the serum potassium concentration is within the normal range and falling. Serum calcium should be monitored and hypocalcaemia treated. Calcium salts should not be given in the same infusion as bicarbonate (to avoid precipitation).

3. In the presence of renal disease, severe acidosis and severe sodium depletion giving rise to uraemia, isotonic sodium bicarbonate should be given by IV infusion along with IV sodium chloride, in a ratio of 1 to 2. A moderately severe case of diabetic ketoacidosis may require as much as 4-6 litres of fluids in the first 24 hours, of which 1-2 litres should be the isotonic sodium bicarbonate solution.

When the plasma bicarbonate level returns to normal, infusion of normal saline alone may be continued if there is still evidence of predominant sodium depletion.

In severe shock or cardiac arrest
Acidosis develops without sodium depletion. Hence 50-100 ml of 7.5 per cent solution of sodium bicarbonate is given IV as a bolus.

In lactic acidosis due to biguanide treatment
The patient is not profoundly dehydrated as in diabetic ketosis nor does the breath smell of acetone. Ketonuria is no more than mild yet the plasma bicarbonate and pH are markedly reduced.

Diagnosis can be confirmed by > 5 mmol/L of lactic acid in blood. Large amounts of IV bicarbonate are needed (as much as 2500 mmol, along with insulin drip till the glucose falls to about 10 mmol/L (180 mg/dl).

Dialysis may be required in very severe cases (pH less than 7) if large quantities of sodium bicarbonate result in volume overload. Despite such measures the mortality in this condition is greater than 50 per cent.

For methyl alcohol poisoning
After gastric lavage, water with sodium bicarbonate (20 g/L) should be left in the stomach.

As ethyl alcohol inhibits the metabolism of methyl alcohol, 1.5 ml/kg of 50 per cent ethyl alcohol diluted to a 5 per cent solution is given orally at 2 hourly intervals, or the same quantity may be given IV for 4-5 days, along with large doses of IV sodium bicarbonate infusion.

Dialysis, if available, is extremely useful.

For salicylate poisoning
Large doses of IV sodium bicarbonate are given to produce forced alkaline diuresis which enhances salicylate excretion by the kidney. In the presence of cardiac and renal involvement, peritoneal or haemodialysis are indicated.

Metabolic Alkalosis

The causes of metabolic alkalosis are given in **Table 14.3**.

Alkalosis is commonly unattended by specific clinical manifestations. However, acute alkalosis causes tetany, which may occur spontaneously or may be induced by the Trousseau manoeuvre.

This is due to a reduction in the concentration of plasma ionized calcium.

Severe alkalosis of some duration is often associated with significant depression of renal function with uraemia; protein and casts are found in the urine. Hence the vomiting due to pyloric stenosis may be erroneously misdiagnosed as due to primary renal disease.

The diagnosis of alkalosis is established by estimation of plasma bicarbonate. In moderately severe alkalosis it is elevated to 35 mmol/L. The pH of the blood is also elevated.

Treatment of Metabolic Alkalosis
1. If the renal function is normal, IV infusion of 2-4 litres of normal saline in 24 hours is enough to correct the alkalosis, if the plasma bicarbonate is not above 35 mmol/L. The chloride is retained by the body and the excess bicarbonate is excreted in the urine.

TABLE 14.3 CAUSES OF METABOLIC ALKALOSIS

A. *Chlorie depletion* (urine chloride 10 mEq/L)
   GI loss of hydrochloric acid:
      vomiting
      nasogastric suction
      villous adenoma
      congenital chloridorrhoea
   Renal loss of chloride:
      loop diuretics
      thiazide diuretics
      (in conjunction with salt restriction)

B. *Mineralocorticoid excess* (urine chloride > 10 mEq/L
   Cushing's syndrome

C. *Severe potassium depletion*
   Laxative abuse (urine K^+ < 30 mEq/L)
   Bartter's syndrome
   Bulimia with vomiting   } (urine K^+ > 30 mEq/L)
   Recent diureticabuse
   Magnesium depletion

2. In severe cases, one litre of a solution containing 63 mmol/L of NaCl, 17 mmol/L of KCl and 70 mmol/L of NH_4Cl is given intravenously over 4-6 hours, and repeated as indicated by blood bicarbonate level. The use of this solution – 'gastric solution' is of particular benefit in those patients who are being prepared for operation to relieve gastric outlet obstruction and in whom continuous gastric aspiration is needed to prevent vomiting and reduce the size of a dilated stomach.

Respiratory Acidosis

Respiratory acidosis arises when the effective alveolar ventilation does not keep pace with the rate of production of carbon dioxide. This results in hypercapnia as indicated by rise in the pressure of CO_2 in the arterial blood ($PaCO_2$) above the upper limit of the normal (45 mm Hg at rest). The carbonic acid concentration of the blood increases and the pH falls. Causes are given in **Table 14.4**.

The kidneys try to compensate for this acidosis by excreting an acid urine and by retaining more bicarbonate over a period of hours or days. Looking at the plasma bicarbonate level alone may give the impression of 'metabolic alkalosis', but the pH of the blood is *low*, indicating that it really is respiratory acidosis. The clinical setting of metabolic alkalosis as described earlier, is quite different from that of respiratory acidosis, and should prevent the misinterpretation of a high blood bicarbonate.

Clinical manifestations include agitation, flapping tremors (asterixis), headache, somnolence, papilloedema, tachycardia, cardiac arrhythmias and heart failure.

The diagnosis is made by an elevated PCO_2 and decreased pH. If the pH change is greater than that expected from a change in PCO_2, a mixed acid-base disorder is present.

TABLE 14.4 CAUSES OF RESPIRATORY ACIDOSIS

Hypoventilation with CO_2 retention:

1. CNS depression:	brain injury infection drugs
2. Neuromuscular disorder	Guillain Barré syndrome myopathy
3. Pulmonary disease	COPD asthma kyphoscoliosis pneumothorax

The treatment of respiratory acidosis is to improve alveolar ventilation (See Chapter 17 on Respiratory Failure).

Respiratory alkalosis

This occurs when there is excessive loss of carbon dioxide by over-ventilation of the lungs. This happens most commonly in hysterical over-breathing or in over-ventilation during the course of assisted ventilation. Clinical manifestations include lightheadedness, paraesthesias, tetany, syncope, seizures and cardiac arrhythmias. The diagnosis is made by an increased pH and decreased PCO_2. In chronic cases the kidneys try to compensate by excreting more bicarbonate in the urine, which mitigates the rise in the pH. The low blood level of bicarbonate alone may give the impression of 'metabolic acidosis', but the pH is clearly indicative of alkalosis. Again the clinical setting is quite different and should prevent the erroneous interpretation of the low bicarbonate level. Causes are given in **Table 14.5**.

TABLE **14.5 CAUSES OF RESPIRATORY ALKALOSIS**

Increased rate of pulmonary CO_2 excretion	
CNS causes:	anxiety
	brainstem tumours
	infection: encephalitis, meningitis
Drug toxicity:	salicylates
	theophylline
	catecholamines
	progestational drugs
Lung diseases with tachypnoea:	pneumonia
	pulmonary emboli
	pulmonary oedema
	restrictive lung disease
	early destructive lung disease
High altitude	
Hyperthyroidism	
Sepsis	
Liver failure	
Mechanical ventilators	

Treatment of respiratory alkalosis

Hysterical over-breathing: A simple procedure is to make the patient breathe his own expired air (which contains 20 per cent CO_2) from a suitable paper bag. Alternatively, inhalation of 5 per cent carbon dioxide in oxygen may be given, with the use of a CO_2 breathing apparatus.

The hysterical patient should be guided for appropriate psychotherapy.

For other causes of respiratory alkalosis, treatment is directed at the underlying disorder. No treatment is usually required unless the pH is greater than 7.5.

When continued hyperventilation occurs (as in CNS disease with compensatory metabolic acidosis with a fall in serum bicarbonate) the use of a CO_2 breathing apparatus may be warranted.

15   Haemoptysis

Haemoptysis means the spitting of blood or coughing blood. Coughing blood is a terrifying experience for the patient and his family members, and produces a great deal of anxiety and apprehension.

When a patient comes with a history of having 'brought up blood', it is necessary to determine whether the blood has come from the lungs, or from the stomach (haematemesis) or from the nose, throat, or gums. Although in most cases the bleeding is genuine, the possibility of malingering should be borne in mind.

Blood coming from the lungs is bright red (vs coffee ground or dark red from the stomach), often with froth (not present in haematemesis), alkaline in reaction (vs acid in haematemesis). It is not infreqently preceded and accompanied by a tickling cough (vs vomiting associated with haematemesis). The patterns of haemoptysis are given in **Table 15.1**.

Haemoptysis may occur as the initial or only manifestation of underlying lung disease or as part of a more general symptom complex. History is of enormous value in determining the probable cause in a given patient from among the several causes of haemoptysis listed in **Tables 15.2** and **15.3**.

Assessment of Severity

Haemoptysis may range from a small amount of blood-stained sputum to a massive amount of bleeding that causes asphyxiation or exsanguination.

Mild haemoptysis is the term used to describe 15-30 ml of blood loss over 24 hours.

Massive haemoptysis is loss of more than 600 ml/24 hours.

Gross haemoptysis refers to a quantity more than mild but less than massive.

Considering that the anatomic dead space in the airway is 100-200 ml in most individuals, an amount of more than 300 ml poses the risk of aspiration into the lungs. The threat to life is either by asphyxiation or exsanguination.

The commonest causes of massive haemoptysis are bronchiectasis, tuberculosis, mycetoma, lung abscess and bronchogenic carcinoma.

The four major concerns in evaluating haemoptysis are:

1. Rule out bronchogenic carcinoma, the most sinister of all causes.

TABLE 15.1 PATTERNS OF HAEMOPTYSIS

Frank blood	Trauma-lung contusion Pulmonary tuberculosis Pulmonary infarction
Blood-streaked sputum	Acute bronchitis, pneumonia Tuberculosis Tropical eosinophilia Bronchogenic carcinoma Bronchial adenoma
Blood with purulent sputum	Lung abscess Bronchiectasis
Anchovy sauce sputum	Ruptured amoebic liver abscess in the lung
Haemoptysis as part of generalized bleeding	Purpura, leukaemia Hereditary haemorrhagic telangiectasia
Recurrent haemoptysis	Bronchial adenoma Bronchogenic carcinoma Bronchiectasis Hereditary haemorrhagic telangiectasia

2. Determine if the underlying cause is treatable, such as tuberculosis

3. Localize the site of bleeding in case further therapeutic intervention is needed.

4. Decide which treatment to implement if bleeding persists, recurs or is massive, and when to treat.

Associated Features

Recent history of blunt trauma: lung contusion.

Acute onset of pleuritic pain, tachypnoea with haemoptysis: pulmonary infarct; pulmonary vasculitis.

History of shortness of breath in a young patient with haemoptysis: mitral stenosis.

Recurrent haemoptysis with plenty of sputum: bronchiectasis.

Anorexia, weight loss in a male smoker over age 40 years: bronchogenic carcinoma.

Anorexia, fever and weight loss in a young person with haemoptysis: pulmonary tuberculosis, fungal infections.

Recurrent haemoptysis in an otherwise young woman: bronchial adenoma.

Accompanying haematuria: Goodpasture's syndrome; PAN; Wegener's granulomatosis.

Physical Examination

One should look carefully for evidence of pleural rub, signs of consolidation or cavitation, crepitations or unilateral wheeze suggestive of partial bronchial obstruction (due to an adenoma or carcinoma). Clubbing of fingers suggests bronchiectasis, lung abscess or bronchogenic carcinoma.

One should carefully auscultate the heart for evidence of accentuated M1, mid-diastolic murmur, and split P2 (evidence of mitral stenosis), and also for loud P2 and systolic murmur in the tricuspid area (pulmonary hypertension). One should also look carefully for evidence of bleeding elsewhere to exclude a bleeding disorder. Examination of the lips, nose and tongue for telangiectasia should be part of routine inspection (to exclude Osler-Weber-Rendu syndrome).

A chest X-ray (PA and lateral) is useful in suggesting many of the possible causes. These are listed in **Table 15.4**.

Problem case: Normal physical findings; normal chest X-ray

It is a challenging task to identify the site of bleeding in a patient with haemoptysis with normal physical findings in the chest or heart or elsewhere, and a normal chest X-ray.

In patients with suspected brochiectasis high resolution CT (HRCT) is now the diagnostic procedure of choice, having replaced bronchography.

The next step should be bronchoscopy.

A rigid bronchoscope permits visualization of the more central airways. It is of particular value if the source of bleeding is in this part of the airways, the degree of haemoptysis is massive, and selective endobronchial intubation is being considered.

A fibreoptic bronchoscope permits visualization of small peripheral airways (as small as a few millimetres in diameter), biopsy and cytologic information to be obtained from these areas. Indeed haemoptysis is one of the most common indications for bronchoscopy.

Idiopathic or cryptogenic haemoptysis has been reported in 2-18 per cent of patients in large series. The typical presentation is a single bout of haemoptysis with minimal or no respiratory symptoms, a normal chest X-ray, normal bronchoscopy and negative bronchial washings for evidence of infection or malignancy. Fortunately the prognosis is usually good.

Therapy of Haemoptysis

A. *Minor haemoptysis:* Therapy for minor bleeding or blood-streaked sputum should be directed to the underlying cause.

B. *Massive haemoptysis* (greater than 600 ml over 48 hours, or quantities sufficient to impair gas exchange): call for urgent surgical consultation.

1. Put the patient to complete bed rest. While awaiting surgical consultation, sedate the patient with codeine 60-120 mg parenterally. This is helpful in allaying anxiety, aids patient cooperation, and suppresses cough. Excessive sedation should be avoided since it may suppress airway protection and mask signs of respiratory decompensation.

TABLE 15.2 DIAGNOSTIC FEATURES OF IMPORTANT CAUSES OF HAEMOPTYSIS

Tuberculosis	Young adult May be presenting symptom Weight loss, cough and fever Sputum for AFB Chest X-ray mandatory
Acute bronchitis	Acute onset with cough
Bronchiectasis	Cough with profuse purulent sputum Clubbing of fingers
Lung abscess	Fever, chest pain, putrid sputum Clubbing of fingers
Pneumonia	Fever with chills, cough, chest pain, signs of consolidation
Lung cancer	Middle-aged or elderly male History of smoking Weight loss Localized wheeze + X-ray chest/CT Bronchoscopy
Bronchial adenoma	Young woman with recurrent haemoptysis Localized wheeze No weight loss or fever Confirmed by bronchoscopy
Pulmonary embolism and infarction	Bed-ridden patient Sudden onset Tachypr.oea, pleural rub Leg vein thrombosis Chest X-ray may be normal VQ lung scan-mismatch/CT Pulmonary angiography
Mitral stenosis	Young patient May be presenting symptom or history of shortness of breath on exertion Accentuation M1, mid-diastolic murmur
Primary pulmonary hypertension	Young woman Gradual onset of dyspnoea Parasternal heaving-RVH Normal VQ scan
Idiopathic pulmonary haemosiderosis	Children and young adults Recurrent haemoptysis Lung biopsy necessary to establish diagnosis
Wegener's granulomatosis	History of nosebleed, sinus infection, fever, weight loss, urine RBCs
Goodpasture's syndrome	Glomerulonephritis with pulmonary haemorrhage Rapidly progressive renal failure
Haemorrhagic diathesis including anticoagulant therapy	Bleeding time, clotting time, PT, PTT, platelet count

TABLE 15.3 CAUSES OF HAEMOPTYSIS ACCORDING TO AGE

Young patient	adenoma
	bronchiectasis
	mitral stenosis
	tuberculosis
	AV malformation
Age over 40	bronchogenic carcinoma
Female during menses	endometriosis
	(catamenial haemoptysis)
Recurrence over years	adenoma
	bronchiectasis

TABLE 15.4 CAUSES OF HAEMOPTYSIS SUGGESTED BY CHEST X-RAY

Chest-X-ray

Abnormal

– *Tuberculosis*
  infiltrations, cavitation (usually upper lobe).
– Fungal infections same as tuberculosis.
– *Bronchiectasis*
  ring shadows, cyst formation, abnormal air bronchograms.
– *Lung abscess*
  air and fluid level.
– *Tumour*
  mass lesion, shift of mediastinum due to atelectasis or pleural effusion.
– *'Blood pneumonitis'*
  due to aspirated blood;
  usually clears in one week;
  repeat chest-X-ray.
– *Mitral stenosis*
  LA enlargement;
  Kerley's lines.

Normal

Possibilities:
– Endobronchial tuberculosis (sputum for AFB).
– Neoplasm:
  adenoma/carcinoma (CT of thorax, bronchoscopy).
– Telangiectasia (bronchoscopy).
– Localized bronchiectasis (bronchogram, high resolution CT lung).
– Pulmonary infarction (radio nuclide lung scanning, ventilation-perfusion mismatch in lung). CT pulmonary arteriography.
– Goodpasture's syndrome (urine for RBCs).
– Idiopathic (No cause found in spite of extensive investigations).

The patient lies with the bleeding side (if known) in a dependent position to reduce chances of aspiration of blood into the contralateral lung.

2. Intubation and suctioning equipment should be available at the bedside since there is always a danger of asphyxiation by flooding of the lung contralateral to the side of bleeding. Asphyxiation is the major cause of mortality in patients with massive haemoptysis. This can be prevented by strategic location of a balloon catheter by direct visualization through a fibreoptic bronchoscope.

3. Prompt surgical resection of the bleeding lesion is the therapy of choice. Contraindications to surgery include inoperable lung cancer, and previous lung function studies which predicted postoperative FEV1 of less than 800 ml.

Undiagnosed haemoptysis
Despite the most extensive investigations, about 10 per cent cases of haemoptysis remain undiagnosed. Such patients should be followed closely for a period of time sufficient to exclude significant underlying disease such as early bronchogenic carcinoma.

Whenever 'poisoning' is mentioned, the general belief (and expectation) is that treatment will be based upon the use of a specific antidote. Actually there are very few effective antidotes (less than 5 per cent of all poisonings). Hence a common pattern of basic life support management is to be applied to all forms of acute poisoning.

As in any other form of clinical medicine, an adequate history is important in the effective management of poisoning, but urgency may dictate that this is deferred pending the institution of emergency resuscitative measures. The history may be less readily available since the patient may be drowsy or comatose and often a certain amount of Sherlock Holmes-type detective work is required. Valuable details may be obtained from relatives, neighbours, workmates or the police, and it is important to question all of them. Suicide notes and information about past or recent mental health are obviously important. The setting in which the patient was found can provide clues e.g. accidental carbon monoxide poisoning.

The physical examination in the first instance should be summarily performed so as not to unduly delay treatment. There are very few clinical signs which are diagnostic for particular poisons (**Table 16.1**). Several toxic syndromes are described in **Table 16.2** and antidotes in **Table 16.3**.

Emergency Treatment

I. *Supportive care:* ABC (Airway, Breathing, Circulation)

    Endotracheal intubation may be required to protect the airway in drowsy or comatose patients.

    Hypotension responds to IV fluids, although vasopressors (dopamine drip) may be needed in refractory cases or in the presence of pulmonary oedema. Cardiac arrhythmias should be monitored and promptly treated.

    If opiate poisoning is suspected naloxone hydrochloride IV 2 mg should be given straight away. Reversal of symptoms is diagnostic of opioid overdose. There is no harm done by giving this injection in non-opioid poisoning.

II. *Prevention of further drug absorption*

    Gastric emptying procedures are useful only if initiated within one hour of the ingestion of poison. Since most adult poisoning cases present several hours after toxic ingestion, gastric lavage has no benefit in them.

    Gastric lavage: In patients with depressed consciousness endotracheal intubation should be done prior to gastric lavage. A large bore orogastric tube (larger than 28 F) should be introduced and 300 ml of normal saline at body temperature should be put in via repeated boluses and sucked out till the return is clear. The orogastric tube also facilitates subsequent administration of activated charcoal.

    Activated charcoal: absorbs most drugs, preventing further absorption from the gastrointestinal tract (exceptions include alkalis, cyanide, ferrous sulphate and mineral acids). It may also promote efflux of the drug from the blood into the bowel lumen by creating a concentration gradient across the bowel wall. The usual dose is 50-100 g diluted in water given rapidly as soon as possible after the toxic ingestion. Pre-hospital administration of charcoal by the GP further enhances drug recovery. Repeated dosing and the use of superactivated charcoal preparations (30 g superactivated charcoal is equivalent to 90 g regular charcoal), also improves efficacy. Cathartics should not be concurrently

TABLE 16.1 CLINICAL CLUES IN POISONING

Pink colour of skin and mucosa	Carbon monoxide
Cyanosis (MetHb)	Nitrates, aniline
Burns around lips and buccal cavity	Corrosive poisons (including paraquat)
Smell of breath Alcohol Methyl alcohol Kerosine Solvents (toluene, xylene, acetone)	 'Tick 20' (organophosphorus)
Needle marks on skin over veins	IV drug abuse
Pin-point pupils and respiratory depression	Opioids, carbamates
Muscle fasciculations	Organophosphorus
Dilated pupils and tachycardia	Anticholinergics (including tricyclic antidepressants)
Jaundice	Paracetamol, phosphorus
Bullous skin rash	Barbiturates
Involuntary movements	Phenothiazines
Delirium	Dhattura, LSD, amphetamine, ecstacy, cocaine
Coma	Narcotics, benzodiazepines, barbiturates phenothiazines, alcohol, insulin and sulfonylureas.

administered since they do not improve the clinical outcome and may decrease the effectiveness of charcoal.

Removal of Absorbed Drug/Poison

1. *Enhancement of renal excretion by forced alkaline diuresis* is useful to treat poisoning with barbital, phenobarbital and salicylates (weak acids). Sodium bicarbonate 50-100 mEq added to 1 litre of half normal saline (0.45 per cent) is given IV at the rate of 250-500 ml per hour. This is usually effective in alkalinizing the urine (pH 7.5-8.5). Additional normal saline and diuretics (e.g. IV frusemide 40-80 mg) may be administered to maintain a urinary output of 3-6 ml/kg/minute.

2. *Forced acid diuresis*, lowering the urine pH to 4.5-6.0, can augment the excretion of weak bases such as amphetamine, phencyclidine (angle dust) and quinine. IV administration of normal saline with ammonium chloride (1-2 g IV or PO of 6 hr) or ascorbic acid (1-2 g IV or PO of 4 hr) is effective.

   An essential pre-requisite for forced diuresis is normal renal and cardiac function.

3. *Extracorporeal removal of specific toxins* Dialysis or haemoperfusion is required when
   (a) There is clinical deterioration despite intensive supportive therapy as outlined above.
   (b) Blood levels reach potentially lethal concentration. (This information is not available to most physicians in the developing world).
   (c) There is a risk of delayed toxic effects.
   (d) Renal or hepatic failure impairs clearance of the poison and precludes forced diuresis as therapy.

4. *Peritoneal or haemodialysis* is most useful for low-molecular weight water-soluble toxins that are minimally bound to plasma proteins (e.g. bromides, ethanol, ethylene glycol, lithium, methyl alcohol, salicylate).

   For drugs or poisons with high protein-binding and low renal clearance, peritoneal dialysis with salt-free albumin is a better option, as for example in copper sulphate poisoning.

   Dialysis will also correct electrolyte, acid-base and osmolar derangements that may accompany toxic ingestions.

5. *Haemopeifusion* removes poisons by direct absorption to the large surface area of the sorbent material (charcoal or polysterine resins) and is generally more effective than either peritoneal or haemodialysis. It is useful in overdose with barbiturates, sedative-hypnotics and lipid-soluble drugs. The technique is effective in copper sulphate, barbiturate, carbamazepine, phenytoin, or theophylline overdose. It has an advantage over chelation therapy (which requires good renal function and by itself may cause toxic effects).

TABLE 16.2 TOXIC SYNDROMES AND POSSIBLE CAUSES

Syndrome	Manifestations	Possible causes
1. Anticholinergic	Dry mouth and skin, blurred vision, dilated pupils, tachycardia, flushing of skin, hyperthermia, abdominal distension, urine retention/incontinence, confusion, excitation, hallucinations, delusions, coma	Atropine, Other belladona alkaloids, Antihistamines, Phenothiazines, Tricyclic antidepressants
2. Cholinergic	Hypersalivation, bronchospasm, bronchorrhoea, bradycardia, urination/defaecation, neuromuscular paralysis esp. respiratory muscle, pin-point pupils	Acetylcholine. Organophosphorus compounds, Bethanechol, Methacholurea Wild mushrooms, (Amanita muscaria).
3. Inhibition of cytochrome oxidase (block respiratory chain)	Metabolic effect in various organs GI tract, Respiratory: pulm, oedema, ARDS Cardiovascular: tachycardia, arrhythmias, CNS	Aluminium phosphide (phosphine gas), 'Cell Phos', 'quickphos'
4. Extrapyramidal	Dysphagia, dysphoria, trismus, oculogyric crisis, rigidity, torticollis, laryngospasm	Prochlorperazine, Haloperidol, Chlorpromazine & other anti-psychotics, Other phenothiazines
5. Haemoglobinopathies	Dyspnoea, cyanosis (unrelieved by oxygen tr.) confusion, lethargy headache, bullae	Carbon monoxide, Methaemoglo-binuria (aniline dyes, sulfa drugs)
6. Metal fume fever	Malaise, myalgia, headache, nausea, vomiting	Fumes of various metals (brass, copper, iron, nickel, zinc).
7. Narcotic	CNS depression, respiratory depression, pin-point pupil, hypotension	Morphine, Heroin, Codeine, Propoxyphene Other synthetic and semisynthetic opiates.
8. Sympathomimetic	Excitation, hypertension, cardiac arrhythmias, seizures	Amphetamines, Cocaine, Caffeine, Aminophylline, B agonists, inhaled or injected
9. Withdrawal	Anxiety, tremulousness, pilo-erection, lacrimation, tachycardia, hypertension, diarrhoea, yawning	Ethyl alcohol, Barbiturates, Cocaine, Benzodiazepines, Opiates, Meprobamate

Specific Antidotes

Specific Antidotes are available that neutralize or prevent the toxic effects of certain drugs (e.g. naloxone for opioids). A poison index should be available in every emergency room of a hospital, and should be consulted for management.

Table 16.3 lists some of the important antidotes.

Follow–up

Conscious patients should be observed for at least four hours, or hospitalized until free of toxic effects. Patients with on-going toxic manifestations should be observed on a medical service until such effects abate. Admission to an intensive care unit is warranted for patients requiring cardiac monitoring, intensive nursing care, or respiratory or circulatory support.

Patients with chronic drug abuse or attempted suicide should be referred to a psychiatrist before discharging them from hospital. This serves two purposes: (1) to detect those patients who are likely to repeat the attempt; and (2) to ventilate the feelings and problems of those who threatened to commit suicide not really intending to die but merely to draw

TABLE 16.3 ANTIDOTES

Poison/toxic sign	Antidote	Dosage (Adult)
Acetaminophen	N-acetyl cystein (within 16 hours upto 24 hours)	140 mg/kg PO followed by 70 mg/kg 4 hrly x 17 doses.
Anticholinergics	Physostigmine salicylate	0.5-2 mg/IV (IM) over 2 minutes; repeat if necessary after 30-60 min.
Anticholinesterases	Atropine sulfate Pralidoxime (I g IV given over 30 min).	1-5 mg IV (IM, SC); repeat if necessary every 15 min. (500-1500 mg/day) may be needed; 100% hyperbaric.
Carbon monoxide	Oxygen	
Cyanide	Amylnitrite or Sodium nitrite (to convert Hb to met-Hb which combines with free cyanide to form cyan-met-Hb)	Inhalation pearls for 15-30 secs every minute 300 mg (10 ml of 3% sol) IV over 3 minutes. Repeat half dose in 2 hrs if persistent or recurrent signs of toxicity.
	Sodium thiosulfate (which combines with cyan-met-Hb to form met-sodium thiocyanate which is excreted in urine)	12.5 g (50 ml of 25% sol) IV over 10 minutes. Repeat half dose in 2 hrs if persistent or recurrent signs of toxicity.
	Hydroxycobalamine (conversion to cyanocobalamine)	1000 µg Inj/d.
Ethyleneglycol and Methyl alcohol (methanol)	Ethanol	0.6 g/kg ethanol in 5% D/W IV over 30 minutes followed by 110 mg/kg/hr to maintain a blood level of 100-150 mg/dl.
Extrapyramidal signs	Diphenhydramine hydrochloride Benztropine mesylate	25-50 mg IV (IM, PO) Repeat if necessary. 1-2 mg IV (IM, PO) Prn.
Heavy metals (arsenic, copper gold, lead, mercury)	Chelators Calcium disodium edetate (EDTA) Dimercaprol (BAL) Penicillamine	I g IV(IM) over 1/hr of 12 hrs. 2.5 to 5 mg/kg/IM every 6 hrs. 250-500 mg PO every hr.
Iron	Deferoxamine mesylate	1 g IV (IM).
Methaemoglobinuria	Methylene blue	1-2 mg/kg (0.1-0. 2 ml/ kg of 1% solution) IV over 5 min. repeated in 1 hour prn.
Opioids	Nalaxone hydrochloride	0.4-2 mg IV (IM, SC) or endotracheally, prn.
Organophosphorus compounds	PAM Atropine	I g IV given over 30 min. every 8-12 hr, 3 doses. 1-5 mg IV. Repeat if necessary every 15 min.; 500-1500 mg per day may be required.
Aluminium phosphide	Magnesium sulphate (for membrane stabilization)	Continuous IV infusion 3 g in first 3 hours; 6 g in next 24 hours (serum Mg level 3.1-7 mEq/L).
Copper sulphate	Potassium ferrocyanide	Via orogastric tube 1 g/l litre of water or milk/egg white.

attention to their predicament. These cases need help to sort out their problems. Till recently, a failed suicide attempt was an offence liable for criminal prosecution, which only made matters worse for the already miserable person. This legal provision happily has been struck down by the Indian Supreme Court.

17 Respiratory Failure

The major function of the respiratory system is gas exchange-to get enough oxygen in and get enough CO_2 out. Normally sufficient O_2 is transferred to fully saturated circulating haemoglobin, and adequate CO_2 is eliminated to maintain a normal arterial pH.

Respiratory failure results when one or more components of the respiratory system fail: (1) the lungs including the airways, lung parenchyma and pulmonary vasculature; (2) the ventilatory apparatus (or the bellows or pump) which includes the thoracic cage and abdomen, respiratory muscles and elements of both central and peripheral nervous systems.

Common causes of acute respiratory failure (ARF) are listed in **Table 17.1**.

Failure of the gas exchange function of the lung usually causes hypoxaemia, with either normal CO_2 (normocapnia) or low CO_2 (hypocapnia).

Failure of the ventilatory apparatus results in hypoventilation manifested primarily by CO_2 retention (hypercapnia) and to a lesser extent, hypoxaemia.

The detection of acute respiratory failure (ARF) requires a high index of suspicion. Any symptoms or signs of respiratory impairment should prompt the analysis of arterial blood gases (ABGs).

Respiratory failure may be separated into oxygenation failure and ventilation failure. Although the two may occur together, it is useful to separate them to understand their pathophysiology and management. In addition, critical tissue hypoxia may result from non-pulmonary factors that influence oxygen delivery and these must also be considered in making a treatment plan.

TABLE 17.1 COMMON CAUSES OF ACUTE RESPIRATORY FAILURE

A. *The lungs* (gas exchange apparatus)	
Airway obstruction	Laryngospasm
	Asthma acute attack
	COPD
	Foreign body
Lung parenchyma	Pneumonia
	Fibrosing alveolitis
	Emphyseam
	ARDS
Pulmonary vasculature	Pulmonary embolism
	Pulmonary oedema:
	Cardiogenic
	Non-cardiogenic
B. *The bellows* (ventilatory apparatus)	
Respiratory centre depression	Drug overdose
	Cerebrovascular accident
	Hypothyroidism
	Cervical spinal cord injury
Paralysis of respiratory muscles	Guillain-Barré syndrome
	Acute intermittent porphyria
	Myasthenia gravis
	Tetanus
C. *Thoracic cage and abdomen*	Trauma-multiple rib fractures
	Thoracic/upper abdominal surgery
	Kyphoscoliosis

Oxygenation Failure

Low PaO_2 can result from:

1. low inspired oxygen tension (e.g. at high attitude);
2. alveolar hypo ventilation;

3. diffusion impairment;
4. mismatch between ventilation and perfusion;
5. right to left intra-pulmonary shunting.
The last two are the most common mechanisms of hypoxaemia.

Ventilation Failure

Elevated $PaCO_2$ with pH less than 7.35 can result from the following mechanisms:

1. Decrease in total minute ventilation resulting from CNS depression, neuromuscular disease or respiratory muscle fatigue.
2. Increased dead space ventilation not compensated by increase in minute ventilation-which occurs when areas of lung are ventilated but not perfused or when decrease in regional perfusion exceeds decrease in ventilation.
3. Increased CO_2 production not matched by rise in alveolar ventilation, due to fever, sepsis, seizures and excessive carbohydrate loading during parenteral alimentation.

Early recognition of inspiratory muscle fatigue or weakness is important. Clinical manifestations usually precede a significant decrease in alveolar ventilation and increase in $PaCO_2$. The clinician should carefully watch for (1) rapid shallow breathing; (2) uncoordinated inspiratory muscle activity (alternating rib-cage and abdominal breathing); and (3) paradoxical abdominal motion (inward movement of the abdominal wall during inspiration).

These signs are important to observe especially for clinicians in developing countries who have no ready access to arterial gas analysis.

Principles of Therapy of ARF

Specific therapy is dictated by the underlying process that precipitated ARF, but some common supportive measures apply to most situations.

Table 17.2 outlines the treatment of ARF

Improving oxygenation:
1. Hypoxaemia caused by mild to moderate V/Q mismatch (e.g. asthma, pneumonia, pulmonary embolism) is usually reversed with supplemental oxygen.
2. Hypoxaemia caused by severe V/Q mismatch and intrapulmonary shunting (e.g. ARDS,

TABLE 17.2 TREATMENT OF ACUTE RESPIRATORY FAILURE

Upper airway obstruction
  Inhaled foreign body
  (usually in children)
	Try to dislodge it by turning child upside down forcibly compressing the thoracic cage or by Heimlich manoeuvre in adults. If ineffective, extract foreign body by laryngoscopy or bronchoscopy.

Acute epiglottitsis *Laryngeal oedema* *Diphtheritic latyngitis* *Vocal cord paralysis* }	Treatment of cause. If medical treatment is ineffective, tracheal intubation or tracheostomy.
Severe/acute asthma	If not rapidly effective, then tracheal intubation and IPPV.
Chest injuries Tension pneumothorax	Pleural decompression by intercostal tube.
Massive/haemothorax	Drainage of blood through intercostal tube. Thoracotomy if necessary for evacuation of clot and ligation of bleeding points.
Flail chest	Tracheal intubation and IPPV. Treatment of cause, where possible.
Poisoning with narcotics and other drugs	Measures to eliminate the poison specific antidotes (e.g. naloxone for opium poisoning). Tracheal intubation and IPPV.

TABLE 17.3 GUIDELINES FOR ELECTIVE INTUBATION AND MECHANICAL VENTILATION IN ARF

Indications	Parameters	Comments
1. Imminent failure of respiratory bellows function (e.g Guillain-Barré, myasthenia gravis)	Respiration rate > 30-40; Vital capacity < 15 ml/kg	Watch carefully for muscle weakness and keep ventilator ready.
2. Respiratory stridor	Tracheostomy may be needed.	
3. ARDS	PaO_2 < 60 mm Hg; $PaCO_2$ > 50 mm Hg; pH < 7.3	Hypercapnia is often a late manifestation.
4. Cardiogenic shock (inadequate gas exchange increases 02 consumption)	PaO_2 < 60 mm Hg; $PaCO_2$ > 50 mm Hg; pH < 7.3	Decreased work load for the ischaemic or failing heart can be critical.
5. Stupor/coma drug overdose: to protect airways	Poor gag reflex; Ineffective cough	Onset of apnoea may be abrupt.
6. Acute or chronic failure e.g. acute exacerbation of COPD	PaO_2 < 35-45 mm Hg despite oxygen; Respiration rate > 30-40 p.m.; pH < 7.2 or 7.25	Oxygen therapy resulting in progressive respiratory acidosis is an indication for mechanical ventilator.

severe pulmonary oedema) is refractory to supplemental oxygen, and needs mechanical ventilation.

3. Hypoxaemia caused by moderate V/Q mismatch associated with ventilation failure (e.g. exacerbation of COPD) maybe improved by supplemental oxygen but it may worsen the hypercapnia and respiratory acidosis for which intubation and mechanical ventilation are required.

Hazards of oxygen therapy

1. Drying of secretions: this can be avoided by adequate humidification via bubble jet or aerosol humidifiers.

2. Atelectasis due to elimination of nitrogen (normally present in alveoli) by high concentration of oxygen.

3. Oxygen toxicity: in intubated patients exposure to greater than 60 per cent oxygen for longer than 48 hours poses a significant risk. In non-intubated patients breathing oxygen by face mask, the risk is less.

Assisted mechanical ventilation

If the conventional management of patients with respiratory failure (supplemental oxygen, antibiotics, control of secretions and airway obstructions) fails to improve the condition, some forms of mechanical respiratory support become necessary to improve ventilation. **Table 17.3** gives the guidelines for elective intubation and mechanical ventilation. **Table 17.4** lists the techniques of ventilatory support currently available. A clear understanding of the potential beneficial effects as well as the dangers of intermittent positive pressure ventilation (IPPV) will permit a rational use this technique.

Benefits:

1. By adjusting the volume of ventilation the $PaCO_2$ can be brought down to normal limits.

2. The work of breathing is relieved and the consequent danger of extreme exhaustion (which may culminate in respiratory arrest) is removed.

3. Because ventilated patients are connected to a leak-free circuit, a high concentration of oxygen (upto 100 per cent) can be given. A positive

Table 17.4 TECHNIQUES OF VENTILATORY SUPPORT

Technique	Comments
1. Intermittent positive pressure ventilation (IPPV)	May be given with positive end-expiratory pressure (PEEP).
2. Continuous positive airway pressure (CPAP)	Given via an endotracheal tube or mask.
3. Intermittent frequency jet ventilation (HFJV)	May be given with PEEP.
4. High frequency jet ventilation (HFJV)	Useful in those with lung leak e.g. bronchopleural fistula.
5. Low volume pressure-limited inverse ratio mechanical ventilation with low level PEEP	May achieve improved oxygenation while minimizing peak airway pressure.
6. Extracorporeal respiratory assistance	Reduces ventilation requirements and rests the lung.

end-expiratory pressure (PEEP) may reduce shunting and increase PaO_2. PEEP should be considered if IPPV alone cannot achieve more than 90 per cent oxygen saturation without raising the inspired oxygen concentration to a potentially dangerous level (> 50 per cent).

4. In cardiogenic pulmonary oedema with severe respiratory distress and exaustion, IPPV may improve cardiac output and BP.

Dangers:

1. Complications of endotracheal intubation of tracheostomy.

2. Mechanical failure. Manual back-up with ambubag and oxygen must always be available.

3. Barotrauma overdistension of alveoli-pneumothorax.

4. Impeded venous return due to PEEP and increased pulmonary vascular resistance may reduce cardiac output (which can be ameliorated by expanding the circulating volume and inotropic support).

Table 17.5 GUIDELINES FOR WITHDRAWAL OF MECHANICAL VENTILATION

1. An awake and alert patient.
2. PaO_2 > 60 mm Hg, pH in normal range.
3. PEEP < 5 cm H_2O.
4. Vital capacity > 10-15 ml/kg.
5. Minute ventilation < 10 litre/minute.
6. Respiratory rate < 25/minute.
7. Maximum voluntary ventilation double that of minute ventilation.
8. Peak inspiratory pressure more negative than - 25 cm H_2O.
9. Spontaneous ventilation via T tube for 1-4 hours with acceptable blood gases and without marked increase in respiratory rate or heart rate, or change in general status.

Criteria for weaning patients from artificial ventilation are given in **Table 17.5**. Patients who have received artificial ventilation for less than 24 hours (e.g. elective IPPV after major surgery) can usually resume spontaneous respiration immediately and no weaning process is required.

Synchronized intermittent mandatory ventilation (SIMV) which allow the patient to breathe spontaneously between mandatory tidal volumes delivered by the ventilator, can be used to provide a smoother, more controlled method of weaning. Extubation should not be considered until the patient can cough, swallow and protect his own airway, and is sufficiently alert to be cooperative.

During a trial of spontaneous breathing through the endotracheal tube the patient should be closely observed for any signs of respiratory distress.

18 Scorpion Sting

Scorpion Sting is an important and at times life threatening problem in tropical and sub-tropical countries like India, South Africa, Middle East and Latin America.

1500 Scorpion species have been described, 50 of which are venomous and dangerous to humans. Apart from excruciating pain at sting site, neurological, respiratory and Cardio Vascular collapse can occur needing urgent treatment.

Scorpion toxins target Na, K, Ca + Cl Channels, of which Na^+ neuronal channels are studied in detail - prolonged neuronal excitement and release of Neurotransmitter such as acetylchorine + catecholamines.

Sting by Hemiscorpous lepturus, Mesobuthus Tamulus (Indian red scorpion), produce iberiotoxin and Tamulotoxin are selective inhibitors of K^+ channels causing intense and persistent depolarization of autonomic nerves evoking An "autonomic storm" accompanied by a rise in serum calicholamine levels, myocardial dysfunction and pulmonary edema.

Several ECG abnormalities are observed in patients after scorpion sting all due to suddenly liberated catecholamines. Myocardial Perfusion Scintigraphy shows perfusion defects due to compromised myocardial microcirculation.

Priapism is seen in 80% children and 20% adult victims of scorpion sting, providing premonitory signals for cardiac effects.

Hypertension is commonly observed in children Alpha 1 adrenergic receptor stimulation is similar to pheochromocytoma.

Dr. Bavaskar showed the beneficial effects of prazocin – α receptor blocker, given orally in 619 patients. Similar beneficial effects from different parts of India and Middle East demonstrated the role of prazocin as a universal antidote for the autonomic storm evoked by scorpion sting irrespective of the species.

Scorpion Antivenom

Todd (1909) prepared scorpion antivenom to combat the high death rate in Cairo. After subcutances injection of venom, injection of large dose of scorpion antivenom 60 minutes later, induced an immediate and complete neutralization of circulatory venom (Krifi MN).

Belghith M et al from Tunisia reported that SAV did not alter the outcome in scorpion victims treated with SAV.

References

Bawaskar HS & Bawaskar PH. Prazocin for vasodilator treatment of acute pulmonary edema due to scorpion sting. Ann. Trop Med and Parasitol 1987; 81: 19-23.

Bawaskar HS, Bawaskar PH. Scorpion Sting Review Medicine Update 2014 Vol 24.1. 2014 PP 841-45 with 186 references.

Nearly one forth of species of snakes in India are poisonous. In rural India (500 million), 10 percent (50 million) population is at risk of snake bite any time of their life.

The infrastructure of medical profession in India is such that we cannot adequately protect our poor rural population against snake bite where immediate medical attention is not available.

In 2004 WHO established Snakebite Treatment Group, to develop recommendations to reduce mortality according to international norms. In July 2006 a National Snake Bite Conference was convened including Indian and International experts. David A Warrell in 2005 edited a single protocol for both first aid and treatment of snakebite - associated complications.

First Aid Treatment

The most commonly used first-aid technique is the tourniquet which carries the risk of ischemic damage and increasing the necrotic action of the venom, the dangers of neurotoxic blockage and clotting when the tourniquet is released and the ineffectiveness of the technique in retarding venom flow.

Pressure Immobilization Method (PIM) is a newer technique - tying crepe bandage around the limb including an integral splint, as for a sprain - to inhibit venom flow into the system. Currently both tourniquet and PIM are rejected for use in India.

Syndromic Approach

Syndrome 1 Local swelling with bleeding/clotting disturbance   =   Viperidae

Syndrome 2 Local swelling with shock or renal failure   =   Russell's Viper

Syndrome 3 Local swelling with Paralysis Cobra or King Cobra

Syndrome 4 Paralysis with minimal or no local envenoming

Bite on land while sleeping - Krait - Bite in the sea - Sea Snake

Syndrome 5 Paralysis with dark brown urine and renal failure

Bite on Land - Russell's Viper

Bite in Sea   - Sea Snake

The 20 minute whole bleed clotting list is simple to carryout and given reliable indication of consumption coagulopathy - indicating that the biting species is vipering.

Confusion, ptosis, altered consciousness, fasciculation and other neurological manifestation should be monitored. Edrophonium test followed by neostigmine may be useful.

If ASV is not available, and can still treat haematologic complications by blood and blood product use.

The neurotoxic poisoning also can be treated by neostigmine (after edrophonium test) and mechanical ventilation.

ASV administration Criteria

ASV is a scarce commodity with known accompanying risks of anaphylaxis.

The recommended initial doses in 100 ml of polyvalent ASV for adults and childrens.

The 100 ml should be administered over one hour preferably diluted with 100 ml normal saline over one hour.

Urticaria, itching, fever, chills, nausea vomiting, diarrhea, abdominal cramps, tachycardia, hypotension, bronchospasm, angioedema suggest anaphylaxis. ASV should be discontinued and IV hydrocortisone and H1 H2 blockers used.

Special Situations

A. Acute renal failure

B. Cardio vascular abnormalities
Acute hypotension, fatal tachyarrhythmias

C. Hyperkalemia

Viperidae snake

The Viperidae are a family of venomous snakes found all over the world, except in Antarctica, Australia, New Zealand, Ireland, Madagascar, Hawaii, various other isolated islands, and north of the Arctic Circle.

Elapidae includes the most venomous land snakes in the country, with three highly venomous snakes (The Indian Cobra and two Kraits) and a single moderately venomous, little known snake, the Sri Lankan Coral snake or Calliophis melanurus sinhaleyus. The actual toxicity of this species is unknown to a great extent, but some herpetologists consider it to have potential lethal envenoming, thus categories it as a highly venomous snake. The Blood-bellied coralsnake (Calliophis haematoetron) was the last elapid to be described from Sri Lanka and is found in the Wasgomuwa and Knuckles regions. The two subspecies of the Sri Lankan Krait (Bungarus ceylonicus) are endemic to the island. Other than for the Coral snake, which is sub-fossorial, the other species are terrestrial and are found within close proximity of human habituations. The Cobra is predominantly diurnal but the two Bungarus species are largely nocturnal.

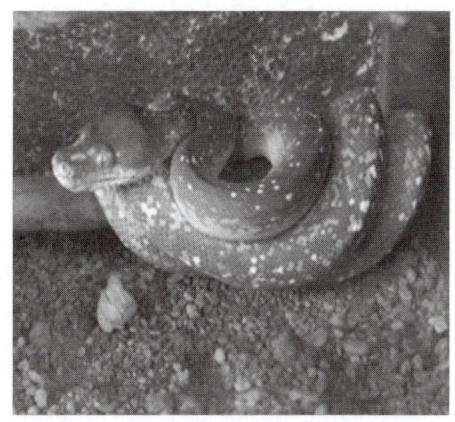

Family Elapidae (Cobras, Kraits, Coral snakes and Sea snakes)

Order Squamata; Suborder Serpentes

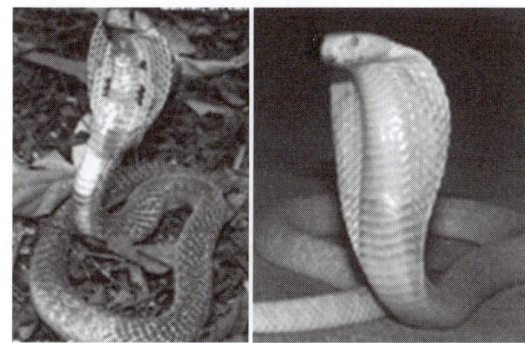

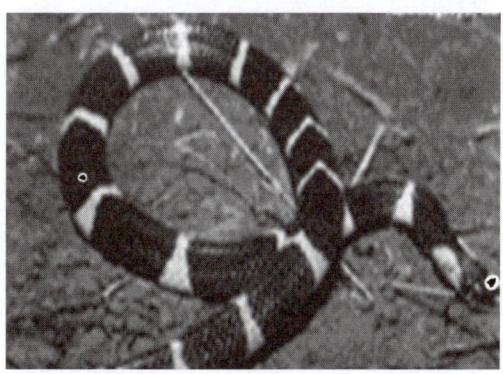

Reference

H S Bawaskar. Snake Venoms and Antivenoms - Critical Supply issues JAPI. 2004; 52: 788-92.

Shibendu Ghosh API medicine Update 2014 Vol. 1. Section 12 Snake bite Critical Care Medicine.

Shock

Shock is a life-threatening syndrome that represents the clinical endpoint of a variety of diseases with a common denominator of poor organ perfusion and tissue ischaemia. Clinically this is manifest by systolic arterial pressure less than 80 mm Hg, cold clammy extremities with poor capillary refill, oliguria, and often impairment of consciousness.

Prompt recognition of the underlying pathophysiology is essential in order to ensure optimal treatment. If the treatment is not prompt and effective, serious consequences will ensue.

Oliguria progresses to acute tubular necrosis and anuria; a rising plasma potassium and lactic acidosis (both from renal failure and ischaemic necrosis of skeletal muscles) may lead to cardiac arrhythmias which can be fatal. Even if recovery occurs, permanent cerebral damage or loss of peripheral tissue (due to gangrene) may be inevitable.

The *mechanisms* underlying the shock syndrome include:

1. *Oligaemic or hypovolaemic shock:* reduced cardiac filling due to reduced circulatory volume.

2. *Cardiogenic shock:* reduced cardiac output in spite of normal filling volume.

3. *Distributive shock:* maldistribution of blood flow and decreased vascular resistance lead to reduced organ flow despite normal or increased cardiac output.

The important causes of shock are given in **Table 20.1**. Identification of the underlying mechanism in the individual patient requires meticulous assessment of the history and physical signs, and efficient use of investigations such as central venous pressure and Swan Ganz catheter.

A *low* central venous pressure (CVP) is characteristic of oligaemic shock, while a *high* CVP is characteristic of cardiogenic shock. CVP is *variable* in distributive shock (septic shock, anaphylactic shock).

Table 20.2 lists the likely causes of shock associated with severe abdominal pain. The possible conditions in which shock is not accompanied by severe abdominal pain are given in **Table 20.3**.

TABLE 20.1 CAUSES OF SHOCK

I. *Hypovolaemic Shock*
  A. *Loss of blood*
      Gastrointestinal bleeding (See Chapter 4).
      Intra-abdominal bleeding
          Leaking aneurysm
          Ruptured spleen
          Ruptured ectopic pregnancy
  B. *Loss of plasma*
      through the skin: severe burns
      in the abdominal cavity: acute pancreatitis
  C. *Loss of fluids*
      Gastrointestinal tract: e.g. cholera

II. *Cardiogenic Shock*
  A. *Myocardial pump failure*
      Acute myocardial infarct
      Acute myocarditis
      Cardiomyopathy
      Sudden aortic or mitral regurgitation
      Sudden rupture of interventricular septum
  B. *Tachyarrhythmias:* refractory, sustained
  C. *Pericardial tamponade*
  D. *Massive pulmonary embolism*

III. *Distributive shock*
      Septic shock (endotoxin)
      Anaphylactic shock

Emergency Therapeutic Measures

1. Keep the patient warm to avoid hypothermia.

2. For pain and anxiety, sedate with IV morphine.

Table 20.2 SHOCK WITH SEVERE ABDOMINAL PAIN

History	Likely causes
History of trauma	Ruptured spleen/kidney
Elderly patient	Mesenteric vascular occlusion
Female patient in reproductive age	Septic abortion
	Ruptured ectopic pregnancy
	Ante-partum haemorrhage
Known diabetes	Ketoacidosis
Known sickle cell disease	Sickle cell crisis

Table 20.3 SHOCK WITHOUT SEVERE ABDOMINAL PAIN

History	Likely causes
History of haematemesis	Cirrhosis of liver
History of injection (penicillin, antivenins)	Anaphylactic shock
Known diabetic	Hypoglycaemia
Acute onset of wheezing urticaria	Anaphylactic shock
History of snakebite	Snake poisoning
History of fever with chills	Septicaemia, malaria

3. Oxygen administration with face mask or nasal prongs.

4. Insert in-dwelling catheter to monitor hourly urine output.

5. Insert a central venous catheter to monitor CVP.

6. Protect ischaemic skin from damage.

Therapy is aimed at the rapid restoration of tissue perfusion as indicated by resolution of oliguria, improvement in mental status, and correction of the metabolic lactic acidosis. A patent airway is essential and mechanical ventilation may be required to provide adequate oxygenation and CO_2 elimination.

Hypovolaemic Shock

For replacement of blood, plasma, plasma substitutes or fluids, see GI bleeding (p. 31), electrolyte disturbances (p. 90), treatment of Addisonian crisis (p. 90), treatment of lactic acidosis (p. 97).

Cardiogenic Shock or Hypovolaemic Shock in Pre-existing Cardiac Disease

When hypovolaemic shock occurs in patients with pre-existing cardiac disease, CVP or right atrial pressure may be an unreliable guide to fluid replacement. It is essential to obtain an estimate of pulmonary venous or left atrial pressure by introducing a Swan-Ganz catheter (a flexible double lumen tube with a small balloon at the distal end). The catheter is introduced into a vein and advanced to the right atrium. One lumen is then used to inflate the balloon with about 1 cm³ of air. The force of the blood stream carries the balloon and the attached catheter through the right ventricle to the pulmonary artery, the changing pressures measured through the other lumen indicating its progress. The tip of the catheter is positioned in a peripheral branch of the pulmonary artery. When the balloon is deflated, it records pulmonary artery pressure; when the balloon is inflated, the tip is isolated from the main pulmonary artery and instead registers the left atrial pressure (normal 5-10 mm Hg). In left sided cardiac failure, it may rise as high as 30 mm Hg. In managing cardiogenic shock, a left atrial pressure of about 15 mm Hg is usually aimed at; this is high enough to give good left ventricular filling, but carries a low risk of pulmonary oedema.

Acute pulmonary oedema is managed by:

1. Oxygen therapy at high concentration.

2. An IV bolus of frusemide 40-80 mg for its powerful diuretic effect as well as vasodilator effect.

3. IV morphine to alleviate breathlessness and reverse reflex peripheral vasoconstriction.

4. Inotropic agents dopamine or dobutamine. Dopamine 2-4 mg/kg/minute has a selective renal vasodilator effect.

Aortic counterpulsation

In cardiogenic shock, mechanical assistance with an intra-aortic balloon pump (IABP), capable of augmenting both arterial diastolic pressure and cardiac out put is helpful in rapidly stabilizing patients. A sausage-shaped balloon at the end of a catheter is introduced into the aorta percutaneously via the femoral artery and the balloon is automatically inflated during early diastole, augmenting coronary blood flow. The balloon collapses in early systole reducing the after load against which the left ventricle ejects. IABP improves haemodynamic status at least temporarily in the majority of patients. Unlike inotropic and vasopressor agents, IABP reduced myocardial oxygen consumption, leading to amelioration of ischemia. IABP buys time prior to and during cardiac catheterization and percutaneous coronary intervention (PCI) or surgery.

IABP is contraindicated if aortic regurgitation or aortic dissection is suspected.

In young eligible patients with refractory shock for cardiac transplantation, ventricular assist device may be considered to buy time.

Septic or Endotoxin Shock

Septic shock is usually caused by bacteraemia, although it may complicate fungaemia or viraemia. Early recognition of bacteraemic shock is critical since delay in treatment increases mortality.

Host factors and comorbid conditions may enhance the risk of infection with certain organisms or of a more fulminant course than is usually seen. Lack of splenic function (prior splenectomy), alcoholism with significant liver disease, I.V. drug abuse, HIV infection, diabetes, malignancy and chemotherapy all predispose to specific infections and increased severity. The primary site of infection (pneumonia, pyelonephritis, cholangitis) may not be evident initially. Petechial rashes on the skin require urgent attention (e.g. meningococcal septicaemia). Hypotension with petiechiae for less than 12 hours is a harbinger of DIC and high mortality (90 per cent). Wide spread vascular endothelial injury is the major mechanism for multiorgan dysfunction. Prominent hypotensive molecules include nitric oxide, β endorphin, bradykinin, PAF and prostacyclin. Decreased peripheral vascular resistance occurs despite increased levels of vasopressor catecholamines. The loss of sensitivity to catecholamines can be restored by infusion of hydrocortisone in many patients of septic shock.

Hypotension and DIC predispose to acrocyanosis and ischaemic necrosis of peripheral tissues most commonly the digits.

Superantigen producing staph. aureus or streptococcus pyogenes cause T cell activation producing a cytokine profile that differs substantially from that elicited by gram-negative bacterial infection.

Cardiovascular collapse occurs in about 40 per cent of gram negative bacillary bacteraemias and has an overall mortality of 40 per cent. Clinically there are two stages of bacteraemic shock.

In the early (hyperdynamic or warm) phase the cardiac output is elevated, peripheral vascular resistance is decreased, despite increased levels of vasopressure catecholamines and the patient is warm, sweating, and peripherally vasodilated. This may proceed to the second hypodynamic phase (cold shock) that is manifested by normal or increased peripheral vascular resistance, cold vasoconstricted skin, and ultimately decreased cardiac output.

Early bactericidal treatment is essential in the therapy of septicaemia. If no obvious source of infection is detected, specimens of potentially infected body fluids (e.g. pleural fluid, CSF) should be examined and sent for culture before therapy is instituted. Several blood cultures should be sent before starting empirically a beta-lactam antibiotic plus an aminoglycoside (gentamicin or tobramycin). Imipenem may be used where aminoglycosides are contraindicated (e.g. poor renal function).

Crystalloid fluids should be administered initially to achieve normal blood pressure. If this is unsuccessful, vasopressor drugs should be used.

DIC (Disseminated intra-vascular coagulation) is a dreaded complication of septic shock. Restoration of blood pressure and appropriate antimicrobial therapy are usually adequate to reverse this problem. Laboratory findings in DIC often include thrombocytopenia, hypofibrinogenaemia, increased fibrin degradation products (FDPs), and prolongation of TT and PTT. Unless serious haemorrhagic or thrombotic complications occur, specific therapy with heparin should be withheld.

Prevention offers the best opportunity to reduce the high morbidity and mortality (40-60%) in spetic shock, by reducing the number of invasive procedures, by limiting the use and duration of indwelling vascular and bladder catheters, by reducing the incidence and duration of profound neutropenia (< 500 neutrophils/μL).

Association between allelic polymorphism in TNFα and interferon γ genes and risk of developing severe sepsis have been identified in patients who have sustained major trauma. Such information could be used prospectively to identify high risk patients and to target preventive and/or therapeutic measures to them.

Anaphylactic Shock

Anaphylaxis is an acute allergic reaction following antigen exposure in a sensitized person. It is usually mediated by IgE antibodies, and involves the release of chemical mediators from mast cells mand basophils.

Common antigens giving rise to anaphylaxis are drugs (e.g. antibiotics, local anaesthetics), foreign serum, insect stings, diagnostic agents (e.g. iodinated contrast media, fluorescine for retinal angiography, BSP for liver function testing).

A history of known sensitivity should be elicited.

Clinical manifestations include apprehension, pruritus, urticaria, angio-oedema, bronchospasm with respiratory distress and hypotension. Respiratory compromise may be caused by laryngeal oedema or laryngeal spasm. Shock is the result of profound peripheral vasodilatation and peripheral capillary leak leading to drop in circulating volume. Vascular collapse may develop in the absence of respiratory symptoms and death may occur within minutes.

Treatment
Epinephrine is the drug of choice for the initial treatment of anaphylaxis. For life-threatening reactions 0.5 mg (5 ml of a 1:10,000 solution) should be given IV and repeated after 5-10 minutes as needed. A continuous infusion of epinephrine may allow more careful titration of dosage and may be preferable to bolus injection.

Sublingual or endotracheal administration may be effective if an IV line cannot be established.

For less severe reactions 0.3-0.5 mg (0.3 to 0.5 ml of a 1:1000 solution) may be given SC and repeated after 20-30 minutes if necessary for up to 3 doses.

Maintenance of airway is essential. Endotracheal intubation and assisted ventilation may be necessary for severe bronchospasm. In case of laryngeal oedema, tracheostomy is indicated.

Oxygen should be administered to all patients in respiratory distress.

Aminophilline 6 mg/kg as a loading dose may be infused IV over 20-30 minutes to treat bronchospasm. This should be followed by an initial maintenance infusion of 0.5-0.6 mg/kg per hour.

A nebulized inhaled beta agonist (e.g. metaproterenol) may also be effective in the treatment of bronchospasm.

Volume expansion with normal saline or Ringer lactate solution may be needed for restoring and maintaining tissue perfusion. Large losses of fluid from the intravascular compartment commonly occur and must be replaced.

Hydrocortisone sodium succinate 500 mg IV 6 hourly or its equivalent should be administered for severe and prolonged reactions. Corticosteroids, however, *are not first line drugs* since their peak effect occurs in 6-12 hours and their major role is in *preventing* later redevelopment of the clinical syndrome.

Anthihistaminics have no role in the treatment of anaphylaxis. However, they may block further histamine-binding to target tissues, shortening the duration of the reaction and preventing relapses. Diphenhydramine hydrochloride 25-50 mg oral, IM or IV may be given. H_2 receptor blockers such as Cimetidine 300 mg IV may have an additive effect.

Observation

All patients with anaphylaxis should be observed for at least 6 hours. Careful monitoring is needed for these patients with hypotension, upper airway obstruction, or persistent bronchospasm.

21   Stroke

The pithy and commonly used term 'stroke' describes the sudden neurological deficit that often ensues following cerebrovascular lesions. In the population over the age of 65, the annual incidence of strokes of various types is more than 1 per cent. In anyone year, in every 1,000 of the population two persons will suffer an initial stroke and one will die from a stroke. The large number of hospital beds occupied by stroke patients reflect the high morbidity caused by cerebrovascular disease.

Cerebrovascular disease most commonly arises in the arteries, but the veins and the capillaries may also be affected, especially in the younger age group. Vascular malformations and vascular tumours may also present as 'stroke'. The causes of stroke are listed in **Table 21.1**.

There are two encouraging new facts regarding stroke:

1. There has been a steady decline over the last two decades, in the incidence of atherosclerotic stroke, probably due to control of risk factors (cigarette smoking and hypertension).

2. If prompt treatment can be initiated within the first six hours following stroke (window period) the damage to the neurones can be minimized.

Assessment of a Patient with Stroke

The clinical spectrum of stroke is described in **Table 21.2**. The clinical picture depends upon the vascular bed of the brain involved–carotid territory or vertebro-basilar territory. Since the internal carotid and middle cerebral arteries are commonly involved, hemiplegia is the commonest manifestation of a stroke. But acute changes in behaviour can occur in stroke without hemiplegia, as described in **Table 21.3**. Embolic and thrombotic hemiplegic strokes probably cause the majority of these cases.

Strokes can be considered clinically under the following five categories: (1) thrombosis of large arteries; (2) lacunar strokes; (3) embolism; (4) intracerebral bleed usually hypertensive; and (5) subarachnoid haemorrhage (SAH) due to ruptured aneurysm or arteriovenous malformation.

How far can the clinician succeed, based on history and physical examination, in arriving at the correct aetiological diagnosis? The usefulness and limitations of a purely clinical approach must be appreciated. One can attempt a guess based on the type of onset (sudden stuttering, smooth, gradual or fluctuating), accompanying symptoms (headache, seizures, vomiting, etc.) and the clinical milieu (diabetes, hypertension, cardiac valvular disease, atrial fibrillation, etc) with the full realization that one can be wrong in the assessment in a given patient. Hence the importance of a CT/MRI when available.

A stepwise, stuttering onset is characteristic of thrombotic stroke, while an abrupt onset– 'a bolt from the blue' –is more suggestive of embolic strokes or SAH.

The combination of headache and vomiting, followed by coma is most often seen with intracerebral bleed or SAH. Headache can occur before, during or after the stroke.

Abrupt onset of focal neurologic deficit without a change in the level of consciousness suggests an ischaemic infarct.

NOTE: All these lesions (mostly embolic or ischaemic infarcts) can be shown as perfusion defects in Brain SPECT blood flow studies, immediately after onset or by means of Perfusion CT/MR Angiography.

TABLE 21.1 CAUSES OF STROKE

I.	Arterial lesions	
	A.Atherosclerosis	Most common after age 40 Associated hypertension, diabetes, history of smoking
	B. Arteritis & vasculitis	Polyarteritis nodosa, SLE, cranial arteritis, Takayashu disease, tuberculosis, syphilis
	C. Embolism	• Heart Acute myocardial infarct Vertricular aneurysm with mural thrombus: Atrial fibrillation Prolapsed mitral valve Endocarditis Prosthetic valve Cardiomyopathy Left atrial myxoma • Aorta and carotid arteries during surgery, catheterization • Fat embol-long bone fracture
	D. Aneurysms & AV malformations	(Vascular tumours may also present as 'stroke')
II.	Venous lesions	
	A. Superior sagittal sinus	Puerperium
	B. Cortical or venous thrombosis	Oral contraceptive pills
	C. Lateral sinus thrombosis	Septicaemia Polycythaemia (Hct > 60%) Dehydration Marasmus Hyperviscocity syndrome Behcet's Disease
III.	Capillary lesions	Falciparum malaria Sickle cell disease Thrombotic thrombocytopenic purpura Disseminated intravascular coagulation
IV.	Haemodynamic changes Causing low cerebral blood flow	Brady-tachy arrhythmias Sick sinus syndrome (diffuse symptoms: dizziness vertigo, visual blurring generalized seizures)

TABLE 21.2 CLINICAL SPECTRUM OF STROKE

	Condition	Description
1.	Completed stroke	Rapid development of focal cerebral dysfunction due to infarction.
2.	Stroke in evolution	Relatively slow, stepwise extension of neurologic deficit–full extent not exhibited for 3-4 days, occasionally 1-2 weeks. Commonly due to occlusion of internal carotid artery; occasionally due to tumour.
3.	Transient ischaemic attack (TIA)	Sudden neurologic deficit, followed, within the hour, by complete recovery of function. Frequency and duration variable. Possible harbinger of a more severe & permanent deficit within the next 6 months.
4.	Reversible ischaemic neurologic deficit (RIND)	Signs of neurologic deficit lasting longer than 24 hours and less than 7 days. Approximately one-third of cases will experience infarct within next 5 years.
5.	Subclavian steal (stenosis of subclavian artery proximal to origin of vertebral artery)	When arm is exercised, ataxia and diplopia occur (due to diversion of blood flow from vertebral territory). Bruit over supraclavicular fossa. Significant difference in BP in the two arms.
6.	Multi-infarct dementia	Gradual & progressive brain atrophy due to gradual reduction in cerebral blood flow. Bilateral pyramidal signs with supranuclear bulbar palsy. Dysphagia, dysarthria. Sudden transient acceleration of deficit and debility.

TABLE 21.3 ACUTE BEHAVIOURAL CHANGES OCCURRING WITHOUT HEMIPLEGIA IN STROKE

Behaviour	Location of ischaemia
1. Incoherent language, confusion, disorientation, appearing acutely	Cardiogenic emboli to left temporoparietal area
2. Apathy, paucity of speech, slow motor response, slow motor activity	Pre-frontal infarction
3. Agitated delirium, excitement, disorientation, visual field defect and memory impairment.	Medial occipito-temporal infarct with involvement of hippocampus and optic radiations
4. Acute memory loss	Infarct in area of posterior cerebral artery involving medial temporal lobe (hippocampus)
5. Acute confusion without agitation, inattention	Right pre-frontal or parietal infarction
6. Acute onset of derangement of judgement and insight	Right temporo-parietal infarct

Physical Examination

Determining the presence of diseases which predispose to thromboembolism or haemorrhage–hypertension, diabetes, cardiac disease–is an important part of the evaluation of the stroke patient. In patients who do not show evidence of these disorders and in younger patients, a search must be made for the manifestations of the nonatherosclerotic causes of stroke–Polyarteritis nodosa, SLE, Wegener's granulomatosis, Takayashu arteritis etc. Tuberculosis, syphilis and fungal infections can involve cerebral vessels.

Disorders of coagulation (oral contraceptives, Polycythaemia, hyperviscocity syndrome, thrombotic thrombocytopenic purpura etc.) usually manifest in a systemic manner and are not confined to the cerebral circulation.

Extra-cranial mechanical arterial compression (e.g. atlanto-axial dislocation), rheumatoid arthritis, cervical spondylosis, which cause vertebral artery compression or occlusion, can be diagnosed by physical signs.

Palpation of the pulses may be revealing: Begin with the common carotid artery, being careful in the elderly patient not to occlude it. One often cannot tell if the internal carotid artery is pulseless, due to transmitted pulsation from the external carotid artery. Palpation of the external carotid branches in the head–superficial temporal and supraorbital arteries–may reveal increased flow or diminished pulses. Palpation of the radial and brachial pulses and comparison of the two sides is useful in detecting Takayashu disease and subclavian steal.

Bruits may be listened for over the head, orbits, mastoids, along the carotid artery in the neck (most common site is at the bifurcation), in the supraclavicular fossa and over the neck posteriorly. Bruits increase in loudness and pitch until the lumen of the vessel is about two-thirds occluded, then they diminish. Interpretation of the presence or absence of bruits and pulses must be done cautiously. Absence of a bruit over the neck vessels is not sufficient to rule out significant internal carotid artery stenosis. On the other hand, a bruit may be present due to excessive flow in a normal artery (to compensate for diminished flow on the contralateral side), hence the importance of a colour doppler study if available.

Blood pressure must be recorded on both arms and compared for a difference of more than 10 mm Hg. It is also useful to listen for femoral and abdominal bruits and evaluate for abdominal aortic aneurysm.

Examination of the fundus is useful in indicating changes due to hypertensive or diabetic retinopathy. Occasionally, emboli may be seen in the retinal vessels–bright cholesterol crystals suggest origin from the carotid artery; white emboli suggest emboli from scarred heart valves.

Since cardiogenic emboli account for 20 per cent of all strokes, evaluation of the heart for a possible source of emboli is important. Apart from clinical evaluation, ECG and 2D echocardiography provide valuable clues.

Since haemodynamic changes critically determine the occurrence of strokes ('low flow infarcts') one should look for evidence of tachybrady arrhythmias or conditions which lead to a critical fall in blood pressure (GI bleed, myocardial infarct).

Strokes caused by other conditions are not common, but there are a large number of causes which must be considered in young patients and in older ones who do not have the risk factors such as hypertension, diabetes and smoking. Fortunately, most of these causes are accompanied by a variety of other systemic symptoms and signs, or they occur in a clinical setting (e.g. the puerperium for cortical vein thrombosis) that suggest the diagnosis.

Hypercoagulable disorders (thrombophilia) such as Protein C deficiency, Protein S deficiency, Anti-thrombin III deficiency, anti-phospholipid syndrome dysproteinemia, Homocysteinemia can be investigated by appropriate laboratory tests.

Nevertheless nearly 30% of stroke remain unexplained despite extensive evaluation. Surprisingly migraine can mimic cerebral ischaemia, even in patients without a significant migraine history (acephalgic migraine). This can occur even after age 65.

Management of Stroke

The first six hours: 'window period'
Following a stroke, the damage results from destruction of neurones caused either by disruption of cerebral blood flow or by haemorrhage into or around the brain. Each hour of ischaemia and tissue injury increases the degree of irreversible tissue damage. Initiating acute stroke care within a 6-hour minimal period is a goal that can be accomplished with proper organization of health services.

The stroke patient should be transported as rapidly and safely as possible to the nearest hospital which has facilities for a CT scan, because that answers the most critical question: 'Is it an ischaemic infarct Or is it a haemorrhage?' The answer to this question determines the subsequent management.

At the time of the first medical contact, the patient should be evaluated for ABC (airway patency, adequate breathing and intact circulation). During transportation, intravenous access should be established, supplemental oxygen administered and advance intimation be sent to the admitting hospital for emergency CT scanning, to save time.

After the patient arrives, neurological evaluation should be performed as indicated in the section on evaluation of the patient. The evaluation should include an ECG, chest-X-ray film, complete blood count, platelet count, prothrombin time (PT) and partial thromboplastin time (PTT), serum electrolyte and blood glucose estimation. For patients with a strong suspicion

of SAH not confirmed by imaging techniques, a lumbar puncture should be done immediately.

The purpose of emergency non-contrast CT scanning on arrival is to determine whether the stroke is haemorrhagic or ischaemic. CT scan will show haemorrhage if present. It will also show a tumour if it is presenting as a stroke. If the stroke is haemorrhagic, CT will indicate if the haemorhage is intracerebral, or subarachnoid, or a combination of both. CT is normal for the first 2 days in ischaemic infarcts. When there is suspicion that carotid artery disease is the underlying problem, an emergency doppler study should be arranged if available.

The National Stroke Association (USA) consensus recommendations on the management of stroke in the first six hours are reproduced in **Fig. 21.1**. The management of acute ischaemic stroke during the first 6 hours is given in **Table 21.4**, that of intracerebral haemorrhage in **Table 21.5** and that of subarachnoid haemorrhage in **Table 21.6**. The various graders of SAH are given in **Table 21.7**.

Promising future developments for ischaemic strokes are

1. Thrombolytic therapy with recombinant TPA (tissue plasminogen activator) is successful if given within a very short time (1½ hours) after symptoms of cerebral ischaemia begin. There must be certainty that the stroke is not haemorrhagic. The dose of rtPA is 0.9 mg/kg to a maximum 90 mg; 10% as an I.V. bolus and the remainder as a drip over 60 minutes.

Table 21.4 MANAGEMENT OF ACUTE ISCHAEMIC STROKE

1. Correct any compromise of airway, breathing or circulation.

2. Do not treat elevation in blood pressure in the absence of specific indications (e.g. myocardial infarction, arterial dissection), or unless systolic BP is ≥ 220 mm Hg or diastolic BP ≥ 120 mm Hg on repeated measurements over 30 to 60 minutes.

3. If seizures occur, administer anticonvulsant therapy, including a full loading dose of phenytoin.

4. If a cerebellar infarct is diagnosed, obtain neurosurgical consultation. Evidence of brainstem compression necessitates urgent surgical decompression.

Table 21.5 MANAGEMENT OF INTRACEREBRAL HAEMORRHAGE

1. Correct any compromise of airway, breathing or circulation.
2. Obtain urgent neurosurgical consultation if the need for surgical intervention is identified (cerebellar haemorrhage, cerebellar infarct, epidural or subdural haematomas, acute hydrocephalus).
3. Treat severe elevation of BP ($\geq$ 200 mm Hg systolic or $\geq$ 120 mm Hg diastolic).
4. If raised intracranial pressure is suspected
   (a) Hyperventilation using endotracheal intubation to reduce $PaCO_2$ to 25-30 mm Hg.
   (b) Mannitol 20% sol (100 g in 500 ml) IV infusion over 10-20 minutes (l-1.5g/kg).

Contraindications to thrombolytic therapy are:
a. sustained high BP > 185/110 despite treatment.
b. Platelets < 100,000
c. CT scan showing haemorrhage
d. Major surgery in preceeding two weeks
e. GI bleeding in preceeding three weeks
f. Recent myocardial infarction
g. Stupor or coma
h. Intra-arterial route of thrombolytics is more effective to increase the concentration of the drug at the clot and to minimise systemic bleeding complications (seen in 6.4% patients after IV γtPA). Intra-arterial pro-urokinase has been given upto the 6th hour following onset of stroke.

2. Calcium channel blockers (nimodipine and nicardipine) help to prevent calcium entry into neurones during ischaemia; calcium activates a number of proteolytic enzymes resulting in production of free radicals which cause neuronal toxicity.

3. Scavengers of free radicals such as 21 amino-steroids ('Lazaroids') have been effective experimentally and are being evaluated clinically.

Table 21.6 MANAGEMENT OF SUBARACHNOID HAEMORRHAGE

1. Correct any compromise of airway, breathing or circulation.
2. Obtain urgent neurosurgical consultation.
3. If patient was previously normotensive, treat elevation of BP if present.
4. Start nimodipine 60 mg PO qrid in patients grade 1, 2 and 3 (**Table 21.7**).
5. If seizures occur, give anticonvulsant therapy including full doses of phenytoin.
6. Give analgesics & sedatives as needed.
7. Emergency angiography, invasive haemodynamic monitoring and early surgery should be considered for aneurysmal SAH.

Table 21.7 CLINICAL GRADES OF SAH

Grade 1: Asymptomatic or minimum headache or neck stiffness

Grade 2: More severe headache and neck stitlness

Grade 3: Drowsy or confused, may have mild hemiparesis

Grade 4: Deeply stuporous, may have moderate to severe hemiparesis, early decerebrate signs

Grade 5: Deeply comatose

Management of embolic strokes

Cardiogenic embolus is a strong indication for full systemic anticoagulation, except that arising from infective endocarditis of native valves. If the prothrombin time is kept at 2-2.5 times normal control, the risk of bleeding is less than I per cent per year, as against the benefit of 70 per cent reduction of ischaemic stroke recurrence. The risk of bleeding is greater in patients above age 75 (3 per cent) hence the important decision for the physician is to weigh the risks versus the benefits. Patients with atrial fibrillation (AF), enlarged left atrium and poor left ventricular function are at high risk of embolic stroke with about 33 per cent mortality during the acute episode, with a 65-80 per cent chance of recurrence of embolus in the survivors. Hence oral warfarin is indicated in these high risk patients.

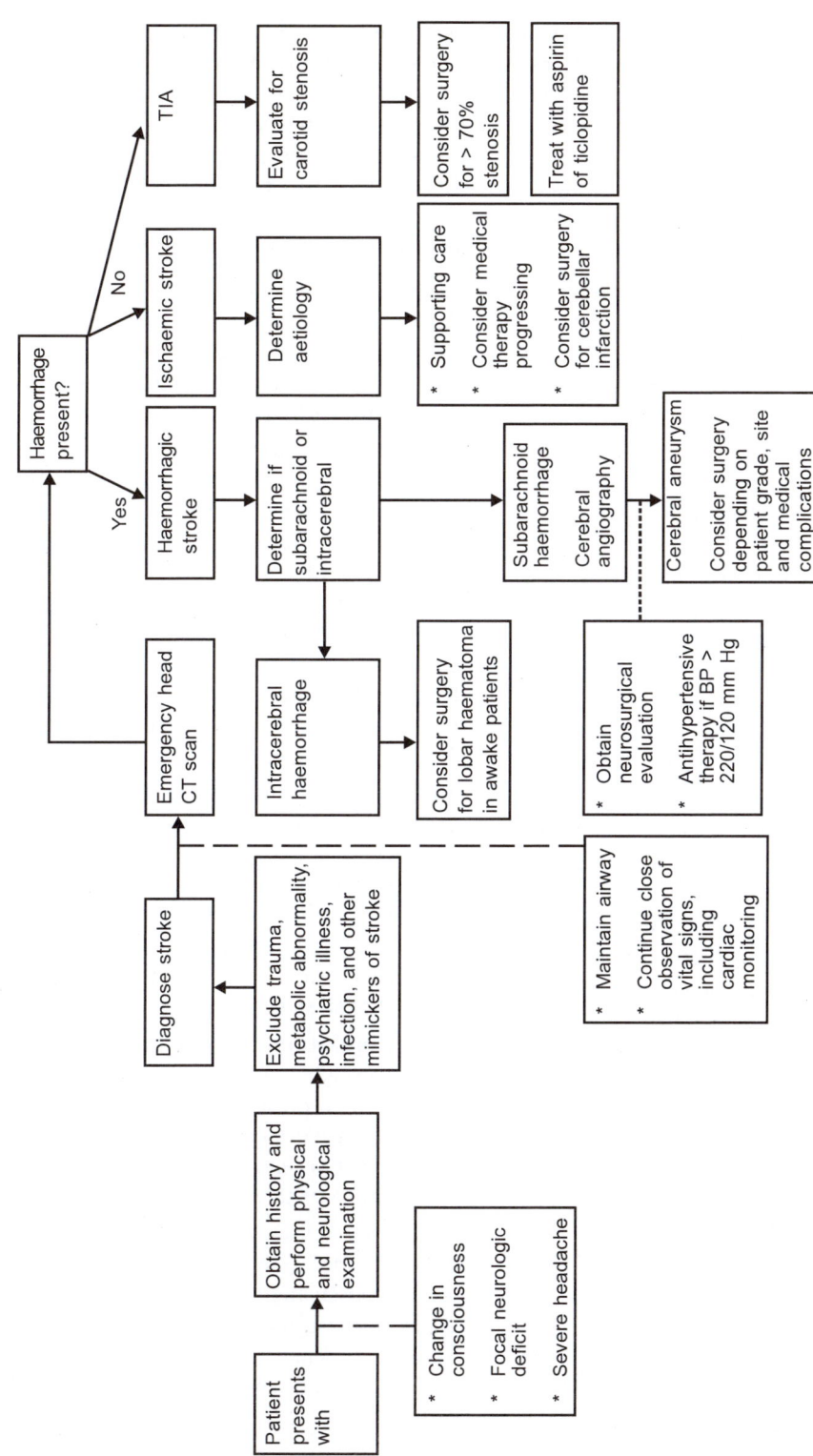

Fig. 21.1: Management of stroke

2D echocardiography should be done in all cases of suspected emboli especially in patients with AF. Trans-oesophageal echocardiography more reliably detects clots in the left atrium and its appendix than precordial echocardiography.

Dipyridamol and warfarin in combination are more effective than warfarin alone in the prevention of embolism from prosthetic heart valves.

The efficacy of aspirin alone in low doses is less than warfarin but since it is inexpensive, easily administered and less risky than warfarin for bleeding, physicians and patients are both more likely to prefer it.

Aspirin is the only anti-platelet agent that has been prospectively studied in the treatment of acute ischaemic stroke. The use is safe and produces a small net benefit.

Glycoprotein IIb/III a receptor inhibitors (e.g. abciximab) given intravenous within 6 hours of stroke onset is safe and may be effective. Trials do not support the use of heparin or low molecular heparin in acute ischemic stroke.

MR Venography has revealed cerebral venous Thrombosis (CVT) to be far more common than previously thought of. The mode of onset and clinical spectrum are highly variable – acute onset with sudden hemiplegia may simulate arterial stroke. Focal signs are present in upto 50 per cent of cases. Headache vomiting, papilloedema and 6th nerve palsy may mimic benign intracranial hypertension.

Inspite of the possibility of haemorrhagic infarct anticoagulant therapy with heparin for 1-2 weeks followed by oral antocoagulants for 6 months of thrombophilitic factors are present.

Aspirin is more effective in preventing non-cardiac emboli (arising in the aortic arch and carotid arteries). Some experts advocate high doses (600-1500 mg/day) for stroke prevention from these sources.

Ticlopidine 250 mg bid is indicated when patients cannot tolerate aspirin, or continue to have disturbing ischaemic events despite aspirin.

Cerebral venous thrombosis
This condition is known to produce haemorhagic infarction hence on the face of it anticoagulants would appear to be contraindicated. Nevertheless, a series of careful observations made by Bousser indicated that the extension of the infarction and the severity of the neurological deficit was decreased rather than increased by anticoagulation therapy. Hence when this condition is diagnosed, which is most reliably done by MRI, warfarin must be considered as desirable therapy.

Carotid endarterectomy
Patients with symptomatic severe carotid stenosis have significantly fewer strokes when treated with carotid endarterectomy, compared to conservative treatment (9% vs 26%).

In persons with asymptomatic carotid bruit, followed up for 8 years in the Framingham study, 28 per cent had TIA, 48 per cent had cerebral infarction, 14 per cent had cerebral embolism and 10 per cent had subarachnoid haemorrhage. Asymptomatic Carotid Atheroslerosis Study (ACAS) over 5 years showed that carotid endarterectomy lowered the risk of ipsilateral stroke to 5.1% compared to medical group (11%). Nearly half of the strokes in the surgery group were caused by preoperative arteriograms. Now MR Angiography provides a safe altenative.

Balloon angioplasty coupled with stenting is being used with increasing frequency to open stenotic carotid vessels and maintain their patency. Many new devices designed to prevent distal embolisation are undergoing clinical trials. Extracranial intracranial (ECIC) bypass surgery has been proven ineffective for atherosclerotic stenosis that is inaccessible to conventional endarterectomy.

Anticoagulation therapy of TIA and RIND is controversial. Randomized, prospective studies have failed to show prevention of stroke or death. Chronic anticoagulation increases the risk of intracerebral haemorhage several-fold and the risk increases with the duration of therapy.

Progressive stroke refers to a stepwise increase in neurologic deficit due to ischaemia, while the patient is under observation. Occlusion of the internal carotid artery is the usual underlying cause. IV heparin is likely to be beneficial in this situation, after tumour is excluded by CT scanning as a cause of this kind of presentation.

Syncope is a transient loss of consciousness that results from a sudden reduction of cerebral blood flow usually brought about by hypotension.

Episodic faintness, light headedness and reduced alertness are frequently difficult to distinguish, tending to shade into one another.

The following features are characteristic of syncope:

1. At the beginning of a syncopal attack, the patient is nearly always in an upright position (either sitting or standing). The exception is Stokes-Adams attack which could occur in any position.

2. Usually the patient is warned of the impending faint by a sense of 'feeling bad'. Nausea and sometimes vomiting may occur.

3. There is a striking pallor or ashen grey colour of the face.

4. Very often the face and body are bathed in cold perspiration.

5. The usual duration is seconds to one or two minutes, but it may last as long as half an hour.

6. Usually the patient lies motionless with the skeletal muscles relaxed.

7. Sphincter control is usually maintained.

8. The pulse is feeble or cannot be felt. The blood pressure may be low or undetectable. Breathing may be almost imperceptible.

9. Once horizontal position is adopted (either by a fall or deliberately), blood flow to the brain is restored: colour begins to return to the face, the strength of the pulse improves, breathing becomes quicker and deeper, and consciousness is regained.

10. There are no residual symptoms like headache, drowsiness or mental confusion (the usual sequelae of a convulsion).

Points of differentiation between syncope and epilepsy are given in Chapter 10 on Convulsions.

Types of Syncope

Table 22.1 gives the different causes of syncope under headings (I) reduced cerebral blood flow and (II) altered cerebral metabolism.

1. *Vasovagal:* Common faint that may be experienced by normal persons during emotional stress, especially in a warm, crowded room, after an injury, shocking accident, and during pain. Mild blood loss, prolonged bed rest, anaemia, fever, fasting and organic heart disease increase the possibility in susceptible individuals. Vagal activity leads to marked *bradycardia* (instead of tachycardia in response to hypotension and vasodilatation). While both components of the abnormal reflex (vasodilatation and bradycardia) are active in most patients, in some individuals one component may predominate accounting for the range of clinical presentations of this syndrome.

2. *Postural hypotension:* This may occur:
   (i) After prolonged illness with recumbency, especially in the elderly, with reduced muscle tone
   (ii) In diabetic, alcoholic, or nutritional neuropathy usually associated with disturbance of sweating, impotence and sphincter difficulties.
   (iii) In patients receiving antihypertensive and vasodilator drugs.
   (iv) Micturition syncope, usually seen in the elderly is a special type of postural hypotension. There may also be a mechanical diminution of venous return.

(v) In otherwise normal persons who for some unknown reasons have defective postural reflexes (which may be familial).

(vi) With primary autonomic insufficiency and dysautonomias.

3. *Carotid sinus syncope:* This may be initiated by turning of the head to one side, by a tight collar, or by shaving over the region of the sinus.

Differential diagnosis of conditions involving episodic weakness and faintness but not syncope:

1. *Anxiety attacks and hyperventilation syndrome:* This is not accompanied by facial pallor and is not relieved by recumbency. Hyperventilation results in hypocapnia, alkalosis, increased cerebrovascular resistance and decreased cerebral blood flow.

2. *Hypoglycaemia:* Mild hypoglycaemia is often of the reactive type, occurring 2 to 5 hours after eating.

3. *Hysterical fainting:* usually occurs under dramatic circumstances. The attack is unattended by any outward display of anxiety. The evident lack of change in the pulse and blood pressure or colour of the skin and mucosa distinguishes it from the vasodepressor faint. The diagnosis is based on the bizarre nature of the attack in a person who exhibits the general personality and behaviour characteristics of the hysteric.

Type of Onset of Syncope

Over period of a few seconds:

Carotid sinus syncope
Postural hypotension
Asystole
Sudden A-V block
Ventricular tachycardia

Gradual onset over several minutes:

Hyperventilation
Hypoglycaemia

Onset during exertion:

Tight stenotic lesions
of heart valves

TABLE 22.1 CAUSES OF SYNCOPE

I. *Reduced cerebral blood flow*
    A. Inadequate vasoconstrictor mechanism
        1. Vasovagal attack
        2. Postural hypotension
        3. Primary autonomic insufficiency
        4. Drugs: antihypertensive and vasodilator
        5. Carotid sinus syncope
    B. Hypovolaemia
        1. Blood loss GI bleed
        2. Addison's disease
    C. Mechanical reduction of venous return
        1. Valsalva manoeuvre (defecation syncope)
        2. Cough syncope
        3. Micturition syncope
    D. Reduced cardiac output
        1. Tight aortic/mitral stenosis, hypertrophic subaortic stenosis
        2. Pulmonary hypertension, PE
        3. Massive myocardial infarct
        4. Cardiac tamponade-pericardial effusion
    E. Arrhythmias
        1. AV block with Stokes-Adams attack
        2. Supraventricular tachycardia
        3. Ventricular tachycardia

II. *Altered state of metabolism of the brain*
    A. Anaemia
        Hypoxia
        Hypoglycaemia
        Hyperventilation & CO_2 washout
    B. Emotional disturbances: anxiety attacks, hysterical seizures

Investigations

Always record the pulse rate and blood pressure in the recumbent, sitting, and standing positions.

Normally, slow heart rates up to 35-40 per minute or rapid heart rates not exceeding 180 beats per minute do not reduce cerebral blood flow, especially when the patient is in the supine position. There are three important syndromes which must be kept in mind: Stokes-Adams syndrome; sick sinus syndrome; and Wolff Parkinson White (WPW) syndrome.

Routine ECG should be performed in almost all patients. It may show conduction abnormalities (prolonged P-R, bundle branch block) suggestive of bradyarrhythmia; pathological Q waves or prolonged QT interval suggest ventricular tachyarrhythmia. The presence of late potentials on a signal averaged ECG suggests increasing risk for ventricular tachyarrhythmias in patients with a prior myocardial infarction. Low-voltage (visually inapparent) T wave alternans is also associated with development of sustained ventricular arrhythmias.

Stokes-Adams Syndrome

This results from transient cerebral ischaemia that follows a sudden decrease in cardiac output owing to a change in cardiac rate or rhythm. The attacks of fainting may occur:

1. During episodes of ventricular tachycardia (VT), ventricular fibrillation (VF), with extreme tachycardia.
2. In complete heart block with extremely slow ventricular rate or transient asystole.
3. With sick sinus syndrome.
4. In carotid sinus hypersensitivity.
5. In subclavian steal syndrome.

Symptoms of impaired consciousness begin 3-10 seconds after circulatory arrest. The onset is often sudden, duration is seldom longer than 1-2 minutes, and generally there are no neurologic sequelae.

In a middle-aged or elderly person with repeated episodes of unexplained fainting, *Holter monitoring* is a useful investigation to document the cause of the attacks.

Sick Sinus Syndrome (SSS)

This includes a spectrum of disorders of impulse initiation and conduction, including marked sinus bradycardia, sinus arrest, sino-atrial block, AV nodal dysfunction, and recurrent supraventricular tachyarrhythmias. It can occur with ischaemic, hypertensive, rheumatic or idiopathic heart disease.

Evidence of SSS can be elicited with provocative tests such as (1) failure of appropriate acceleration of heart rate after atropine (1-2 mg IV) or isoproterenol (1-2 µg/minute IV infusion; (2) a prolonged sinus recovery time following over drive atrial stimulation; or (3) an accentuated cardioinhibitory response to carotid sinus massage.

Wolff Parkinson White Syndrome

Patients with Wolff Parkinson White Syndrome (WPW) are susceptible to several forms of supraventricular tachycardia, the most dangerous of which is atrial fibrillation with rapid ante-grade conduction to the ventricles over an accessory atrioventricular connection which may result in syncope, and in rare instances, sudden death.

Ambulatory ECG monitoring is especially required in patients with recurrent syncope (asystole, extreme bradycardia, tachyarrhythmia). When supraventricular tachycardia is suspected as a cause of syncope, electrophysiological testing is indicated to define the mechanism and pathway of the tachycardia and to facilitate the selection of an effective anti-arrhythmic intervention.

Paroxysmal ventricular tachycardia is a relatively common cause of syncope particularly in patients with structural heart disease. Thus, occurrence of unexplained syncope in a patient with structural heart disease is a potentially ominous finding and merits careful evaluation.

Cardiac syncope may also result from massive myocardial infarction particularly when associated with cardiogenic shock.

Not infrequently the cause of syncope is multifactorial. Patients with peripheral neuropathy (alcoholic, diabetic, nutritional), and elderly patients receiving polypharmacy with antihypertensive or antidepressant drugs, get orthostatic hypotension on assumption of upright posture. Many CNS disorders have associated postural hypotension (e.g. Parkinsonism–Shy-Drager Syndrome, Progressive cerebellar degeneration). Prolonged illness with recumbency, especially in elderly individuals with reduce muscle tone leads to physical deconditioning and postural syncope.

The prevention of fainting depends on the mechanism involved. In postural hypotension, patients should be cautioned against rising suddenly from bed. Instead, they should first exercise their legs for a few seconds, then sit on the edge of the bed and make sure they are not lightheaded or dizzy before standing and starting to walk.

The chief hazard of a faint in most elderly persons occurs when walking from their bed to the toilet. Carpeting the floor and rubber mats in the bathroom are desirable. Outdoor walking should be on soft ground rather than on a hard surface and the patient should avoid standing still, which is more likely than walking to induce an attack.

Upright tilt table testing is indicated for recurrent syncope, a single syncope that caused injury, or a single syncopeal event in a "high risk" setting (pilots, commercial vehicle drivers). In susceptible patients upright tilt at an angle of between 60° to 80° for 30-60 minutes induces a vasovagal episode. The reproducibility of a negative test is 85-100%.

Treatment of Syncope

First, think of the causes of fainting that constitute a therapeutic emergency; among them are:

- Massive internal haemorrhage
- Myocardial infarction (which may be painless)
- Cardiac arrhythmias

In elderly persons a sudden faint without obvious cause should arouse the suspicion of complete heart block or a tachyarrhythmia even though the clinical findings are negative when the patient is seen. Repeated episodes of fainting without apparent reason need investigation with Holter monitoring.

1. Patients seen during syncope should be placed in a supine position, with the legs raised to facilitate venous return.

2. All tight clothing and other constriction should be loosened and the head turned so that the tongue does not fall back blocking the airway.

3. Since emesis is frequent, nothing should be given by mouth until the patient has regained consciousness.

4. The patient should not be permitted to rise until the sense of physical weakness has passed, and should be watched carefully for a few minutes after rising.

23   Vertigo

Approach to a Patient with Vertigo

Vertigo consists of a sensation of rotation or turning either of the patient's body or its surroundings. The patient experiences, following an attack of vertigo, a sense of uncertainty of equilibrium and unsteadiness of the legs on walking. The patient tends to keep his head immobile out of his fear of a fresh attack, and is disinclined to walk, especially across the street. This experience is very demoralizing to the patient. Depending upon the cause the attack (i) may come in paroxysms as brief as a few seconds; (ii) may last for several hours at a time; (iii) the attack may be recurrent in some diseases; (iv) it may be brought on transiently only by certain movements or postures.

To the clinician, vertigo indicates a disturbance of (1) the labyrinth; (2) the 8th nerve; or (3) the central connections in the brains tern vestibular nucleus. The accompanying symptoms of headache, pallor, sweating, nausea, vomiting and occasional diarrhoea, point to a spread of the impulse from the vestibular nucleus to the other brainstem nuclei including the vagus.

Vertigo or Syncope?

The first question to be decided by the clinician is– Does the complaint represent true vertigo or is it syncope (giddiness, dizziness)? The following points will help to determine a true vertigo:

1. Element of rotation.
2. Associated headache, nausea, vomiting, nystagmus, ataxia.
3. Attack reproduced by movements of the head rapidly in one direction.

The causes of vertigo are listed in **Table 23.1**. By a systematic approach in history taking and physical examination (**Tables 23.2 and 23.3**), the clinician can locate the site of the trouble in one of three regions. These three types of vertigo may overlap and may occur in combinations.

> Is it in the labyrinth?
> Is it in the 8th nerve?
> Is it in the brainstem?

It is always worthwhile to get an answer so that the prognosis and treatment can be determined (**Table 23.4**). If the patient can be reassured that the trouble is peripherally located in the organ of balance and not in the brain, he can bear the nuisance of vertigo without the accompanying anxiety that something might be seriously wrong in the brain, threatening loss of life or paralysis.

Brief paroxysms usually suggest a peripheral mechanism. Longer duration suggests progressive lesions of the vestibular pathway or brainstem lesions such as multiple sclerosis or arterial occlusion.

Vertigo may be a manifestation of aura of migraine, but some patients with migraine have episodes of vertigo unassociated with their headaches. Anti-migraine treatment may be considered in such patients with otherwise enigmatic episodes of vertigo.

Vertigo secondary to temporal lobe epilepsy (vestibular epilepsy) is rare and almost always intermixed with other epilepitic manifestations.

Psychogenic vertigo is usually a concomitant of panic attacks or agoraphobia (fear of large open spaces, crowds or leaving the safety of home) Organic vertigo is accompanied by nystagmus which is absent in psychogenic vertigo.

Benign paroxysmal positional vertigo (BPPV) of the posterior semicircular canal is particularly common.

TABLE 23.1 CAUSES OF VERTIGO

A. *Labyrinthine*
   Wax in the ear
   Spread of middle ear suppuration
   'Neuronitis'? Viral
   Specific illness e.g. mumps complicated by neuro-labyrinthitis
   Benign positional vertigo
   Ménière's syndrome
   Occlusion of internal auditory artery

B. *8th nerve lesions*
   Acoustic neuroma
   Aneurysm
   Syphilitic pachymeningitis
   Arachnoiditis (could be tuberculous)

C. *Brainstem lesions*
   Vascular occlusion-vertebro-basilar territory
   Tumour
   Demyelination (multiple sclerosis)

D. *Cerebellar haemorrhage*

E. *Parietal and temporal lobe epilepsy*

F. *Drugs*
   Quinine, Streptomycin, Salicylates, Nicotine

The vertigo and accompanying nystagrmus have a distinct pattern of latency, fatiguability, and habituation that differ from the less common central positional vertigo. Moreover the pattern of nystagmus in posterior canal BPPV is distinctive.

Caloric Test

This is useful for testing the vestibular apparatus. The standard procedure is for the patient to lie down with his head raised about 30° above the horizontal. This position brings the lateral semicircular canal into the vertical plane and this is the position of maximal sensitivity to thermal stimuli. The labyrinth is stimulated by syringing the ear with water at 30°C, and then at 44°C each for 40 seconds. The cold water initiates nystagmus to the opposite side, and the warm water to the same side. The patient fixes his gaze on a point straight ahead, and the doctor records the time interval from the beginning of the syringing to the disappearance of the induced nystagmus. Delayed, brief, diminished or absent response indicates labyrinthine disease.

TABLE 23.2 QUESTIONS TO BE ASKED OF EVERY PATIENT OF VERTIGO

1. Is it the first attack or were there previous attacks? How many?

2. Was the onset sudden? Any recent throat infection?

3. Is it brought on or aggravated by movements of the head or change of position in bed?

4. Any ringing noises in the ears? Is the hearing normal?

5. Any difficulty in swallowing? Nasal regurgitation?

6. Any difficulty in walking? Tendency to fall on one side?

7. Any history of taking drugs: Streptomycin? Salicylates? Quinine? Nicotinic acid?

Treatment of Vertigo

Immediate symptomatic relief is most important for the patient

1. Phenothiazine derivatives.
   Stemetil 5 mg 1M injection *or* Siquil 10 mg IM injection.
   Phenothiazines : Prochlorperazine 5 mg IM Inj. 25 mg Suppository

2. Antihistaminic drugs
   Dramamine (50 mg tid) Betahistine (8 mg tid)
   Antihistamines : Meclizine 25-50 mg tid
                     Promethazine 25 mg IM inj. Or suppository 25 mg

3. GABA –ergic   Diazepam 2.5 mg tid
                         Clonazepam 0.25 mg Tid

When the underlying mechanism is known or suspected e.g. hydrops of the endolymph in Ménière's syndrome, salt restriction in diet and acetazolamide (Diamox) 250 mg qid may be tried.

In intractable cases of vertigo, destruction of the labyrinth by surgery or ultrasound is the only way to obtain relief from symptoms.

In cases of cerebellar haemorrhage, surgical evacuation of the haematoma is the necessary treatment.

TABLE 23.3 POINTS IN PHYSICAL EXAMINATION WHICH MUST BE NOTED IN A CASE OF VERTIGO

1. Take blood pressure: Is it high?

2. Examine the ear with a speculum: Any wax? 'Foreign body? Suppuration? Perforated drum?

3. Test the hearing: Weber's Test; Rinne's Test.

4. Test the corneal reflex on both sides: Look for nystagmus.

5. Test the facial nerve (seven); test movements of soft palate.

6. Test for cerebellar dysfunction: Finger-nose test.

7. Test for knee jerks, ankle jerks, plantars.

TABLE 23.4 DIAGNOSTIC APPROACH TO VERTIGO

Condition	Clinical picture	Confirmation by tests
A. *Labyrinthine*		
Inflammation? viral	Acute onset Benign course Recovery within days or weeks Hearing normal	Vertigo induced or aggravated by movements of head or change of position. Reduced or absent response to caloric test.
Vestibular neuronitis	No tinnitus or deafness	Vertigo induced or aggravated by movements of head, or change of position Reduced or absent response to caloric test.
Ménière's syndrome (non-inflammatory)	Repeated attacks of vertigo Progressive deafness with interval of hours to years	Audiometry: deafness of perceptive type especially for low frequency sounds.
Occlusion of internal auditory artery	Abrupt onset of vertigo and deafness Permanent loss of function	Dead labyrinth on caloric test.
B. *8th Nerve*		
Acoustic neuroma	Insidious onset Vertigo with tinnitus Perceptive deafness Decreased corneal reflex Facial paresis same side Nystagmus Cerebellar signs	Abnormal caloric response. Abnormal audiagram. X-ray: internal auditory meatus widening. CSF increased protein. CT/MRI.
C. *Brainstem*		
Multiple sclerosis	Sudden onset of vertigo and vomiting, lasting several days	Other neurological signs showing paralysis of palate.
Posterior inferior cerebellar artery thrombosis	Horizontal or vertical nystagmus	No tinnitus or deafness.

Vomiting is a protective reflex which has been utilized since antiquity by doctors to prevent further absorption of drugs or poisons in situations of poisoning or drug overdose, if detected within an hour.

But the clinician encounters vomiting and nausea as common symptoms in a wide variety of conditions: primary gastrointestinal and hepatobiliary disease, central nervous system diseases, from systemic illness, and as side effects of medications. It may also be a manifestation of hysteria and anxiety.

A careful history and physical examination will often point to a specific cause (**Fig. 24.1** and **Table 24.1**).

Analysis of History

In the otherwise healthy individual the most common cause of vomiting is an infectious illness, which is

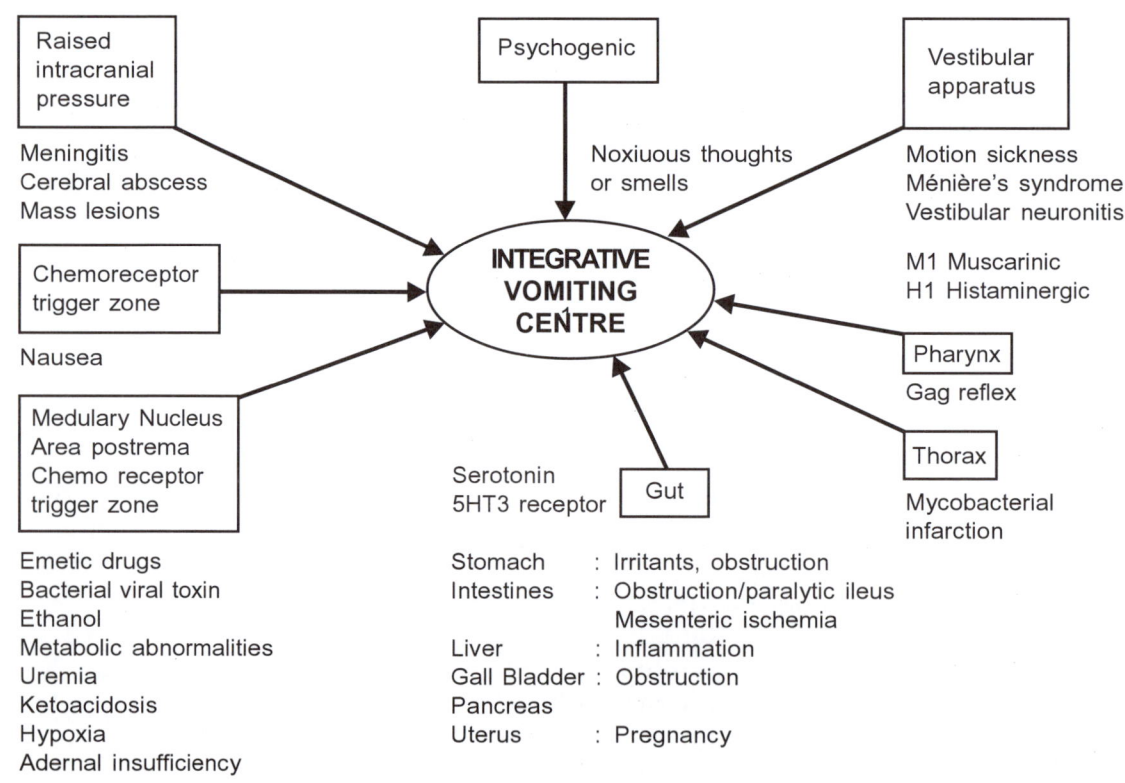

Fig. 24.1: Mechanisms of vomiting and sites of action of anti-emetic drugs

TABLE 24.1 DIAGNOSTIC FEATURES OF IMPORTANT CAUSES OF VOMITING

	Clues		Clues
A. *Local causes in stomach*		D. *Vestibular disturbances*	Vomiting associated with vertigo, nystagmus.
Gastric irritants	Drugs e.g. cisplatin	E. *Systemic illness*	
Acute dilatation of stomach	Distension of stomach.	Diabetic ketosis	Urine for sugar, acetone
Acute volvulus of stomach	History of similar previous attacks.	Renal failure	BUN, creatinine high.
Acute duodenal ileus	Dilated stomach.	Diabetic gastropathy	Other features of diabetic autonomic neuropathy.
After gastrectomy/ vagotomy	Vomiting after meals.		
Dumping syndrome	Post-prandial sinking feeling.	Addison's disease– crisis	Hypotension. Pigmentation.
B. *Reflex from other abdominal organs*		Hypercalcaemia	High serum Ca
		F. *Acute infections*	Influenza, Pertussis Malaria, Viral hepatitis.
Acute viral hepatitis	Total anorexia, urine + for bilirubin and urobilinogen.		
Inflammatory lesions	Pain and tenderness,	G. *Psychogenic*	Noxious thoughts or smells
Obstructive lesions (see also Chapter 3)	muscle guarding, rebound tenderness.	H. *Alcohol excess*	
Hyperemesis gravidarum	Signs of pregnancy.	I. *Drugs causing vomiting*	Drug history: Digitalis, Oestrogens, Ferrous sulphate,
C. *Central vomiting*			Levodopa, Opiates,
Meningitis & encephalitis	Headache, neck stiffness,		Potassium chloride, Theophylline, Anti-
Cerebral abscess Neoplasm.	papilloedema.		cancer drugs. Cisplatin.

usually of viral origin. In children, any infection may present as vomiting.

In a young married woman, presenting with nausea and vomiting in the morning the wise mother-in-law correctly diagnoses pregnancy while her doctor husband may think of viral hepatitis! Always ask for the date of the last menstrual period.

In hospitalized patients, vomiting may frequently represent drug toxicity such as with digoxin or aminophylline. Vomiting is a major symptom of cytotoxic drugs used in the treatment of malignancy.

In the post-operative period vomiting is commonly due to the anaesthetic effect.

In previously well patients sudden onset of vomiting may be due to ingested food items (shell fish, infected food, rancid fats). Excess of alcohol intake will also produce vomiting.

In patients who have had prior abdominal surgery, mechanical causes such as small bowel obstruction due to adhesions may present as vomiting.

Sudden vomiting without preceding nausea may be due to direct stimulation of the vomiting centre in the medulla, and thus may be an indication of intracranial disease.

Vomiting associated with vertigo is seen in labyrinthine disease (See Chapter 23).

Vomiting of large quantities of food and secretions late in the day or night indicates gastric outlet obstruction.

Vomiting which relieves pain is often due to a peptic ulcer.

Vomiting of blood is discussed separately (See Chapter 4).

Vomiting is common in severe myocardial infarction, and in the absence of pain ('silent' infarct) its significance may be missed. The alert clinician should elicit other symptoms like breathlessness, syncope and tiredness which may be 'angina equivalents'.

Anorexia, nausea and vomiting may be the presenting features of diabetic ketoacidosis, Addison's disease with crisis, chronic renal failure and hypercalcaemia due to various causes.

Psychogenic vomiting
Gastric secretion, motility of the alimentary tract, and blood flow are influenced by emotion. Commonly, psychological factors cause oesophageal and gastrointestinal disorders, some of which mimic organic disease.

Psychogenic vomiting is not an uncommon manifestation of anxiety neurosis. It occurs usually on waking or immediately after breakfast. Only rarely does it occur later in the day. It is probably a reaction of awakening and facing up to the realities and worries of everyday life which 'cannot be stomached'.

There may be retching alone, or the vomiting of gastric secretions or of food. Although psychogenic vomiting may occur regularly over long periods, there is little or no weight loss, and this helps to distinguish it from organic disease of the alimentary tract.

Early morning vomiting also occurs in pregnancy, alcohol abuse and depression.

Physical Examination

The main aim is to find our whether :
1. There is any evidence of an obstructed or inflammed organ.
2. There is evidence of a systemic disease.
3. There is evidence of CNS disease.

Table 24.1 gives the diagnostic features of important causes in these three categories.

Orthostatic hypotension and poor skin turgor indicate intravascular fluid depletion.

Pulmonary abnormalities raise the suspicion that the vomitus is aspirated.

Abdominal ausculation may reveal absent bowel sounds due to ileus. High pitched rushes suggest bowel obstruction, while a succession splash on abrupt lateral movement of the patient suggest gastroparesis, or pyloric obstruction.

Tenderness or involuntary guarding raises the suspicion of inflammation.

Fecal vomiting suggests gastrocolic fistula (Crohn's Disease).

Fundus examination showing papilloedema, or visual field loss or focal neurological abnormalities suggest intracranial mass lesions. (tumour, abscess, haemorrhage or hydrocephalus).

Appropriate investigation may include endoscopy, US, CT/MRI.

With this methodical approach the doctor will avoid labelling a child with incessant vomiting due to raised intra-cranial pressure, as 'gastritis' or 'pyloric obstruction'. He will also be alert in a middle-aged person with vomiting not to miss a 'silent' myocardial infarction.

Knowledge of the physiological mechanisms controlling nausea and vomiting is being used to improve anti-emetic therapy especially for patients of cancer receiving cytotoxic drugs (**Fig. 24.1**).

Neurotransmitters that mediate induction of vomiting are selective for these anatomic sites.

Lzabyrinthine disorders stimulate vestibular cholinergic muscarinic M1 and histaminergic H1 receptors, whereas gastroduodenal vagal afferent stimuli activate serotonin 5HT3 receptors. The area postrema, a medullary nucleus is richly served by nerve fibres acting on 5HT3, M1, H1 and Dopamine D2 receptor subtypes. Optimal pharmacological management is based on the understanding of these pathways.

Management

Supportive measures include nil by mouth and electral solution if tolerated. Many patients with self-limiting illness such as viral gastroenteritis will require no further treatment.

Pregnant women with hyperemesis gravidarum pose a special problem with drug treatment for fear of possible teratogenic effects. Simple measures like pyridoxine and sucking ginger may be tried preferentially to drugs.

TABLE 24.2 Treatment of nausea and vomiting

Treatment	Clinical indications	Mechanism	Example
Anti-emetic	Motion sickness Inner ear disease	Anti-histamine	meclizine 25 mg PO Dimenhydrinate 50 mg IM
		Anticholinergic antidopaminergic	Scopolamine 0.3 mg IM Prochlorperazine 5 mg PO droperidol 5 mg IM
	Medication, toxin or metabolic induced		
	Chemotherapy/radiation induced emesis	$5HT_3$ antagonists	Ondansetron 0.15 mg/kg IV granisetron 1 mg PO
	Functional nausea	Tricyclic anti- depressants	Amitriptyline 75 mg PO Nortriptyline 25 mg PO
Prokinetic Agents	Gatroparesis Intestinal pseudo- Obstruction	$5HT_4$ agonist	Cisapride
	Functionsl dyspesia	$5HT_4$ Dopamine and Dopamine antagonist	Metoclopramide 10 mg PO
		peripheral antidopaminergic	Dopamine
		Motilin agonist Somatostatin analogue	erythromycin 250 mg Octreotide 100 μg SC
Special Settings	Anti-emetic nausea Chemotherapy - induced emesis	Beuzodiazepines cannabinoid receptor Glucocorticoids	Lorazepam 2-6 mg PO Tetrahydro cannabinol 5 mg/m^2 PO Methyl Predinsolone 4 mg PO Dexamethasone 10-20 mg IV

Childrens with cyclical vomiting syndrome may be treated with seritonin 5HT3 antagonists. Considering the possible link to migrane headaches, anti-migrane therapy with 5HT1 agonist sumatriptan may be tried.

Drugs used in symptomatic relief of nausea and vomiting are described along with doses in **Table 24.2**.

GENERAL MEDICAL PROBLEMS

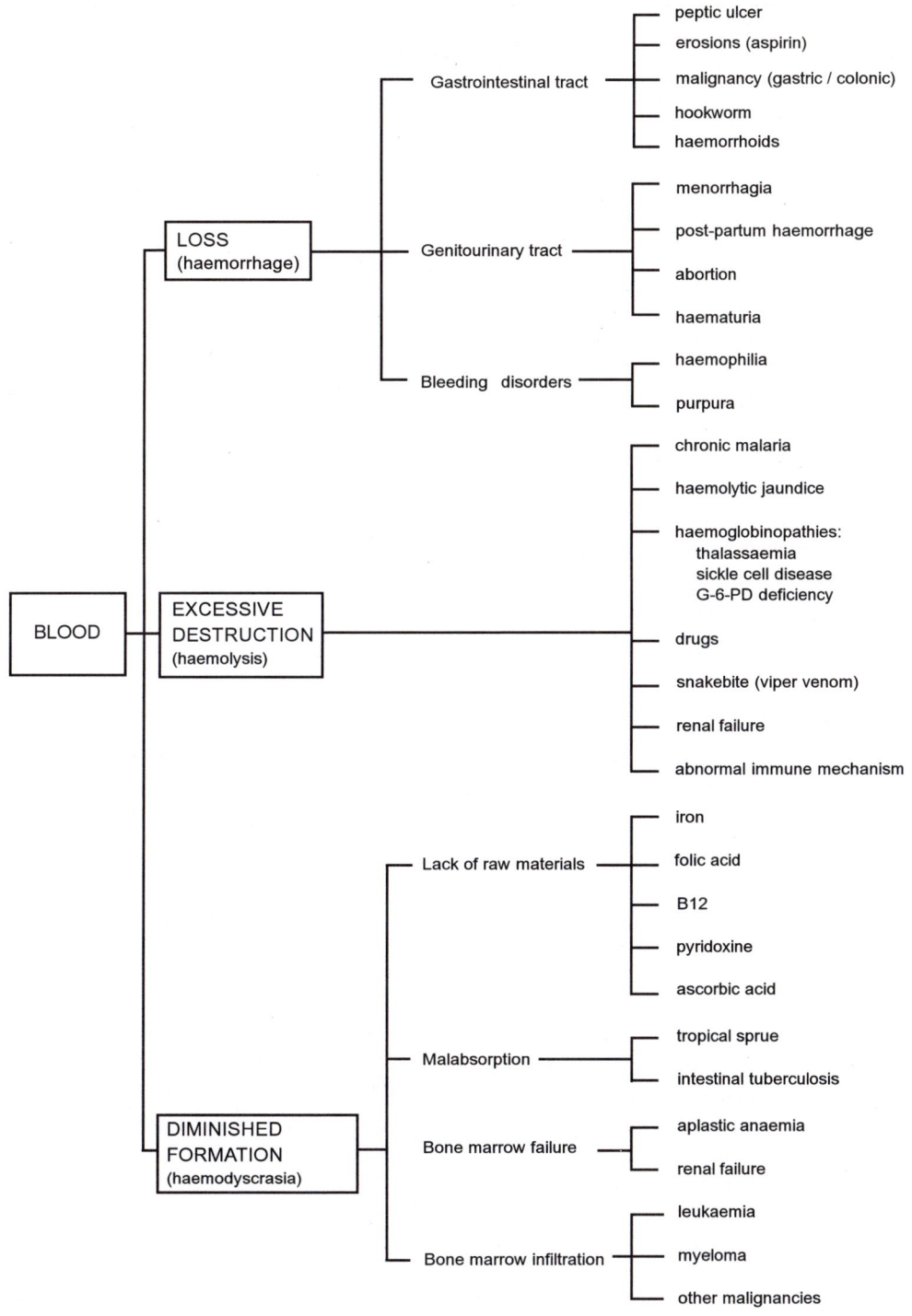

Fig. 25.1: Causes of anaemia

The clinical suspicion of anaemia is aroused by merely inspecting the colour of the skin and mucosa, and by finding *pallor*. Although this inference will be generally correct, it must be remembered that pallor can exist *without* anaemia, and anaemia can exist without pallor. The colour of the skin depends on many factors including the thickness of the epidermis, the quantity of pigment (melanin and carotene) therein, the number and degree of patency of blood vessels, and the quantity of oxyhaemoglobin and reduced haemoglobin carried within them.

Thus, the clinician should remember the following situations where pallor can give a *false* impression of anaemia:

1. Oedema of the skin or increased thickness of the skin:
   nephrotic syndrome
   scleroderma
   myxoedema.

2. Decreased melanin pigment, e.g. In the Parsi community in India.

3. Increased carotenoid pigment.

4. Decreased cutaneous blood flow:
   hypogonadism, panhypopituitarism.

On the other hand, local cutaneous vasodilatation (blushing, exercise, exposure to sun and wind) may mask an underlying anaemia. In dark persons, the palms and soles, finger nails, the lips and palpebral conjunctiva should be inspected for assessment of pallor because of minimal interference by melanin pigment in these areas. If the conjuctivae are pale, the Hb is below 10 g per cent. If the creases of the palms are pale, then the Hb is below 5 g per cent.

A combination of pallor and icterus (lemon yellow tint) suggests a haemolytic anaemia. Excess of carotene may also produce a yellow colour, especially in the palms and soles (areas with a heavy layer of stratum corneum) or forehead, nose and cheeks (rich in sebaceous glands). Unlike bilirubin, carotene and mepacrine (an antimalarial drug) do not produce a yellow colour in the sclera, bulbar conjunctiva and oral mucosa, and can thus be differentiated clinically from jaundice.

Importance of establishing the cause of anaemia (Fig. 25.1)

Anaemia is not a diagnosis by itself. It is essential to establish the cause; hence the physician must get answers to the following questions:

1. Is there *loss* of blood?

2. Is there *excessive destruction* of blood?

3. Is there *diminished formation* of blood? If so,
   - is it due to lack of raw materials in the diet?
   - is it due to malabsorption?
   - is it due to bone marrow failure?
   - is it due to bone marrow infiltration?
   - is some other disease interfering with normal marrow function?

All efforts in history-taking and physical examination should be directed at answering these questions. In a given case, more than one mechanism might be operating to produce anaemia. Multifactorial anaemia is common in clinical practice.

The importance of establishing the cause can be appreciated by looking at **Table 25.1** which indicates the diverse range of therapeutic possibilities in anaemia. It is worth appreciating that a type of therapy which is appropriate for one type of anaemia (and therefore will produce a striking response within a short period of time), may be entirely inappropriate for another type, therefore leading to waste of time waste of time and money and worsening of the

Table 25.1 THERAPEUTIC POSSIBILITIES IN ANAEMIA

Mechanism	Treatment	
I. Deficiency of raw materials: Absolute deficiency or Conditioned deficiency due to increased demand of pregnancy, growth, blood loss, haemolysis	Iron, B_{12}, Folic Acid	Common
	Pyridoxine, Ascorbic acid, Thyroxine	Rare
II. Diminished absorption: (a) Malabsorption syndrome		
(b) Blind loop syndrome competition for B_{12} by bacteria	Oral antibiotics e.g. tetracycline, doxycycline	
III. Anaemia of infection	Appropriate chemotherapy of infection	
IV. Drug-induced anaemia	Stop the drug	
V. Hypersequestration of RBCs by the spleen	Splenectomy	
VI. Immune haemolysis	Corticosteroids Immuno-suppressive drugs ± splenectomy	
VII. Bone marrow failure	Corticosteroids Androgens Oxymethalone Blood transfusion	
VIII. Bone marrow infiltration	Cytotoxic drugs Blood transfusions	
IX. Haemoglobinopathies and thalassaemia	Blood transfusion Bone marrow transplant	
X. Anaemia of chronic renal failure	Inj. erythropoietin	

Table 25.2 COMMON ERRORS IN TREATING ANAEMIA

1. Treating an adult male patient as 'iron deficiency' anaemia without making efforts to locate a source of blood loss, which may be treatable (peptic ulcer, hiatus hernia, hookworm) or sinister (gastric or colonic carcinoma) or gastric erosions (aspirin).

2. Continuing futile prescription of 'haematinics' (iron, B_{12} and folic acid) over months, while an underlying bacterial endocarditis, pyelonephritis, or tuberculosis is missed; appropriate treatment for the underlying infection would automatically lead to improvement in the anaemia.

3. Missing a thalassaemia or haemoglobinopathy and giving the patient parenteral iron when he is already overloaded with iron.

Table 25.3 COMMON CAUSES OF ANAEMIA

1. Iron deficiency
   Chronic blood loss:
   GI tract in males
   Genital tract in females

2. B_{12} and folic acid deficiency
   Nutritional deficiency
   Malabsorption
   Mixed deficiency is common

3. Anaemia of
   Infection
   Malignancy
   Chronic renal failure
   Collagen diseases (e.g. SLE, RA, PAN)

4. Haemolytic anaemia:
   Thalassaemia
   Sickle cell disease
   G-6-PD deficiency (Parsi, Bohra & Mahar communities in India)
   Chronic malaria

untreated underlying condition (of which anaemia was only one manifestation).

The so-called 'refractory' anaemia which fails to respond to treatment may in fact represent 'refractoriness of the doctor's mind'. Three common errors are observed in general practice, as shown in Table 25.2. Common causes of anaemia are given in Table 25.3; causes of sudden or rapid onset of anaemia are given in Table 25.4.

Additional factors should be suspected in any anaemic patient with worsening of a previously stable anaemia, increased blood transfusion requirements, or a poor therapeutic response to what otherwise should be adequate treatment.

Table 25.5 lists the important diagnostic clues for various causes or anaemia.

Evaluation of a Patient with Anaemia

I. *Peripheral blood smear examination*

Peripheral blood smear examination is the single most important study. in the evaluation of a patient with anaemia. If the treating physician cannot perform this himself, he should at least insist on a full report from the haematologist/pathologist, on the following:

1. Abnormal red cell morphology (e.g. microcytes, macrocytes, spherocytes, schistocytes, sickle cells, target cells, burr cells): this is informative for ascertaning the underlying cause and mechanism of anaemia.

2. Reticulocytosis and nucleated RBCs: give evidence of intense marrow stimulation.

3. Abnormal white cells: e.g. hypersegmented neutrophils in megaloblastic anaemia; or myeloblasts in leukaemia should always be sought.

Reticulocyte count essentially reflects the rate of RBC production. The laboratory reports the number of reticulocytes per 100 RBCs. This value should be corrected for the patient's degree of anaemia according to the following formula.

RPI (reticulocyte production index) =

Retic. count x $\dfrac{Hct^2}{45}$

When anaemia develops in an individual with a normally functioning bone marrow, the RPI will be increased (more than 2 per cent) in proportion to the degree of Hb deficit. A low corrected value suggests an *inadequate bone marrow response* and suggests a hypoproliferative component for the anaemia.

II. *Indices*

MCV (mean corpuscular volume) provides a useful basis in establishing a differential diagnosis. However proper interpretation of MCV requires an inspection of the peripheral smear because

1. A small number of small or large cells may be present without affecting MCV.

2. Microcytes and macrocytes may be present simultaneously, producing an MCV in the 'normal range'.

3. A high reticulocyte count will elevate MCV as those cells are larger than mature RBCs.

MCH and MCHC are derived values and usually provide little additional information.

RDW (*red cell distribution width*) is a quantitative estimation of anisocytosis that is useful in identifying cell populations of different sizes; e.g.

iron deficiency anaemia and thalassaemia are both characterized by microcytosis but the RDW is typically *elevated* in iron deficiency while it is *normal* in thalassaemia.

According to morphology, the doctor can further investigate for aetiology (**Table 25.6**). Further check-lists for microcytic hypochromic anaemia (**Table 25.7**), macrocytic anaemia (**Table 25.8**), 'refractory anaemias' (**Table 25.9**), and bone marrow failure (**Table 25.10**), will enable a final decision as to the exact cause and mechanism of anaemia.

If the pallor is associated with icterus, **Table 25.11** will give the approach to such a problem. **Table 25.12** contains a list of drugs causing anaemia.

Pyridoxine - Responsive Anemia is characterized by hypochromic microcytic RBCs with reduced life-span, high Serum iron (300 µg), normoblastic bone marrow hyperplasia with positive hemosiderin reaction. With pyridoxine 100 mg/d IM injection for a month there is a prompt reticulocyte response and Hb rises from 8 gm% to 14.5 gm% with fall in Serum Iron to 150 µg. Liver biopsy does not show any evidence of haemochromatosis. There is no evidence of Thalassemia triat or Hb A2. Indian clinicians should be aware of this treatable anemia.

Dr. R. D. Lele JIMA 1963, 41(4) 199-202. JAPI 1963, 41, 199-202; JAPI 1965 19. 215-217; IJMSc 1965 19, 215-217

TABLE 25.4 SUDDEN OR RAPID ONSET OF ANAEMIA

A. Severe blood loss (history obvious)
B. Severe haemolysis (icterus obvious)
C. Acute leukaemia (purpura, bone tenderness)
D. Aplastic anaemia (accompanying leucopenia and thrombocytopenia-purpura, oral ulcers)

TABLE 25.5 DIAGNOSTIC CLUES FROM SIGNS AND SYMPTOMS OF ANAEMIA

System	Clues common to all anaemias	Clues that suggest specific cause	Consider
I. Skin and mucosa	Pallor	Bruising	Aplastic anaemia, Leukaemia.
		Lemon yellow tinge	Meghtloblastic A, Haemolytic A.
		Pigmentation	B12 deficiency.
		Glossitis	Deficiency of iron, B12, folic acid.
		Flat or spoon-shaped nails	Iron deficiency.
		Leg ulcers	Sickle cell disease, Ch. haemolytic A.
		Follicular petechiae	Scurvy.
II. Alimentary tract and abdomen		Dysphagia	Iron deficiency.
		Diarrhoea	B12, Folic acid deficiency.
		Abdominal pain	Haemolytic A, in crisis.
		Splenomegaly	Haemolytic A, Iron deficiency, Leukaemia, Myelofibrosis.
III. Cardiovascular	Dyspnoea Tachycardia Palpitation Angina	Heart failure	Chronic haemolytic A. e. g. sickle cell, thalassaemia major, any severe chronic A.
IV. Neurological	Dizziness Fatigue Headache Irritability Tinnitus Tychopsis	Delirium	Bl2 deficiency, Thrombotic thrombocytopenic purpura.
		Peripheral neuropathy	B12 deficiency.
V. Fundus oculi		Retinal haemorrhage Tortuous vessels	Bl2 & folic acid deficiency, Sickle cell disease.
VI. Bones & joints		Pain and tenderness	Sickle cell disease, Leukaemia, Myelomatosis.

TABLE 25.6 RED CELL MORPHOLOGY RELATED TO AETIOLOGY

I. Hypochromic microcytic (**Table 25.7**) Small size of red cells Low Hb content	Iron deficiency, Chronic blood loss. Thalassaemia. Pyridoxine-responsive anaemia Sideroblastic A.
II. Macrocytic (**Table 25.8**) Large size of red cells	Vit. B12 deficiency, Folic acid deficiency, Liver disease, High reticulocytosis (blood loss, haemolysis).
III. Normocytic (**Table 25.9**) Normal size of red cells	Acute blood loss, Acute haemolysis, Bone marrow failure, Chronic infection, Malignancy.
IV. Spherocytes (**Table 25.11**) 'Cricket ball' appearance	Hereditary spherocytosis (Coomb's test negative). Acquired spherocytosis (Coomb's test positive).
V. Sickling	Sickle cell disease.
VI. Burr cells	Renal failure.
VII. Target cells	Thalassaemia.

TABLE 25.7 HYPOCHROMIC MICROCYTIC ANAEMIA:
CHECK-LIST TO ESTABLISH CAUSES

Question	Conditions	Confirmation
1. Is there obvious blood loss?	In females: menorrhagia; post-partum bleeding; abortion. In males and females: bleeding piles; haematemesis-melaena; epistaxis; haematuria; bleeding disorders.	History. Other evidence of cirrhosis liver with portal hypertension, peptic ulcer, purpura, haemophilia.
2. Is there a possibility of *hidden* blood loss?	Hookworm; habitual ingestion of aspirin; hiatus hernia; peptic ulcer; gastric carcinoma; colonic carcinoma.	Routine examination of the stools for: 1. Hookworm ova 2. Occult blood. If occult blood test is repeatedly positive and hookworm negative, then ask for: 3. Endoscopy 4. Barium meal and enema.

Laboratory confirmation of iron-deficiency anaemia

Early: MCV and MCH normal (MCV: 80-97 μm; MCH: 26.7-33.7 pg/cell)

Late: Microcytes, anisocytes, increase in RDW

Serum iron below 60 μg/dl

TIBC more than 360 μg/dl

Transferrin saturation less than 15 per cent

Serum ferritin: Less than 12 μg/dl (reflects decreased or absent stainable bone marrow haemosiderin).

Caution: Ferritin is an acute phase reactant and in inflammatory states, liver disease, and malignancy, its levels may be 'normal' even in the presence of iron deficiency.

Table 25.8 APPROACH TO DIAGNOSIS OF MEGALOBLASTIC ANAEMIA

Question	Clinical clues	Tests for confirmation
1. Is there clinical evidence of B12 deficiency?	Skin pigmentation; Glossitis; Peripheral neuropathy; Lateral and posterior column involvement; Personality changes; Psychosis.	Hypersegmented polymorphs in peripheral blood smear; Low serum B12 < 80 µg; Reticulocytic response to microdose of B12 (1 µg inj).
2. What is the pathogenesis of B12 deficiency?		
(a) Poor diet?	History of poor intake of meat, eggs, milk, cheese.	Normal absorption of radioactive B12.
(b) Lack of intrinsic factor in stomach?	Total gastrectomy; Gastric carcinoma; Pernicious anaemia (rare in India); Antibodies to gastric IF.	Low absorption of radioactive B12 improves on adding intrinsic factor RIA of IF. Associated condition with primary hypothyroidism.
(c) Malabsorption?	Tuberculosis of ileum; Tropical sprue; Small bowel resection.	Low absorption of radioactive B12. No improvement with intrinsic factor or antibiotics.
(d) Competition for B12?	Blind loop syndrome; Jejunal diverticula; Stricture; Gastro-jejunostomy.	Low absorption of radioactive B12. Improvement on oral antibiotics.
3. Is there clinical evidence of folic acid deficiency?	Glossitis; No neurological involvement (unlike in B12 deficiency).	Low serum folic acid. Normal B12. Reticulocytic response to small dose of folic acid (1 mg/day).
4. What is the pathogenesis of folic acid deficiency?		
(a) Poor diet?	History of poor intake of meat, yeast, leafy vegetables, cereals, nuts.	
(b) Alcoholism?	Tropical sprue accompanying deficiency of Vito A, D, K.	High faecal fat > 6 g.
(c) Malabsorption?		Poor absorption of D-Xylose. Flat glucose tolerance curve.
(d) Excessive demand?	Pregnancy.	Rapid response to folic acid.
(e) Antagonists to folic acid?	History of prolonged therapy with anticonvulsant drugs: diphenylhydantoin, phenobarbitone.	Improvement of anaemia on stopping drugs or giving folic acid.

Table 25.9 IMPORTANT CONDITIONS WHICH INTERFERE WITH NORMAL BONE MARROW FUNCTION

(Normochromic, normocytic anaemia or hypochromic anaemia)

Common features:	Poor response to haematinics. Low serum iron, low TIBC, high transferrin saturation. Serum ferritin levels high or normal.
I. Anaemia of infection:	Important examples: Tuberculosis (any part of the body). Pyelonephritis. Subacute bacterial endocarditis.
II. Anaemia of collagen disease:	Rheumatoid arthritis. Systemic lupus erythematosus. Polyarteritis nodosa.
III. Anaemia of renal failure:	BUN, Creatinine high, Bicarbonate low (acidosis)
IV. Anaemia of malignancy:	Multi-factorial

Table 25.10 FEATURES SUGGESTIVE OF BONE MARROW FAILURE

I. No evidence of blood loss or haemolysis, that are sufficient to account for the degree of anaemia.

II. Absent or decreased reticulocytes.

III. Associated granulocytopenia (sore throat, mouth ulcers) and thrombocytopenia Rarely pure red cell aplasia (purpuric spots).

IV. Failure of response to iron, B12, folic acid and pyridoxine.

Table 25.11 APPROACH TO A CASE OF HAEMOLYTIC ANAEMIA

Question	Clinical clues	Confirmatory tests
1. What is the evidence of haemolysis?	Icterus; Dark coloured urine and dark coloured stools; Previous episodes of jaundice.	Reticulocytosis Urine: urobilinogen++ bilirubin – High serum bilirubin (indirect).
2. Is there a precipitating factor?	History of drugs (**Table 25.12**); Malaria; Septicaemia; Lead poisoning; Snakebite.	G-6-PD level of RBCs Peripheral blood suear for MP Blood culture Lead level in blood.
3. Is haemolysis part of an underlying disorder?	Fever, joint pains other system involvement– SLE, RA. Lymph node enlargement; splenomegaly (lymphoma, leukaemia). Renal failure.	LE test, ANF and DNA antibodies Bone marrow examination BUN, Creatinine, Burr cells in the peripheral smear.
4. Is this a chronic haemolysis?	Repeated episodes of jaundice; Pigmentation. Pigment gallstones.	See tests under 5.
5. Is there any inherent defect of RBCs?	Stunted growth; Prominent cheek bones; Prominent, upper teeth (hypertrophy of maxilla); splenomegaly; Leg ulcer.	(1) Peripheral smear: spherocytes (2) Sickling test (3) Haemoglobin electrophoresis (4) Osmotic fragility (5) Autohaemolysis
6. Is there a family history/community history?	Similar episodes in siblings, parents, uncles, aunts etc. Parsi Mahar, Bengali (G-6-PD), HbE, Sickle.	Study other members for tests under 5.
7. Is it an acquired defect (AIHA)?	Diagnosis by exclusion of secondary causes (SLE), loymphoma, lukaemia, drugs, etc.	Coomb's test positive, Warm (IgG) Cold (IgM) Ab Auto immune thrombocytopenia and/or neutropenia may be present (Evan's syndrome)
8. Non-immune haemolysis PNH (paroxysmal nocturnal haemoglobinuria)	Haemolysis precipitated by infection or surgery; Thrombotic episodes (acute abdominal pain, myocardial infarcts, stroke)	Urine haemosiderin positive Ham's test-cell lysis in acid serum Bone marrow hypoplastic despite haemolysis

TABLE 25.12 ANAEMIA DUE TO DRUGS

	Mechanism	Important drugs	Confirmatory tests	Remarks
I.	Erosion or ulceration of gastrointestinal mucosa	Aspirin, NSAIDs (e.g. Butazolidin), Corticosteroids, Reserpine, Enteric coated potassium chloride tabs.	Stools for occult blood, repeated examination.	1. Avoid the drug. 2. If unavoidable, then take it on a *full* stomach along with antacids & H_2 blockers. 3. Watch for occult blood in stools.
II.	Depresssion of the bone marrow		Acompanying leucopenia; thrombocytopenia; High serum iron.	Drugs have to be discontinued temporarily and blood transfusion may become necessary.
	(a) Predicatable: dose-related	Ionizing radiation, Antimetabolites, Alkylating agents, Benzene, Heavy metals e.g. gold.		
	(b) Unpredictable: not dose-related; immune mechanism possible	Chloramphenicol, Chlorpromazine, Phenyl-butazone, Thiouracil, Sulphonamides, Streptomycin, Gold, Meprobamate, Phenytoin, Troxidone.		Effects may occur weeks or months after therapy is stopped. Prognosis poor, but some patients may recover.
III.	Haemolysis of red cells			
	(a) Glucose-6-phosphate dehydrogenase enzyme deficiency in the RBCs	Primaquine, Pamaquin Nitrofurantoin Sulphonamides, PAS, Sulphones, Phenacetin, Aspirin, Vit. K substitutes.	Low level of G-6-PD in RBCs. Coomb's test negative.	20% of the Bohra and the Parsi community and a still higher number in the Mahar community have G-6-PD deficiency.
	(b) Chemical effect of drug: dose-related No enzyme deficiency No immune mechanism	Industrial solvents, Benzene, Toluene, Phenacetin, Acetanilid.	Normal G-6-PD level, Coomb's test negative.	
	(c) Antigen-antibody reactions			
	i. Hapten type ii. 'Innocent by-stander'	Penicillin, Quinidine, Quinine, Phenacetin.	Coomb's test positive.	Stop drug. Self-limiting.
	iii. Autoimmune	Alpha-methyl dopa.	Coomb's test positive.	On stopping drug, anaemia disappears.

26 Arthralgia and Arthritis

Arthralgia, pain in the joints and *arthritis*, pain and swelling (with other features of inflammation such as heat, tenderness and limitation of movement)– are common clinical conditions. Over a hundred different types of arthritis are recognized by now. The challenge before the clinician is to use history and physical examination as his two most important tools, to come to the most probable diagnosis. The age of onset, sex, type of onset (acute or insidious), number of joints affected, (monoarticular; pauciarticular i.e. three or less joints; polyarticular i.e. four or more joints), distribution of joint involvement (symmetrical or asymmetrical, small joints or big joints) presence or absence of general constitutional symptoms (fever, anaemia, weight loss), the presence or absence of features other than in the joints, the course of the illness (single episode or recurrent episodes), precipitating factors (recent infection, trauma, drug use, sexual exposure, excessive alcohol, or exertion), presence or absence of deformities of the joints and wasting of adjacent muscles–all these features help to make a tentative diagnosis.

One should remember that with the *passage of time* the clinical picture will unfold, which may not be recognizable in the first encounter with the patient. For instance, early in the course of disease, the joint manifestations of rheumatoid arthritis and systemic lupus erythematosus (SLE) will be identical. Only when new findings suggestive of multiorgan involvement outside of the joints develop, will the true nature of the arthralgia become known. Similarly what may begin as a monoarthritis may in course of time become polyarthritis, thereby necessitating a review of the alternative diagnostic possibilities.

Causes of polyarthritis are listed in **Table 26.1**, and their diagnostic features in **Tables 26.2** and **26.3**.

The systemic clues in the physical examination are listed in **Table 26.4**. Causes of monoarthritis are listed in **Table 26.5**, along with the distinguishing features in **Table 26.6**; causes according to age are listed in **Table 26.7**, and according to sex in **Table 26.8**. Drugs causing arthralgia/arthritis are listed in **Table 26.9**.

Laboratory Tests

Hb and ESR provide a general guide regarding the presence or absence of systemic effects of arthritis. For instance in osteoarthritis Hb and ESR are normal.

Leucocytosis indicates infection or inflammation including gouty arthritis. In haemophilia and haemarthrosis the warmth and swelling in the joint along with leucocytosis may lead to a misdiagnosis of septic arthritis, hence it is always necessary to inquire about a past history of bleeding tendency.

Rheumatoid Factor (RF) test is now routinely available but since a typical clinical picture of rheumatoid arthritis (RA) can occur both in the presence or absence of RF positivity, and since the management is not altered by the test result, too much importance should not be given to this test (which furthermore can be positive in other non-rheumatic conditions such as subacute bacterial endocarditis).

ANF is useful as a screening test for SLE.

Since the outlook of SLE is more serious than RA in terms of systemic complications, it is a good practice to have this test done in every case of so-called 'rheumatoid arthritis'.

HLA B27 is mainly a research tool. Since typical SSA syndrome can occur in the absence of test positivity, and since a large number of healthy people without SSA are positive, this test should not be employed for diagnostic decisions in an individual patient.

TABLE 26.1 CAUSES OF POLYARTHRITIS

	Aetiology	Acute	Chronic
I.	Infection	Gonococcal	
		Meningococcal	Meningococcal septicaemia
		Staphylococcal	
		Streptococcal	
		Viral-dengue, rubella etc.	
		Lymphogranuloma	
		Syphilis	
		Yersinia	
		Lyme's disease	May be recurrent
		Acute lepra reaction	May be recurrent
II.	Immune-mediated	Rheumatic fever	May be recurrent
		Serum sickness	
		Drug reactions	
		Henoch-Schonlein purpura	May be recurrent
III.	Collagen disease	Rheumatoid arthritis	Remission & relapses
		Systemic lupus erythematosis	Remission & relapses
		Polyarteritis nodosa	
		Progressive systemic sclerosis	
		Sjögren's syndrome	
		Polymyalgia rheumatica	
		Relapsing polychondritis	May be recurrent
IV.	Reactive arthritis	Bacillary dysentery (Shigella)	
		Ulcerative colitis	
		Crohn's disease	
		Whipple's disease	
V.	Metabolic	Gout	May be recurrent
		Crystal arthritis	May be recurrent
VI.	Haematologic	Haemophilia	May be recurrent
		Sickle cell disease	
VII.	Malignancy	Pulmonary osteoarthropathy	
VIII.	Miscellaneous	Sarcoidosis	
		Amyloidosis	

X-ray of the joint may be normal in the early stages of most acute arthritis patients. Its main use is in chronic arthritis to assess the extent of damage to the joint cartilages.

Radionuclide joint scanning is the most sensitive modality to demonstrate active sacroiliac disease, and. to indicate asymptomatic involvement of several joints in the so-called 'monoarthritis'.

TABLE 26.2 DIAGNOSTIC FEATURES OF IMPORTANT DISEASES CAUSING POLYARTHRITIS

Disease	Clinical	Laboratory
Rheumatic fever with arthritis (RF)	Children or young adults; Previous history strepto-tonsillitis or skin lesions; Acute onset with fever; Pain & swelling in several joints one after another.	ASO titre > 400 units
Rheumatoid Arthritis (RA)	Females : Males 2:1; Most common age at onset 30-50; Symmetrical involvement of small joints (hands, feet); Chronic, progressive, deforming; Systemic manifestations can occur but rarer than other groups (e.g. SLE).	Rheumatoid factor RF + (80%) ANA + (30%)
Juvenile RA 5 sub-groups	Children and young adults: i. Systemic onset (Still's disease) ii. Polyarthritis (more than 4) ≡ adult RA iii. Polyarthritis iv. Oligoarthritis < 3) early age of onset. v. Oligoarthritis : late onset.	RF + RF − ANA + HLA B27
Sjögren's syndrome (SS)	Dry mouth and dry eyes (Sicca syndrome); Parotid enlargement (a) occurs alone or (b) with RA, SLE, SS Non-articular manifestations.	
Felty's syndrome	Triad of RA Splenomegaly Granulocytopenia Anaemia, thrombocytopenia may also be present. Frequent infections Chronic leg ulcers.	
Systemic Lupus Erythematosus (SLE)	Females > Males 8:1; Most common age at onset 15-40; Arthritis/arthralgia ≡ RA Skin lesions (85%); Nephritis (60%); Pleurisy or pericarditis.	ANA + high titre (95%) LE cells + (65-75%) Anti ds DNA Ab + Anti Sm Ab +
Polyarteritis Nodosa (PAN)	Males : Females 3:1; Most common age at onset 30-50; Arthralgia/arthritis ≡ RA Systemic manifestations: fever, weight loss, nephritis, hypertension, pulmonary, hepatic, CNS, mononeuritis multiplex.	RF +ve in only 37% ANA −ve Muscle biopsy: vasculitis

Table 26.3 SPONDYLOARTHROPATHIES

Disease	Clinical	Laboratory
Ankylosing Spondylitis (AS)	Males: Females 3:1; Commonest age at onset 12-40; Systemic symptoms ±; Insidious onset of low back pain: lumbar or buttock areas; Tender sacroiliac joints; Loss of lumbar lordosis; Limitation of movement; Hip and shoulder involvement; Chest expansion less than 3.75 cm (1.5").	RF (-) HLA B27 (+) in 90% X-ray obliteration of sacroiliac joint Radionuclide scan sacroiliac: sacrum ratio > 1.8
Reiters' Syndrome (RS)	Males: Females 9:1; Young adults; Systemic symptoms: acute onset; Monoarticular or polyarticular; Urethritis; Conjunctivitis; Skin lesions: keratoderma blenorrhagica.	RF (-) HLA B27 (+) in 75% asymmetrical, e.g. one knee, opposite ankle, single PIP of one hand; low back pain in 30%
Reactive arthritis	No urethritis or conjuctivitis but other prior episodes of Shigella dysentery, ulcerative colitis; Asymmetric joint involvement; Large joints more commonly affected; Lower limb joints (80-90%) upper limb joints (50%); Typically oligoarthritis; Enthesopathy (35%).	
Psoriatic Arthritis	Both sexes; Common age of onset 20-40; Pauciarticular or polyarticular ≡ RA Distal phalangeal joint; Nail involvement correlates better with joint involvement.	RF (-) HLA B27 (+) in 50%

Table 26.5 CAUSES OF MONOARTHRITIS

	Distribution
Acute monoarthritis	
Trauma	
	Any joint
Infection (e.g. gonoccocal)	Any joint: usually large
Gout	Big toe
Pseudo-gout (Crystal disease)	
Haemarthrosis (Haemophilia)	Large joints e.g. knee
Henoch-Schönlein purpura	Knee
Chronic monoarthritis	
Degenerative joint disease	Weightbearing joints: hips, knees, spine, shoulder (bus conductor's), fingers (spin bowler's)
Tuberculosis	Any joint big or small (dactilitis)
Atypical rheumatoid arthritis	
Neurogenic arthropathy (Charcot's joint)	
Diabetic neuropathy	Ankle, foot
Syringomyelia	Shoulder, elbow
Tabes dorsalis	Knee
Leprosy	Metatarsal joint, interphalangeal joints

TABLE 26.4 CLUES IN POLYARTHRITIS FROM EXTRA-ARTICULAR MANIFESTATIONS

System	Findings	Disease Association
1. Eyes	Conjuctivitis;	Gonococcal
		Reiter's syndrome
	Episcleritis;	Rheumatoid arthritis
		Polyarteritis nodosa
	Uveitis;	Ankylosing spondylitis
		Ulcerative colitis
		Sarcoidosis
	Keratitis sicca;	Sjögren's syndrome
	Visual changes: band keratopathy.	Juvenile Rheumatoid Arthritis
2. Skin	Hypopigmented anaesthetic patch;	Leprosy: Acute lepra reaction
	Butterfly rash on face;	Systemic lupus erythematosus
	Small, red, non-blanching spots on upper limbs; Keratoderma blenorrhagica palms and soles; Brown papules; Chronic lesions resemble psoriasis;	Gonococcal arthritis
	Petechiae & purpura;	Henoch-Schönlein purpura
	Urticaria, Erythema multiforme;	Serum sickness drug allergy
		Systemic lupus erythematosus.
	Nodules over pressure points & extensor surface;	Rheumatic fever
		Rheumatoid A
	Olecranon bursa; Tophi;	Gout
	Psoriasis of skin & nails;	Psoriasis arthropathy
		SLE
		PAN
		Systemic sclerosis
	Raynaud's phenomenon.	
3. Oral cavity	Transient, painless superficial ulcers.	Behcet's syndrome
		SLE
4. Haemopoietic	Splenomegaly' & lymphadenopathy;	Still's disease, SLE, Sarcoidosis
	Bleeding disorder.	Haemophilia, SLE
5. Genito-urinary	Urethritis;	Gonococcal arthritis
	Prostatitis;	Reiter's syndrome
	Cervicitis;	
	Vaginitis;	
	Calculi;	Gout
	Nephropathy;	SLE
	Proteinuria;	Polyarteritis nodosa
	Abnormal sediments.	Subacute bact. endocarditis
6. Respiraory	Pleuritis;	Tuberculosis
		SLE
		Rheumatoid arthritis
	Parenchymal lung infiltrates;	Sarcoidosis
		Rheumatoid arthritis
		Polyarteritis nodosa
		SLE.
	Hilar lymphadenopathy.	Sarcoidosis
		SLE

(Contd)

TABLE **26.4** (Contd)

System	Findings	Disease Association
7. Cardio-vascular	Pericarditis	Rheumatic fever
	Myocarditis	Rheumatoid arthritis
	Conduction defects	SLE
	Endocarditis	Rheumatic fever
		SLE
		Subacute bacterial endocarditis
	Aortic incompetence	Ankylosing spondylitis
		Reiter's syndrome
		Rheumatoid arthritis
	Raynaud's phenomena	SLE
		Polyarteritis
		Systemic sclerosis
8. Gastro-intestinal	Enteritis	Bacillary dysentery (Shigella)
	Colitis	Ulcerative colitis
	Malabsorption	Tuberculosis
		Whipple's disease
9. Neurologic	Loss of pain and deep sensation	Neurogenic arthropathy
	Absent ankle jerk	Tabes
		Diabetes
		Hansen's disease
		PAN
	Meningoencephalitis	
	Collagen diseases	
	Optic neuritis	
	Proximal neuropathy	
	Peripheral neuropathy	

TABLE **26.6** DISTINGUISHING FEATURES OF MONOARTICULAR ARTHRITIS

Disease	Diagnostic features	Confirmatory tests
1. Trauma	Abrupt onset; History of significant injury; Lack of systemic signs; Self-limiting course; If prolonged consider tuberculosis.	Normal Hb% & ESR Synovial fluid non-inflammatory, may be haemorrhagic.
2. Infection	Acute onset; Focus of infection elsewhere; Fever with chills; Large joints usually affected.	Synovial fluid Exudate: 50,000 WBCs with low sugar Response to antibiotics
i. Gonococcal	Acute monoarticular or history of urethritis 3-4 weeks previously (knee, small carpal/tarsal joints) or evanescent polyarticular tenosynovitis with cutaneous lesions.	Urethral/endocervical smears and culture ELISA test for gonococcal antigen joint aspiration

(Contd)

TABLE 26.6 (Contd)

	Disease	Diagnostic features	Confirmatory tests
ii.	Non-gonococcal	Usually Staphylococcus aureus (70%) & Streptococcus; Gram negative organisms in IV drug abuse; brucellosis.	Brucella agglutination
iii.	Non-bacterial septic arthritis:	Many viral infections.	
iv.	Lyme disease	Tickborne spirochaete Borrelia burghdorferi: Arthritis preceded by annular rash; Knee joint alone or diffuse arthralgia: may be recurrent; Meningoencephalitis; Cardiac conduction abnormalities.	ELISA Test for antibodies Confirmed by Western blotting
3.	Tuberculosis	Insidious onset (may be preceded by trauma); knee, hip or wrist tenosynovitis.	Synovial fluid exudate Biopsy characteristic Response to anti-TB drugs
4.	Degenerative joint disease	Middle-aged or elderly persons; Pain with weight-bearing and exercise; Hip, knee; Minimal or absent inflammation; No contractures or ankylosis: General health not affected.	X-ray characteristic: subchondral sclerosis Marginal spur Hb and ESR normal
5.	Osteochondritis dessicans	Adolescents & young adults; Acute & chronic symptoms; Knee joint predominantly affected; Non-inflammatory effusion.	X-ray characteristic: density or defect of articular surface of femoral condyle
6.	Gout	Acute onset; Family history; Predominantly middle-aged men (postmenopausal women); Recurrent attacks; Single joint, usually big toe; Intense inflammation; Fever and leucocytosis 20,000 or more.	Ear tophi; olecranon bursa Serum uric acid high Uric acid crystals in synovial fluid Response to colchicine
7.	Pseudo-gout (chondro-calcinosis)	Mimics gout in acuteness and intensity of inflammation; Fever, leucocytosis, calcification joint cartilage, knee, wrist, pubic symphysis.	Serum uric acid normal Calcium pyrophosphate crystals in synovial fluid
8.	Intermittent hydrarthrosis	Primarily young women; One or both knees; Effusion in joints, exacerbated with menses; No systemic features; Subsequent rheumatoid arthritis in a small minority.	X-ray negative Synovial fluid non-inflammatory
9.	Pigmented villonodular synovitis	Primarily knee joint; Recurrent effusions.	Synovial fluid haemorrhagic Synovial biopsy characteristic Surgical removal necessary

(Contd)

TABLE 26.6 (Contd)

Disease	Diagnostic features	Confirmatory tests
10. Haemophilia (with haemarthrosis)	Acute onset; Usually knee; Local signs may be confused for acute infective arthritis; Confounded by leucocytosis and fever; Previous history of bleeding usually obtained.	Prolonged clotting time (CT) Prolonged partial thromboplastin time (PIT) Fresh blood transfusion or cryoprecipate controls the conditions.
11. Neurogenic (Charcot's joint)	Diabetes mellitus; Leprosy; Tabes dorsalis; Syringomyelia.	Painless destroyed joints on X-ray Other features of these disorders
12. Henoch-Schonlein purpura	Children & young adults; Knee pain and swelling along with fever; Abdominal pain; Skin purpuric rash.	Increased fragility of capillaries Urine for RBCs Platelets, BT, CT normal

TABLE 26.7 CAUSES OF ARTHRITIS ACCORDING TO AGE

Young children	Trauma
	Rheumatic fever & arthritis
	Juvenile rheumatoid arthritis
	Haemophilia
Adolescents	SSA, Rheumatic fever & arthritis
Young Adults	Gonococcal arthritis
	SLE
	SSA
	Reactive arthritis
	Psoriatic arthritis
Middle age	Gout
	Osteoarthritis
	Rheumatoid arthritis

TABLE 26.8 SEX PREDOMINANCE IN ARTHRITIS

Male pre-dominance	Gout (9:1)
	Reiter's syndrome (9:1)
	Polyarteritis nodosa (3:1)
	Ankylosing spondylitis (3:1)
Female pre-dominance	SLE (8:1)
	Rheumatoid arthritis (2:1)
	Gonococcal arthritis (males get prompt treatment for gonorrhoea, while it remains undetected in females)

TABLE 26.9 DRUGS CAUSING ARTHRALGIA/ARTHRITIS

Penicillin	Hydralazine
Sulfonamides	Procainamide
Iodides	Thiouracil
Hydantoin	

TABLE 26.10 DRUGS USED IN THE TREATMENT OF ARTHRITIS

A. *Non-steroidal anti-inflammatory drugs*

Aspirin (acetylsalicylate)	650-1300 mg qid	
Choline salicylate	650 mg/ teaspoonful	
Diclofenac	50-75 mg bid	
Flurbiprofen	350-400 mg tid	
Ibuprofen	400 mg qid	
Indomethacin	25 mg bid	
Naproxen	50 mg tid-qid	
Phenylbutazone	100 mg tid	
Piroxicam	20 mg qid	
Sulindac	150-200 mg bid	
Tolmetin sodium	400 mg tid	

B. *Glucocorticoid preparations*

Prednisolone	20-40 mg/d	Max. 60-100 mg/d
Methyl-prednisolone	16-32 mg/d	Max. 48-80 mg/d
Dexamethasone	3-6 mg/d	Max. 9-15 mg/d
Betamethasone	2.4-4.8 mg/d	Max. 7.2-12 mg/d

TABLE 26.11 DISEASE-MODIFYING ANTI-RHEUMATIC DRUGS (DMARD)

	Drug	Dosage and maximum	Side-effects	Comments
1.	Chloroquine	250 mg/d	Nausea, vomiting, abdominal pain, corneal deposits, retinopathy.	Commonly used drug; regular eye check necessary.
2.	Hydroxychloroquine	400 mg/d	Nausea, vomiting, abdominal pain, corneal deposits, retinopathy.	Initial drug for less severe disease.
3.	Sulphasalazine	2 g/d	Skin rash, GI disturbance, granulocytopenia, megaloblastic A.	Induced remission in short-term studies.
4.	Injectable gold (sodium aurothiomalate, sodium aurothioglucose)	50 mg IM/wk	Dermatitis, stomatitis, leucopenia, thrombocytopenia, proteinuria, nephrotic syndrome.	Regular follow-up essential; test urine and blood before each injection.
5.	Oral gold	6 mg/d	Diarrhoea, skin rash.	Haematological and renal complications less than with injectable gold.
6.	D. Penicillamine	500 mg/d	Dermatitis, stomatitis, leucopenia, thrombocytopenia, proteinuria, nephrotic syndrome.	Start with low dose; increase slowly; toxicity high at higher dose. Check urine & blood.
7.	Methotrexate	7.5-15 mg/wk oral or IV	GI side-effects, hepatic & pulmonary.	Monitor hepatic and pulmonary function.
8.	Azathioprine	100-150 mg/d	GI side effects, leucopenia.	All cytotoxic drugs have a small but significant increase in the occurrence of neoplasia.
9.	Cyclophosphamide	100 mg/d	GI side-effects, alopecia, haemorrhagic cystitis.	
10.	Cyclosporine	10 mg/kg/d	Hypertension, nephrotoxicity.	

Note: • The appearance of benefit from DMARD therapy is usually delayed for weeks or months, hence NSAIDs must be continued during their administration • Careful monitoring for toxicity is needed • Failure to respond to one drug does not preclude responsiveness to another, and it is not possible to determine the drug of first choice • For severe erosive disease with vasculitis, DMARD may be given early in the course of the disease.

GLUCOSTEROIDS ARE INDICATED *ONLY* IN:
1. Patients with RA who continue to have active synovitis in multiple joints despite sufficient trial of NSAIDs, gold, hydroxychloroquine or penicillamine.
2. Patients with severe constitutional symptoms (e.g. fever and weight loss), anaemia or vasculitis.
3. Occasionally a patient incapacitated by arthritis and at risk for complications from immobility may be given glucosteroids in an attempt to control the disease while awaiting a response to slower-acting, disease-modifying agents.
4. Intra-articular steroid therapy of the most painful 2 or 3 joints may delay or negate the need for systemic glucocorticoids.

Management of Arthritis and Rheumatological Disease (Tables 26.10 and 26.11)

Disease	Management goals
Rheumatoid arthritis	Aspirin, NSAIDs: routine use Corticosteroids: emergency use 1) Suppression of inflammation in joints and other tissues. 2) Maintenance of joint and muscle function and prevention of deformities. 3) Repair of joint damage when such repair will relieve pain or improve function.
Ankylosing spondylitis	Indomethacin 25 mg bid or tid. Progression of spinal disease currently cannot be prevented. Therapeutic goal is to maximize the opportunity for the apophyseal joints to fuse in a straight line. Such fusion minimizes eventual postural defect and respiratory compromise. Sleep supine on a firm bed without a pillow. Practise postural and deep breathing exercises regularly.
Infective	Typically acute monoarticular arthritis with fever; haematogenous spread may affect multiple joints e.g. gonococcal. 1) Intravenous antibiotics ensure good serum and synovial fluid levels of drug (intra-articular not needed). 2) Repeated arthrocentesis to remove destructive by-products of inflammation when swelling persists. 3) Surgical drainage in Septic hip, Shoulder. Joints that do not respond in 5-7 days to appropriate antibiotics and arthrocentesis. 4) NSAIDs to relieve pain and increase joint mobility.

Newer Drugs

TNFα Ab : Infliximab and Adalimumab are available for treatment of severe rheumatoid arthritis and ankylosing spondylitis with dramatic effects. Low dose - less than 3 mg/kg of infliximab once in 4 to 8 weeks, or 20 mg adalimumab weekly, high dose > 6 mg/kg infliximab every 8 weeks or 40 mg adalimumab every other week. But there is a serious increased risk of infection (e.g. flare-up of latent tuberculosis) and malignancy. This is because TNF plays an important role in host defense against infection & tumor growth control (JAMA 2013, 309(16), 1973.

Etanercept, a fusion protein TNF inhibitor induces apoptosis in synovial macrophages. It is marketed as Enbrel. It has similar disadvantages like TNFα mAbs such as flare-up of latent infection including Hepatitis B. The cost of Embrel for RA is about $ 20,000 a year. Cipla's Etacept is a biosimilar of Etanercept launched in April 2013, with 30% less cost. Indian guidelines on screening and prophylaxis prior to biological therapy are available (Handa R et al APLAR J. Rheum. 2006, 9, 181-83) chest radiograph/CT. TNFα mA induced tuberculosis).

Anti-Il-6 receptor mAb-Tocilizumab is equally effective in RA, but free from the risk of flare-up of infection.

Reference : Malaviya AN et al J. Rheum 2010, 37, 1.

Backache is one of the most common problems in general medicine. It is second only to upper respiratory infections as a cause of days lost from work.

It is convenient to distinguish those patients who have an acute onset of back pain from those with a more chronic course.

Acute backache often begins after an injury or strain such as a fall, lifting a heavy object or twisting suddenly. Sometimes there may be no preceding event. Symptoms are often in the lower back and consist of pain, spasm of the paravertebral muscles, and an inability to bend. Coughing, straining, or bending may aggravate the pain. The most likely causes are (1) a prolapse of the intervertebral disc; (2) 'lumbago' arising from the fascial covering of the lumbar muscles; or (3) collapse of a vertebra also causes sudden severe pain not necessarily located in the lumbosacral region; it may occur anywhere, usually in the mid-dorsal region. In women, low back pain may be referred from acute gynaecological lesions.

In the cervical region, acute onset of pain usually follows a 'whip lash' (sudden extension-flexion movement) of the neck, or is due to spondylosis. The pain is usually over the lower portion of the neck with palpable spasm of the posterior cervical muscles.

Chronic backache usually arises from poor posture, indolence, weak paravertebral muscles and obesity, often in combination. In women low back pain, especially over the sacral region, can result from pelvic inflammatory disease, or pelvic tumours. The three main questions the doctor should raise in his mind are:

Is the pain arising in the vertebral column? (**Table 27.1**)

Is the pain referred from other organs? (**Table 27.2**)

Is the pain psychogenic?

A thorough physical examination will help to answer these questions.

Systematic palpation for tenderness is important.

The information obtained thereby is summarized in **Table 27.3**. Apart from tenderness, limitation of movement and deformity should be noted.

If the pain is suggestive of root compression (pain aggravated by coughing, sneezing or straining) one should look for hyperaesthesia or hypo aesthesia, and neurological signs.

If no local evidence is found in the back, the question arises: is the pain referred from other organs? For this a thorough abdominal, rectal and vaginal examination is necessary. In middle-aged and elderly persons, assessment of the peripheral vascular system is essential. In these persons, vascular, neoplastic and inflammatory causes are to be considered.

Referred pain is not accompanied by local tenderness. Upper abdominal disease is referred to the lower thoracic region (8th thoracic to 1-2 lumbar).

Lower abdominal disease is referred to the lumbar region (2-4 lumbar).

Pelvic disease is referred to the sacral region.

In elderly patients with lumbar canal stenosis, there is encroachment on the roots of the cauda equina. Patients complain of low back pain, often bilateral, along the sciatic distribution, aggravated by standing or walking, and relieved by rest. Motor, reflex and sensory changes may be present. The peripheral pulses are felt, which differentiate 'lumbar claudication' from that due to peripheral vascular disease.

TABLE 27.1 CAUSES OF BACK PAIN

Cause	Diagnostic features
I. *Intervertebral disc prolapse*	
Most common lesion: L_5-S_1	Acute onset of pain.
	Pain in mid-gluteal region, posterior part of thigh, posterior calf & heel, plantar surface of foot, 4th and 5th toe.
	Absent ankle jerk.
Next most common lesion: L_4-L_5	Pain in hip, groin, posterolateral thigh, lateral calf, dorsum of foot, 1st, 2nd and 3rd toe.
Less common lesion: L_3-L_4	Pain in anterior part of thigh and knee.
Least common lesion: L_2-L_3	Inverted Lasègue's sign (pain with hyperextension of limb with patient prone).
II. *Collapse of vertebra*	Acute onset of pain.
Trauma	Local tenderness, deformity.
Metabolic bone disease	Limitation of movement.
Metastatic bone disease	See **Table 27.3**.
Myeloma Lymphoma	
III. *Tuberculosis of spine or sacroiliac joint*	Insidious onset.
	Duration more than a month.
	Weight loss, fever, raised ESR, local tenderness, usually middorsal or sacroiliac.
IV. *Spinal cord tumour*	Pyramidal, posterior column signs.
V. *Osteoarthritis of spine*	Chronic nature of pain.
	Pain centred over the spine.
	Stiffness, limitation of movement, relief by rest. No systemic signs (fever, malaise). Normal ESR.
VI. *Spondyloarthropathy*	Younger age group.
SSA	Morning stiffness of back.
Reiter's syndrome	Tenderness over sacroiliac joint.
Reactive arthritis	Limitation of chest expansion.
	High ESR.
VII. *Lumbar Canal Stenosis*	Pain in one or both legs on walking, relieved by rest.
	Signs of root compression.
	Confirmed by CT/MRI.
	Surgical decompression.

Plain X-ray of the vertebrae will show degenerative changes of osteoarthritis, collapse of the vertebrae, and narrowing of the intervertebral disc space in the cervical and lumbar region.

Degenerative changes are seen in the bone X-rays of most people (90 per cent) after the age of 40, but only a small proportion of them (5 per cent) develop symptoms. Hence it is important to be sure that the symptoms complained of are due to osteoarthritis and not to other causes.

CT is more helpful in demonstrating herniated discs. MRI clearly shows the root compression by the bulging disc fragment, thereby eliminating the need for contrast myelography.

Metabolic Bone Disease

This includes the following 4 groups:
Nutritional rickets and osteomalacia.
Involutional (post-menopausal) osteoporosis.
Hyperparathyroidism.
Renal osteodystrophy.

TABLE 27.2 CAUSES OF REFERRED BACK PAIN

I. *Retroperitoneal lesions*
   Lymphoma
   Sarcoma
   Carcinoma
   Retroperitoneal haemorrhage
      (anticoagulant therapy)

II. *Aneurysm of abdominal aorta*

III. *Abdominal organ disease*
   Upper abdomen
      Posterior wall peptic ulcer
      Pancreatitis
      Pancreatic carcinoma
   Lower abdomen
      Colitis
      Diverticulitis
      Colon cancer
      Renal tumours

IV. *Pelvic organ disease*
   Menstrual pain
   Last weeks of pregnancy
   Pelvic inflammatory disease
   Endometriosis
   Carcinoma of uterus & cervix
   Sigmoid colon cancer
   Carcinoma prostate
   Chronic prostatitis

TABLE 27.3 PALPATION FOR TENDERNESS ASSOCIATED WITH BACK PAIN

Cervical vertebrae
   $\left. \begin{array}{l} C_5\text{-}C_6 \\ C_6\text{-}C_7 \end{array} \right\}$ DISC prolapse
   C_1-C_3, Rheumatoid arthritis
   Any level, Tuberculosis

Upper thoracic vertebrae
   Tuberculosis
   Metastasis from carcinoma
   Osteoporosis

Costo-vertebral angle
   Renal/adrenal disease
   Injury to transverse process of L_1, L_2

Spinous process
   L_5, S_1 Faulty posture
   Occasionally, spina bifida occulta

Sacroiliac ligaments
   L_5, S_1 disc prolapse
   Tuberculosis (usually unilateral)

Sacrococcygeal junction
   Sacrococcygeal injury, sprain/fracture

Sacrosciatic notch
   L_4-L_5 disc rupture
   Sacroiliac sprain

Sciatic nerve trunk
   Ruptured lumbar disc or sciatic nerve lesion

Osteomalacia due to combined calcium and vitamin D deficiency is common in women in developing countries, in whom repeated pregnancy and lactation deplete the bone minerals and vitamin D reserves. Hence any woman with two or more children, presenting with low back pain, muscular weakness, and difficulty in rising up from the squatting position unaided, should be regarded as a case of osteomalacia unless proved otherwise. It is a pity if the doctor misses such a treatable condition.

Osteoporosis is common in post-menopausal women. The reduced volume of bone tissue leads to compression of the trabecular bone in the vertebrae, and causes back pain.

Primary hyperparathyroidism is commonly caused by a parathyroid adenoma (more in young women than in men). Secondary hyperparathyroidism results from disturbance of vitamin D metabolism from renal disease. Patients with long-standing secondary hyperparathyroidism may develop tertiary (autonomous) hyperparathyroidism with absolute and persistent hypercalcaemia. Occasionally, tertiary hyperparathyroidism may develop in long-standing nutritional osteomalacia.

Renal osteodystrophy usually presents as a combination of osteomalacia and secondary hyperparathyroidism resulting from 1.25 $(OH)_2$ D3 deficiency and hyperphosphataemia.

Today most doctors have the facility of routinely having the serum calcium, phosphorus, alkaline phosphatase and urinary calcium and phosphorus estimations carried out. In addition, many laboratories provide RIA of parathyroid hormone (PTH) and urinary hydroxyproline. These tests help to categorize metabolic bone disorders as shown in **Table 27.4**.

Table 27.4 LABORATORY EVALUATION OF METABOLIC BONE DISEASE

	Nutritional osteomalacia	Osteoporosis	Renal osteodystrophy	Primary hyperparathyroidism
Plasma				
Calcium	N/L	N	N/L	H
Phosphorus	L/N	N	H	L
Alkaline phosphatase	H	N	H	H
PTH	H	N/H	H	H
Urine				
Calcium	L	N/H	L	H
Phosphorus	L	N	H	H
Hydroxyproline	H (GA)	N	H	H

N = Normal   L = Low   H = High
GA = Generalized aminoaciduria

Features that Suggest that Back Pain is Serious

Recent onset
Weight loss
Symptoms elsewhere e.g. cough
Localized pain in the dorsal spine
Fever Raised ESR

Investigations to Consider in a Patient with Back Pain

Plain X-rays
Blood count and ESR
Serum calcium, phosphorus and alkaline phosphatase
Serum acid phosphate and prostate–specific antigen
Serum protein electrophoresis, immunoglobulins
Radionuclide bone scan
MRI

Management of Backache

1. Sprains and strains: NSAIDs, heat massage.

2. Sacroiliac strain: Bed rest and NSAIDs.

3. Disc disease:

   Acute disc prolapse [usually in age group (20-40)]
   Rest for a few days on a firm bed.

   Corsets may be used in the acute stage for support.

   Analgesics and NSAIDs for pain relief.

Diazepan 5 mg bid. for short periods as a muscle relaxant.

Surgery only for severe or increasing neurologic impairment e.g. footdrop or bladder symptoms.

Physiotherapy in recovery stage to relieve pain, correct posture, and restore movement–Back exercises.

Chronic disc degeneration

Analgesics and NSAIDs – Transcutaneous nerve stimulation; acupuncture.

Physiotherapy – back exercises.

Advice about way of life, lifting weights, firm beds, weight reduction for abused patients.

Surgery for severe pain despite conservative measures.

4. *Spondylolisthesis:* for large displacement causing severe pain especially in a younger patient without associated degenerative changes–surgery (spinal fusion).

5. *Spinal canal stenosis:* Surgical decompression.

6. *Spinal tuberculosis:* INAH, rifampicin, pyrazinamide, for 6-8 months.

Obscure Type of Low Back Pain

The practitioner is frequently consulted by persons who complain of low back pain of obscure origin. Usually the disorder is benign in nature, and results from some minor derangement, muscular strain or disc prolapse. This is particularly true for pain of acute onset, aggravated by movement and relieved by rest.

Even after exhaustive studies including CT and MRI, some patients continue to have pain without any evidence of anatomic or pathologic lesions. Poor posture may be the cause of pain brought about by prolonged sitting or standing. The pain is *diffuse* in nature, and is relieved by bed rest. Exercises to strengthen the paraspinal and abdominal muscles are sometimes beneficial to these patients.

Low back pain is common in chronic anxiety states and depression, and in patients with compensation neurosis, hysteria and malingering.

In depressed patients, the pain is often continuous in nature and obscure in origin. There are associated symptoms of fatigue, insomnia etc. Antidepressants may have an important role in the management of chronic pain whether in the back or elsewhere.

Back Pain as a Somatoform Disorder

Somatoform disorders are those in which symptoms suggest an organic disease but there is no evidence of a physical disorder that might explain these symptoms. Patients with this diagnosis do not have depressive symptoms and do not usually respond to antidepressant drugs. Anxiolytics and muscle relaxants are usually prescribed for them, with little or no benefit. Many patients have had multiple operations for discogenic disease with or without orthodesis of the lumbar vertebrae but the pain and disability persist, raising doubts about the indications for the original surgery, especially with non-neurologic signs. When a new physician sees them for the first time, they often have unrealistic expectations. Frequently they state that none of their previous doctors was competent and that this is their last hope for relief from their suffering. *A group approach* (a physician, physiotherapist and psychiatrist) is more likely to avoid another treatment failure. Drug therapy should be minimum and major emphasis should be on massage, transcutaneous electrical nerve stimulation (TENS) and functional rehabilitation.

Prevention of Backache

There would be fewer back and neck problems if adults kept their trunk muscles in optimal condition by regular exercise. For patients with chronic back discomfort, weight reduction and a programme to strengthen the abdominal and paraspinal muscles is helpful. Correct sitting posture is facilitated by well-designed furniture and auto seats. It is estimated that pressures between discs are increased 200 per cent by changing from a recumbent to a standing position, and 400 per cent by sitting slumped in an easy chair. Long trips in a car or plane without change in position put maximum strain on discs and ligamentous structures in the spine. Professionals who are required to bend frequently e.g. nurses, dock workers, should be taught the correct way of lifting weights. Lifting from a position of a flexed trunk, as in removing a suitcase from the holding of a car, is dangerous. One should always lift the object holding it close to the body. Sudden strenuous activity without conditioning and warm-up is always likely to cause trouble to discs and ligaments. Simple measures for house wives like raised platforms for cooking, long handles for brooms and mops for sweeping the floor, will go a long way in preventing backaches in women.

Chest pain is a frequent presenting complaint. To the patient its significance is usually more ominous than that of other symptoms; he is apprehensive that it indicates a 'heart attack'. The major concern of the clinician is therefore to establish or exclude chest pain of cardiac origin, with its propensity to produce sudden unexpected death.

The physician may see the patient in one of two settings:

(1) Severe chest pain, suddenly appearing for the first time, which is prolonged, which does not have any obvious initiating factors; the patient appears very ill and probably a medical emergency is on hand (such as acute myocardial infarction, pulmonary embolism or dissecting aneurysm).

(2) History of brief episodes of pain in a patient who is reasonably healthy between episodes.

The main tools of a clinician are history taking and physical examination. When chest pain is a presenting symptom, the physical examination often does not reveal any abnormality, hence a good history and analysis of the characteristics of the chest pain become all the more important.

The following characteristics of chest pain must be identified in each and every case;

1. Location (origin and radiation)
2. Quality (sharp or dull etc.)
3. Quantity (severity and duration in minutes)
4. Chronology (periodicity to date)
5. Setting in which pain occurs
6. Aggravating and relieving factors
7. Associated symptoms (dyspnoea, cough, sweating etc.)

With this analysis the clinician is able to distinguish acute from chronic disease processes, and to determine if a life-threatening process is involved. The analysis also prompts the clinician to check for appropriate findings in physical examination and laboratory tests, as indicated below.

Causes and Mechanisms of Chest Pain

Table 28.1 lists the important causes of chest pain and **Table 28.2** gives their characteristic clinical features. It will be noted that chest pain may have its origin in the *intrathoracic structures* (heart and pericardium, aorta and pulmonary artery, pleura and oesophagus) or in the various tissues of the *chest wall* (skin, muscle, ribs and cartilages, sternum, vertebrae, nerve roots, mammary gland), or in *structures below the diaphragm* (gallbladder, pancreas, splenic flexure of colon, stomach and duodenum). When the pain arises in the skin or superficial structures, it can usually be localized accurately by the patient. When it arises in deeper structures it may be diffuse and difficult to localize, or it may radiate in such a pattern as to mislead both patient and physician into believing that the lesion lies elsewhere. A typical example is the referred pain of ischaemic heart disease to the jaw, leading to a visit to the dental surgeon.

Many thoracic structures, including the heart and aorta, the pleura and oesophagus are supplied by sensory fibres which originate in the same segment of the spinal cord. Pain fibres from the heart and pericardium are carried principally in the sympathetic nerves, but some reach the central nervous system via the vagus and phrenic nerves; the latter also carry the pain fibres from the pericardium, diaphragm and diaphragmatic pleura. This pathway accounts for the referral of pericardial pain to the trapezius and shoulder.

TABLE 28.1 CAUSES OF CHEST PAIN

I. *Cardiovascular system*

    A. *Angina pectoris:* Ischaemia

    (a) Diminished supply due to coronary artery disease

        Atherosclerotic coronary artery disease

        Coronary artery spasm

        Coronary vasculitis Coronary embolism

    (b) Increased myocardial demand due to hypertrophy

        Severe valvular disease e.g. aortic stenosis

        Severe hypertension

        Obstructive cardiomyopathy

        Dilated cardiomyopathy

    (c) Anginal syndrome with no identifiable cause

    B. *Acute pericarditis*

    C. *Pulmonary embolism and infarct*

    D. *Dissecting aneurysm of aorta*

II. *Respiratory system*

    Pleurisy and pneumonia

    Bornholm disease (Coxsackie B viral infection)

    Pneumothorax Carcinoma lung

III. *Chest wall causes*

    Thoracic outlet syndrome

    Herpes zoster involving thoracic nerve roots

    Nerve root pressure: TB spine, vertebral metastases

    Mondor's disease (Phlebitis of subcutaneous anterior thoracic veins)

    Costo-chondritis: Tietze's syndrome, Xiphoidodynia

IV. *Alimentary system*

    Oesophageal reflux, Oesophageal spasm

    Perforation of thoracic· oesophagus (mediastinal emphysema)

    Gallbladder disease

    Pancreatitis

    Splenic flexure syndrome

V. *Anxiety neurosis*

    Commonest problem in differentiation from organic pain

Pain arising from the oesophagus, biliary tract (acute cholecystitis, passage of gallstone) and less frequently the stomach and duodenum, is often confused with cardiac pain. To confuse matters further, oesophageal spasm which often accompanies reflux oesophagitis, may be relieved by nitroglycerin. ECG changes may accompany these gastrointestinal disorders, and disease in the gastrointestinal tract may serve as a trigger for acute cardiac events.

Typical anginal pain which radiates to the left arm and neck may occur in patients with normal coronary angiograms. There is no clear explanation for this, but probably about 50 per cent of them may have an oesophageal cause which can be confirmed by a supine hydrochloric acid perfusion test which typically reproduces the heartburn or chest pain. In 30 per cent of these patients, IV edrophonium (80 µg per kilogram body weight), by increasing oesophageal contractility, reproduces the chest pain. Because coronary artery disease and oesophageal disease may frequently coexist in older patients, the former should be excluded before testing for the latter. Demonstrating to the patient that his pain is definitely due to an oesophageal (and not cardiac) cause is reassuring and anxiety-relieving.

The basic mechanism of chest pain due to anxiety neurosis is poorly understood. Experimentally, chest pain, palpitations, dyspnoea, tremors, and sweating have been produced by infusion of adrenaline and nor-adrenaline.

Ischaemic Cardiac Pain

Myocardial ischaemia is defined as a condition of myocardial oxygen deprivation secondary to diminished perfusion of blood. During exercise, in response to increased cardiac work and increased demand for oxygen, the normal coronary vascular bed dilates to increase the blood supply five-fold. Angina pectoris (chest pain) produced by exertion and relieved by rest occurs most commonly because an atherosclerotic obstruction of the coronary arteries prevents an increase in blood flow. In simple terms it is a demand–supply problem, with the trouble at the supply end.

TABLE 28.2 CHARACTERISTIC FEATURES OF VARIOUS CAUSES OF CHEST PAIN

Condition	Origin & radiation	Quality	Duration	Aggravating factors	Relieving factors	Associated features	Comments
1. Angina pectoris	Retrosternal: neck, jaw, upper limbs.	Tightness, pressure, squeezing, crushing, heaviness, aching, burning, 'indigestion'	5 to 10 mins or shorter if precipitating factors are relieved.	Stress; physical, emotional, heavy meal, cold weather, smoking, sexual intercourse.	Rest, Nitroglycerin within 1-2 mins.	Transient systolic murmur; S_3 or S_4 gallop may be heard during episode.	Pain relieved within 1-5 mins usually; 5-15 mins if precipitated by emotional stress; pain lasting longer than 20 mins is always serious.
2. Variant angina	Same as in angina pectoris.	Same as in angina pectoris but more severe.	More prolonged 10-20 mins.	May occur at rest or on mild exertion.	Nitroglycerin, nifedipine.	Weakness, dizziness, dyspnoea, sweating, arrhythmia.	Coronary spasm alone (25%) or in addition to atherosclerosis (75%) decided by coronary angiography.
3. Pericarditis	Precordial; neck, shoulder.	Sharp, occasionally crushing.	Several hours or days.	Breathing, swallowing, lying flat.	Sitting up.	Pericardial rub, local tenderness may be present.	Can be confused with musculoskeletal pain, because of local tenderness.
4. Mitral valve prolapse	Precordial.	Sharp and brief.	Few seconds.	Not related to exertion.	Not relieved by nitroglycerin.	Palpitations, dyspnoea, fatigue, systolic click & murmur.	Exercise ECG may show ST depression in upto 60% patients but mostly benign condition, occasionally sudden unexpected death.
5. Pulmonary embolism	Substernal.	Pressure; choking, simulates angina.	Several minutes.	Breathing: chest movements.	Lying flat.	Haemoptysis ±, dyspnoea, tachypnoea.	Must be suspected in post-operative, post-traumatic or postpartum patients confined to bed.

(Contd)

TABLE 28.2 (Contd)

	Condition	Origin & radiation	Quality	Duration	Aggravating factors	Relieving factors	Associated features	Comments
6.	Dissecting aneurysm	Chest, neck, upper back, interscapular, lower back, abdomen, legs.	Ripping, tearing, boring.	Hours; severity maximum at onset, unlike myocardial which increases	Unusual physical exertion, hypertension.	None.	Diminished or absent radial pulse	X-ray chest will show widening of the superior mediastinum; aortography confirms dissection.
7.	Oesophageal pain	Retrosternal, shoulders, arms.	Burning.	5–10 mins or shorter if precipitating factor relieved.	Lying/flat, bending forward, citrous juice.	Sitting up, Antacid, Nitroglycerin.	Hiatus hernia, Gallbladder disease.	Pain reproduced by acid infusion in gullet or IV edrophonium.
8.	Mediastinal emphysema (e.g. thoracic oesophageal perforation)	Substernal, radiating to epigastrium, neck, back.	Severe, tearing pain mimicking myocardial infarction.	Several hours.		None.	Fever, dysphagia, palpable subcutaneous crepitations.	X-ray chest shows mediastinal air, pneumothorax, pleural effusion.
9.	Pleural pain (pleurisy, pneumothorax)	Side of the chest, shoulder, upper abdomen.	Sharp, stabbing.	Several hours or days.	Breathing, coughing.	Lying down on affected side.	Fever, cough, pleural rub, dyspnoea.	X-ray chest may show pleural effusion or pneumothorax.
10.	Chest wall pain	Costochondral, sternochondral junctions, chest wall muscles.	Dull ache, sometimes, acute, sharp.	Few seconds or several hours or days.	Movements: turning, twisting, deep breathing, shoulder and arm movements.	Not relieved by nitroglycerin, relieved by aspirin.	Local tenderness.	Cardiac surgery may be followed by many types of chest wall pain which create fear about fresh heart trouble.
11.	Anxiety neurosis	Left inframammary or any other area across the sternum.	Usually sharp, tightness, aching.	A few seconds or several hours or days.	Emotional, tension, no relationship to exertion.	Reassurance, tranquillizers, not relieved by nitroglycerin.	Emotional disorders, deep sighing breathing. choking feeling in throat.	Frequently confused with ischaemic cardiac pain.

Increased myocardial demand due to ventricular hypertrophy (severe valvular disease, hypertension, obstructive cardiomyopathy) can lead to ischaemic cardiac pain with normal coronary arteries. In some situations increased demand and decreased supply coexist (as in severe aortic stenosis or hypertension with coronary atherosclerosis).

Coronary artery spasm mediated by alpha adrenergic receptors can cause ischaemia even at rest or during mild physical activity. Coronary spasm can occur in normal vessels (25 per cent) or in atherosclerotic vessels (75 per cent). In Prinzmetal's syndrome or variant angina, the pain is more intense and lasts longer than in angina of effort. The attacks often occur at approximately the same time each day and may recur in a cyclic waxing and waning fashion. Possible explanations include hyper-reactivity of the vessel wall, increase in circulating. catecholamines, and local release of vasospastic substances such as thromboxane A_2 from local platelet aggregation. Tobacco smoking also contributes to coronary artery spasm and is therefore a definite health hazard.

Coronary angiography alone can decide if the syndrome is caused only by coronary spasm, or is caused by spasm in addition to high grade fixed atherosclerotic lesions. Spasm may occur in a major feeder vessel or in the collateral vessels.

Stable and Unstable Angina

Stable angina implies that there has been no change in the angina in the previous 60 days. The pain has been present for some time (months to years), occurs predictably with exertion, and is alleviated rapidly with rest and nitroglycerin. There is always some event that is responsible for in creasing the myocardial oxygen demands.

Unstable angina implies that (1) the angina has started or has increased within the previous 60 days; (2) the pain may occur at rest without obvious provoking factors; (3) it may last *longer than* 10 minutes; and (4) nitroglycerin may offer no relief or incomplete relief.

The distinction between stable and unstable angina is useful since the prognosis and management strategies are different for the two conditions.

Rupture or erosions of a vulnerable plaque causes acute coronary syndrome. Patients with unstable. angina are at a much higher risk for early myocardial infarction and early death. Hence it is good practice to refer these patients for hospitalization and observation in an intensive coronary care unit and further investigation with coronary arteriography for more aggressive therapy (bypass or angioplasty). (see also chapter : Acute myocardial infarct).

Limitations of History

The importance of history-taking and a careful analysis of the symptoms has been emphasized earlier, but it is equally important to appreciate its limitations. While a typical history of angina pectoris, i.e. pain in the chest brought on by exercise and relieved by rest or nitroglycerin, is a highly sensitive and specific indicator of ischaemic coronary artery disease, the converse is not true. *Absence of angina* does not mean absence of severe or significant coronary artery disease. Wide experience with exercise radionuclide ventriculography (Ex-RNV) has shown that marked changes in global and regional ventricular function due to ischaemia during exercise occur *in the absence of pain*. Silent myocardial infarction has been detected by special investigations in the absence of pain. Sudden unexpected death may be the first and only symptom in as many as 25 per cent of patients with coronary artery disease. One should recognize *angina equivalents* in patients without angina pectoris. Some patients may experience *dyspnoea* at rest or with mild effort; this is due to transient myocardial ischaemia resulting in acute decrease in left ventricular compliance and transient left ventricular failure. Palpitations at rest and exhaustion at times may be angina equivalents. Another point to be appreciated in relation to anginal pain is that *severity* of pain is not related to prognosis, while *duration* is. A patient may have severe and terrifying angina due to a high grade obstruction of the right coronary artery, yet this has a fairly good long-term prognosis; while another patient with only a mild angina may have high grade obstruction of the left main coronary artery with a very poor long-term prognosis.

Limitations of Physical Examination

Physical examination helps to identify many of the causes of chest pain listed in **Table 28.1**. Palpation for local tenderness over muscles, ribs, cartilages, sternum and vertebral column, gives valuable clues. Percussion and auscultation reveal clues for respiratory causes. Cardiac auscultation may reveal pericardial rub, cardiac murmurs and systolic click of mitral valve prolapse. But most cases of angina pectoris do not reveal any abnormal physical signs in the chest.

Chest X-ray may be considered now as an integral part of physical examination and will give clues for many conditions listed in **Table 28.1**. It must be remembered that carcinoma of the lung may present with chest pain and may be detected only on radiological examination, with no physical signs.

With the increasing use of 2D echocardiography the condition of mitral valve prolapse is being diagnosed more often. Most patients with this syndrome do not have symptoms, and just because chest pain and prolapse coexist does not mean that the two are causally related.

Utility and Limitations of ECG

When coronary artery disease is suspected and cannot be ruled out as a cause of angina, additional diagnostic procedures must be considered. The *rest ECG* may be normal in as many as 50-70 per cent of patients with stable angina pectoris, when they are not experiencing angina. Hence the importance of *exercise ECG* which has, however, false positive and false negative results in 20-30 per cent. When the history is classical, a positive exercise test does not increase the predictive value that already exists and a negative stress ECG does not eliminate the possibility of the disease being present. Exercise radionuclide ventriculography (Ex-RNV) (or the ECG-gated equilibrium blood pool study) by showing exercise-induced fall in LVEF with regional wall motion abnormality which is reversed by nitroglycerin, improves the sensitivity and specificity of the stress ECG diagnosis by 20 per cent. For instance, if the pre-test probability of coronary artery disease is 40-50 per cent, then a negative stress ECG and negative Ex-RNV together reduce the post-test probability to less than 5 per cent. On the other hand, a positive stress ECG and Ex-RNV increases the probability to more than 97 per cent. Ex-RNV, apart from helping to confirm or exclude the diagnosis, helps to assess risk stratification based on exercise ejection fraction (high, low or intermediate risk for future coronary events and death); assesses the functional significance of angiographically proved lesions in the coronary arteries; predicts which patients will benefit by bypass surgery or angioplasty; and evaluates the results of these procedures. Stress myocardial perfusion imaging helps to determine the culprit lesions from among those seen on angiography, and also helps to assess the viability of the myocardium.

Patient Education

A large number of anxious patients with chest pain spend a large amount of money making hundreds of visits to doctors and having innumerable ECGs and laboratory tests. Frequently these patients have minor or irrelevant physical findings. An adequate history and physical examination with appropriate tests followed by an explanation to the patient about the nature of the problem, may be reassuring. Supportive psychotherapy may be needed for the large number of patients with anxiety neurosis.

Once the diagnosis of angina pectoris has been established, the patient should be advised about the natural history of the illness, the possible complications of the disease, and the side effects of drug therapy. Advice about lifestyle and health-related behaviour (diet, exercise, weight control, abstinence from smoking and alcohol) should be given. In cases of unstable angina or variant angina the need for hospitalization of angina lasting for longer than 20 minutes and the need for coronary arteriography must be explained. If coronary bypass or angioplasty are planned, the patient must know about the possible results and complications of the procedure so that he can be helped to make an appropriate choice. After bypass, patients may develop chest pain due to a variety of noncardiac causes which may upset or demoralize them. Here again proper analysis of the history will help in the assessment of the real situation.

Approach to a Patient with Cough

Coughing is a normal respiratory defence reflex and as such occurs intermittently in all individuals. Cough is also the most common and important respiratory symptom. The diagnosis of 'abnormal cough' necessitates further diagnostic work-up. The history is the most important aspect of this work-up. Information elicited by questions regarding its onset, duration, severity, sputum production, association with exercise, meals, posture, season, exposure to environmental agents, and association with other respiratory or systemic complaints, is important and in a majority of cases leads to the correct diagnosis.

Some patients, especially females, are inclined to swallow sputum and not expectorate it. This may lead to the erroneous conclusion that the cough is not productive and thus may lead to a consideration of a different set of diseases (such as interstitial pulmonary fibrosis or endobronchial tumour).

Some patients are at high risk for disease. These need special attention:

- Cigarette smoking
- Environmental pollution
- HIV infection-for PCP and tuberculosis
- Immobilization-hypostatic pneumonia, pulmonary embolism

Many drugs can produce or aggravate cough hence drug history is also important; e.g. ACE inhibitors or beta-adrenergic blockers given for the treatment of hypertension may cause troublesome cough.

The important clues in relation to the diagnosis of cough are given in **Table 29.1**.

Looking at the sputum is very informative. For instance there may be only saliva, or copious foul smelling sputum, or it may show blood streaks. Clues obtained from sputum are given in **Table 29.2**.

Physical Examination

Tables 29.3 and **29.4** list the physical signs of important respiratory diseases causing cough. Apart from the examination of the chest, the doctor should examine the paranasal sinuses and nasopharynx for congestion, polyps and post-nasal drip. The ear canals and tympanic membrane should be examined for rare foreign body or cerumen which may reflexly stimulate cough. The neck should be palpated for lymph nodes and the fingers examined for clubbing. **Fig. 29.1** indicates the clues from general examination in respiratory diseases.

If the physical examination does not reveal any findings, a chest X-ray is mandatory. In developing countries pulmonary tuberculosis is common and in the present context of AIDS, tuberculosis has become universally important. Anyone coughing for more than a month must have an X-ray of the chest even if there are no physical findings in the chest.

Total and differential WBC count showing eosinophilia is useful in diagnosis of tropical eosinophilia, asthma and hypersensitivity reactions.

If the physical examination and chest X-ray are normal, a follow-up visit in 4-6 weeks should be arranged to ensure that the cough has gone. This is particularly true for a post-viral or infectious cough and smoker's cough. Smokers should be urged to stop smoking, as this may frequently rid them of the cough. If the coughing persists, a progressive work-up should begin, for rare or unusual causes of cough.

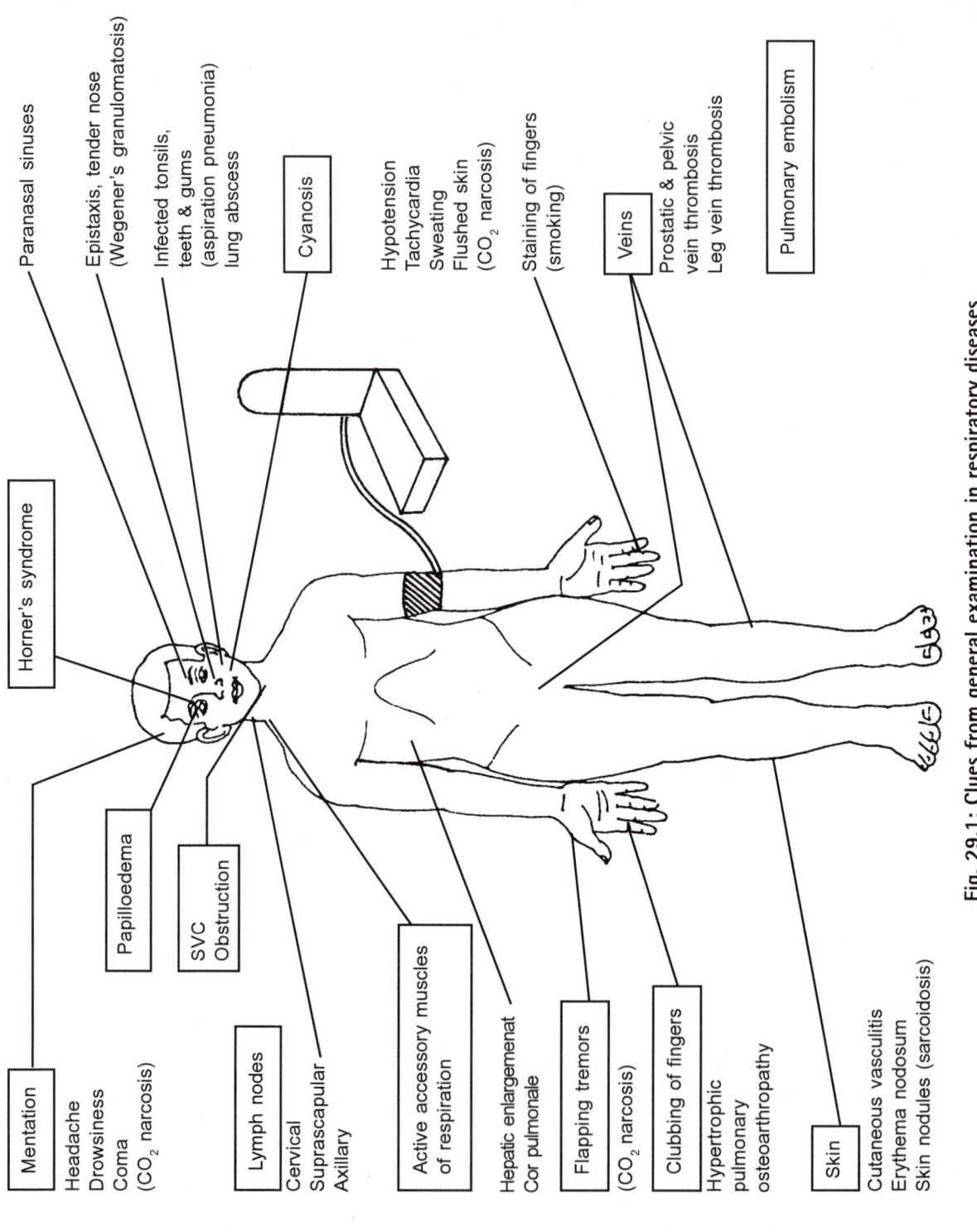

Paranasal sinuses

Epistaxis, tender nose
(Wegener's granulomatosis)

Infected tonsils,
teeth & gums
(aspiration pneumonia)
lung abscess

Cyanosis

Hypotension
Tachycardia
Sweating
Flushed skin
(CO_2 narcosis)

Staining of fingers
(smoking)

Veins

Prostatic & pelvic
vein thrombosis
Leg vein thrombosis

Pulmonary embolism

Horner's syndrome

Mentation

Headache
Drowsiness
Coma
(CO_2 narcosis)

Papilloedema

SVC
Obstruction

Lymph nodes

Cervical
Suprascapular
Axillary

Active accessory muscles
of respiration

Hepatic enlargemenat
Cor pulmonale

Flapping tremors

(CO_2 narcosis)

Clubbing of fingers

Hypertrophic
pulmonary
osteoarthropathy

Skin

Cutaneous vasculitis
Erythema nodosum
Skin nodules (sarcoidosis)

Fig. 29.1: Clues from general examination in respiratory diseases

Cough

TABLE 29.1 CLUES FROM HISTORY REGARDING CAUSE OF COUGH

Complaints	Possible Cause
A. Acute Cough	
Acute onset in previously well person	Foreign body aspiration; Acute episode of asthma; Acute bronchitis.
Acute onset with fever	Viral/bacterial pneumonia.
Acute onset with dyspnoea	Pulmonary embolism; Left ventricular failure.
B. Chronic cough	
Cough more than a month	Pulmonary tuberculosis; Post-nasal drip from sinus infection.
Cough associated with fever, weight loss and other systemic manifestations	Tuberculosis; Collagen vascular disease; Lung cancer.
Cough related to posture	Bronchiectasis; Lung abscess; Pressure of mediastinal mass on bronchi.
Cough related to meals	Oesophageal diverticulum; Oesophageal reflux with aspiration; Tracheo-oesophageal fistula.
Cough worse at night	Mitral stenosis; Left ventricular failure; Bronchial asthma; Tropical eosinophilia.
Cough related to work	'Monday morning cough'; Byssinosis.
Cough related to seasonal exposures	Allergic asthma.
Cough related to exercise	Bronchial asthma; Cardiac decompensation.
Cough present throughout patient's life	Chronic bronchitis; Asthma; Bronchiectasis.
Cough non-productive	Endobronchial tumour; Diffuse pulmonary fibrosis.
Barking cough	Whooping cough; Psychological cough.
Brassy cough	Trachea or major bronchus compression.

NOTE: Any change in the nature or character of a chronic cough in a cigarette smoker should lead to a fresh diagnostic evaluation, particularly to exclude malignancy.

TABLE 29.2 INFORMATION FROM SPUTUM EXAMINATION

Colour	
White	Mucoid: does not need antibiotics.
Yellow Green Brown	Bacterial infection: requires antibiotics.
Anchovy sauce	Amoebic abscess of liver ruptured into lung.
Black	Atmospheric pollution: coal workers.
Rusty	Pneumonia.
Frothy	Pulmonary oedema.
Serous frothy	Bronchoalveolar carcinoma.
Consistency	
Solid	Bronchial asthma.
Casts	Aspergillosis.
Quantity	
Profuse	Chronic bronchitis.
Profuse + purulent	Bronchiectasis, lung abscess.
Smell	
Foetid	Anaerobic infection in lung abscess or bronchiectasis.

NOTE: Microscopic examination and culture of sputum should be carried out in all cases.

Mediastinal lymph nodes or masses causing cough may be better shown on a CT scan.

Bronchoscopy is often indicated in persistent undiagnosed cough (malignant or stenosing bronchial lesions, foreign body which is non-opaque). Transbronchial lung biopsy could be obtained through a bronchoscope.

The Problem of Persistent Unexplained Cough

Most chronic coughs are associated with established disease such as chronic bronchitis or bronchogenic carcinoma. There remains a small group of patients with a normal chest X-ray and spirometry, who have a persistent unexplained cough. In these patients one should consider the following possibilities.

Bronchial asthma: Chronic cough rather than wheezing may be the only manifestation of bronchial asthma. This can be confirmed by methacholine challenge. The cough can be relieved by bronchodilators e. g. salbutamol.

TABLE 29.3 PHYSICAL SIGNS IN RESPIRATORY DISEASES

Condition	Movements of chest wall	Trachea	Percussion note	Breath sounds	VF/VR	Accompanying sounds
Bronchitis acute & chronic	Normal or symmetrically reduced	Central	Normal	Vesicular with prolonged expiration	Normal	Rhonchi; coarse crepitations.
Bronchial asthma	Symmetrically reduced	Central	Normal	Vesicular with prolonged expiration	Normal or reduced	Rhonchi, mainly expiratory, sibilant.
Emphysema	Symmetrically reduced	Central	Normal	Diminished, vesicular with prolonged expiration	Normal or reduced	Rhonchi and creps due to associated chr. bronchitis.
Interstitial lung disease	Symmetrically reduced	Central	Normal	Harsh vesicular with prolonged expiration	Normal or increased	Coarse crepitations, uninfluenced by coughing.
Broncho-pneumonia	Symmetrically reduced	Central	May be impaired	Usually harsh vesicular with prolonged expiration	Normal or increased	Rhonchi & coarse crepitations.
Lobar pneumonia	Reduced on affected side	Central	Dull	High pitched, bronchial pectoriloquy (WP) +	Increased; whispering	Early-fine, later-coarse crepitations.
Collapse: peripheral bronchus obstruction	Reduced on affected side	Towards lesion	Dull	High pitched, bronchial	Increased WP +	Early-none, later-coarse crepitations.
Collapse: obstruction to major bronchus.	Reduced on affected side	Towards lesion	Dull	Diminished or absent	Reduced or absent	None.
Cavity	Slightly reduced on affected side	Central or towards lesion	Impaired	Amphoric, bronchial	Increased WP+	Coarse crepitations.
Localized fibrosis and/or bronchiectasis	Slightly reduced on affected side with retraction	Towards lesion	Impaired	Low pitched, bronchial	Increased	Coarse crepitations.
Pleural effusion, empyema	Reduced or absent with oedema of chest wall	Towards opposite side of lesion	Stony, dull	Diminished or absent, occasionally high pitched, bronchial	Reduced or absent, occasionally increased with egopathy	Pleural rub in some cases.
Pneumothorax—complete:	Absent	Towards opposite side	Hyper-resonant	Absent	Absent	Nil.
partial:	Reduced	Central	Normal	Reduced	Reduced	Nil.

Left ventricular failure: This can be confirmed by 2D echocardiography, which may reveal chamber enlargement with poor EF.

Sinus infection with post-nasal drip: This can be confirmed by X-ray of the paranasal sinuses.

Oesophageal reflux with aspiration: This can be confirmed by barium swallow and radionuclide studies.

Unsuspected bronchiectasis and cystic fibrosis: This can be confirmed by bronchography CT.

Psychological cough: This is characteristically non-productive of sputum, and has a barking quality.

Therapeutic Plan

Coughing is a symptom and treatment is directed at its aetiology (tuberculosis, asthma, allergic bronchitis, bronchiectasis, bronchogenic carcinoma etc). It must be remembered that bronchial asthma may present as cough rather than wheezing; this cough responds to bronchodilators e.g. salbutamol 2 mg tid or terbutaline 2 mg tid.

As a general rule substantially productive coughs obviously play a role in airway clearance and should not be suppressed. Treatment is based on enhancing secretion, clearance by bronchodilators, chest physiotherapy, postural drainage, aerosols with humidifiers and mucolytics.

Troublesome and minimally productive cough may be treated with codeine 10 mg orally 3-4 times daily. Many over-the-counter cough remedies contain antihistaminics which may act as central nervous system cough suppressants.

TABLE **29.4** 'ATYPICAL PNEUMONIAS'

Diagnostic possibilities	Findings and tests
1. Mycoplasma (erythromycin, tetracycline)	Usually introduced into the family by small children. Cold agglutinins not specific but 1:64 + suggestive.
2. Viruses (none except amantadine for influenza A)	Influenza, parainfluenza, adenovirus, RSV. Acute and convalescent serology.
3. Legionella pneumophilia (erythromycin C, rifampicin)	Endemic or epidemic form. Disease progresses in face of penicillin, cephalosporin and aminoglycoside therapy. Lung biopsy–direct immuno-fluorescent antibody diagnostic.
4. Q fever (tetracycline)	Inhalation of dust near infected animals. May be accompanied by hepatitis. Rising antibody titre diagnostic.
5. Psittacosis (tetracycline)	Inhalation of dust of faeces of infected birds. Splenomegaly, serological tests positive
6. Plague pneumonia (streptomycin plus tetracycline)	Acute onset with haemoptysis. Sputum + for P. pestis.

Dementia

Dementia is a syndrome defined by a general deterioration of intellectual function in the conscious person. This definition differentiates dementia from other syndromes that affect cognition (such as acute confusional states and delirium).

Dementia affects 5 to 10 per cent of the general population over age 65, and 20 to 30 per cent over age 85. As the population ages, dementia will become an increasingly serious public health problem.

The main concern of the doctor is to find out if there are any *treatable causes* which should not be missed. **Table 30.1** lists the diagnostic features of the various causes of dementia and indicates which are the treatable ones.

Clinical Evaluation

The history of the present illness is best obtained from informants other than the patient. Information about the onset and progression of dementia should be obtained from the relatives, asking for specific examples of the abnormalities (loss of memory, difficulty with using language, capacity to understand and communicate, capacity to use common objects such as the telephone and pen, mood disturbances especially depression and anxiety, difficulty in walking, bladder control, seizures, myoclonus) and any other difficulties that are especially troublesome to the patient and his family.

The family history often reveals relatives affected by Alzheimer's disease–ask about parents and grandparents and how they spent their last years of life.

The educational history is important to evaluate the patient's cognitive disability. A diagnosis of dementia requires evidence of deterioration from a previous normal level (unlike mental retardation where the impairment is lifelong).

The medical history of a patient with dementia may reveal precipitating factors (hypoglycaemia, hypoxia, hypotension, drugs, and alcohol) or associated medical disorders that require management.

A past history of depressive illness would be of particular importance, because dementia may be a manifestation of severe depression. Details of the patient's personality are important when considering the difficulties that may be encountered during his care and in planning activities for him.

A gradual decline in cognitive function is characteristic of Alzheimer's disease.

Dramatic, sharp changes in the intellectual function are more likely to represent a vascular cause or an infectious process.

Physical Examination

The physical and neurological examination provides helpful information for differential diagnosis and also reveals medical conditions coexisting with dementia.

Clinical clues for multi-infarct dementia may be sought in the cardiovascular system for possible sources of emboli. The skin and mucous membranes should be carefully checked for evidence of vitamin deficiency (thiamine, niacin, Vit. B12). In patients leading an indoor life there may be no skin lesions typical of pellagra and the patient may present only with dementia.

Laboratory tests for investigation of dementia are described in **Table 30.2**. The most common problem of differential diagnosis is the distinction between Alzheimer's disease and multi-infarct dementia. Today the most cost-effective test for this purpose is HMPAO-SPECT perfusion imaging of the brain.

TABLE 30.1 CAUSES OF DEMENTIA

A. *Primary dementia:*
     Alzheimer's disease
     Pick's disease
     Frontal lobe degeneration

    Vascular disease
     Multi-infarct dementia (preventable)
     Vasculitis: SLE, PAN (treatable)

    Infection
     HIV (preventable)
     Syphilis (treatable)
     Tuberculosis (Preventable; treatable)
     Fungal & protozoal infections (treatable)

B. *Secondary dementia with signs of underlying neurologic
     disorder:*
     Tumours: primary and secondary (some are
     treatable)
     Carcinomatous meningitis

    Chronic subdural haematoma (treatable)

    Normal pressure hydrocephalus (NPH) (treatable)
     Parkinson's disease
     Huntington's disease
     Progressive supranuclear palsy
     Wilson's disease
     Progressive myoclonic epilepsy

C. *Endocrine & nutritional deficiencies (treatable):*
     Hypothyroidism
     Vit. B12 deficiency
     Thiamine deficiency
     Niacin deficiency (pellagra)
     Adrenocortical insufficiency
     Cushing's syndrome
     Hypo and hyperparathyroidism
     Chronic hypoglycaemia (preventable)

D. *Toxic disorders:*
     Drugs and narcotics (preventable)
     Alcoholic dementia (preventable)
     Heavy metal intoxication (treatable)
     Dialysis dementia (treatable)
     Chronic hepatic encephalopathy (treatable)

TABLE 30.2 INVESTIGATION OF DEMENTIA

In all cases:
  Blood count and ESR
  Blood sugar
  Serum Na, K, Ca, BUN and creatinine
  Liver function tests
  Thyroid function tests – T_3 T_4 TSH
  RIA of serum B12
  Serology for syphilis
  Chest X-ray
  EEG
  CT/MRI to exclude intracranial mass lesion, and to
  document atrophic changes in Alzheimer's and multi-
  infarct dementia
  SPECT brain perfusion imaging

In selected cases:
  CSF examination
  HIV antibodies
  Serum copper and ceruloplasmin
  Arterial blood gases
  In very selected cases: brain biopsy

In suspected metabolic disease:
  White cell enzyme screen
  Plasma and urinary aminoacids
  Plasma pyruvate and lactate
  Urine and faecal porphyrins
  Bone marrow, liver, nerve, muscle, rectal biopsy

Management

Currently there is no cure for Alzheimer's disease, or
multi-infarct dementia.

The treatable causes of dementia are listed in
Table 30.1. Removal of a subdural haematoma or a
mass lesion, and ventriculo-peritoneal shunt for NPH
are the surgically curable dementias. Hypothyroidism
and various vitamin and mineral deficiences can be
treated medically and can also be prevented. HIV
dementia improves with azidothimidine therapy.

31   Diabetes Mellitus

The word doctor is derived from the Latin *docere* to teach. Patient education in diabetes mellitus provides the best example of the crucial role of the doctor as a teacher. Patients should be made to realize as early as possible that it is upon themselves that the success or failure of treatment will depend. Patient education aims at helping the diabetic patient 'to become his own physician' as Joslin put it more than 50 years ago. This does not imply that a diabetic patient should not keep in touch with his attending physician at regular intervals. The main aim of intensive education is the patient's self-control of his metabolic condition. As adherence to a diabetic regimen demands from the patient self-discipline and a sense of purpose, every effort should be made to ensure that the object of each aspect of management is understood by the patient. Self-monitoring of urine glucose and blood glucose (easily performed with enzymatic test strips) is particularly important in insulin-injecting patients. Self-monitoring by the diabetic patient is a valuable support to the family doctor and the diabetologist consultant in achieving optimum care.

A number of studies have clearly demonstrated that patient education significantly lowers the period of hospitalization and the duration of incapacity of working, especially in patients without late diabetic complications. If a diabetic patient can follow a regular diet, monitor his blood sugar, develop an understanding of hypoglycaemia and the circumstances when it may occur, and learn to recognize its warning signals, he can do his job well. Experience has indicated that a diabetic is generally a good employee and may have a better work motivation than non-diabetic employees.

Regular Surveillance

Apart from patient education, the family doctor has the important task of patient surveillance at regular intervals. The object is to check the degree of control and if necessary to make appropriate alterations in treatment and to ensure early detection of complications and their proper management. The check-list for surveillance is given in **Table 31.1**.

Although the relationship between the degree of control of blood sugar and the development of serious complications is not a simple one, it would appear that the vascular abnormalities are secondary to metabolic abnormalities occurring in diabetes. It is therefore incumbent on the physician to strive in every way to achieve as good control as is practicable in terms of blood sugar and lipids.

Maintenance of a proper record will alert the doctor immediately if any change in health status has occurred. The frequency of visits is determined by the severity of the disability and the reliability of the patient. Many hospitals run diabetic clinics and patients should be encouraged to avail of their services. These clinics provide cards to the patients to be carried with them all the time, stating the name and address of the patient, the nature and dose of medication the patient is receiving, the telephone number of the family doctor or any special diabetic clinic where the patient should report during an emergency.

Factors that Promote Hyperglycaemia

When the family doctor finds that the blood sugar is not adequately controlled (post-meal blood sugar more than 200 mg per cent, glycosylated Hb more than 8.5 per cent), he should consider the factors that promote hyperglycaemia, as listed in **Table 31.2**, and search for their presence in the patient.

TABLE 31.1 CHECK-LIST FOR URVEILLANCE OF A DIABETIC PATIENT

- Record weight at each examination, determine departure from ideal weight, and plan for correction accordingly.

- Inquire about effort tolerance, shortness of breath, angina.

- Encourage regular physical exercise.

- Record blood pressure in supine and erect positions (for evidence of postural hypotension).

- Palpate all peripheral pulses and compare both sides: carotid, brachial, radial; femoral, posterior tibial, dorsalis pedis.

- Look for foci of infection: gums and teeth, chest, skin.

- Foot care: properly fitting shoes, care in nail cutting, skin ulcers.

- Vision acuity testing: send for ophthalmoscopic examination once a year or earlier if there is deterioration of vision.

- Test for knee jerks and ankle jerks, vibration sense on shins; inquire about paraesthesia, cramps, pain in limbs.

- Inquire about sexual function (See also **Table 48.1**).

- Scrutinize the blood sugar reports & urine reports for adequacy of control:
  Glycosylated Hb (Hb A1C) - once in 3 months;
  BUN and creatinine-at least once in a year;
  Urine for microalbuminuria - at least once in a year;
  X-ray chest-once in a year;
  ECG & stress test if indicated by history.

Correction of an illness or other factors promoting hyperglycaemia is the most important aspect of successful management.

The three main objectives of management to be constantly remembered, and to be impressed on the patient's mind are:

1. Attain and maintain appropriate body weight for the age and height (See Chapter 45 on Obesity).

2. Control hyperglycaemia, glycosuria and hyperlipidaemia, and abolish the symptoms of diabetes.

3. Avoid hypoglycaemia (See Chapter 39).

TABLE 31.2 FACTORS THAT PROMOTE HYPER GLYCAEMIA IN A DIABETIC

1. Increased dietary intake (especially carbohydrates)
2. Decreased physical activity
3. Drugs that limit insulin production:
   Thiazide diuretics
   Phenytoin
   Diazoxide
4. Drugs that create insulin resistance:
   Glucocorticoids
   Oral contraceptives
   Sympathomimetic agents
   Nicotinic acid
5. Conditions that lead to insulin resistance:
   Infection
   Inflammation
   Pregnancy
   Trauma (including surgery)
6. Antibodies to insulin (rare)
7. Antibodies to insulin receptors (rare)

Advice Regarding Diet

Dietary modification is important in all types of DM and may also be beneficial to patients with impaired glucose tolerance. The objectives of dietary therapy differ according to the diagnostic subclass of DM, the extent of obesity, the presence of diabetic complications and the concurrent drug therapy. Dietary objectives should be understood by the patient and the help of a dietician should be taken to make a meal plan considering the individual patient preferences, resources and needs.

1. *Calories* will be determined according to the need to achieve and maintain ideal body weight. Normal weight individuals with moderate physical activity need about 35 kcal/kg/day. Obese, sedentary patients will need 20-25 kcal/kg/day to bring down their weight.

2. *Composition and timing of meals* are particularly important for patients using insulin or oral hypoglycaemic drugs. The onset of action, peak effect and duration of action of various types of insulin are given in **Table 31.3** and those of the oral hypoglycaemic drugs are given in **Table 31.4**. Timing and quantities of meals should coincide with the peak effects of the drugs to avoid periods of hypogylcaemia.

It is prudent to balance the daily distribution of carbohydrates, proteins and fats.

Carbohydrates (50-60 per cent) are essential to maintain caloric intake. Complex carbohydrates (contained in the normal vegetarian diet) have a low glycaemic index and hence have a different effect on post-prandial blood glucose than refined sugar which should be totally avoided (except to treat or avert hypoglycaemia).

NOTE: Activity of sulfonylureas is prolonged in both hepatic and renal failure.

Proteins (10-15 per cent) should be sufficient to maintain positive nitrogen balance and to promote growth. In patients with diabetic nephropathy protein intake is limited to 30 g/day.

Fats should be restricted to less than 30 per cent of total calories, and saturated fat should be less than one-third of the total fat intake, polyunsaturated fat one-third, and mono-unsaturated fat (omega 3 and 6) one-third.

Fibre in the food prolongs the absorption of glucose and prevents reabsorption of cholesterol thereby lowering LDL and total cholesterol.

Fruits and green vegetables at least 400 g per day are encouraged because of their content of free radical scavengers (vitamin C, E, carotenoids). Fenugreek seeds are encouraged to be taken (30 g/day) for the fibre and myoinositol content.

Artificial sweeteners– aspartame (18 mg tab) and saccharin- are helpful in reducing sucrose intake (with tea, coffee etc.) while maintaining a palatable diet.

Alcohol may promote hypoglycaemia in patients receiving insulin or oral hypoglycaemic drugs. Patients with diabetic neuropathy should avoid alcohol totally.

Physical exercise promotes glucose utilization by muscles and enhances sensitivity to insulin. A graded exercise programme should be used in untrained patients only after medical evaluation. In patients older than 40 years of age or with a duration of DM greater than 10 years, the evaluation should include a rest and stress ECG.

Exercise programmes may be detrimental to patients with labile hyperglycaemia, or to patients on insulin or oral hypoglycaemic drugs who experience severe hypoglycaemia.

Chronic Complications of Diabetes Mellitus

Eyes
Ophthalmic complications of DM include diabetic retinopathy and diseases of the anterior chamber that affect vision.

Diabetic retinopathy includes:
(1) background retinopathy (microaneurysms, intraretinal blot haemorrhages, retinal infarcts and hard exudates;
(2) proliferative retinopathy (neovascularization) which may lead to retinal detachment and acute visual loss.

Visual loss
i. Transient blurring of vision caused by lens swelling due to fluctuating blood sugar levels, may be seen in diabetics in poor control. This does not implicate a serious visual threat, although it may take several weeks to resolve.

ii. A refractive error can occur in a diabetic as in all others, and can be corrected by glasses.

iii. Cataract. DM affects the development, progression and severity of a cataract due to increased sorbitol content of the lens.

iv. Glaucoma (either open angle or narrow angle) can lead to sudden onset of pain and visual loss which could be permanent with uncontrolled elevation of intraocular pressure.

v. Acute monocular visual loss can be due to vitreous haemorrhage, retinal detachment or embolic retinal infarction following central retinal artery occlusion.

vi. Bilateral acute visual loss suggests stroke but may also result from a dominant monocular loss when vision in the non-dominant eye is insidiously impaired.

vii. If the DM patient has carotid artery atherosclerosis, he may get transient recurrent visual loss (amaurosis fugax), or total or near total visual loss, usually permanent. Visual symptoms and signs observed in the presence of a systolic bruit and decreased pulsation over the carotid artery establishes the diagnosis.

If marked asymmetry between the findings of the two eyes of a patient with diabetic or hypertensive retinopathy is noted, carotid occlusive disease should be suspected (the eye on the ischaemic side being protected from retinopathy).

Yearly examination by an ophthalmologist is a minimum requirement for detection of diabetic retinopathy and is recommended at 5 years after onset in type I (IDDM) and at the time of diagnosis in type II (NIDDM). Although vision may be affected, visual acuity changes are not a reliable indicator of the presence or absence of diabetic retinopathy. Frequently a patient of diabetic retinopathy can progress to intermediate or even advanced stages without visual impairment. On the other hand, visual impairment can occur gradually when the macula is involved, or suddenly when vitreous haemorrhage occurs.

Both the extent of the retinopathy when initially diagnosed and its progression can be important in determining the prognosis and directing therapy.

Fluorescein angiography can help in determining the extent of retinal ischaemia and uncovering of new vessel growth. Unlike established retinal vessels, new vessels leak the dye which can be photographed with the help of a fundus camera. This requires clear ocular media; in those DM patients who do not have it, ophthalmic ultrasonography can be used to determine the stage of retinopathy and the location of the damage.

Pan-retinal photocoagulation (PRP) with argon laser has been shown to delay the progression of diabetic retinopathy in high risk patients (those with macular oedema and proliferation of new vessels growing on or within the optic disc whether or not haemorrhage is present; and new vessel growth away from the disc when haemorrhage is present or there is a history of haemorrhage).

Vitrectomy is used for severe vitreous haemorrhage not clearing spontaneously and in severe proliferating retinopathy which in turn causes detachment of the retina thereby threatening macular vision. In patients who require this surgery with an operating microscope, damage is already severe and the goal of surgery is to prevent further damage by arresting progression.

In some cases improvement of vision is an added bonus.

Diabetic neuropathy

This complication occurs in over 30 per cent of patients with a duration of DM of more than 10 years. Any nerve or combination of nerves may be affected: cranial, somatosensory, mononeuropathy, polyneuropathy, autonomic neuropathy (atonic bladder, gastroparesis with delayed emptying, diarrhoea, constipation, postural hypotension, gustatory sweating, abnormal pulse rate response to the erect stance and Valsalva manoeuvre). The differential diagnosis includes entrapment neuropathy, degenerative disc disease, cord tumour, alcoholic and uraemic neuropathy, Vit. B12 deficiency, hypothyroidism, Paget's disease of the spine and syphilis.

Motor deficit may result in muscular weakness and atrophy. Physical therapy may be helpful to patients with disability.

There is no effective and specific therapy for painful diabetic neuropathy Potent analgesics may be needed for severe pain. Amitriptyline 25-100 mg PO has been found useful in relief of chronic pain but it may aggravate the symptoms of autonomic neuropathy.

Diabetic nephropathy

This may cause proteinuria, hypertension and renal failure.

Hypertension is a manifestation of diabetic nephropathy and if left untreated, will promote further retinal, renal and cardiovascular impairment. ACE inhibitors reduce proteinuria, reduce blood pressure and preserve renal function and should be routinely used in this situation.

Urinary tract infection should be treated aggressively.

Diabetic peripheral vascular disease

There is 40 times greater prevalence of macrovascular lesions in the lower limbs of DM patients compared to non-diabetics. The lesions are more diffuse and extensive and involve *distal* blood vessels (tibial and peroneal). About 25 per cent of those with peripheral vascular disease also have peripheral neuropathy. Intermittent claudication, or pain in the calf, thigh or buttock after walking, which is relieved by rest, is the first subjective finding; this may progress to rest pain.

Objective findings include weak or absent pulses, tight shiny skin, hair loss, delayed venous filling and delayed capillary flush when the leg returns to the dependent position after several minutes of elevation, localized pallor and/or cyanosis, callus formation, muscle atrophy, ulceration, gangrene, diminished sensation and absent reflexes.

Doppler ultrasonography and limb plethysmography are two non-invasive tests to evaluate circulation in the lower limbs. Surgical treatment is often warranted in the management of symptomatic peripheral vascular disease. Pentoxifylline 400 mg PO tid may be helpful when surgery is not advisable. Hyperlipidaemia and hypertension should be treated. Smoking should be discouraged.

Coronary artery disease and myocardial infarct
These occur with increased frequency in DM. Heart disease must be considered when dyspnoea and unexplained hyperglycaemia occur even when other symptoms of angina pectoris are atypical or absent. Young age should not preclude the diagnosis coronary heart disease. Yearly ECG is part of routine diabetic care.

The diabetic foot
Chronic neuropathy, vascular insufficiency and infection contribute to this problem. Sensory loss allows tolerance of repeated trauma from tight shoes and improper weight-bearing, which leads to skin breakdown, skin ulceration, tissue necrosis and fracture. Specialized treatment is needed to prevent and to manage foot disease.

Patients with foot ulcers must totally avoid local pressure to allow healing; this is preferably achieved by hospitalization. Infection is common and osteomyelitis can complicate deep ulcers. Antibiotics effective against anaerobic bacteria (e.g.

metronidazole, clindamycin) should be included as part of combination antibiotic therapy in the management of infected ulcers. Surgical debridement and treatment of vascular disease may aid healing. Amputation may be necessary to prevent recurrent septicaemia and death.

Many amputations in DM could be prevented or delayed by more effective patient education regarding the principles of foot care and medical supervision. Appropriately designed footwear can be made available.

Surgery in Diabetic Patients

Surgery poses a significant stress to diabetic patients and often perturbs dietary management. Careful control of blood sugar is necessary to avoid symptomatic hyperglycaemia and ketoacidosis, and to allow a normal inflammatory response and wound healing. Elective surgery should be done on cases of well-controlled DM.

Patients managed with diet alone usually require no additional measures. Purified human (or porcine) insulin should be used to manage fasting glucose greater than 250 mg/dl.

Patients using oral hypoglycaemic drugs should discontinue them on the day preceding surgery. Insulin should be used for control of hyperglycaemia.

Insulin-treated patients require dose adjustments. On the morning of surgery a dextrose infusion should be given with the administration of half of the usual total daily insulin dose as long-acting or intermediate-acting insulin. The reduced dosage may be continued as long as oral intake is limited, or can be titrated when IV dextrose or parenteral alimentation is used post-operatively.

Endo PAT, a new device, better than FMD (flow-mediated dilation) for non invasive assessment of endothelial function in peripheral vessels. Which should become part of regular health check up. Simultaneous recording is done on both arms - while endothelial function is tested in one arm, the contralateral arm is used to monitor systemic vascular changes e.g . alteration in anatomical tone, transient environmental effects etc.

The fingers have an inherently larger ability to vary local vascular tone, enabling assessment of small conduit vessels as well as resistance vessels. Since 2003 the Framingham Heart Study has included endothelial function measurement with ENDOPAT. In a study of 500 subjects there was significant inverse correlation between Endo PAT index and multiple cardiovascular risk factors. Response to treatment and lifestyle modification can be documented by Endo PAT.

Sudo scan

It is a new diagnostic modality for early detection of diabetic complications, related to peripheral and autonomic neuropathy. Small nerve fibres are impaired at early stage because they are long, thin and amyelinic. Functional evaluation of these fibres can be useful in preventing complications caused by diabetic neuropathies.

There is reduced sweat gland fibre density. It is a non invasive dynamic measurement of the ability of sweat glands to release chloride ions in response to electrochemical activation in relation to their sweat gland innervations.

Low voltage is applied to nickel electrodes in contact with the hands and feet, areas with highest sweat gland density. The voltage extracts ions (chloride, hydrogen ions) which reach the electrodes, passing solely via the sweat gland ducts. At low voltage, the stratum corneum acts as a capacitor and sweat ducts only allow transmission of ions to the skin. This ensures that the measurements taken correspond solely to the sweat gland function.

Reaction - there is an observable electrochemical reaction between 1. The chloride ions and the anode, and 2. The H^+ ions and the cathode.

The device records electrochemical conductance related to the pH and the concentration of the chloride ions supplied from the sweat glands and detected by the electrodes (on hands and feet).

Helps in immediate early diagnosis of complications relating to micro angiopathies.

1. Diabetic peripheral neuropathy: Effective in screening for the risk of diabetic foot. A study involving 150 diabetic patients to be highly correlated with symmetrical neuropathy.

2. Cardiac autonomic neuropathy- the detection of cardiac autonomic neuropathy correlated with two abnormal Ewing tests which according to ADA is confirmatory for cardiac autonomic neuropathy1.

3. Diabetic Retinopathy - Correlated well with retinopathy.

4. Diabetic nephropathy- Sudoscan scores are highly correlated with e GFR values and albumin creatinine ratio in the diagnosis of nephropathy.

Diabetes in Pregnancy

Patients with pre-existing DM become pregnant are particularly vulnerable to complications; maternal health can be compromised when diabetic complications occur. Optimum care includes the initiation of intensive therapy prior to conception. Caloric requirements in pregnancy are roughly 5 kcal/kg greater than in the nonpregnant adult. Insulin requirements vary during pregnancy–lower in the first trimester. increases after 24 weeks and suddenly drops in the immediate postpartum period.

New Concept: Alzheimer's Disease is Type 3 Diabetes

Since 2005 a new concept has arisen that Alzheimer's disease (AD) is intrinsically a neuroendocrine disorder caused by selective impairment of insulin and IGF signaling. This idea was fuelled by evidence that gene expression and phosphorylation of Tau protein are regulated through insulin and IGF signaling cascades. Many key aspects of the central nervous system (CNS) degeneration that occurs in AD can be effectuated by impaired insulin signaling. Insulin and IGF–1 mediate their effects by activating complex intracellular signaling pathways starting with ligand binding to cell surface receptors followed by autophosphorylation and activation of the intrinsic receptor tyrosine kinases which eventually activate extracellular signal-regulated kinases/mitogen-activated protein kinases (ERK/MAPK) and Insulin Receptor Substrate/PI3K/AKT pathways. Major biological responses to Insulin Receptor Substrate signaling include increased cell growth, survival, energy metabolism and cholinergic gene expression, inhibition of oxidative stress and apoptosis. These very same signaling pathways are activated in various cell types, tissue and target organs including the brain. Oligodendroglia requires intact insulin/IGF signaling mechanism for myelin synthesis. Reduced insulin and IGF-1 receptor expression in neurons begins early and progresses as disease becomes severe and global. Growth factor withdrawal is a well-established mechanism of neuronal death. Post mortem studies of advanced AD patients have shown significant abnormality in the expression of genes coding insulin, IGF-1 and IGF-2 peptides and their receptors and down-stream signaling molecules. These abnormalities can occur with or without T2DM. Epidemiological data indicate increased risk of developing mild cognitive impairment, dementia or AD in individuals with T2DM and metabolic syndrome. Peroxisome proliferator-activated receptors (PPARs)

(PPARα, PPARδ and PPARγ) are expressed in adult human brain and function at the level of the nucleus to activate insulin-response genes and signaling pathways. PPARδ agonists preserve insulin and IGF receptor bearing cells including neurons and oligodendroglia. Deficient insulin/IGF signaling decreases expression of choline acetyl transferase leading to reduced acetyl choline production. Insulin resistance in AD patients is associated with IGF-1 resistance, Insulin Receptor Substrate-1 dysregulation and cognitive decline.

Referring to AD as type 3 diabetes mellitus (T3DM) is justified because the fundamental molecular and biochemical abnormalities overlap with insulin-resistance and T2DM. This is confirmed by demonstration of cognitive improvement and/or stabilization of cognitive impairment in subjects with early AD following treatment with intranasal insulin or a PP AR agonist (**Table 31.3, 4 & 5**).

TABLE 31.3 CLASSIFICATION OF VARIOUS ORAL AGENTS USED FOR THE TREATMENT OF DIABETES MELLITUS

Sr No	Drug group	Mechanism of action	Examples	Dosage
1.	**Insulin sensitizers**			
	A. Biguanides	↓Hepatic glucose production	Metformin	500mg OD-1250mg OD
	B. Thiazolidinediones (TZDs)	↓Insulin resistance, ↑Glucose utilization	Pioglitazone Rosiglitazone	15-45mg OD 2-8mg OD
2.	Insulin secretagogues			
	A. Sulfonylureas	↑Insulin secretion		
	i) First generation		Tolbutamide Chiorpropamide	Not used these days Not used these days
	ii) Second generation		Glimeopiride Glipizide Glyburide Gliclazide	1-8 mg OD 2.5mg-20mg OD 1.25mg OD-10mg BD 40-160mg BD
	B. Non-sulfonylureas (Meglitinides)	↑Insulin secretion	Nateginide Repaglinide	60-120mg TDS 0.5-4mg TDS
3.	Alpha-glucosidase inhibitors	↓GI glucose absorption	Acarbose Miglitol Voglibose	25-100 mg TDS 25-100 mg TDS 0.2-0.3 mg TDS
4.	Dipeptidyl peptidase 4 (DPP4) inhibitors	Prolong endogenous GLP-1 action Suppression of glucagon	Saxagliptin Sitagliptin Vildagliptin Linagliptin	2.5-5 mg OD 50-200 mg OD 50-200 mg OD 5 mg OD
5.	Selective sodium glucose transporter-2 inhibitors (SGLT2 inhibitors or glycosurics)	↑Renal excretion of glucose	Canagliflozin Dapagliflozin	100 to 300 mg OD 5-10 mg OD
6.	Bile acid sequestrants	Bind bile acids, mechanism of glucose lowering not known	Colesevelam	1875mg BD or 3750mg OD
7.	Dopamine agonists	Resetting abnormally elevated hypothalamic drive for increased plasma glucose, FFA and TG in insulin resistant patients	Bromocriptine (quick release formulation)	0.8-4.8 mg OD

Table 31.4 CLASSIFICATION OF VARIOUS PARENTERAL AGENTS USED FOR THE TREATMENT OF DIABETES MELLITUS

Sr No	Drug group	Mechanism of action	Examples	Dosage
1.	**Insulins**	↑Glucose utilization ↓Hepatic glucose production and other anabolic action	See table **Table 31.5**	
2.	Glucagon-like peptide-1 (GLP-1) receptor agonists	↑Insulin, ↓Glucagon, slow gastric emptying, satiety	Exenatide Liraglutide	2 mg SC once weekly 0.6-1.8 mg SC OD
3.	Amylin agonists	Slow gastric emptying, ↓Glucagon	Pramlintide	15-120mcg SC premeals

Table 31.5 INSULINS

Type	Onset of action	Peak action	Duration of action
1. Rapid acting			
Lispro (Humalog)	< 30 minutes	30-90 minutes	3-5 hours
Aspart (Novorapid)	< 15 minutes	3 hours	3-5 hours
Glulisine (Apidra)	10-20 minutes	30-90 minutes	4-6 hours
2. Short acting			
Regular Human Actrapid Insulin (HAI)	0.5-1 hour	2-4 hours	6-12 hours
3. Intermediate			
Neutral Protamine Hagedorn (NPH)	1-2 hours	4-14 hours	10-24 hours
Lente	1-3 hours	6-12 hours	12-24 hours
4. Long acting			
Glargine (Lantus)	1 hour	No peak	24 hours
Determir (Levemir)	1-4 hours	No peak	12-20 hours
Ultralente (Human Insulin)	4-8 hours	10-30 hours	18-36 hours
5. Ultralong acting			
Degludec (Tresiba)	30-90 minutes	No peak	> 42 hours
6. Mixtures (Premix)			
a. Human premix			
70% NPH + 30% Regular	30 minutes	4-8 hours	16-24 hours
50% NPH + 50% Regular	30 minutes	7-12 hours	16-24 hours
b. Lispro premix			
75% Protaminated Lispro + 25% Lispro	< 30 minutes	30-90 minutes	18-24 hours
c. Aspart premix			
70% Protaminated Aspart + 30% Aspart (BIAsp 70/30)	10-20 minutes	1-4 hours	18-24 hours

Diarrhoea is defined as 'too frequent passage of too fluid stools'.

Careful analysis of the history is useful in determining what is causing the diarrhoea. A clinical classification of diarrhoea may be done on the following criteria: acute; chronic or recurrent.

1. Acute Diarrhoea

Usually of sudden onset and short duration. Infection due to viral, bacterial and parasitic agents, toxins, poisons and drugs are the major causes of acute diarrhoea (**Table 32.1**).

Acute diarrhoea with blood and mucus: indicates infection like amoebic or bacillary dysentery, and inflammatory bowel disease (ulcerative colitis).

Acute diarrhoea which is profuse, watery and soon followed by dehydration and collapse: indicates cholera.

2. Chronic Diarrhoea

This is defined as frequent fluid stools persisting beyond 4 weeks.

Since chronic diarrhoea can occur in diseases of the small intestine, large intestine and pancreas, it is essential to clinically suspect the diseased organ so that appropriate investigations can be planned (**Table 32.2** and **Fig. 32.1**).

It is useful to understand the causative mechanism of chronic diarrhoea so that appropriate treatment can be planned (**Table 32.3**).

Osmotic diarrhoea
Since the diarrhoea depends upon the solute content of the intestine, fasting for 48 hours controls osmotic diarrhoea. Examples of this kind of diarrhoea are lactose intolerance, tropical sprue, coeliac disease, and intestinal resection (reduced absorptive surface).

Secretory diarrhoea
Excessive secretion of anions (chloride and bicarbonate) leading to excessive secretion may be caused by bacterial endotoxins, bile acids, laxative abuse or gut hormones (Zollinger-Ellison syndrome due to excessive gastrin secretion, carcinoid syndrome, VIPoma).

Mucosal injury
Causing impairment of absorption, and ulceration leading to exudation of plasma with or without bleeding. Giardia lamblia, Yersinia enterocolitis, tropical sprue, inflammatory bowel disease (Crohn's disease) and ileocaecal tuberculosis are important examples.

Altered motility
Altered motility is the cause of diarrhoea in thyrotoxicosis, pellagra, diabetic neuropathy, and psychogenic stress (irritable bowel syndrome).

Nocturnal diarrhoea
Nocturnal diarrhoea always indicates organic disease. Any severe diarrhoea may have a nocturnal component but diabetic autonomic neuropathy, thyrotoxicosis and ulcerative colitis are important causes. In diabetics of more than 7 years' duration, peripheral neuropathy may be accompanied by autonomic neuropathy. Loss of ileal innervation and bile acid malabsorption may be the mechanism of nocturnal diarrhoea.

Diarrhoea in AIDS
Unexplained diarrhoea may be the first presenting symptom for a patient with HIV infection. Various opportunistic infections like cryptosporidosis, Isospora belli, Giardia lamblia, Kaposi's sarcoma involving the intestine, and lymphoma may all present as diarrhoea in an immunocompromised patient. Large voluminous diarrhoea which fails to

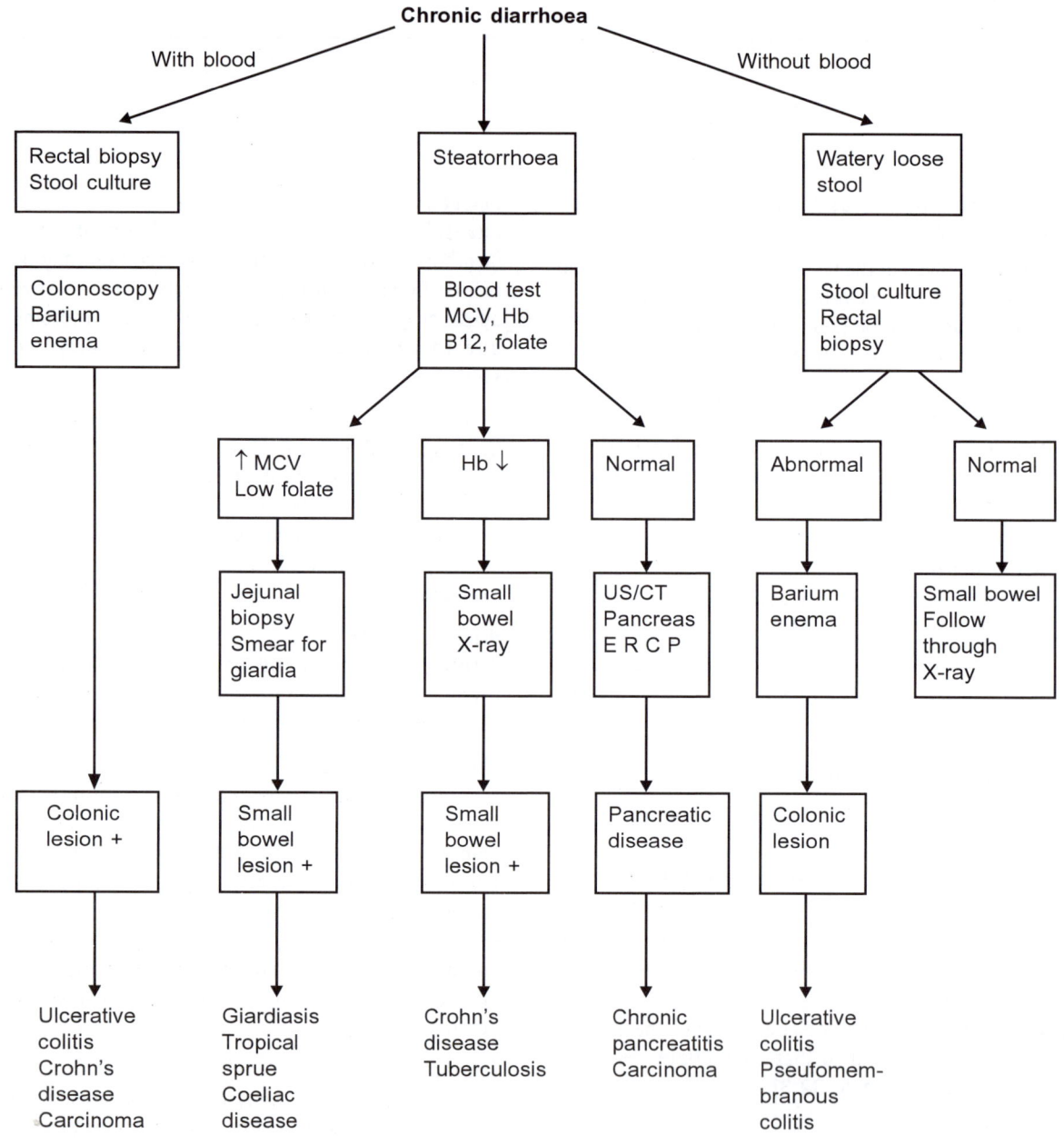

Fig. 32.1: Investigation of chronic diarrhoea

TABLE 32.1 DIAGNOSIS OF ACUTE DIARRHOEA

Cause	Associated symptoms	Features in stool	Management
Viral enteritis	No fever; abdominal pain; particularly in infants and children; may be epidemic esp. summer.	No blood or pus in stools	Symptomatic
Viral gastroenteritis	Vomiting; abdominal pain; low grade or no fever; respiratory symptoms.	No blood or pus in stools	Symptomatic
Staphylococcus toxin	Vomiting; abdominal pain; no fever; onset 6-12 hours after eating; lasts less than 24 hours.	No blood or pus in stools	Symptomatic
Clostridium welchii infection	Diarrhoea; pain; tenesmus; no fever.	No blood or pus in stools	Symptomatic
Salmonella enteritis	Pain; tenesmus; fever; 8-24 hours after eating.	Blood and mucus in stools; stool culture positive	Tetracycline, chloramphenicol, ampicillin
Shigella enteritis	Pain; tenesmus; fever.	Blood, mucus and pus in stools	Tetracycline, chloramphenicol
Amoebic colitis	Pain; tenesmus; fever.	Blood and mucus in stools; E.h. trophozoites in stools	Metronidazole
Ulcerative colitis	Fever; pain; tenesmus.	Blood and mucus in stools; no E.h.	Glucosteroids Sulphathalazine
Giardiasis	Pain.	Giardia in stools	Mepacrine, metronidazole
Cholera	Painless passage of watery stools; rapid dehydration; collapse.	'Rice water' stools	Fluid and electrolyte replacement (ORT), tetracycline
Compylobacter enteritis	Fever; constitutional disturbance; abdominal X-ray: megacolon.	Stool culture	Erythromycin 0.5-1 g PO qid for 1-4 weeks
Pseudomembranous colitis	Prior use of antibiotics.	Stool culture Clostridrium difficile	Stop suspected antibiotic, Vancomycin 120 mg PO qid x 10 days, metronidazole less expensive
Malaria	Fever with chills. Can present as 'gastroenteritis'		Chloroquine '10-tab in 3 days'
AIDS	Weight loss; lymphopenia.	Negative stool culture	Symptomatic

E.h. = *Entamoeba histolytica*

TABLE 32.2 FEATURES OF DIARRHOEA ACCORDING TO ORGAN OF INVOLVEMENT

Disease site	Small intestine	Large intestine	Pancreas
No. of stools/day	3–6	> 6	1–3
Volume	Large	Small	Large
Consistency	Semisolid	Liquid	Semisolid
Tenesmus	Absent	Present	Absent
Blood & mucus	Absent	Present	Absent
Pain site	Periumbilical	Lower abdomen	Upper abdomen radiating to back
Weight loss	+ +	±	+ + +
Sigmoidoscopy	Normal	Abnormal	Normal
Faecal fat	Higher than normal	Normal	Very high
D-xylose test	Abnormal	Normal	Normal
Vit. B12 absorption	Abnormal in ileal disease	Normal	Normal
Plain X-ray abdomen	Normal	Normal or may show toxic megacolon	May show pancreatic calcification
Barium studies	Abnormal	Abnormal	May show widening of the C-loop (rare)

TABLE 32.3 CAUSES OF CHRONIC OR RECURRENT DIARRHOEA

	Confirmatory tests
Small bowel	
Intestinal giardiasis	Stools or duodenal aspirate for trophozoites
Hookworm disease	Stool examination
Ileocaecal tuberculosis	Barium enema of small bowel; colonoscopic biopsy of ileocaecal region
Crohn's disease	Endoscopy
Tropical sprue	Faecal fat estimation; D-xylose absorption test
Pellagra	Other features of pellagra: skin & mental changes
Addison's disease	Plasma cortisol < 5 μg/ml and ACTH > 80 units
Large bowel	
Ulcerative colitis	Sigmoidoscopy: continuous multiple shallow ulcers, contact bleeding
Crohn's disease of colon	Sigmoidoscopy: continuous or patchy
Amoebic colitis	Sigmoidoscopy: ulcers with intervening mucosa normal
Irritable bowel syndrome	Normal sigmoidoscopy

respond to metronidazole or doxycyline should raise the suspicion of AIDS in a 'high-risk' individual (homosexual, promiscuous heterosexual, drug addict, recipient of untested blood transfusion). The average survival from the onset of diarrhoea is 9–12 months.

AIDS with superimposed CMV colitis can produce bloody diarrhoea clinically and is sigmoidoscopically indistinguishable from ulcerative colitis; but biopsy shows no crypt abscesses.

Irritable bowel syndrome

In spite of repeated episodes of diarrhoea and abdominal pain and distension, the patient looks well. A discussion of his lifestyle and reassurance are often enough. Over investigation and drug therapy should be avoided.

33 Dyspepsia

The terms dyspepsia and indigestion are difficult to define. Patients use these terms variously to express a feeling of epigastric fullness, discomfort or pain, heartburn or acidity (which is relieved by antacids), nausea, vomiting, belching, or flatulence.

With the availability of oesophago-gastroduodenoscopy it has become possible to directly visualize this part of the alimentary tract, take colour pictures for documentation of lesions, and obtain biopsy for histological information. Endoscopic studies are not useful in assessing GI motility disorder which may be more accurately determined by barium studies or radionuclide studies.

In as many as 50 per cent of patients presenting with epigastric pain or discomfort, it is not possible to arrive at a specific pathological diagnosis even after a complete work-up. Endoscopic findings of inflammation- 'gastritis or duodenitis' –have a poor correlation with the symptoms of dyspepsia. These changes may be seen in totally asymptomatic persons, while patients with classic dyspeptic symptoms may have an absolutely normal endoscopic appearance of the stomach and duodenum. A poor correlation is also found between histologic changes and symptoms. The subject then resolves into considering:

A. conditions in which organic disease is present in the alimentary tract (e.g. peptic ulcer, gastric carcinoma, gallbladder disease) or elsewhere (e.g. pulmonary or intestinal tuberculosis, Addison's disease, cirrhosis, congestive heart failure); and

B. conditions in which the alimentary tract is structurally intact but functionally disturbed.

Table 33.1 lists the important causes of dyspepsia.

TABLE 33.1 CAUSES OF DYSPEPSIA

	Clinical picture	Comments
Non-ulcer dyspepsia	Suggestive of peptic ulcer but none found on barium meal/ endoscopy	Twice as common as peptic ulcer; may affect 20-30% of population; disordered motility.
H. pylori infection	Suggestive of peptic ulcer but none found	Delayed gastric emptying shown on radionuclide studies.
Food intolerance e.g. milk	Flatulence, distension, abdominal cramps, diarrhoea	Deficiency of enzyme lactase– congenital or acquired.
Gluten enteropathy	Abdominal distension, diarrhoea	Sensitivity to gluten; treated with gluten-free diet.
Functional biliary dyskinesis	Fatty or fried food leads to pain and distension; no gallstones or cholecystitis seen on investigation	Cholecystectomy seldom cures the patient with normal gallbladder function.
Aerophagy	Bloating, belching, abdominal distension, flatulence	Motility disturbance.
Increased gas production in colon by bacteria	Consumption of legumes, some grains, beans, cause distension & flatulence	Common in giardiasis and amoebiasis.
Decreased gas absorption	Hepatomegaly, ascites, stigmata of cirrhosis, raised JVP	Congestive heart failure; cirrhosis with portal hypertension.

Non-ulcer Dyspepsia (NUD)

This term is used to describe symptoms suggestive of peptic ulcer but with no evidence of peptic ulcer on endoscopy. Some cases may have H. pylori infection and a prolonged gastric emptying time has been seen in many of them.

Gallstones and Chronic Cholecystitis

The relationship of dyspepsia and gallstones can be coincidental rather than cause-and-effect. If gallstones are associated with poor gallbladder function on HIDA scintigraphy, dyspepsia is less likely to be cured by cholecystectomy than if the gallbladder is functioning well.

Disordered Gastrointestinal Motility

The motility of the alimentary tract is controlled by the autonomic nervous system and gut hormones including cholecystokinin, thereby ensuring the orderly progression of nutrients through the system so that the stage of digestion and absorption is appropriate to a given region of the tract. The complexity of both local and distant neural and endocrine factors that regulate intestinal motility is only now becoming fully appreciated. Disruption of normal motility is quite common, with functional bowel complaints afflicting as many as 15 per cent of adult individuals.

Disordered gastrointestinal motility may occur post-vagotomy, or in diabetic autonomic neuropathy or idiopathic gastroparesis (gastric atony). Gastric electrical activity can be determined by placing electrodes on the abdominal wall—('electrogastrogram'). Some patients with otherwise unexplained nausea and vomiting have shown accelerated gastric movements ('tachygastria') or irregular movement ('gastric tachyarrhythmia'). Some patients with functional indigestion also have features of irritable bowel syndrome suggesting a diffuse intestinal motility disturbance. The role of emotional factors in producing these changes is well-recognized. Since the epigastrium is a frequent location for 'functional' pain, it would be worth studying the correlation of depression, anxiety. and chronic stress with the patterns in the electrogastrogram, and studying the effect of prokinetic drugs such as metoclopramide, cisapride and erythromycin.

Functional Biliary Dyskinesia

Although gallbladder disease typically causes pain limited to the right upper quadrant, about half of the patients with this condition experience only epigastric pain. In the absence of gallstones, demonstration of abnormal gallbladder function (low ejection fraction, delayed emptying due to spasm of sphincter of Oddi by CCK-augmented HIDA scintigraphy can identify a subset of patients who will benefit by cholecystectomy or papillotomy of the sphincter of Oddi.

Intestinal Gas

Gas in the gastrointestinal tract may be derived from three sources: swallowed air, production in the intestines, and diffusion from the blood into the gut lumen.

Normally 2 to 3 ml of air is taken in with each swallow, particularly of liquids. The stomach contains about 50 ml of gas. Many patients increase this amount as well as increase the number of swallows to obtain a feeling of relief from symptomatic gastro-oesophageal reflux frequently associated with a decrease in lower oesophageal sphincter pressure. This unrecognized habit may lead to accumulation of air within the stomach too rapidly for its passage on into the small intestine, and belching may occur, with each eructation consisting of 20 to 80 ml of gas. The stomach is emptied in one to six belches. Hypersalivation may lead to excessive air swallowing.

The normal small intestine does not contain any gas. Gas not eructed from the stomach passes into the small bowel where most of it is rapidly diffused into the blood. Due to the absence of bacterial flora in the small intestine, very little gas is formed by bacterial fermentation. In the presence of intestinal obstruction, fermentation may produce 3500 ml of gas in 24 hours in the small intestine.

The normal colonic bacterial flora produce gas by fermentation, the amount depending on the nature of unabsorbed residue. Of this, 14 per cent is absorbed and excreted through the lungs, the rest escapes in flatus. Undigestible oligosaccharides (raffinose, stachyose) contained in beans may increase the passage of flatus from the basal 20 ml an hour to as much as 200 ml an hour. A person with lactase deficiency, on ingesting lactose-containing foods, can produce 240 ml gas per hour. Odourless gas is carbon dioxide or hydrogen; gas with a foetid odour is hydrogen sulfide.

Diffusion of gas from the blood into the lumen of the gut can occur in conditions of increased portal venous pressure as in cirrhosis or congestive heart failure which may also retard diffusion of CO_2 from the gut lumen into the blood. This explains the abdominal distension in these patients in the absence of ascites.

Approach to a Patient with Dyspepsia

The main concern of the doctor is to establish that the symptoms are not due to primary gastrointestinal disease but are rather a functional response of an organically normal alimentary tract, probably to emotionally stressful situations. The fear of peptic ulcer, gastric cancer or gallbladder disease has to be allayed by the standard work-up of gastrointestinal barium meal studies and/or endoscopy. Lactose intolerance must be considered in every case and is usually detected by a careful history.

As our knowledge base expands, we have to revise our concepts of the 'typical textbook picture' of disease. Horrocks and de Dombal reported a prospective study of 350 patients suffering from dyspepsia. Surprisingly, 53 per cent of those with peptic ulcer seen endoscopically, *did not* have pain related to meals. They just had bellyache localized to the epigastrium and occurring in attacks with pain-free intervals in between. 32 per cent of patients with non-ulcer dyspepsia had discomfort soon after eating. Loss of weight may not occur in cancer of the stomach and may occur in non-ulcer dyspepsia, thus upsetting our previous knowledge base.

Gastric cancer, when superficial and surgically curable, usually produces no symptoms. As the tumour becomes more expansive, patients may complain of an insidious upper abdominal discomfort varying in intensity from a vague postprandial fullness to a severe steady pain. Anorexia and nausea come much later and are not the presenting complaints. There are no early physical signs, and the finding of a palpable mass is a late sign, probably indicating regional spread. Gastroscopy and biopsy and brush cytology are required for all patients with a gastric ulcer in order to exclude malignancy.

Management of Dyspepsia

Patients with lactose intolerance should avoid milk, butter, cream, cheese etc. Yogurt is low in lactose and is generally well tolerated.

H. pylori infection may be treated with colloidal bismuth subsalicylate 30 ml qid and amoxicillin 150 mg qid for 1-8 weeks. Eradication of the organisms results in disappearance of inflammatory changes in the gastric mucosa but recurrence is frequent.

Approach to a Case of Dysphagia

Dysphagia or difficulty in swallowing is one of the most reliable of all indicators of disorders in the alimentary tract. The patient often locates the pain or discomfort or difficulty of the passage of the bolus on swallowing, anywhere from the oropharynx to the epigastrium. For clinical purposes it is useful to separate oropharyngeal from oesophageal dysphagia since the symptoms, causes, and management strategies are different.

It is important to ascertain if the difficulty is in swallowing *liquids* or *solids* or *both*.

If the patient has difficulty in swallowing both liquids and solids, he is likely to have a *motility disorder* of the oesophagus.

If the patient has progressive dysphagia to solids but relatively little difficulty for liquids, then an *obstructive lesion* is most likely.

Painful swallowing (odynophagia) may reflect diffuse oesophageal spasm, or an inflammatory lesion like candida oesophagitis, or malignancy, or peptic ulcer of the oesophagus (Barrett's ulcer).

Chest pain induced by swallowing hot or cold liquids is suggestive of diffuse oesophageal spasm.

Intermittent dysphagia to solids is suggestive of a Schatzki's ring (lower oesophageal mucosal ring).

Rapid weight loss along with dysphagia is highly suggestive of malignancy of the oesophagus.

The crucial clinical features of the various important causes of oropharyngeal dysphagia are given in **Table 34.1** and those of oesophageal dysphagia are given in **Table 34.2**.

Extrinsic pressure on the oesophagus due to aneurysm of the aorta, giant left auricle, massive pericardial effusion, or mediastinal tumours may all

TABLE 34.1 CRUCIAL FEATURES OF OROPHARYNGEAL CAUSES OF DYSPHAGIA

Cause	Diagnostic clues
Ulcers on the tongue	Lesions obvious on examination of the mouth and pharynx.
Vincent's angina Tonsillar abscess Pharyngitis Retropharyngeal abscess	
Plummer Vinson syndrome (Sideropaenic dysphagia) due to iron deficiency	Pallor, Koilonychia, Hypochromic microcytic anaemia.
Neuromuscular disorders Bulbar poliomyelitis Motor neurone disease Diphtheritic neuritis	Choking or coughing during swallowing. Nasal regurgitation.
Myasthenia gravis	Chewing and swallowing become more difficult as meal progresses, Diplopia, Ptosis, Improvement with inj. prostigmine 1 mg.
Pharyngeal pouch	Palpable mass medial to sternomastoid.
Retrosternal goitre	Neck goitre visible, Tracheal compression, Arm raising test.
Tumour/granuloma	Palpable mass· causing extrinsic pressure.
Cancer of hypopharynx	Usually superimposed on Plummer Vinson syndrome.

cause dysphagia but other features of these conditions are also present and make the diagnosis clear.

TABLE 34.2 CRUCIAL FEATURES OF OESOPHAGEAL CAUSES OF DYSPHAGIA

	Clinical features
Obstructive lesions	
• Benign stricture of mid-oesophagus	History of corrosive poisons, foreign body, or prolonged intubation.
• Reflux oesophagitis	History of heartburn and water brash, or angina-like pain aggravated by lying flat or bending forward, relieved by sitting up or antacids.
• Inflammatory lesions Candida CMV Herpes simplex	Candida in oral cavity also, immunosuppressed patient; odynophagia, weight loss.
• Radiation oesophagitis	Dysphagia for solids.
• Malignancy of oesophagus	Dysphagia for solids, odynophagia, weight loss, hoarseness of voice (recurrent laryngeal palsy), cough (aspiration into lungs, tracheooesophageal fistula).
Motility disorders	
• Achalasia cardia	Initial dysphagia for liquids, later on for solids, no pain, heartburn, aspiration into lungs.
• Diffuse oesophageal spasm	Painful swallowing brought on by cold liquids & solids, chest pain, independent of swallowing-mimics angina but not brought on by exertion, relieved by nitroglycerin or nifedipine.
• Scleroderma oesophagus	Difficulty in swallowing liquids & solids, heartburn, reflux oesophagitis, may go on to stricture formation, skin showing scleroderma, Raynaud's phenomenon.
• Extrinsic pressure on the oesophagus	Other features of aneurysm, pericardial effusion, mediastinal tumour etc.

Physical Examination

1. Examine the mouth and pharynx for any ulcerative lesions or tonsillar abscess which can cause difficulty in swallowing.

2. Ask the patient to say 'Ah!' and observe the movement of the soft palate. Check for a history of nasal regurgitation. If there is paralysis of the palate, look for other neurological signs (**Table 34.1**).

3. If the thyroid is enlarged, palpate its lower poles while the patient swallows a sip of water, to make sure that there is no retrosternal extension of the goitre which may press on the oesophagus.

4. If the voice is hoarse, get the larynx examined by indirect laryngoscopy for evidence of tuberculosis or malignancy, which can cause painful dysphagia.

Diagnostic Confirmation

Barium swallow: oesophageal X-ray in upright and head low positions.

Motility studies: for achalasia, diffuse spasm scleroderma.

Oesophagoscopy: Mainly scleroderma for confirmation of peptic oesophagitis and Barrett's ulcer or exclusion of malignancy. The malignant tumour of the oesophagus or tumours invading the oesophagus often spread beneath the mucosa and therefore might not be seen endoscopically or reached by a superficial biopsy. Hence malignancy is not ruled out by a report of 'only inflammatory cells'.

Oesophageal Pain versus Angina Pectoris

The pain of oesophageal disease (spasm, reflux oesophagitis) may mimic angina pectoris (due to ischaemic coronary artery disease) in every respect-site (retrosternal), radiation (neck and jaw, dorsal spine, shoulder, arm, epigastrium). It may be described as crushing or burning. The pain is promptly relieved by nitroglycerin or sublingual nifedipine, as in angina pectoris.

The duration of oesophageal pain may be much longer than that of angina–30 minutes or more, which may resemble pre-infarction angina, but the ECG is normal in oesophageal pain.

The crucial differentiating point is that oesophageal pain has no relation to exertion.

Oesophageal spasm may occur at rest or may be related to emotional duress. Diffuse oesophageal spasm may be associated with vasovagal phenomena (sweating, tachycardia, pallor), again mimicking rest angina (Prinzmetal) but the ECG is normal.

To make matters more complicated, both oesophageal and coronary artery disease may coexist, hence it is prudent to exclude significant coronary artery disease by a more definitive test (stress thallium myocardial perfusion).

Heartburn is the common symptom of reflux oesophagitis. The patient points to the entire region from the suprasternal notch to the epigastrium (while in angina the heartburn is localized to one spot retrosternally). Oesophageal symptoms are aggravated by lying flat or bending forward (unlike angina) and are relieved by assuming an upright position or by antacid. Patients with angina-like chest pain in whom CAD has been excluded may be investigated by 24 hours ambulatory oesophageal pH and motility recording. Most of these patients are found to have reflux oesophagitis.

Management Plan

Reflux oesophagitis: The goals of treatment are to decrease gastro-oesophageal reflux, neutralize the refluxed acid, improve oesophageal clearance and protect oesophageal mucosa. These can be achieved by:

- weight reduction;
- sleeping with elevation of the head of the bed;
- avoiding smoking, alcohol, coffee, orange juice, and fatty foods;
- avoiding anticholinergic drugs, calcium channel blockers and smooth muscle relaxants;
- sucralfate to protect the mucosa;
- antacids, H2 blockers (ranitidine 150 mg tid, or famotidine 20 mg at bedtime for 6 months;
- prokinetic agents (metoclopramide, 10 mg qid, or cisapride or domperidone).

Candida oesphagitis: Ketoconazole (200-400 mg in a single oral dose) is the treatment of choice.

Achalasia cardia: is treated with pneumatic dilatation of the lower oesophageal sphincter.

Cancer of oesophagus:

- palliation with surgical resection followed by radiation therapy;
- repeated endoscopic dilatations;
- gastrostomy for hydration and feeding;
- endoscopic fulguration of the obstructive tumour with lasers appears to be the most promising technique.

35 Fever

Fever is one of the commonest complaints with which a doctor is faced. Fever indicates that the thermoregulatory centre in the hypothalamus is disturbed by some product or products of tissue injury. Infection is the most frequent cause of such tissue injury, hence many doctors, faced with a patient with fever give a 'knee jerk' response with antimicrobial therapy. It is, therefore, worth emphasizing that there are other causes of tissue injury apart from infection. These are listed in **Table 35.1**. In tropical countries the atmospheric temperature in summer months often goes beyond 115°F (45°C) giving rise to heat hyperpyrexia, a good example of fever in the absence of infection.

It is also worth emphasizing that fever by itself (except when it exceeds 105°F/40.5°C) is a *beneficial* response of the body in combating infection.

For instance gonococci, Treponema pallida and the schizonts of malarial parasites are killed at a temperature of 40°C. Antibody production is increased five-fold at a temperature of 39.5°C than at 37°C. Hence there is no need to panic and rush into speculative antimicrobial therapy until sufficient evidence is collected regarding the possible cause of fever. Many fevers due to viral infection are short-lived and self-limited (3-5 days). Except in an emergency, there is no need to start specific antimicrobial therapy till the report of a simple peripheral blood smear, CBC, urine examination, throat swab or sputum are available.

It is also worth stressing that samples for urine culture and blood culture should be sent *before* any antimicrobial therapy is started. A single capsule of 500 mg ampicillin will successfully vitiate an attempt to get a positive blood culture for Salmonella typhi.

TABLE 35.1 FEVER IN THE ABSENCE OF INFECTION

1. Heat stroke.
2. Infarction: myocardial, pulmonary, cerebral, mesenteric.
3. Antigen-antibody reactions: rheumatic fever, allergic fever, drugs, & serum therapy, autoimmune mechanism e.g. SLE, polyarteritis nodosa.
4. Malignancy: leukaemia, Hodgkin's disease, hypernephroma, gastric and pancreatic carcinoma.
5. Thyrotoxicosis, especially thyroid crisis, thyroiditis (tenderness over the gland).
6. Metabolic factors: gout, porphyria, steroids.
7. Anaesthetic agents: halothane with succinyl choline, malignant hyperthermia.
8. Pontine lesions: embolism, haemorrhage.
9. Familial Mediterranean fever.
10. Habitual hyperthermia (in young females).
11. Fictitious (patient-induced) fever.

Hyperpyrexia (temperature over 105°F) by itself demands measures to bring it down, apart from specific therapy against the causative agent. Living tissues are irreversibly damaged when the body temperature goes beyond 46°C (114°F). There are a number of reports of recovery from a body temperature of 112-113°F.

Prolonged fever has detrimental effects on the body, through excessive catabolism (mediated by several lymphokines and cytokines), mild acidosis, and increased work for the heart.

In elderly patients, or in patients on high dose corticosteroids, there may be no fever in spite of a life-threatening infection such as gram negative septicaemia. Tachycardia, tachypnoea, mental confusion and hypotension are the only clues for infection in such patients.

Pyrexia of uncertain origin (PUO) is a common problem in clinical practice. The criterion of PUO is any fever of more than 4 weeks' duration with failure to reach a diagnosis after one week of study in the hospital. This definition excludes many common causes of fever either because they are self-limiting or because they can be readily diagnosed by proper methodology (e.g. *repeated* thick and thin smears for malaria parasites instead of a single random sample, a blood culture drawn without prior antibiotics, *repeated* blood cultures for subacute bacterial endocarditis). The important causes of PUQ are given in **Table 35.2**. A wise physician will consider *common diseases* presenting in unusual fashion (e.g. tuberculosis, typhoid and malaria) just as he would consider rarer disorders like brucellosis and sarcoidosis.

Diagnostic Approach

When a doctor is called upon to see a case of fever, he may or may not be able to reach a conclusion at the first visit. The approach to a case of fever is given in a schematic form in **Fig. 35.1**. History, physical examination, complete blood count (CBC) and blood smear, urine examination (pus cells, RBCs, bilirubin and urobilinogen) and chest X-ray, and simple microbiological tests like sputum, throat swab or urethral smear, are sufficient to establish a presumptive diagnosis in the majority of patients with fever.

At the first visit the doctor should seek *localizing signs* (**Fig. 35.2** and **Table 35.3**) which will enable him to suspect the offending organism and start specific therapy. The time factor in the diagnosis of fever is illustrated in **Table 35.4**. Clues from simple laboratory tests are given in **Table 35.5**. Fever with chills also gives useful diagnostic clues (**Table 35.6**).

The doctor may find a rash at his first visit or later during the course of the illness. This will facilitate diagnosis of many fevers (**Table 35.7**). A rash not related particularly to the time table of fever raises the possibility of drug rash (**Table 35.8**). For counting purposes, if a patient took ill on a Monday and the rash appeared on Thursday, it would be the 4th day, suggestive of measles. If the diagnosis is not obvious by these steps, repeated clinical examinations will be necessary for seeking new clues (**Table 35.9**). A study of the temperature chart will also be helpful in suggesting various possibilities (**Table 35.10**).

Guessing the Offending Agent

One could take advantage of the fact that certain micro-organisms tend to locate in certain cells or organs and produce damage there. For example, the pneumococcus usually causes infection of the lung but not in the kidney. Haemophilus influenzae infection is confined almost solely to the respiratory tract and the meninges. Similarly the presence of a lesion known to be produced by a particular organism like staphylococcus may enable an intelligent search for haematogenous spread to predictable sites like the bones and the lungs. Drugs of choice for various infections are listed in **Table 35.11**.

Fever Due to Infection

The following characteristics are highly suggestive of an acute infection:

1. Abrupt onset.

2. High fever: 102°-105°F with or without chills.

3. Respiratory symptoms: sore throat, cough, rhinorrhoea.

4. Nausea, vomiting, diarrhoea.

5. Malaise, headache, backache, muscle and joint pains.

6. Splenomegaly and lymph node enlargement.

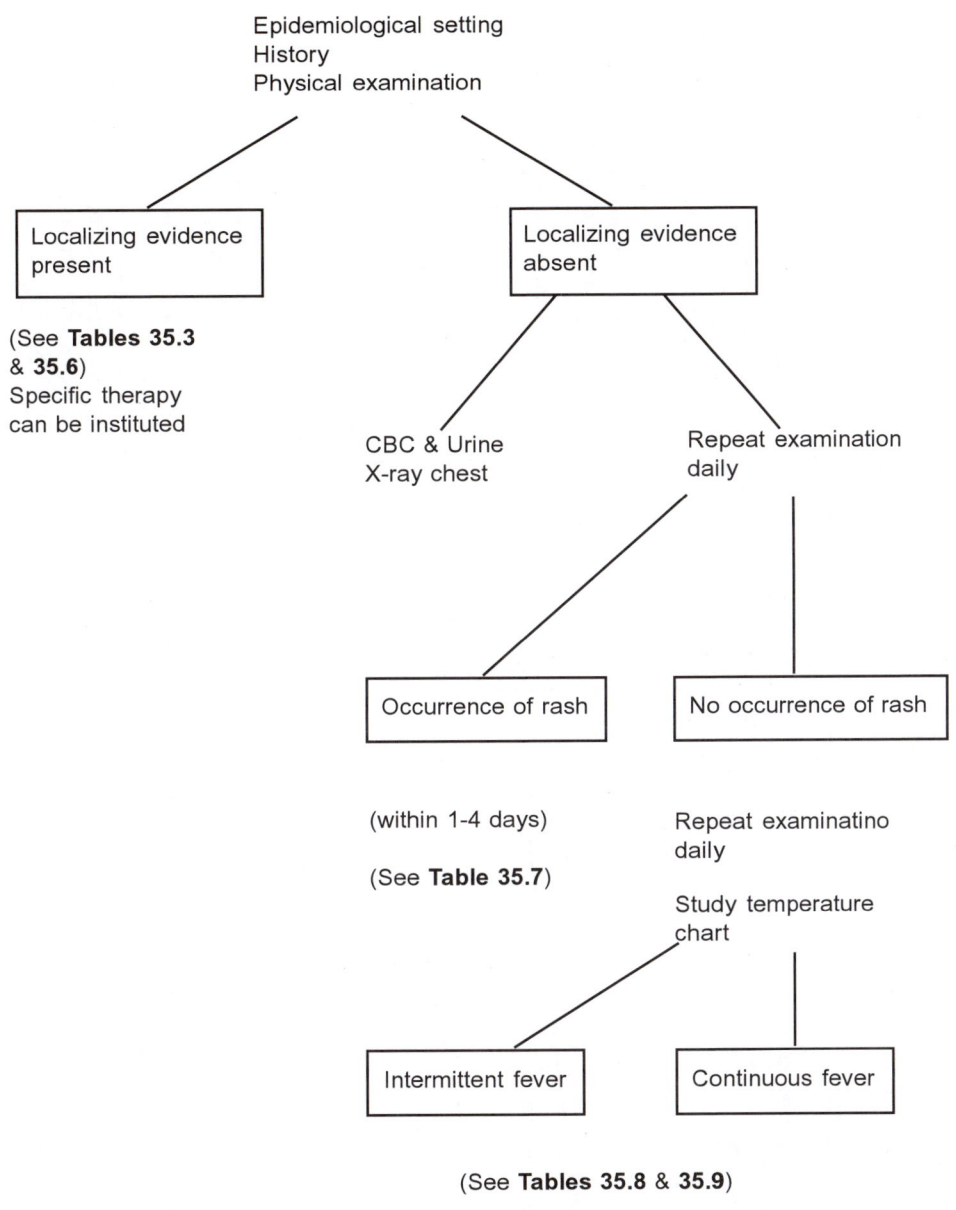

Fig. 35.1: Clinical approach to a case of fever

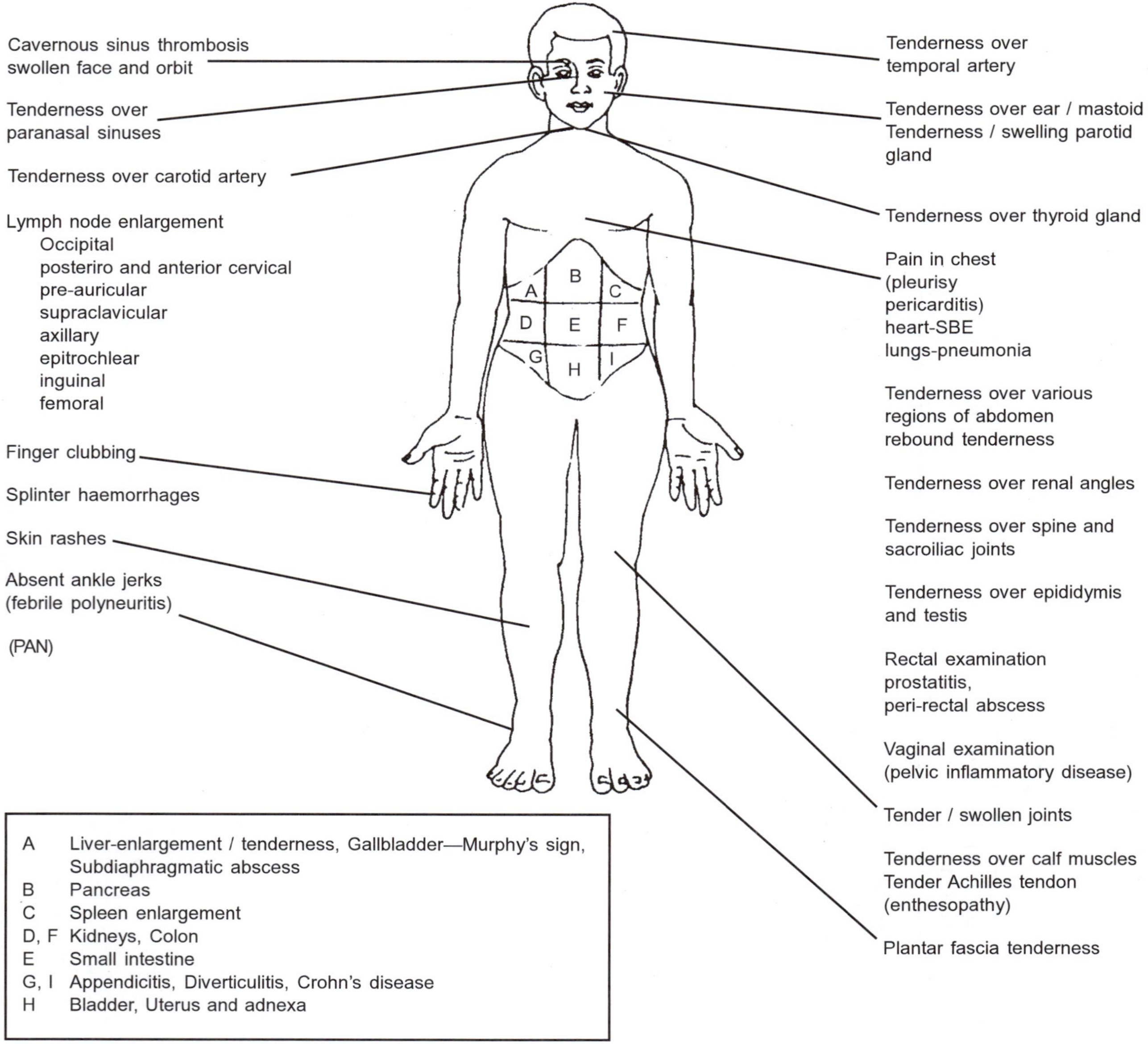

Fever

Fig. 35.2: Localizing signs in a patient with fever

Tenderness over temporal artery

Tenderness over ear / mastoid
Tenderness / swelling parotid gland

Tenderness over thyroid gland

Pain in chest
(pleurisy
pericarditis)
heart-SBE
lungs-pneumonia

Tenderness over various regions of abdomen
rebound tenderness

Tenderness over renal angles

Tenderness over spine and sacroiliac joints

Tenderness over epididymis and testis

Rectal examination
prostatitis,
peri-rectal abscess

Vaginal examination
(pelvic inflammatory disease)

Tender / swollen joints

Tenderness over calf muscles
Tender Achilles tendon
(enthesopathy)

Plantar fascia tenderness

Cavernous sinus thrombosis
swollen face and orbit

Tenderness over paranasal sinuses

Tenderness over carotid artery

Lymph node enlargement
Occipital
posteriro and anterior cervical
pre-auricular
supraclavicular
axillary
epitrochlear
inguinal
femoral

Finger clubbing

Splinter haemorrhages

Skin rashes

Absent ankle jerks
(febrile polyneuritis)

(PAN)

A   Liver-enlargement / tenderness, Gallbladder—Murphy's sign,
      Subdiaphragmatic abscess
B   Pancreas
C   Spleen enlargement
D, F Kidneys, Colon
E   Small intestine
G, I Appendicitis, Diverticulitis, Crohn's disease
H   Bladder, Uterus and adnexa

TABLE 35.2 PYREXIA OF UNCERTAIN ORIGIN

			Comments
A.	*Infections*		
	Tuberculosis:	Renal	Urine culture for AFB
		Bone	Gallium scanning
		Liver	Liver biopsy
	Bacterial endocarditis		2D echo, if blood culture -ve
	Brucellosis		Agglutination test
	HIV		ELISA and Western blot tests
B.	*Malignancy*		
	Hodgkin's Disease		Gallium scanning
	Lymphoma		
	Leukaemias		
	Solid tumours:	Kidneys	CT/MRI, Endoscopy
		Pancreas	
		Liver	
		Stomach	
C.	*Collagen disease*		
	SLE		NA, DNA Ab (double stranded)
	PAN		Muscle biopsy
	Polymyalgia rheumatica with temporal arteritis		Temporal artery biopsy High ESR. Dramatic response to low dose steroids.
	Retroperitoneal fibrosis		IVP: medial displacement of ureter on one or both sides
D.	*Thyroiditis* May be 'silent'		Tenderness on palpation Radionuclide scan: no uptake of tracer
E.	*Sarcoidosis*		Gallium scan, ↑ ACE in serum
F.	*Inflammatory bowel disease* Crohn's disease Whipple's disease		Colonoscopy, Ba studies
G.	*Drug Fever*		Fever disappears on stopping drug

TABLE 35.3 FEVER WITH LOCALIZING SIGNS

1.	Face	Suppurative sinusitis, Parotitis, Cavernous sinus thrombophlebitis.
2.	Ears	Otitis media, Mastoiditis.
3.	Mouth & throat	Candida-Vincent's Angina (bleeding gums), Koplik's spots (measles) Ulcers (SLE, Behcet's syndrome) Tonsillitis-streptococcal, diphtheria, Pharyngitis-viral, bacterial, gonococcal, retropharyngeal abscess.
4.	Neck	Meningitis (neck stiffness), Thyroiditis (tenderness over gland).
5.	Skin	Generalized skin rash (**Table 35.7**). Pustules & boils, paronychia, carbuncles, cellulitis, cellulitis with crepitus (Clostridium welchii).
6.	Lymph node enlarge- ment	Infectious mononucleosis, Secondary syphilis, Tuberculosis, Lymphogranuloma venereum, Filariasis, Lymphomas, Bubonic plague.
7.	Chest	Pleurisy, Tuberculosis, Pneumonia, lung abscess, bronchiectasis, Bacterial endocarditis, pericarditis.
8.	Abdomen	Appendicitis, diverticulitis, Cholecystitis-empyema of gallbladder, Liver abscess-hepatitis, Perinephric abscess, Retroperitoneal fibrosis.
	Rectal & PV: exam.	Prostatitis-perirectal abscess, Uterus and Fallopian tube infection, PID (pelvic inflammatory disease).
9.	Scrotum	Orchitis, Epididymitis.
10.	Back	Sacroiliac arthritis, Spinal epidural abscess (tenderness over spine), Paravertebral abscess, Perinephric abscess, Pyelonephritis (tenderness over costovertebral angle).
11.	Bones	Osteomyelitis, Dengue and chikungunya virus.
12.	Joints	Arthritis (See Chapter 26)
13.	Muscles	Polymyositis, Pyomyositis (very rare), Bornholm Disease (Coxsackie virus).
14.	Chest X-ray	Elevation of right dome of diaphragm, Liver abscess, subdiaphragmatic abscess.
15.	Urine	Pus cells, RBCs (pyelonephritis, cystitis), Bilirubin (viral hepatitis).

TABLE 35.4 TIME FACTOR IN DIAGNOSIS OF FEVER

Duration	Probable Cause
2-4 days	Viral infections.
2-7 days	Bacterial infections. malaria, plague.
7-14 days	Enteric group (typhoid), malaria.
15-30 days	Enteric group, tuberculosis, malaria.
1-6 months	Tuberculosis, Subacute bacterial endocarditis, Brucellosis, Drug-resistant malaria, HIV, Collagen disease, SLE, Polyarteritis nodosa, Malignancy e.g. hypernephroma, Hodgkin's-lymphoma.
One to several years	Habitual hyperthermia (needs no treatment), Familial Mediterranean fever (responds to colchicine).

TABLE 35.5 CLUES FROM SIMPLE LABORATORY TESTS FOR FEVER

- Urine — albumin, pus cells, RBCs bilirubin (pre-icteric phase of viral hepatitis).
- Blood smear — malarial parasites.
- WBC count — leucopenia: viral infections, typhoid, kala azar, tuberculosis my infection (lymphopenia)
  Leucocytosis:
    with neutrophil pred.:
      pyogenic infection, plague.
    with lymphocyte pred.:
      whooping cough, TB.
  Atypical lymphocytes: infectious mononucleosis.

NOTE: Any white cell count is compatible with malaria.

TABLE 35.6 FEVER WITH CHILLS

A single chill at onset
  Malaria
  Filariasis
  Viral infection (e.g. influenza)
  Pneumococcal pneumonia
  Streptococcal infections (cellulitis, puerperal sepsis)
  Osteomyelitis Leptospirosis

Repeated chills
  Pyogenic abscess
  Septicaemia
  Bacterial endocarditis (esp. staphylococcal)
  Pyelonephritis
  Intermittent biliary duct obstruction
  Malaria
  Brucellosis Phlebitis (pyelophlebitis, pelvic vein thrombosis, lateral sinus thrombosis)
  Intermittent aspirin administration

TABLE 35.7 EXANTHEMS WITH DAY OF OCCURRENCE OF RASH

	Common	Rare
1st day	Chickenpox	Dengue, Chikungunya
2nd day	Scarlet fever	
3rd day	Smallpox	
4th day	Measles	Exanthema subitum
5th day	Typhus	

TABLE 35.8 CAUSES OF FEVER WITH RASH APART FROM EXANTHEMS

Drug allergy	e.g. ampicillin.
Erythema nodosum	Tuberculosis, leprosy, fungal infections, streptococcal infection.
Erythema multiforme	Herpes simplex, mycoplasma, drugs.
Butterfly rash	SLE.
Miliaria	Heat rash.
Septicaemia	Meningococcal, gonococcal, gram negative. Toxic shock (menstruating women using tampons). Staphylococcus toxic epidermolysis.
Ecthyma gangrenosum	Pseudomonas infection in immunocompromised patients.

TABLE 35.9 USEFUL DIAGNOSTIC CLUES IN FEVER

Findings	Remarks	Findings	Remarks
1. Wasting	Chronic infection e.g. TB, HIV; or underlying debilitating disease: malignancy; diabetes mellitus; malabsorption; malnutrition.	14. Herpes febrilis on lips	Malaria; Pneumococcal pneumonia; Meningococcal meningitis.
2. Pallor	Severe or chronic infection.	*Findings*	*Remarks*
3. High fever without sweating: Hyperpyrexia (above 105°F) with sweating:	Heat stroke; Meningitis, malaria, typhoid; Gram -ve septicaemia; miliary TB, brucellosis, leptospirosis.	15. Bradycardia relative to temperature (e.g. temp. 39°C, pulse 96 p.m.)	Typhoid fever; viral infection (e.g. influenza); CNS infection.
4. Marked sweating	Septicaemia; amoebic liver abscess; tuberculosis; brucellosis; rheumatic fever.	16. Tachycardia relative to temperature (e.g. temp 38°C pulse 140 p.m.)	Myocarditis (diphtheria, pneumonia, rheumatic); bacterial endocarditis; polyarteritis nodosa.
5. Jaundice	Viral hepatitis, malaria, amoebic hepatitis.	17. Rapid respiration (pulse: respiration ratio less than 4:1)	Bacterial pneumonia; Gram -ve sepsis; pulmonary embolism and infarction.
6. Pruritus	Hodgkin's disease, cholangitis.	18. Dyspnoea	Pneumonia; poliomyelitis; diphtheria.
7. Purpura	Septicaemia, leukaemia, miliary TB.	19. Non-productive cough	Viral upper respiratory infection; viral pneumonia; malaria; typhoid; tuberculosis.
8. Toxic appearance	Typhoid, typhus; miliary tuberculosis; septicaemia.	20. Productive cough	Pneumonic plague; bacterial pneumonia; acute bronchitis; tuberculosis; lung abscess; bronchiectasis.
9. Delirium	Typhoid; typhus; pneumococcal pneumonia; meningo-encephalitis; non-specific in elderly patients.	21. Nausea, vomiting	Viral hepatitis, malaria; cholangitis; staphylococcal enteritis.
10. Severe headache	Typhoid, malaria, meningitis.	22. Hepatomegaly	Viral hepatitis, malaria; amoebic hepatitis; leptospirosis; cholangio-hepatitis; pneumonia.
11. Convulsions	Meningitis; brain absess; non-specific in children.		
12. Coma or stupor	Meningitis, encephalitis; brain abscess, cerebral malaria.	23. Splenomegaly	Typhoid; malaria, kala azar; miliary tuberculosis; brucelosis; bacterial endocarditis; acute pyelonephritis.
13. Severe muscle pain	Dengue & chikungunya virus infection; Influenza; Coxsackie virus infection; Leptospirosis; Meningococcaemia.	24. Lymph node enlargement	Tuberculosis, sarcoidosis; leukaemia, secondary syphilis, HIV.

TABLE 35.10 FEVER PATTERNS IN INFECTION

I. *Continuous or sustained*
   Typhoid fever
   Pneumococcal pneumonia
   Central nervous system infections

II. *Remittent* (more than 1° variation, not touching normal)
   Tuberculosis
   Brucellosis
   Malaria (falciparum)
   Typhoid (occasionally)

III. *Intermittent* (Fever touching normal every day)
   Tuberculosis
   Pyogenic abscess
   Malaria

IV. *Double spikes* (of fever every day)
   Miliary tuberculosis
   Kala azar
   Gonococcal endocarditis

V. *Hectic* (widely and irregularly swinging)
   Pyogenic abscess
   Malaria
   Gram -ve septicaemia
   Disseminated tuberculosis

VI. *Relapsing* (Periods of fever interspersed with period of normal temperature)
   Rat bite fever
   Relapsing fever
   Chronic meningococcaemia
   Brucellosis
   Malaria
   Tuberculosis esp. extrapulmonary

VII. *Hyperpyrexia* (above 105°F)
   Typhoid
   Tuberculosis
   Malaria
   Brucellosis
   Leptospirosis
   Gram negative urinary infection
   Heat hyperpyrexia
   Pontine embolism or haemorrhage

NOTE: Any pattern of fever is compatible with malaria, typhoid and tuberculosis.

The clinical diagnosis of a specific infection is often possible by (1) epidemiological evidence: occurrence of the same fever in other patients; (2) a definite time-course of the fever; and (3) a certain syndrome characteristic for each fever, e.g. skin rashes. It must be remembered that immunologically mediated injury can produce a similar picture (e.g. SLE, polyarterits nodosa).

Temperature Record

Patients vary enormously in their perception of fever. Some individuals can tell accurately whether they have fever, by the sensation of warmth of their skins. Others may be wholly unaware of a rise in temperature even 103°F, especially in an infection like tuberculosis. Others may not pay attention to the fever due to distraction of more troublesome symptoms like headache, pleural pain, joint pain etc.

Hence recording the *mouth temperature* is very essential for detection and follow-up of fever. Axillary temperature is often misleading. In children, rectal temperature is easier to record than mouth temperature.

In a 'shocked' patient the axillary and oral temperature may not represent the true 'core' temperature in the body. In such a case rectal temperature is more reliable.

Very little information can be derived from a single observation of a patient's temperature. In all cases of fever a serial record of temperature is essential. This may be needed hour-to-hour in hyperpyrexia (105°F). Usually it is enough to record 4-hourly temperature in acute cases and twice daily (morning and evening) in every case. A simultaneous record of pulse rate, blood pressure and respiration rate gives a correct assessment of the mischief that is going on.

Table 35.4 has been prepared for the guidance of clinicians, showing common organisms in usual infection sites. **Table 35.11** shows the antibiotic sensitivity of various micro-organisms so as to select the drug of choice.

TABLE 35.11 DRUGS OF CHOICE IN INFECTIONS

Organism	Drugs of choice in order of preference	Remarks
Streptococcus haemolyticus Group A	(1) Penicillin G	6,00,000 units/d procaine PG x 10 12,00,000 units/d benzathine PG. Oral penicillin G 1.2 megaunits/d or penicillin V. In patients allergic to penicillin.
	(2) Erythromycin	Erythromy 0.25-1 g PO qid.
	(3) Cephalothin	Cephalothin 1-2 g IV qid.
Streptococcus viridans	(1) Penicillin G (2) Penicillin + Streptomycin (3) Erythromycin	Bacterial endocarditis 2.4 to 6 megaunits/day IM or IV for 4-6 weeks when no response to penicillin alone. In patients allergic to penicillin.
Streptococcus faecalis (enterococcus)	(1) Penicillin G + Streptomycin	Bacterial endocarditis 20 megaunits IM or IV with streptomycin 1 g/d 4-6 weeks. Urinary tract infection 4 megaunits with 1 g strepto daily x 7-10 days.
Pneumococcus	(1) Penicillin G (2) Erythromycin (3) Tetracycline (4) Chloramphenicol	Pneumonia 60,00,000 units procaine P/d x 7 or until pt. afebrile for 2 days. Meningitis 12-20 megaunits/d for 7 days or till CSF clear.
Staphylococcus aureus (Penicillin-sensitive)	(1) Penicillin 2 (2) Erythromycin (3) Cephalothin	For abscess and cellulitis as for streptococcus above. Bact. endocarditis 6-10 megaunits/day for 4-6 weeks. Meningitis 15-20 megaunits/d. Pneumonia 1.2-2.4 megaunits/d
(Penicillin resistant)	(1) Oxacillin (2) Naficillin	1-2 g IV qid. 0.5-2 g IV qid.
Meningococcus	(1) Penicillin G	Meningitis 12-20 megaunits/d IM or IV for 7 or more days. Meningococcaemia 2.4 megaunits/d until pt. afebrile for 2 days.
Gonococcus	(1) Penicillin G	Venereal infection 6,00,000 units procaine PG/d IM for 3-5 days 2.4 megaunits benzathine PG IM.
Clostridia (tetanus) (gas gangrene)	(1) Penicillin G (2) Erythromycin (3) Tetracycline (4) Chloramphenicol	600,000-1.2 megaunits 1M daily until signs of local infection subside.
Corynebacterium diphtheriae	(1) Penicillin G	Same as above.
Actinomyces	(1) Penicillin G	1.2-2.4 megaunits/d IM until evidence of infection is gone.
E.coli	(1) Tetracycline (2) Streptomycin (3) Chloramphenicol (4) Ampicillin (5) Cephalothin (6) Kanamycin	Bacteraemia 2-4 g /orally daily or 1 g IM or IV combined with 1 g streptomycin. Final selection according to sensitivity testing.

(Contd)

TABLE 35.11 (Contd)

Organism	Drugs of choice in order of preference	Remarks
Klebsiella aerobacter	(1) Chloramphenicol + Streptomycin (2) Tetracycline + Streptomycin	Same as for E. coli.
Pseudomonas aeruginosa	(1) Colistin (2) Polymyxin B	Urinary infection 50-75 mg IM every 12 hours. Bacteraemia 100-150 mg IM every 12 hours for 7-10 days.
Proteus mirabilis	(1) Penicillin G (2) Ampicillin (3) Cephalothin	12-20 megaunits 1M or IV daily for 7-10 days. 0.5 g PO qid.
Proteus (Indole) Positive	(1) Kanamycin	0.5 g IM 2-3 times/day not more than 10 days. Not more than 15 g total.
Haemophilus influenzae Salmonella	(1) Chloramphenicol (2) Tetracycline	Typhoid fever 2-4 g/day for 10-14 days.
Shigella	(1) Tetracycline (2) Chloramphenicol (3) Ampicillin	For resistant strains: Ciprofloxacin or Ofloxacin 500 mg bid for 14 days.
Bacterioides	(1) Tetracycline	Abscesses or bacteraemia 2-4 g/d oral or g IM/d
Brucella	(1) Tetracycline + Streptomycin	2-4 g/d oral plus 1 g IM/d for 10-14 days 500 mg orally/6 hourly for 2 days. 1.5-2 g/d
Vibrio cholera	(1) Tetracycline	
Pasteurella pestis	(1) Tetracycline (2) Streptomycin	

Incubation Periods of Important Infections

1. Influenza — 1-3 days
2. Pneumonia — 1-3 days
3. Cholera — 1-5 days
4. Diphtheria — 1-6 days
5. Gonorrhoea — 2-3 days
6. Plague — 2-7 days
   (Pneumonic) — 2-3 days
7. Measles — 8-12 days
8. Typhoid — 10-15 days
9. Amoebiasis — 9-90 days
10. Syphilis — 15-25 days
11. Tetanus — 3-21 days
12. Malaria — 12-20 days up to several months
13. Hepatitis A — 2-6 weeks
14. Hepatitis B, C — 2-6 months
15. Kala azar — (10 days to 1 year) 3-6 months
16. Filariasis — 3m-2 years
17. Rabies — 1-3 months (to several years)
18. HIV — 2-15 years

It is useful to know the incubation period of common and important infections.

Rickettsial diseases in India

Rickettsial diseases in various parts of India are not so uncommon as believed - both in rural and urban, as there can be small "mite islands" in vegetations around residences.

The clinical presentation can range from a short duration undifferentiated fever to a systemic vasculitis with multiorgan dysfunction and ARDS with significant morbidity and mortality. There are strain variations in the O. tsutsugamushi with various degrees of virulence.

A necrotic eschar - in the inguinal region, thigh, popliteal region, buttock, trunk, axilla is seen in 30% of patients.

The clustering of cases during the month of September to November should be remembered as it demands high index of suspicion.

The weil-felix test is insensitive whereas the IgM and IgE ELISA lists are more sensitive and specific.

Doxycycline is the drug of choice for scrub typhus or spotted fever. Clinical response occurs within 48 hrs hence it can almost be a therapeutic test in sick patients with multi organ dysfunction IV doxycycline is the preferred route although no IV preparation is available in India. For pregnant women, Azithromycin is the current drug of choice. Chloramphenicol is another useful agent.

No reliable vaccine with long term protection is available.

Ebola

The Ebola virus causes an acute, serious illness which is often fatal if untreated. Ebola virus disease (EVD). It occurred in a village near the Ebola river, from which the disease takes lots name.

The virus family Filoviridae includes 3 genera: Cuevavirus, Marburgvirus and Ebolavirus.

Ebola virus is transmitted through fruit bats of the Pteropodidae family where are natural Ebola virus hosts. Ebola is introduced into human population through close contact with the blood, secretions or other body fluids of infected animals. Ebola then spreads through human - to -human transmission via direct contact(through broken skin or mucous membranes)with the blood, secretions, organs or other body fluids in infected people , and with surfaces and materials (e.g. bedding, clothing) contaminated with fluids.

Health care workers have frequently been infected while treating patients with suspected or confirmed EVD.

Men who have recovered from the disease can still transmit the virus for up to 7 weeks after recovery from illness.

Symptoms of Ebola virus disease:

The incubation period, that is, the time interval from infection with the virus to onset of symptoms is 2 to 21 days. Humans are not infectious until the develop symptoms. First symptoms are the sudden onset of fever, fatigue, muscle pain, headache and sore throat. This is followed by vomiting, diarrhea, rash, symptoms of impaired kidney and liver function, and in some cases, both internal and external bleeding (e.g. oozing from gums, blood in the stools)

Diagnosis

It can be difficult to distinguish EVD from other infectious diseases such as malaria, typhoid fever and meningitis.

Samples from patients are an extreme biohazard risk; laboratory testing on non -inactivated samples should be conducted under maximum biological containment conditions.

Treatment:

Supportive care - rehydration with oral or intravenous fluids and treatment of specific symptoms, improves survival. There is as yet no proven treatment available for EVD However, a range of potential treatments including blood products, immune therapies and drug therapies are currently being evaluated .No licensed vaccines are available yet, but 2 potential vaccines are undergoing human safety testing.

Prevention and Control:

Good outbreak control relies on applying a package of interventions, namely case management , surveillance and contact tracing , a good laboratory service, safe burials and social mobilization . Community engagement is the key to successfully controlling the disease.

Drug Fever

A number of drugs may cause fever, important among them being atropine, anti-histamines, barbiturates and bromides, butazolidin, diphenyl hydantoin, iodides, morphine, PAS, penicillin, quinidine, salicylates, streptomycin, sulfonamides and thiouracil. In most cases the mechanism of fever is hypersensitivity, a clue for which is a skin rash along with the fever. Eosinophilia is present in only 50 per cent of patients. The usual response in fevers is eosinopenia, hence the first appearance of eosinophilia during the course of fever is a useful clue for immunologic injury. Stopping all the drugs would be the best policy when the fever continues in the face of full dose and duration of drugs. On

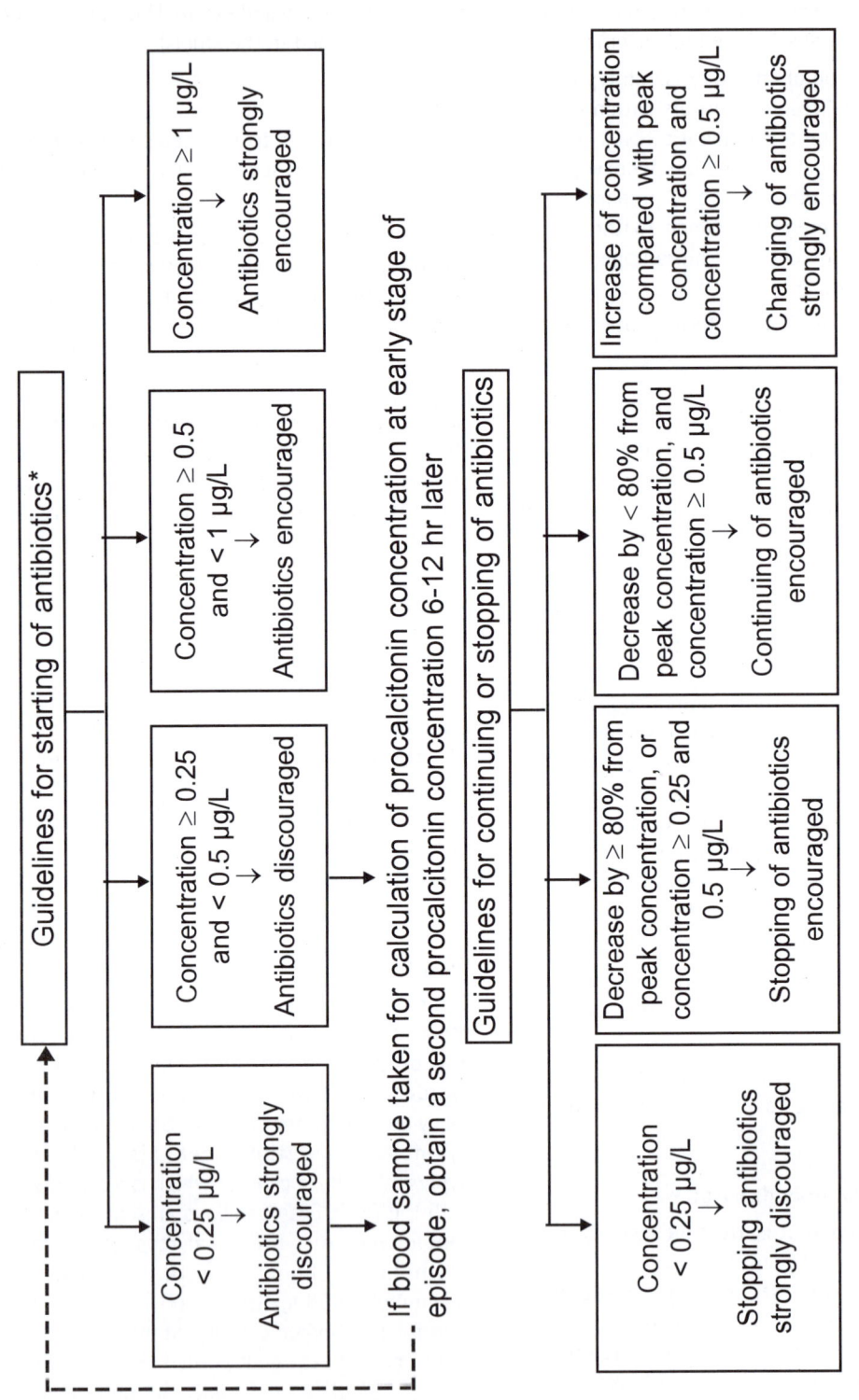

Fig. 35.3 : Guidelines for starting, continuing, or stopping of antibiotics according to procalcitonin concentrations

stopping the drug, the fever disappears within 2-3 days.

Pyrogens

Chills and high fever may follow the intravenous administration of saline solutions, serum and other biological preparations, because of the presence of bacterial pyrogens which gain access through contamination. Special precautions must be taken to avoid pyrogen contamination of any material to be given intravenously. Pyrogens can pass through bacterial filters and can withstand autoclaving. Fortunately their effect is short-lived.

Combination of Drugs

1. Mixed bacterial infections-2 or more organisms Bronchiectasis Peritonitis Otitis (acute and chronic)
2. To delay emergence of resistant strain TB-3 drugs INAH, rifampicin, pyrazinamide Miliary TB and TBM-4 drugs
3. Fixed dose combination may be inadequate due to differing sensitivity. But in places where the facility for testing sensitivity is not available, this approach may work.
4. Severe infection-cause?

   Hope that combination will cover the unknown culprit.

   If short duration, conservatism better because agent is probably a virus.

Examples of beneficial combinations
Enterococcus: Penicillin + Streptomycin
K. pneumoniae: Chloramphenicol + Streptomycin
Brucellosis: Tetracycline + Streptomycin

Examples of inferior performance by combination
Pneumococcal meningitis: Penicillin + tetracycline; Penicillin + chloramphenicol
Streptococcal pharyngitis: Penicillin + erythromycin

Procalcitonin

Procalcitonin (PCT) is produced ubiquitously in response to endotoxin or mediators released in response to bacterial infections (IL-IB, TNF &

IL-6) and strongly correlates with the extent and severity of bacterial infections. IFN a cytokine released in response to viral infections attenuates PCT upregulation, PCT is more specific for bacterial infections, and may help to distinguish bacterial infections from viral illnesses PCT shows a favourable kinetic profile for use as a Clinical marker; it promptly increases within 6-12 hours upon stimulation and circulating PCT levels halve daily when the infection is controlled by the host immune defence or antibiotic therapy, PCT correlates with bacterial load and severity of infection. Thus PCT has prognostic implications and the course of PCT predicts outcome in patients with community acquired pneumonia (CAP) and critically ill patients with sepsis PCT demonstrated a better discriminatory ability compared to WBC and hs CRP. At a cut off of 0.1 mg/L PCT has a very high sensitivity to exclude bacterial infection. A value < 0.25mg/L helps to exclude bacterial infection with a high negative predictive value. This helps to avoid unnecessary antimicrobial therapy.

In Urinary Tract Infection (UTI) especially in paediatric population, PCT correlates with the extent of renal involvement and renal scarring in pyelonephritis, in children with febrile UTI.

Production of PCT is not attenuated by high dose corticosteroids and PCT production does not rely on white blood cells hence it can be useful in febrile neutropenia.

PCT can be used to decide both the need for antibiotics (lug/L) and discontinuation of antibiotics (PTC less than 0.5 mg/L) along with clinical evaluation. This is the most important control against over use and misuse of antibiotics (e.g. 75%) of patients with upper and lower respiratory viral infections and in Surgical ICU.

Emerging bacterial resistance to antimicrobial drugs calls for more effective efforts to reduce the unnecessary and prolonged use of antibiotics (Ref Philips Schuetz etc BMC Medicine 2011, 9, 107 "Procalcitonin for diagnosis of infection and guide to antibiotic decisions: past, present and future".

TABLE 35.12 RADIONUCLIDE IMAGING OF INFECTION/INFLAMMATION

Fluorine18 FDG Fluro-deoxy-glucose taken up excessively by activated leucocytes and macrophages, compared to the surrounding normal tissue.

Galluim-67 Binds to transferin receptors on leucocytes and siderophores on bacteria.

Human Ig-Nonspecific Binds to Fc receptors on leucocytes.

Avidin-biotin Localise to sites of infection/inflammation due to increased vascular permeability.

Leucocyte labelling Direct labelling - Indium-111, Tc HMPAO.

Indirect labelling: Anti-granulocyte Ab

Cytokines IL-1, I1-2, IL-8 Bind to IL-1a type 2 receptors IL-2 and IL-8 receptors on leucocytes and macrophages.

Antimicrobial Peptide Ubiquicidine binds to bacterial wall specific for infection.

Ciprofloxacin Binds to DNA gyrase of bacteria specific for infection.

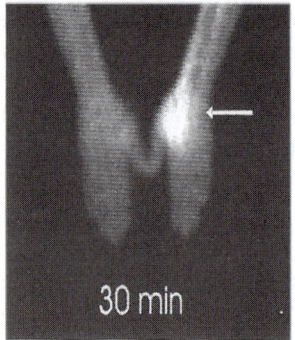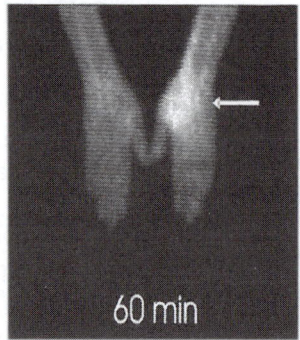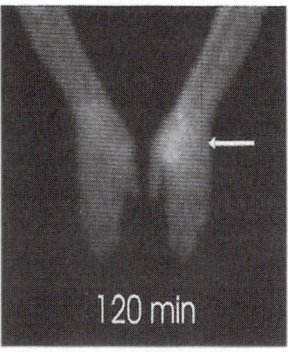

Fig. 35.4 99m Tc–Ubiquicidin images in a man with infection in medial side of left wrist

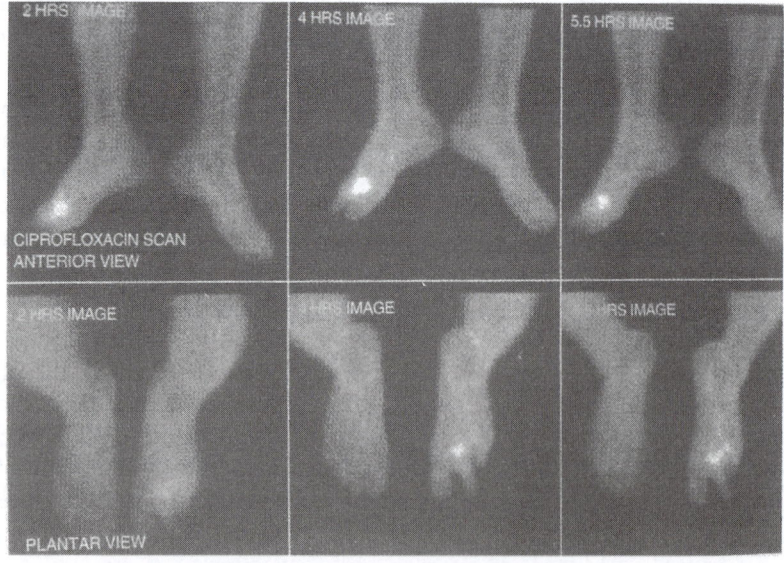

Fig. 35.5 Tc Ciprofloxacin scan showing infection in the right foot

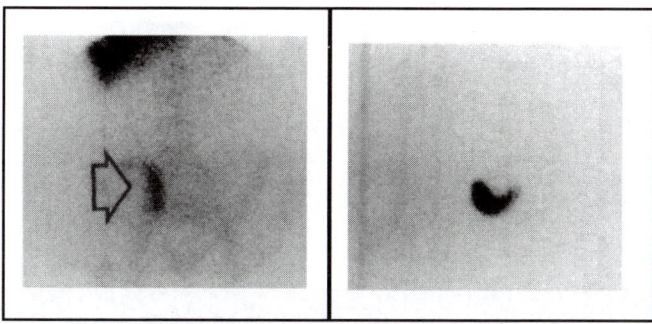

Fig. 35.6 Labelled leukocyte scan showing appendicitis

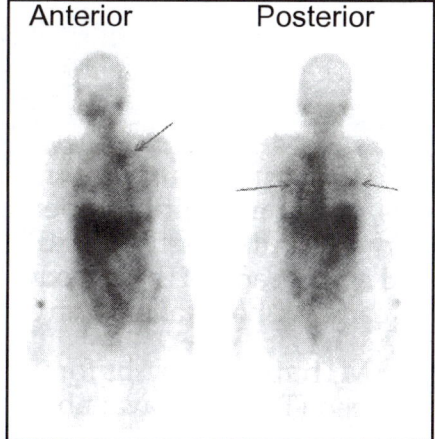

Fig. 35.7 Galluim 67 scan showing tracer concentration in tuberculosis lesions in the lungs

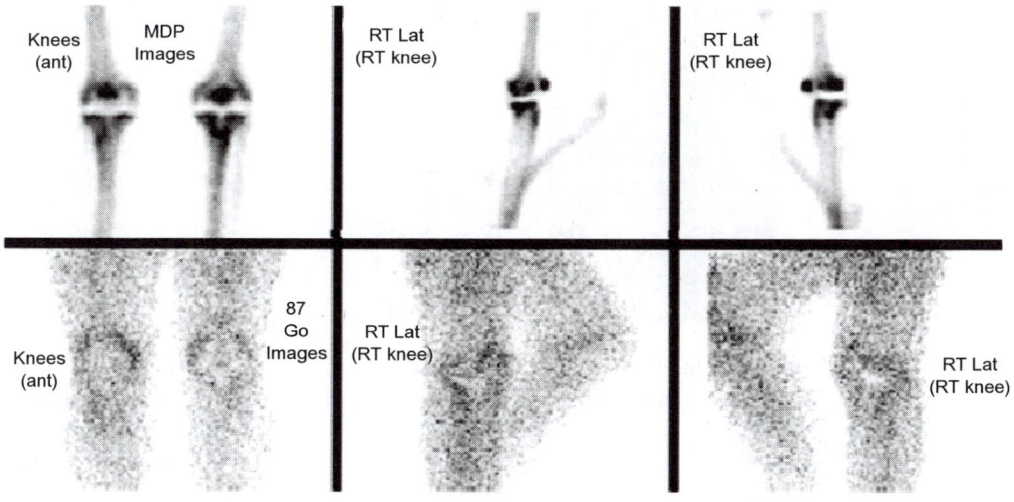

Fig. 35.8 Bone (Tc-MDP) and gallium-67 scans showing increased osteoplastic activity in peri-implant regions but no evidence of active infection

---

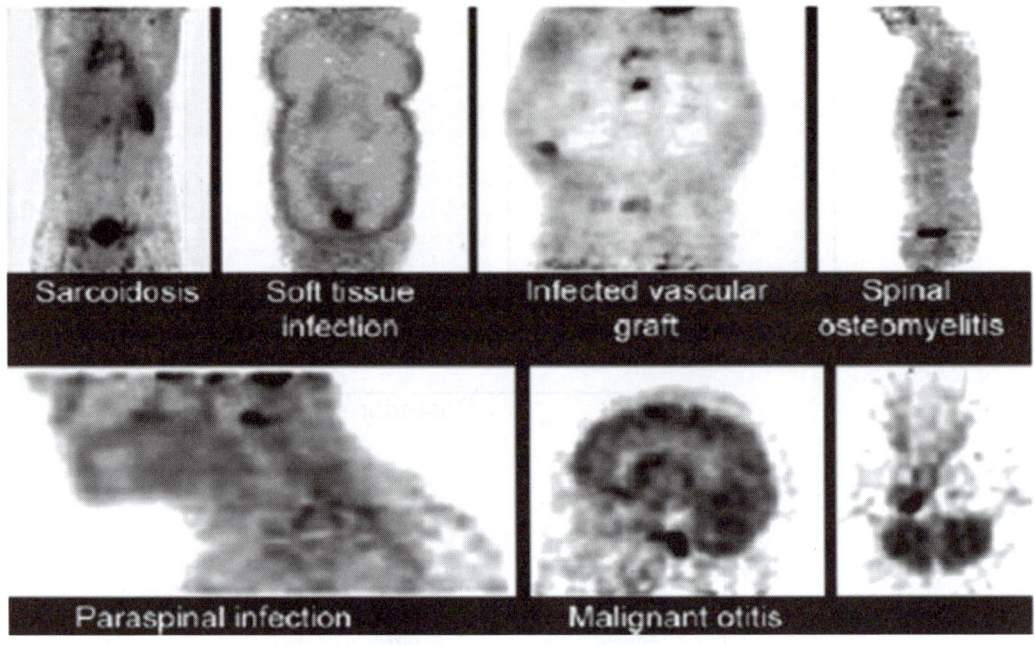

Fig. 35.9 18-F-FDG uptake in various sites of infection

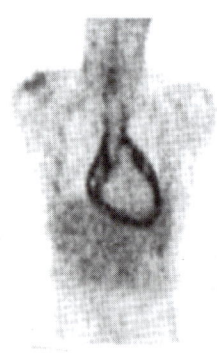

Fig. 35.10 FDG PET scan in a case of infective pericarditis

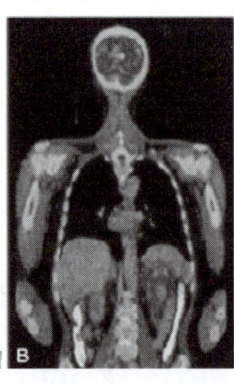

Fig. 35.11 A and B FDG scan in a case of pancolitis

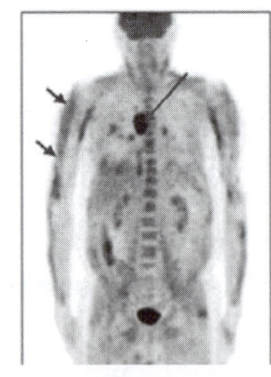

Fig. 35.12 FDG PET in polymyositis (small arrows) in a patient of lymphoma (long arrow)

Headache

Headache is one of the commonest of all symptoms of illness. Headache, like any pain, is a warning that something has gone wrong. This may be due to very serious and life-threatening causes (meningitis, subarachnoid haemorrhage, mass lesions in the skull) or causes that threaten vision (glaucoma, temporal arteritis) which the physician is anxious not to miss. Fortunately these serious causes constitute only a small minority; the commonest cause of headache is tension and fatigue incident to the affairs of day-to-day life. Next most common are the headaches due to vascular mechanism (migraine, hypertension, fever, anaemia) and next in frequency are causes attributable to the paranasal sinuses, eyes, ears and teeth. The physician should develop a clinical methodology which will leave none of the common and treatable causes unexplored.

In the analysis of headache. the importance of a good history cannot be over-emphasized. Many headaches can be diagnosed solely on the basis of the history, there being no physical signs at the time of the physical examination. There are others which enable the diagnosis to be made from the history associated with physical signs. Headache may be only a part of a general symptom complex. These three broad groups of headaches are summarized in **Table 36.1**. The typical location and description, time relationship, precipitating, aggravating and relieving factors, associated signs and symptoms of the important causes of headache are given in **Tables 36.2** and **36.3**. Causes such as dental abscess, otitis media, and mastoiditis usually reveal themselves by readily identifiable evidence of local disease. In contrast, ethmoid and sphenoid sinusitis, nasopharyngeal carcinoma and cranial arteritis may not cause any easily identifiable local manifestations.

Three questions present themselves and need to be answered:

1. Is it the sole symptom?

2. Is it a part of system illness?

3. Does it represent a potentially serious threat to life (meningitis, haemorrhage, mass lesion) or to vision (glaucoma, temporal arteritis)?

TABLE 36.1 CAUSES OF HEADACHE

Diagnosed chiefly by symptoms: No physical signs	Suspected by history: Diagnosed primarily by associated physical signs	Suspected by history: General symptoms and signs confirmatory
Tension headaches	Sinusitis	Fever, esp. typhoid and malaria
Migraine	Ear & mastoid disease	Anaemia, polycythaemia
Cluster headaches	Ocular disease	Hypoxia
Trigeminal neuralgia	Tooth abscess, impacted molar	Hypoglycaemia
Mass lesions (early)	Hypertension	Pre-menstrual
Hypoglycaemia	Temporal arteritis	Syphilis
Pheochromocytoma	Meningitis	Vertigo (See Chapter 23)
Post-traumatic headache	Subarachnoid haemorrhage	Depressive illness

TABLE 36.2 HEADACHES DIAGNOSED BY SYMPTOMS ALONE–NO PHYSICAL SIGNS

Type	Description	Temporal factors and duration	Precipitant factors	Aggravating factors	Relieving factors	Associated symptoms & signs
Tension Headache	Usually bilateral with diffuse extension over top of the skull; 'fullness tightness, pressure'.	Continuous, day & night. May last for weeks, months or years.	Emotional tension.	Worry, emotional tension.	May not be benefited by analgesics.	Anxiety, depression; common in menopausal females. Local tenderness may be present.
Migraine	Unilateral or bilateral; 'dull, boring throbbing'; begins in childhood or adolescence; strong family history.	Episodic: onset usually early morning, lasts over an hour or subsides in 4–24 hours. Patient completely well in between two attacks.	Tension.	Alcohol, smoking.	Carotid pressure; caffeine, ergot, sleep, methysergide.	Aura-scotoma before attack. Nausea & vomiting during attack. Occasionally transient loss of vision (amaurosis fugax).
Cluster Headache	Awakens patient from sleep due to severe throbbing pain in orbit or periorbital area.	Abrupt onset, lasts an hour.		Alcohol.	Ergot, methysergide.	Nasal congestion, rhinorrhoea, sweat, tears, flushing of face.
Trigeminal neuralgia	Brief, repetitive stabs of pain of great severity making the patient wince. Unilateral, localized to one division of 5th cranial nerve, usually maxillary or mandibular.	May recur several times a day; tends to occur in clusters of weeks.	Touching trigger area.		Nerve block, tegretol.	None; occasionally due to an intracranial mass lesion.
Temporomandibular neuralgia	Dull ache or intense stabs.		Chewing, biting.	Opening the mouth wide.		Malocclusion of teeth.
Hypoglycaemia	Associated with tremors, palpitations & sweating.	Never on a full stomach.	May be provoked by starvation.	Muscular exercise; alcohol.	Food, glucose.	Depending upon the mechanism causing hypoglycaemia.
Preochromocytoma	Suddera severe pounding headache; tremors; sweating; feeling of impending doom.	Few minutes; in between attacks patient may be quite normal.	Change of posture; full bladder; straining at stool.	Emotional events; ingestion of cheese.		High BP, postural hypeItension; café-au-lait spots; neurofibromas.
Post-traumatic headache	May mimic any type of headache; chronic, recurrent	May be intermittent or continuous.	Previous head injury.	Emotional tension.	Muscle relaxants.	None

Type	Description and location	Temporal factors and duration	Precipitant factors	Aggravating factors	Relieving factors	Associated symptoms and signs
Hypertension	Usually occipital throbbing; no direct relation to level of blood pressure.	Worse on awakening. Subsides during the day.	Overnight, recumbence.	Anxiety, tension.	Hypotensive drugs, pressure on carotids.	Other evidence of hypertension & retinopathy.
Temporal arteritis	Pain over affected vessel: spreads widely; may be bilateral; burning, dull or throbbing, severe; interferes with sleep; usually in elderly males.	May last for weeks with fluctuations.			Corticosteroids	Tenderness over temporal arteries; fever, leucocytosis, high ESR; visual disturbance; jaw claudication.
Subarachnoid haemorrhage	Abrupt onset of severe pain; 'bolt from the blue'.	Subsides over days or weeks.	Coughing, bending, sudden head movements.			Neck rigidity; Kernig's sign +; Blood in CSF.
Meningitis	Progressively increasing severe generalized headache; deep-seated constant, throbbing.	Unlike the common headache of any fever, the headache becomes worse day-by-day.	Sudden movements.			Fever, neck rigidity, typical CSF findings on LP.
Mass lesion	Generalized throbbing.	Early morning on waking. Also after an afternoon nap.	Coughing, straining, bending, sudden head movements.			Focal neurological deficit, papilloedema, seizures, vomiting, drowsiness.

(Contd)

TABLE 36.3 (Contd)

Type	Description and location	Temporal factors and duration	Precipitant factors	Aggravating factors	Relieving factors	Associated symptoms and signs
Sinusitis	Deep, full, aching pain, non-throbbing; location overlying frontal or maxillary sinuses, over vertex or behind eyes (sphenoid or ethmoid sinuses).	Commonly at 9.00 a.m.; gradually becomes worse by afternoon; ends towards evening or retiring.	Upper respiratory infection; sudden changes of temperature; sexual excitement; alcohol.	Bending forward, sudden changes of temperature, shaking head.	Nasal decongestion, aspirin.	Nasal discharge; Blockage of nose, tenderness over sinuses; opaque sinuses on transillumination and X-rays.
Acute narrow angle glaucoma	Severe deep ocular pain; often with nausea and vomiting. Firm hard eyeball compared to other eye.	Haloes around lights; initially blurred vision, later loss of vision.	Sustained darkness causing dilatation of pupil; angle becomes blocked.	Drugs that dilate pupils.	Pilocarpine drops; inserted every 10 minutes; oral glycerine; IV mannitol; urgent surgery.	Red eye; hazy cornea; shallow anterior chamber; non-reactive pupil.

Causes Which Can be Diagnosed Easily

The headaches associated with corneal abrasions, glaucoma, iridocyclitis, frontal and maxillary sinusitis, mastoiditis and dental abscess, usually reveal themselves by the presence of identifiable local disease, on physical examination.

On the other hand, ethmoid and sphenoid sinusitis, carcinoma of the nasopharynx, chronic mastoiditis (especially with extension to the lateral sinus intracranially) and cervical arthritis may cause little or no localizing manifestations. Hence a thorough plan of clinical examination has to be followed, making a systematic check in all possible areas of interest as shown in **Table 36.4**.

TABLE 36.4 PLAN OF EXAMINATION OF A CASE OF HEADACHE

A. *History taking*: A study of **Table 36.2** will enable the physician to suspect the conditions which can be diagnosed by history alone and indicate possibilities listed in **Table 36.3**.

B. *Physical examination*: Temperature, pulse rate, respiratory rate, pallor, cyanosis.
   1. Look for neck stiffness and Kernig's sign.
   2. Record blood pressure.
   3. Examine fundus oculi.
   4. Examine the eyes for evidence of glaucoma (increased tension), refractive errors (astigmatism, hypermetropia).
   5. Examine paranasal sinuses: tenderness, transillumination.
   6. Examine the teeth for dental abscess (painful swelling), impacted molar.
   7. Examine ear and mastoid.
   8. Examine cervical spine for limitations of movement in all directions, muscle spasm.

A study of **Table 36.3** will enable the physician to diagnose conditions associated with physical signs.

C. *Simple investigations:*   Hb% and ESR.
                               Blood urea & Creatinine.
                               Blood VDRL.
                               CSF for VDRL.
                               X-ray skull.
                               P.A+ lateral.
                               X-ray chest.
                               CT for suspected SOL.

D. *Special investigation:*   The Problem Case

It is common to see patients whose headache does not confirm to a typical pattern, who have no neurological signs, no papilloedema, no evidence of involvement of the eyes, ears, teeth and sinuses, no hypertension, and no other apparent cause for headache. One has then to decide how far to pursue the diagnostic studies. An enthusiastic physician may be tempted to push investigations which themselves may cause some morbidity. A conservative physician may prefer to wait and watch, but an over-anxious patient may force him to do investigations such as CT scan, or MRI.

A good compromise is to do the safe, simple and non-traumatic investigations in a problem case.

If these facilities are not available or affordable, the patient should be examined periodically for fresh evidence of an intracranial mass lesion (e.g. focal neurological deficit, convulsions).

Treatment of Headache

The most important steps in the treatment of headache are those measures which uncover and remove the underlying disease or disturbance of function.

In headache of acute onset with fever, a high index of suspicion is needed for the diagnosis of meningitis at an early stage so that effective treatment can be undertaken. The usual mistake is to postpone lumbar puncture till late, when the patient has already become drowsy.

For the common everyday headache, acetyl salicylic acid 0.6 g will suffice.

Premenstrual headache can be treated, along with acetyl salicylic acid, by a thiazide diuretic a week before the expected period, and phenobarbitone 30 mg.

Some patients have headaches when constipated. They often have associated depression or hypochondriasis. A mild laxative like senna and anti-depressant drugs like tofranil will help them.

Hypertensive headaches respond to agents which lower blood pressure and relieve muscle tension. A thiazide diuretic along with aldomet 250-500 mg twice a day, combined with phenobarbitone 30 mg or meprobamate 200 mg or diazepoxide 5 mg three times a day, give satisfactory results.

Treatment of Migraine

Most drugs effective in migraine treatment are members of one of three classes:

1. Anti-inflammatory agents :
   NSAIDs : aspirin
   Diclofenec,
   Ibuprofen
   Naproxen

2. $5HT_1$ agonists :
   non-selective : ergotamine
   dihydroergotamine
   Selective : Rizatriptan
   Zolmitriptan
   Sumatriptan

3. Dopamine antagonists
   oral : Metoplopramide
   Prochlorperazine
   inj. : Chlorpromazine

Recurrent vascular headaches (migraine type) if of a mild nature, may respond to acetyl salicylic acid 0.6 g alone. More severe attacks need ergotamine three (1 mg) tablets orally (to be held under the tongue till dissolved) and repeated in 2 mg doses every half hour until the headache is relieved. To cut short a severe attack IV Inj. 0.5 mg ergotamine tartrate or 1 mg dihydroergotamine is effective, which can be repeated in 30 minutes if necessary. Ergotamine tartrate 1 mg can also be given sublingually or by aerosol, or by rectal suppositories. The earlier the institution of ergot therapy (within 30-60 minutes of onset), the greater the success. Patients with ischaemic heart disease or peripheral vascular disease or pregnancy should not be given more than an occasional dose of ergot. Unfortunately oral ergotamine causes nausea and vomiting.

Numerous prophylactic measures to prevent migraine are all inconsistently successful. Phenobarbitone, diazepam or pizotifen given thrice daily often reduce the frequency of headaches. Propranolol, Clonidine, MAO inhibitors and tricyclic antidepressants are also sometimes helpful. Methysergide, a serotonin antagonist, is sometimes effective, but is prone to produce peripheral vasoconstriction, and rarely, retroperitoneal fibrosis. Hence it should be reserved for those patients whose attacks are not responsive to simple measures and are very frequent, severe and disabling.

Headaches of muscular tension respond to massage, relaxation and phenobarbitone. The headache of post-traumatic nervous instability needs supportive psychotherapy, reassurance and drugs to allay anxiety and depression.

Acupuncture is a non-drug modality of pain relief which proves effective in 30 per cent of patients, since they have the natural ability to produce sufficient endogenous endorphines in response to a painful stimulus, to obtain pain relief. Since there are no undesirable side effects with this treatment, it may be given a fair trial. In this era of HIV infection, scrupulons sterilization of needles is of paramount importance in this modality.

Hirsutism (male pattern hair growth in females) is a common and perplexing problem both to the patient and the physician. The distribution and growth of hair in normal persons is under complex genetic and endocrine control so that there is considerable *variability in hair growth* in normal men and women. Consequently 'abnormal' hair growth is difficult to define. The central issue in dealing with 'hairy' females is to separate those infrequent instances in which hirsutism is a manifestation of a serious and remediable underlying disorder, from the vast majority of hairy women in whom excess hair is essentially a *cosmetic problem*, and not a medical problem.

Control of Normal Hair Growth and Distribution

In both sexes, androgens are the major determinants of hair distribution. In females there are three principal circulating androgens:

1. Dehydroepiandrosterone (DHEA)-derived from adrenal cortex.
2. Androstenedione-derived equally from adrenal cortex and ovary.
3. Testosterone-formed in peripheral tissues from circulating 1 and 2.

The production of adrenal androgen is regulated by ACTH while ovarian androgen secretion is regulated by LH.

Vellus or soft fine hair on the face and elsewhere and hair on the forearms and lower legs are not sex-hormone dependent. Hair in the beard, moustache, breast, chest, axilla, abdominal midline, pubic and thigh areas are androgen-dependent.

Pathological Hair Growth and Distribution

A central consideration in hirsute females is whether evidence of virilization or de feminization is also present.

Signs of virilization:
Frontal balding
Increase in size of shoulder girdle muscles
Enlargement of clitoris
Acne
Coarsening of the voice, and hair.

Signs of defeminization:
Amenorrhoea
Decrease in breast size
Loss of female body contours.

In patients with *over production of androgens*, defeminizing signs such as amenorrhoea are more frequently present than are signs of virilization.

Causes and Investigations

The causes of hirsutism are listed in **Table 37.1** and the diagnostic approach is given in **Fig. 37.1**.

Drug history: Drugs causing hirsutism include phenytoin, minoxodil, diazoxide, cyclosporin, cortisone, androgens and some progestogens.

Idiopathic hirsutism: Evidence of androgenic excess but *normal* menses, normal-sized ovaries, no evidence of tumour of adrenals or ovaries, and normal adrenal function.

Oestrogens are converted to androgens in adipose tissue which may explain the frequent coexistence of hirsutism and obesity without definable endocrine disease.

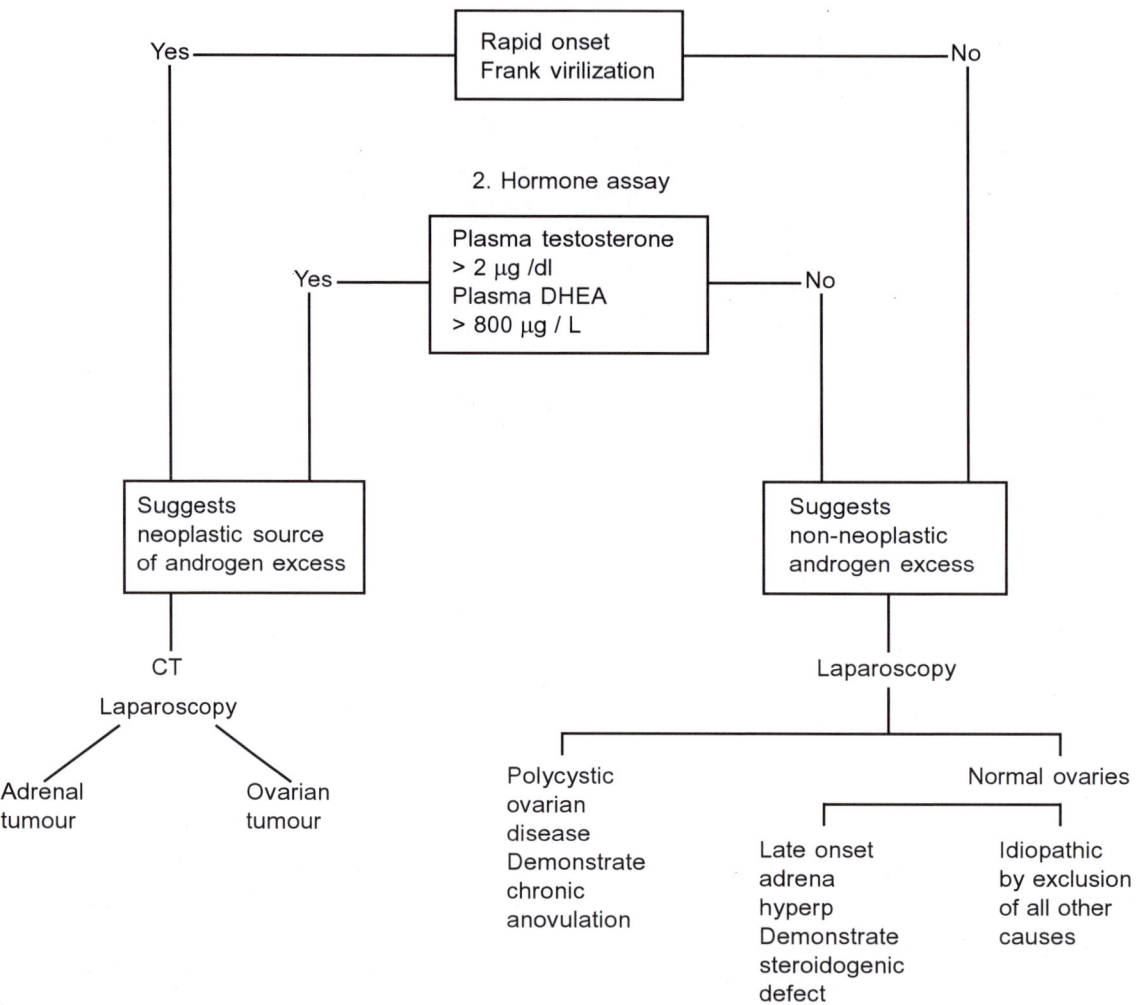

1. History and physical examination

Yes ——————— Rapid onset Frank virilization ——————— No

2. Hormone assay

Yes —— Plasma testosterone > 2 μg /dl Plasma DHEA > 800 μg / L —— No

Suggests neoplastic source of androgen excess

Suggests non-neoplastic androgen excess

CT
Laparoscopy

Adrenal tumour   Ovarian tumour

Laparoscopy

Polycystic ovarian disease Demonstrate chronic anovulation

Normal ovaries

Late onset adrena hyperp Demonstrate steroidogenic defect

Idiopathic by exclusion of all other causes

Fig. 37.1: Diagnostic approach to hirsutism

Table 37.1 CAUSES OF HIRSUTISM

Condition	Clinical presentation	Menstruation	Test results
A. Hirsutism without virilization			
1. Familial	Family history often present Long history after menarche	Normal	Normal
2. Idiopathic	Long history	Normal	Normal
3. Polycystic ovarian syndrome (mild)	Long history after menarche Acne, greasy skin ±	Chaotic	Androgens ↑; LH ↑; Ultrasound of ovary
4. Late onset CAH	Often before menarche Often short-stature	Variable	↑17 hydroxyprogesterone after inj. ACTH
5. Drugs	Drug history; Distribution non-androgenic 'hypertrichosis'		
B. Hirsutism with virilization			
6. Polycystic ovarian syndrome (severe)	Long history beginning after menarche	Amenorrhoea	Same as 3
7. Ovarian tumours	Short-history; Adult age	Amenorrhoea	Ultrasound laparoscopy
8. Congenital adrenal hyperplasia	Infancy, childhood		-17 hydroxyprogesterone
9. Adrenal tumours	Any age	Amenorrhoea	CT of adrenals

Congenital Adrenal Hyperplasia (CAH)

Some enzyme systems are common to the adrenal glands and the gonads, and a deficiency of these enzymes results in abnormal secretion of both adrenal and gonadal steroids.

A good example is 21 hydroxylase deficiency. While a severe enzyme deficiency presents at birth or in early childhood with virilization and often adrenocortical deficiency, a partial mild deficiency of adrenal 21 hydroxylase may remain unrecognized for many years. Glucocorticoid secretion is adequate (due to compensatory adrenocortical hyperplasia), but the excessive androgen biosynthesis leads to hirsutism and menstrual irregularities that may not be readily distinguished from other causes. It is important to recognize 'late onset CAH' from other causes of hyperandrogenism since its treatment is very specific and very effective.

Late onset CAH can now be readily diagnosed by the exaggerated 17 α hydroxyprogesterone response to an injection of ACTH. Late onset CAH may be found in 10 per cent of women with amenorrhoea and hirsutism.

Treatment of Hirsutism

The underlying cause should be removed in the rare instances where it is possible, e.g. drugs, adrenal or ovarian tumours. Other therapy is either local or systemic.

Local therapy: Bleaching, plucking, depilatory cream or wax and shaving may all help. Electrolysis is slow and expensive

Systemic therapy: Oestragen (or oral contraceptives) reduce free androgen by increasing SHBG levels when these are low. Prednisolone given in a reverse circadian manner (5 mg at night, 2.5 mg in the morning) may rarely improve hirsutism in polycystic ovarian syndrome. Cyprotenone acetate is an antiandrogen, given usually from day 1-14 of each menstrual cycle (50-200 mg/day). In women of child-bearing age contraception is necessary in view of its potential teratogenicity.

Spironolactone, bromocryptine and cimetidine have unproven efficacy.

38 Hypertension

The WHO has described hypertension (HTN) as a 'silent killer'. As there are no symptoms pertaining to high blood pressure (BP) *per se* (except when it is very high) there is no way of knowing about its presence except by measuring the BP. Since HTN affects a large segment of the population it is a good practice for all doctors to take the blood pressure (BP) of every patient who comes to consult them for whatever reasons. This is the most cost-effective approach for case finding in the community.

Blood pressure, like height, is a continuous variable hence it is difficult to determine cut-off points beyond which the blood pressure is 'high'. Arbitrarily 140/90 is taken as a cut-off point in adults. In pregnant women 130/90 is taken as HTN.

Continuous ambulatory BP monitoring has revealed that BP within individuals is highly variable. Almost a quarter of patients diagnosed in the doctor's consulting room have normal BP at other times. This is referred to as 'white coat' hypertension or 'office HTN'. The importance of circadian patterns of BP is also gaining interest. BP tends to be at a plateau during the day but falls in the evening to a nadir shortly after midnight. During the early morning hours there is a sharp increase in BP back to the daytime values. This may be part of the arousal process, parallel with the increased activity of the sympathetic nervous system. The greater frequency of myocardial infarction and strokes during the early to mid-morning hours may be related to this phenomenon.

The enthusiasm for early detection and control of HTN is based on the striking decline in the incidence of strokes, myocardial infarctions, heart failure and renal failure in the last two decades. Stoppage of cigarette smoking, regular physical exercise, weight control and HTN control seem to have contributed to this decline.

The proper method of recording BP is described in the next section. The patient's history in different types of HTN is given in **Table 38.1**. The clinical spectrum of essential HTN is given in **Table 38.2**. Causes of isolated systolic hypertension are described in **Table 38.3**. Renovascular hypertension, although forming 5 per cent of the entire HTN group, is an important area since it provides scope for a curative therapeutic modality. The vast majority of patients have to be managed by drugs and non-pharmacological approaches.

Recommendations for proper measurement of blood pressure

1. The patient should sit erect with legs extended for 5 minutes without smoking, moving about or drinking caffeine.

2. The patient's arm should be extended on a surface at heart level, with the palm of the hand turned upward. No constrictive clothing should be worn about the arm.

3. In order to increase audibility during auscultation, the arm should be raised for 30 seconds, thereby increasing venous return.

4. The width of the cuff should be between 1.2 and 1.5 times the diameter of the arm (circumference in cm x 7/22).

5. A mercury sphygmomanometer is dependable. If an aneroid instrument is used it should be checked intermittently for accuracy with a mercury instrument.

6. The cuff should be placed one inch above the natural crease of the inner aspect of the elbow.

7. The bladder of the cuff should be centred over the area of the brachial artery.

Table 38.1 PATIENT'S HISTORY IN DIFFERENT TYPES OF HYPERTENSION

Essential (primary)	Family history; Past history of high BP; Lack of cause.
Renal parenchymal	History of flank pain, glomerulo/pyelonephritis; History of renal stone; History of analgesic abuse.
Renal artery stenosis	Young women (fibromuscular); Abrupt onset or worsening at older age (atherosclerosis).
Pheochromocytoma	Headache, anxiety, palpitation; Tachycardia, tremors, sweating, recent weight loss, 'spells'.
Corticosteroid	Fatigue, muscle weakness, polyuria, polydipsia, nocturia; History of steroid therapy; Excess licorice intake.
Oral contraceptives	Use of oestrogen-containing pills; Lack of other causes.
Conn's syndrome	Paraesthesiae, weakness; Tetany.
Coarctation of aorta	Young age; Lack of other causes.
Aortoarteritis	Young age-claudication in upper limbs.
Hypercalcaemia	History of thiazide diuretics, renal stones, renal disease, known peptic ulcer; Excessive Vit. D intake.
NSAIDs	Prolonged use interferes with vasodilator prostaglandins; interferes with the effect of antihypertensive drugs such as betablockers, captopril and frusemide.

8. Initially the observer should pump the cuff until the radial artery cannot be palpated. This is the pulse obliteration level.

9. When rapidly inflating the cuff, pressure should be raised to 30 mmHg above the pulse obliteration level.

10. In order to increase audibility the patient should rapidly open and close his or her hand.

11. The observer should deflate the cuff at 2 mm per second allowing the reading to fall below the last definite blood pressure sound.

12. The observer should use the bell of the stethoscope to auscultate over the brachial artery. The level at which the first sound is heard is the systolic pressure. The level at which the last sound is heard (fifth phase) is the diastolic pressure.

13. After releasing pressure in the cuff the observer should wait 30 seconds before pumping the cuff again, this provides an opportunity for circulatory flow to equalize.

14. Measure blood pressure on both arms if the radial pulses are found to be unequal.

15. Measure blood pressure in the legs if the femoral pulse is weaker, delayed or absent compared to the radial pulse.

Renovascular Hypertension

About 5 per cent of the hypertensive population have a potentially correctable form of the disease. It is not possible to investigate all hypertensive patients in order to detect the curable forms (since it would be economically unsupportable), hence a cost-effective approach is to concentrate on the most likely group, based on the following clinical considerations.

1. All young hypertensives with onset under age 30 years.

2. All hypertensives in whom recent onset is known to have occurred after age 50.

3. All known hypertensives who have deteriorated suddenly or have failed to respond to treatment.

4. All cases of malignant hypertension.

5. Any patient of hypertension who shows unusual features:

abdominal bruit;
radial-femoral pulse delay;
X-ray chest-rib notching;
inappropriate response to anaesthesia or drugs;
weakness, paraesthesia, muscle cramps;
bizarre complaints;
clinical features of Cushing's syndrome.

TABLE 38.2 ESSENTIAL HYPERTENSION: CLINICAL SPECTRUM

Presentation	Possible symptoms	Common physical signs	Lab tests
I. Symptomless	None	High BP	None
II. Symptomatic but no major complications	Headache Tinnitus Nosebleed Nervousness Palpitations	High BP Slight LVH Ankle oedema	ECG ST-T changes 2 D echo: no LVH
III. Symptomatic with complications Cardiac:	Dyspnoea Orthopnoea Angina pectoris	Enlarged heart $S_3 S_4$ Ankle oedema	ECG LV hypertrophy ST-T changes
CNS:	Occipital headaches Dizziness Vertigo Paraesthesia Deterioration of vision or mental function	Fundus oculi Retinal vessels: narrowing, A V nipping	LVH on 2 D echo
Renal:	Nocturia Polyuria		Urine sp.gr. low Proteinuria High BUN, Creatinine
IV. Malignant Phase	Severe headache Visual impairment Weight loss Symptoms of hypertensive encephalopathy	Fundus oculi Papilloedema Haemorrhages Haemolytic anaemia	Any of above RBCs in urine Heavy proteinuria

NOTE: A patient may present himself for the first time in *any* of the phases hence it is important to record the blood pressure of *every* patient that the doctor sees for *any* reason.

TABLE 38.3 CAUSES OF ISOLATED SYSTOLIC HYPERTENSION (ISH)

Acute exercise	Normal response
Aortic insufficiency	Auscultation of heart
Severe anaemia	Hct < 30
Hyperthyroidism	Clinical & lab. evidence
Arteriovenous fistula	Continuous murmur
Patent ductus arteriosus	Continuous murmur left 2nd space
Hyperkinetic heart	Tachycardia, High pulse pressure
Complete heart block	Heart rate 30-40 per minute
Generalized arteriosclerosis	Older patient

Hypertension: Therapeutic Considerations

Individuals with mild BP elevation should have the BP measurement repeated within 1-2 months; individuals with moderate BP rise should be rechecked within 1-2 weeks of their initial visit. Patients with severe or accelerated malignant HTN should be treated immediately.

The primary goal of treatment is to lower BP to 140/90. Because an increased relative risk for coronary artery disease extends to diastolic pressures below those considered within the normal range < 90 mmHg) it is difficult to specify a BP level that is truly risk-free. Since the need to lower the BP is lifelong, adequate patient education is an essential component of the treatment plan, as it ensures patient compliance. It should be impressed on the patient that symptoms are unreliable gauges of the severity of HTN, and that prognosis improves with adequate blood pressure control.

Effective therapy reduces morbidity and mortality from stroke, heart failure and renal failure for all degrees of HTN, but the effect is modest for mild HTN.

The excess risk for coronary artery disease in HTN patients is concentrated in those with hypercholesterolaemia, impaired glucose tolerance, left ventricular hypertrophy and in cigarette smokers.

If in the initial assessment of mild HTN there IS no evidence of end-organ damage (LVH or strain, fundus changes, kidney function) a short trial (2-4 months) of non-pharmacologic modalities is recommended.

Currently diuretics, beta blockers (with or without intrinsic sympathomimetic activity or alpha-blocking properties), calcium antagonists and ACE inhibitors are all regarded as first step agents The question is whether any drug is suitable for any patient (on the analogy of aspirin to reduce fever) or certain pathophysiological profiles such as the individual renin secretion, sympathetic tone, renal sodium handling, cardiac output, peripheral vascular resistance and extracellular fluid (ECF) volume status should determine the logical therapeutic choice.

Withdrawal symptoms and secondary serum lipid abnormalities are associated with many drugs.

1. Weight reduction-achieved by caloric reduction and regular physical exercise. Improvement in cholesterol: HDL profile and regression of LVH have been achieved by this approach channel blockers labetalol.

2. Magnesium sulfate for pre-eclampsia.

Withdrawal Symptoms

Most patients experience a gradual return of HTN on stopping drugs. If substitution therapy is attempted in those with moderate to severe HTN on an outpatient basis, it is desirable to increase the dose of the new drug in small amounts while decreasing the dose of the previous drug in a similar manner to avoid excessive swings in blood pressure.

In a few patients the blood pressure may rise to levels much greater than the baseline values (overshoot) on acute drug withdrawal. The most severe complications include encephalopathy, cerebrovascular accident, myocardial infarct. and sudden death. Clonidine, methyldopa guanabenz (centrally acting drugs) and beta blockers should be tapered over several days to weeks when discontinuing therapy.

TABLE 38.4 Anti-hypertensive drugs

	Dose (mg)/day		Dose (mg)/day
Diuretics		**β-blockers**	
Hydrochlorothiazide	12.5-50	Propranolol	40-240
Indapamide	1.25-5	Atenolol	25-100
Chlorthalidone	2.5-10	Metoprolol	50-200
Metolazone	2.5-10	Bisopropol	2.5-20
Furosemide	20-240	Nebivolol	5-40
Bumetanide	0.5-4	Pindolol	10-50
Torsemide	0.5-4		
Ethacrynic acid	25-100		
Potassium sparing drugs		**α + β blockers**	
Amiloride	5-10	Labetalol	200-1000
Triamterene	25.100	Carvedilol	12.5-100
Aldosterone antagonists		**α1 blockers**	
Spironolactone	25-100	Prazosin	2-20
Epleronone	50-100	Doxazosin	1-16
		Terazosin	1-20

(Contd)

TABLE 38.4 (Contd)

ACE inhibitors		Central α-agonists	
Benazepril	5-40	Clonidine	0.2-1.0
Captopril	25-150	Methyldopa	500-2500
Emalapril	5-40	Moxonidine	0.2-0.6
Lisinopril	5-40		
Perindopril	4-16	**Peripheral Sympathetic blockers**	
Tirandolapril	1-4	Reserpine	0.05-0.25
		Guanethidine	10-100
Calcium channel blockers		**Angiotensin receptor blockers**	
Amlodipine	2.5-10	Telmisartan	40-80
Felodipine	2.5-20	Valsartan	80-320
Nifedipine	30-120	Losartan	50-100
Nicardipine	60-120	Candesartan	8-32
Cilnidipine	5-20	Eprosartan	400-800
Verapamil	90-480	Irbesartan	150-300
Diazepam	120-480	Omlesartan	20-40
Direct arterial dilators		**Direct renin inhibitor**	
Hydralazine	50-200	Aliskerin	150-300
Minoxidil	5-100		

TABLE **38.5 Special Considerations in the Choice of Drugs**

	Pathophysiologic profile	Suitable drug
Young hypertensive:	Increased sympathetic activity; elevated plasma renin activity; ECF normal/decreased.	ACE inhibitors; Combined β-α blockers; $α_1$ selective blockers; calcium channel blockers.
Middle-aged males:	Smokers; ischaemic heart disease.	Selective $β_1$ blockers reduce coronary events, strokes and total mortality.
Elderly hypertensive (60+):	Increased vascular resistance; peripheral vascular disease; ischaemic heart disease; LVH; COPD; glucose intolerance; renal insufficiency.	Diuretics; $β_1$ selective blockers; ACE inhibitors.
Obese hypertensive:	More modest elevation of vascular resistance; higher cardiac output, lower plasma renin.	Diuretics; Weight reduction.
Hypertensive with diabetic nephropathy:	Diuretics & beta blockers have numerous liabilities in this group. Calcium antagonists may adversely affect insulin secretion.	ACE inhibitors: favourable effect on renal function & proteinuria.

Secondary lipid abnormalities

Thiazide, loop and potassium sparing diuretics have been shown to raise serum total cholesterol, LDL, VLDL and TG, except indapamide. Most non-selective and $β_1$ selective agents increase TO and lower HDL. Beta blockers that possess intrinsic sympathomimetic activity (e. g. oxprenolol, pindolol and acebutolol), or additional a blocking properties (e. g. labetalol) have little or no effect on VLDL and HDL.

Management of HTN during pregnancy

BP above 140/90 associated with peripheral oedema and proteinuria may be a prelude to eclampsia

Pre-eclampsia is treated with bed-rest and hypotensive drugs safe in pregnancy–hydralazine (10-75 mg/day); or methyl dopa (250-1000 mg/day) or atenolol (25-100 mg/day) or nifedipine (30-100 mg/day). Full-blown eclampsia is a hypertensive emergency treated with IV hydralazine (10-50 mg 6 hourly). If BP cannot be reduced, termination of pregnancy becomes necessary which invariably reduces the high BP unless the patient had prior HTN.

Non-drug therapeutic measures

Non-drug intervention is indicated in all patients with sustained HTN and probably most with labile HTN. The general measures employed include relief of stress, diet, regular aerobic exercise and weight control. Relaxation techniques like 'shavasan' also help to lower BP.

A vegetarian diet (e.g. rice, and vegetables and fruits) is low in sodium and high in potassium, and restricted in cholesterol and saturated fats; it is recommended since it may diminish oxidative stress and the incidence of atherosclerotic complications. High fibre content in diet retards absorption glucose and cholesterol and reduces plasma cholesterol. Polyunsaturated fatty acids from corn oil/safflower oil (linoleic acid or omega 6) and linseed, rapseed and soyabean oil (alpha linolenic acid or omega 3) yield derivativeseicosapentaenoic acid (EA) and docosahexaenoic acid (DA) which compete with cell membranebound arachidonic acid in several ways. The net result is a more vasodilatory state with less platelet aggregation and reduced viscocity of the whole blood by increased deformability of red blood cells. Further there is reduced vasoconstrictive response to catchol amines and angiotensin.

Shifting to a vegetarian diet will hopefully reduce the incidence of HTN, strokes and atherosclerosis in the community.

Renal artery sympathectomy for resistant hypertension **Fig. 38.1**.

Molecular Approach to Hypertension

The so-called "essential Hypertension". EHT is not a single entity but a mixed bag with several polygenic quantitative traits acting in consert in different combinations in different individuals. 75 candidate genes for human EHT have been identified with 874 candidate SNPs, connected with the gene expression of several molecules involved in the homeostasis of blood pressure : nitric oxide, superoxide, prostacyclin, EDHF IRS-1, endothelin, selectin, tetreahydro bioptrem (BH_4), renin, angiotensinogen, angiotensin II, AVP, aldosterone, natriuretic peptides (ANP, BNP) bradykinin, bombesin, adducin $\alpha\beta\gamma$, mineralocorticoid receptors, $\beta2$ adrenoreceptors, sodium-lithium cotransporters, epithelial-sodium channel, ENaC, NaCl cotransporters, $Na^+K^+ATPase$ etc.

Within the next five years cDNA microarrays will enable clinicians to obtain a drop of blood from the hypertensive patient, which will reveal polymorphisms in several genes related to hypertension as well as type 2 diabetes mellitus atherosclerosis. This information will help the selection of the appropriate drug from among different drugs-diuretics, β adrenoreceptor blockers, α adrenoreceptor blockers such as prazosin, calcium channel blockers, ACE inhibitors, AT receptor blockers, direct vasodilators such as hydralazine and minoxidil, or centrally acting drugs such as reserpine and clonidine. This scenario will be vastly different from the current "trial and error" method of matching a patient with a drug or drug combination.

The traditional approach to treating resistant hypertension medically is to utilize a combination of conventional antihypertensive drugs at maximally tolerated doses. In many cases, after excluding etiological factors, direct vasodilators (hydralazine/minoxidil) are also tried as a component of combination therapy to manage resistant hypertension. One of the pathophysiological mechanisms attributed to resistant hypertension is excessive activity of the SNS. It has become apparent in recent years that renal afferent and efferent output affects SNS activity and contributes to hypertension. Both the afferent and efferent pathways between the renal artery and brain exacerbate the activity of the SNS, resulting in the development of hypertension.

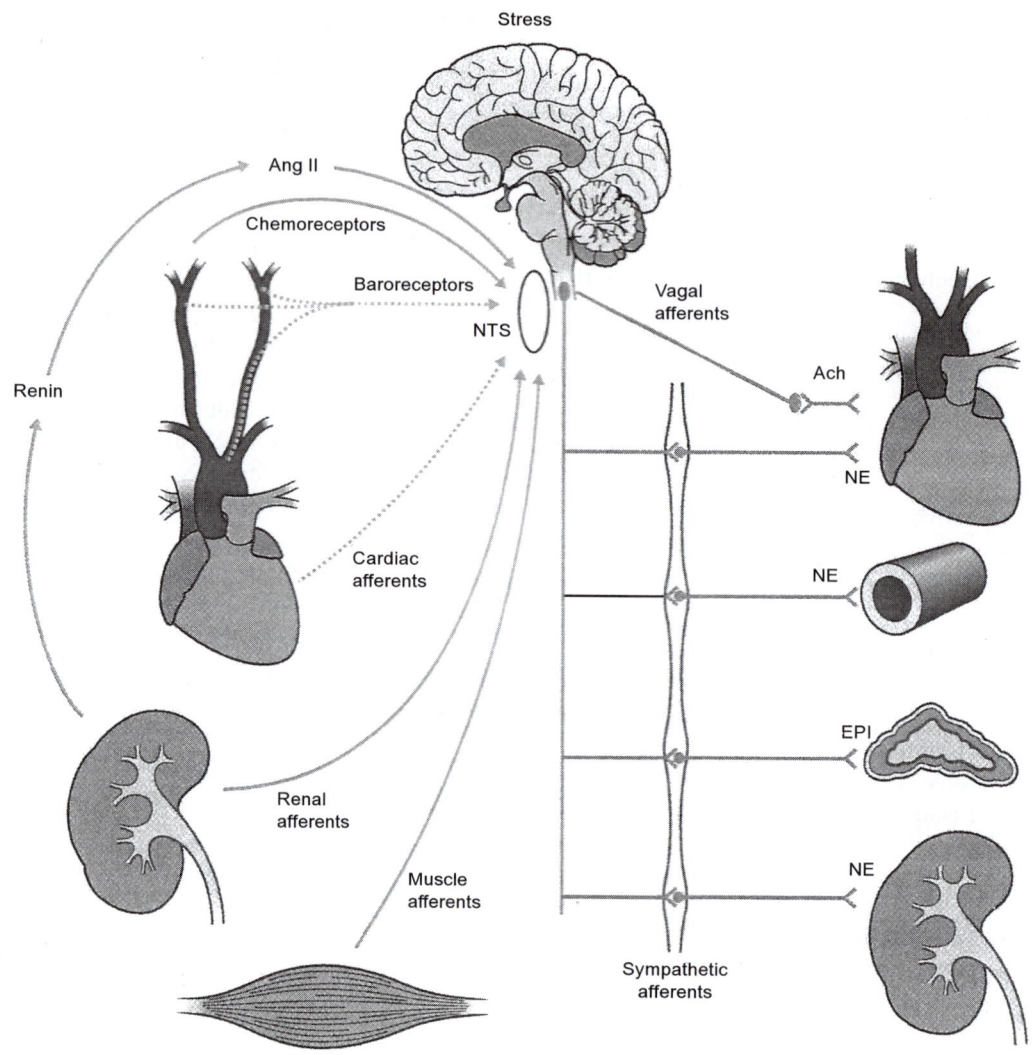

Fig. 38.1 Sympathetic nervous system and blood pressure regulation pathways

Interruption of the connection between brain sympathetic activity and the kidney has been shown to lower BP. Disruption of the renal afferent and efferent nerve traffic lowers the BP. A new novel technique [renal denervation (RDN) therapy] has been shown to improve BP substantially in hypertension. Using a catheter, low frequency ablation of renal nerves is accomplished in a safe manner to control resistant hypertension. RDN as a method of controlling resistant hypertension is currently undergoing extensive investigation; the results so far arc promising. Further experience and additional clinical trials will yield evidence about the future value of RDN in the clinical management of patients with resistant hypertension.

39   Hypoglycaemia

Maintenance of plasma glucose concentration is critical for survival because the central nervous system relies only on glucose as a fuel under most conditions.

In the post-absorptive phase (about 5-6 hours after a night meal) the liver mobilizes its store of glycogen (70 g) which can sustain the plasma glucose level for a short time (8-10 hours).

If glycogenolysis is not enough, hepatic gluconeogenesis begins, with (1) fall in the insulin concentration in plasma, coupled with (2) a rise in the counter–regulatory hormonesglucagon, epinephrine, cortisol and growth hormone. There is a mobilization of substrate from muscle (alanine) and adipose tissue (long chain fatty acids LCFA) to the liver, which produces 2 mg/kg per minute of glucose (over 70 g per hour) in the initial period of fasting. With prolonged fasting the kidney also becomes the site of gluconeogenesis (from the substrate glutamine).

The bulk of LCFA (normally about 120 g/day) is utilized directly by the tissues, and the remainder (about 40 g/day) is oxidized in the liver to acetoacetic acid and β hydroxybutyric acid. The shift of most tissues to lipid (FFA and ketone) spares glucose for the brain during prolonged fasting. When ketones are plentiful in circulation, as during prolonged fasting (40 days), they can support the majority (80-90 per cent) of the needs of the brain and reduce its glucose utilization.

Breakdown in any of the adaptive mechanisms leads to hypoglycaemia. The symptoms of hypoglycaemia are listed in **Table 39.1**.

In non-diabetic persons, acute lowering of plasma glucose to around 2.8 mmol/L (50 mg/dl) produces autonomic nervous system symptoms and induces release of counter-regulatory hormones. However,

utilizing auditory evoked potentials as a sensitive indicator of CNS function, abnormalities can be seen with a drop in plasma glucose from 87 to 72 mg/dl in normal persons. Cerebral atherosclerosis allows symptoms to be produced at higher glucose levels. Poorly controlled diabetics can develop symptoms at a level of 80 mg/dl.

TABLE 39.1 SYMPTOMS OF HYPOGLYCAEMIA

A. *Due to neuroglycopenia per se*
   Headache
   Impaired performance of routine tasks
   Lethargy, fatigue, muscle weakness
   Confusion, mental dullness
   Behaviour changes.
   Paraesthesia, especially circumoral
   Slurred speech
   Incoordination
   Blurring of vision
   Vertigo, dizziness
   Focal neurological deficit: diplopia, hemiparesis
   Convulsions-coma
   Chronic hypoglycaemia: dementia, psychosis

B. *Due to CNS-mediated sympathochromaffin activity*
   Non-specific sense of arousal
   Anxiety and impending doom
   Palpitations
   Tremulousness
   Sweating

(These symptoms are identical with those in pheochromocytoma or those produced by an injection of adrenaline)

C. *Parasympathetic*
   Hunger, nausea, sweating

Exercise increases glucose utilization by muscles several-fold greater than in the postabsorptive state. During exercise both a fall in insulin and a rise in glucagon and epinephrine prevent hypoglycaemia.

Pregnancy, glucosuria, and large tumours consuming sugar can contribute to hypoglycaemia.

Causes of Hypoglycaemia

Causes of hypoglycaemia can best be grouped under two headings;

1. Fasting (or post-absorptive) hypoglycaemia (**Table 39.2**).
2. Post-prandial hypoglycaemia (**Table 39.3**).

The distinction between fasting and postprandial hypoglycaemia is important since the former raises the distinct possibility of a progressive, potentially fatal disorder and demands conclusive diagnostic assessment, treatment, and follow-up. The presence of post-prandial hypoglycaemia is diagnostically irrelevant in the patient who has fasting hypoglycaemia.

In contrast, post-prandial hypoglycaemia (which results from the action of insulin secreted in response to meals) has no life-threatening implications. Symptoms appear within 1½-3 hours after meals (contrast dumping syndrome which occurs in less than one hour after meals), and can be prevented by a change in eating habits, change in dietary components (low sugar, high fat and protein) and small frequent feeds instead of two large meals.

Alcohol (ethanol) does not prevent glycolysis but it inhibits gluconeogenesis. It also inhibits cortisol and growth hormone response to hypoglycaemia and delays epinephrine response. Alcohol-induced hypo glycaemia typically follows (by 6-24 hours) a binge of moderate to heavy alcohol consumption during which very little food is eaten (i.e. in the setting of glycogen depletion).

Hypoglycaemia can be profound, with a mortality as high as 10 per cent (children appear to be particularly susceptible to hypoglycaemia following accidental ingestion of alcohol).

Ethanol is usually still measurable in the blood at the time the patient presents with hypoglycaemia.

However, the ethanol levels may not be markedly elevated and correlate poorly with the plasma glucose level.

The long list of drugs causing hypoglycaemia is given in **Table 39.4**.

TABLE 39.2 CLINICAL CONDITIONS CAUSING FASTING HYPOGLYCAEMIA

A. *Drugs*
1. Insulin, sulfonylurea, alcohol-common.
2. Quinine, pentamidine-(during treatment of malaria, kala azar).
3. Salicylates, sulfonamides-rare.

B. *Critical organ failure*
1. Hepatic disease-Fulminant viral hepatitis, chronic hepatitis, cirrhosis, alcoholic fatty liver, nutritional fatty liver.
2. Cardiac disease.
3. Renal disease.
4. Sepsis-excess interleukin 1.
5. Inanition-prolonged starvation.

C. *Hormonal deficiencies*
1. Glucagon.
2. Epinephrine.
3. Cortisol.
4. Growth hormone.

D. *Non-beta cell tumours*

E. *Endogenous hyperinsulinism*
1. Pancreatic beta cell
   (a) tumour (insulinoma);
   (b) non-tumour.
2. Beta cell secretagogue e.g. sulfonylureas.
3. Autoimmune mechanisms
   (a) insulin antibodies;
   (b) insulin receptor antibodies;
   (c) beta cell antibodies.
4. Ectopic insulin secretion.

F. *Hypoglycaemia of infancy & childhood*
1. Neonatal.
2. Congenital deficiencies of glucogenic enzymes.
3. Ketotic hypo glycaemia of childhood.

Salicylates in high doses (4-6 g/day) can lower blood sugar and can produce hypoglycaemia in children (Reye's syndrome), and rarely, in adults. Sulfonamides may also do the same.

Pentamidine and quinine cause hypoglycaemia via insulin release. In severe malaria, hypoglycaemia can occur in the absence of quinine treatment, and in the absence of hyperinsulinism in quinine-treated patients.

Table 39.3 CLINICAL CONDITIONS CAUSING POST-PRANDIAL HYPOGLYCAEMIA

A. *Congenital deficiencies of enzymes of carbohydrate metabolism*
   1. Galactosaemia.
   2. Hereditary fructose intolerance.

B. *Alimentary hypoglycaemia*
   1. Gastric surgery:
      gastrectomy,
      gastroenterostomy,
      pyloroplasty.
   2. Leucine sensitivity.
   3. Idiopathic alimentary hypo glycaemia.

C. *Ethanol*

Beta-adrenergic blockers (e. g. propranolol) have little effect on glucoregulation when the islet cell function is normal, but in IDDM, where glucagon counter-regulatory response is deficient and hence the patient is entirely dependent on epinephrine response, the drug increases the risk of hypoglycaemia. An alternative to β blockers should be considered for a patient with a history of severe or recurrent hypoglycaemia taking these drugs.

Clinical Approach to a Patient of Hypoglycaemia

In practice, the approach to a patient with hypoglycaemia goes along the following branching.
A. Patient is a diabetic on drug treatment.
B. Patient is not a known diabetic and is not using insulin or oral hypoglycaemic drugs.

In practice the vast majority of episodes of hypo glycaemia are due to insulin, sulfonylureas and alcohol.

Hypoglycaemia is a fact of life for IDDM patients who must take insulin to survive. On conventional insulin therapy, patients experience on an average one episode per week of symptomatic hypo glycaemia, and twice as many with intensive insulin therapy. Such events often include convulsions and loss of consciousness requiring IV glucose or IM glucagon. Four per cent of deaths of IDDM patients are attributed to hypoglycaemia. This is a problem that has not been solved. Symptoms of hypoglycaemia in IDDM are listed in **Table 39.5.**

Table 39.4 ESTABLISHED & PUTATIVE HYPOGLYCAEMIC AGENTS

Established
Used commonly:
Insulin
Salicylates
Sulfonamides
Sulfonylureas
Alcohol

Used rarely:
Quinine Pentamidine

Putative
Antihypertensives: beta-adrenergic antagonists (esp. in IDDM) particularly those that block B2 receptors; Captopril.
Analgesic/anti-inflammatory: indomethacin, acetaminophen, propoxyphene, phenylbutazone, penicillamine.
Anti-gout drugs: colchicine, sulphinpyrazone.
Lipid-lowering drugs: clofibrate, benzafibrate.
Antibiotics: chloramphenicol, ketoconazole, PAS.
Antipsychotics: haloperidol, MAO inhibitors.
Antianginals: perhexilene.

Deficient glucagon and epinephrine counter-regulatory response seems to be acquired within the first few years of IDDM. Some patients with long-standing disease lose the neuroglycopenic symptoms and therefore fail to act (i.e. eat) to prevent hypoglycaemia. The mechanism of 'hypoglycaemia unawareness' is not known but is probably related to deficient epinephrine response.

IDDM patients may suffer from hypoglycaemia due to
i.   medication overdose;
ii. increase in physical activity;
iii. change in content or timing of meals.

Twenty per cent of sulfonylurea-treated patients show at least one episode of hypoglycaemia in a 6-month period. A striking feature is the long duration of hypoglycaemia, sometimes persisting for days, more so in patients with renal insufficiency.

Adjustment of diet, physical activity, and drug dosage will prevent these episodes.

TABLE 39.5 HYPOGLYCAEMIC SYMPTOMS IN ORDER OF FREQUENCY IN IDDM

Symptoms	Per cent
Sweating	49
Tremors	32
Blurred or double vision	29
Weakness	28
Hunger	25
Confusion	13
Vertigo	13
Odd behaviour	13
Paraesthesia of lips & tongue	10
Anxiety	10
Cold feeling	9
Incoordination	9
Fear of losing consciousness	8
Slurred speech	7
Palpitations	6
Nausea	5
Headache	4
Stupor	2
Vomiting	1

Investigation of Hypoglycaemia

The first step is to document that a sample of blood drawn during symptoms of hypo glycaemia is below 60 mg/dl and that the symptoms are promptly relieved by glucose (Whipple's triad). If hypoglycaemia is documented in the absence of an obvious cause, one has to determine if it is post-absorptive, by obtaining a blood sample after an overnight fast (12 hours).

If this is normal, prolonged fast (upto 72 hours) may be necessary to obtain evidence of inappropriate insulin secretion (i.e. blood sugar below 50 mg/dl and insulin above 20 μu, suggest insulinoma).

The blood sample at the height of symptoms should be assayed for insulin, pro-insulin and C-peptide, and cortisol. Sulfonylurea assay in the blood and urine should also be done on the same sample.

Both plasma insulin and C-peptide levels are inappropriately high in patients with sulfonylurea-induced hypoglycaemia, a pattern similar to insulinoma. However, the drug level will be measurable in the plasma and urine.

Exogenous insulin-induced hypoglycaemia is suggested by low C-peptide level and low proinsulin (unlike insulinoma where the levels of both are high). Hypoglycaemia resulting from hormonal deficiency is uncommon but worth looking for, because it is treatable by hormone replacement, e.g. cortisol in Addison's disease.

Insulinoma is an extremely rare disease (1 in a million population) but since it can be cured by surgery, the search for the same is rewarding, and the error of missing it may be tragic. The investigations involve CT/MRI, coeliac arteriography and intraoperative ultrasonography.

Treatment of Hypoglycaemic Episodes

This should be guided by (1) the mental status of the patient; (2) the level of blood sugar; and (3) the anticipated clinical course. Prolonged observation is warranted in sulfonylurea overdose.

1. Oral carbohydrate (glucose, sucrose, or sugar-containing liquids, 1-2 cups of milk, fruit, cheese) is adequate for alert patients when drug overdose is not apparent. Frequent monitoring of blood sugar (e.g. every hour) should verify the efficacy.

2. Intravenous glucose should be given to a patient with impaired mental function, when medication overdose is suspected. 50 ml of 50 per cent dextrose should be given initially, followed by infusion of 5-10 per cent D/W. Blood glucose should be kept greater than 150 mg/dl as verified by frequent measurements.

3. Glucagon 1 mg IM inj. may be given to treat severe hypoglycaemia in outpatients or when IV access is difficult. Patients with recurrent hypoglycaemia should have glucagon available for home use.

4. Diazoxide 50-100 mg PO tid may be used to limit insulin secretion in patients with insulinoma in anticipation of surgical therapy. Prolonged treatment may cause volume overload necessitating diuretics. Thiazide diuretics potentiate the hyperglycaemic effects of diazoxide.

Jaundice (or icterus) is a clinical term describing the yellow appearance of the skin and mucosa, resulting from an increased bilirubin concentration in the body fluids. It is clinically detectable when the serum bilirubin concentration exceeds 50 μmol/L (3 mg/dl). Less marked hyperbilirubinaemia is called 'latent' jaundice. Natural daylight is preferable to appreciate the presence of jaundice. Sclera is rich in elastin which has special affinity for bilirubin, hence it is a good place to look for evidence of jaundice. Other causes of yellow pigmentation (e.g. carotenoid pigments) cause yellow discoloration of the skin but not of the sclera.

Derangement of bilirubin metabolism may occur through *over-production* as in excessive haemolysis, *decreased hepatic uptake* as in sepsis, and *decreased hepatic conjugation* and *decreased excretion* of bilirubin into bile due to both intrahepatic and extrahepatic factors. For the sake of understanding one can consider three groups of jaundice: haemolytic, hepatocellular, and cholestatic or obstructive. Their characteristic clinical and laboratory features are summarized in **Table 40.1**.

TABLE 40.1 CHARACTERISTICS OF THREE TYPES OF JAUNDICE

	Type	Clinical features	Laboratory tests
1.	Haemolytic	Jaundice usually mild; usually bilirubin less than 6 mg/dl. Dark coloured urine; Dark coloured stools; Pallor due to anaemia; Lemon yellow tint due to icterus; Splenomegaly may be present; No itching.	Urine urobilinogen (++); Urine bilirubin (-); Serum bilirubin unconjugated; Anaemia, reticulocytosis; SGOT/SGPT normal.
2.	Hepatocellular	Jaundice ranges from mild to very severe due to concomitant haemolysis and renal insufficiency; may exceed 50-60 mg/dl; clinical features of underlying disease **(Table 40.2)**; anorexia.	Urine bilirubin (+); Urobilinogen varies according to phase of disease; SGOT/SGPT high; Serum bilirubin conjugated plus unconjugated.
3.	Cholestatic	Jaundice becomes progressively severe; plateaus at a level of 30-40 mg/dl due to renal excretion; Dark coloured urine; Pale coloured stools; Pruritus; Metallic taste; Upper abdominal pain. **(Table 40.3)**.	Urine bilirubin (+); Urobilinogen (-); Serum bilirubin conjugated. SGOT/SGPT normal or minimally raised; Alk. phosphatase and GGT raised. Ultrasonography useful.

TABLE 40.2 CAUSES OF HEPATOCELLULAR JAUNDICE

A. *Acute infections*
  I. Acute viral hepatitis
      Common: A, B, C, D, E hepatitis
      Rare: Infectious mononucleosis
      CMV, EBV, Coxsackie, HSV
  II. Leptospirosis.
  III. Malaria, toxoplasmosis.
  IV. Liver abscess (esp. in alcoholics) pyaemic, amoebic.
B. *Drugs:* halothane, phenytoin, INAH, rifampicin etc.
C. *Alcoholic hepatitis*
D. *Chronic active hepatitis* (acute onset)
   Past history of unexplained repeated episodes of acute hepatitis.
E. *Hepatic vein thrombosis*

In practice, multiple mechanisms may be operative simultaneously; for instance in a patient with viral hepatitis there is impairment of uptake, conjugation and excretion of bilirubin. Similarly, in a patient with cirrhosis, jaundice may result both from impaired liver cell function as well as haemolysis.

The causes of haemolytic jaundice and their diagnosis are discussed in the chapter on Anaemia (See Chapter 25, **Table 25.11**).

The causes of hepatocellular jaundice are listed in **Table 40.2**.

The causes of cholestatic jaundice are listed in **Table 40.3**.

Extra-hepatic causes are often amenable to correction by surgery, and are hence called 'surgical jaundice'.

Post-operative jaundice is a problem of increasing importance, because larger numbers of patients are undergoing major surgical procedures (e.g. cardiac surgery, repair of ruptured aneurysms) and surviving. Several factors contribute to the jaundice in this setting, as listed in **Table 40.4**.

Differential Diagnosis

Acute viral hepatitis is the commonest cause of jaundice. A simple approach is to routinely screen for HBsAg, IgM–anti-HAV, and IgM–anti-HBc and HCV (**Table 40.5**). The diagnostic features of infectious causes of jaundice other than viral hepatitis are given in **Table 40.6**.

TABLE 40.3 CLINICAL FEATURES OF DIFFERENT CAUSES OF CHOLESTATIC JAUNDICE

Site	Clinical features	Laboratory tests
Large duct obstruction		
Impacted gallstone	History of recurrent biliary colic or 'dyspepsia' aggravated by fatty food.	X-ray; Ultrasonography; Radionuclide HIDA scans.
Carcinoma of head of pancreas	Pain in abdomen or back.	ERCP (endoscopic
Carcinoma of ampulla of Vater	Painless persistent jaundice	retrograde cholangio-
Stricture of bile duct	History of previous biliary surgery.	pancreatography).
Sclerosing cholangitis	May be associated with ulcerative colitis or Crohn's disease.	
Small duct obstruction		
Cholestatic phase of viral hepatitis	Can mimic 'surgical jaundice'.	Liver biopsy.
Drugs	Can mimic viral hepatitis or surgical jaundice.	
Primary biliary cirrhosis	Female 30-50 years; pruritus; skin xanthomata.	Anti-mitochondrial Ab IgM; Liver biopsy
Widespread liver metastases	Primary may not be obvious; gross nodularity of the liver; tenderness.	CT/MRI.

TABLE 40.4 POST-OPERATIVE JAUNDICE

I. *Increased pigment load*
   A. Haemolytic anaemia
   B. Transfusion (especially of stored blood)
   C. Resorption of haematomas, blood in extravascular spaces

II. *Impaired hepatocellular function*
   A. Hepatitis-like picture
      1. Halothane anaesthesia
      2. Drugs
      3. Shock
      4. Infection with hepatitis viruses
   B. Cholestatic picture
      1. Hypotension, hypoxaemia
      2. Drugs
      3. Sepsis

III. *Extrahepatic obstruction*
   A. Bile duct injury
   B. Choledocholithiasis

Some Problems in Differential Diagnosis of Viral Hepatitis

1. *'Surgical jaundice'*
   Because of RUQ pain, nausea, vomiting, fever and icterus, acute viral hepatitis may be confused with acute cholecystitis, common duct stone or ascending cholangitis. Since patients with acute viral hepatitis may tolerate surgery poorly, it is important to exclude this diagnosis prior to laparotomy.

In confusing cases, a percutaneous liver biopsy may be necessary prior to laparotomy.

2. *Carcinoma of pancreas*
   Viral hepatitis in the elderly is often misdiagnosed as obstructive jaundice resulting from a common duct stone or carcinoma of the pancreas. Because acute hepatitis in the elderly may be quite severe and the operative mortality high, it is necessary to exclude primary parenchymal liver disease before deciding on surgery. This may need evaluation of biochemical tests, radiographic studies of the biliary tree and even liver biopsy.

3. *Drugs*
   Many drugs and certain anaesthetic agents can produce a picture of either acute hepatitis or cholestasis, which can mimic viral hepatitis but the serological tests as outlined in Table 38.5 are negative for viral hepatitis A, B, C. Currently a test has become available for HEV also.

4. *Alcoholic hepatitis*
   This mimics viral hepatitis. Cholestatic jaundice mimicking biliary tract obstruction may also develop in some cases of acute alcoholic hepatitis. Usually the serum aminotransferase levels are not as markedly elevated and other stigmata of alcoholism may be present. Liver biopsy findings of fatty liver, neutrophil inflammatory reaction, and alcoholic hyaline, suggest the diagnosis.

TABLE 40.5 SIMPLIFIED DIAGNOSTIC APPROACH FOR ACUTE HEPATITIS

Test patient's serum for			Diagnostic Conclusion
HBsAg	IgM–anti-HEV	IgM–anti-HBc	
+	–	+	Acute hepatitis B
+	–	–	Chronic hepatitis B
+	+	–	Acute hepatitis A in addition to chronic hepatitis B
+	+	+	Acute hepatitis A and B
–	+	–	Acute hepatitis A
–	+	+	Acute hepatitis A and B
–	–	+	Acute hepatitis B
–	–	–	Suggestive of HCV infection. Test for anti-HCV antibody and for HEV antibody

NOTE: If these tests are negative, look for other clues such as infectious mononucleosis, CMV, HSV, Coxsackie viruses, toxoplasmosis.

TABLE 40.6 DIAGNOSTIC FEATURES OF INFECTIVE JAUNDICE OTHER THAN VIRAL HEPATITIS

Disease	Clinical	Laboratory tests
Infectious mononucleosis (EBV)	Young persons; Sore throat; pharyngitis; Lymphadenopathy; Splenomegaly; Skin rash; Anorexia; nausea; Vomiting ±; Jaundice.	Atypical blood lymphocytosis; Paul Bunnell Test (heterophil antibody); SGOT/SGPT high.
Cytomegalovirus (CMV)	Immunosuppressed patient; Recent blood transfusion.	Virus may be isolated from urine. Liver biopsy: giant cells and intranuclear inclusion.
Weils disease (Leptospirosis)	May be subclinical or mild PUO. Severe infection with headache, myalgia, conjunctival suffusion, anorexia, vomiting, skin rash/ etechiae; Liver & spleen enlargement.	Polymorphonuclear leucocytosis in blood; Protein, RBCs, casts in urine; Leptospira may be isolated from blood or urine; Rise in specific Ab.
Liver abscess (amoebic or pyogenic)	Right upper quadrant pain; Tender hepatomegaly; Fever; History of dysentery; Jaundice uncommon–when present, implies a grave prognosis.	Leucocytosis; IHA test for amoebiasis; Radionuclide liver scanning.
Toxoplasmosis	Cervical lymphadenopathy; 20% have low grade fever, arthralgia, myalgia; Hepatitis is self-limiting except in immunocompromised host.	Atypical lymphocytosis upto 40-50%; Sabin Feldman dye test and indirect fluorescent antibody test.
Malaria	Tender hepatomegaly; vomiting, mild icterus; May mimic viral hepatitis when cholestasis is present especially along with renal failure.	Bilirubin mainly unconjugated due to haemolysis. SGOT/SGPT may be normal or mildly elevated; Blood smear positive for MP.
Typhoid	Especially in children; Tender hepatomegaly; Jaundice due to cholestasis may mimic viral hepatitis.	Blood culture; Rising titre of Widal.

5. *Chronic active hepatitis (CAH)*
    Early in the course of CAH, the disease may resemble typical acute viral hepatitis. However, the persistence of symptoms, including biochemical abnormalities such as elevated bilirubin and aminotransferases, or circulating HBsAg over the ensuing months indicate that a chronic liver disorder is present. A past history of unexplained repeated episodes of acute hepatitis should alert the doctor to the possibility that CAH is the underlying disease. It is important to distinguish between the three forms–chronic active, chronic persistent, and lobular hepatitis, because chronic persistent and lobular hepatitis are not progressive disorders, rarely if ever result in cirrhosis, and require no therapy.

TABLE 40.7 RARER TYPES OF JAUNDICE

Condition	Mechanism	Comments
Gilbert's Syndrome	Decreased bilirubin clearance by hepatocytes due to deficiency of bilirubinglucuronyl transferase enzyme. Liver function tests are all normal. Some patients may have additional, evidence of haemolysis (often occult).	Asymptomatic, mild, persistent, unconjugated hyperbilirubinaemia (1.2 to 3 mg/dl rarely exceeds 5 mg/dl). Increase on prolonged fasting, surgery, infection, or alcohol ingestion. Benign condition needs no treatment. Patient often unaware of jaundice.
Crigler-Najjar Syndrome	Absence of glucuronyl transferase. No conjugated bilirubin formed by the liver.	High unconjugated bilirubin in blood 20-45 mg/dl. Death in infancy from
Type I	Bile is colourless. Liver function tests and liver histology are normal.	kernicterus. Some patients have survived 10-20 years.
Type II	Partial deficiency of glucuronyl transferase. Bile contains variable amounts of conjugated bilirubin. Liver function tests and liver histology are normal.	Serum unconjugated levels 6-20 mg/dl. Kernicterus rare. Phenobarbitone effective in lowering serum bilirubin level. Relatively benign disorder.
Dubin Johnson Syndrome	Defect in biliary excretion. Part of conjugated bilirubin is deconjugated and refluxed into the plasma. BSP late rise in plasma at 90 minutes. Brown or black pigment accumulation in hepatocytes.	Asymptomatic: serum bilirubin 3-15 mg/dl (conjugated and unconjugated components). Serum alkaline phosphatase not elevated. Excellent prognosis.
Rotor Syndrome	Impairment of hepatic storage capacity. No pigment in liver cells.	
Benign Familial	Unknown.	Benign disorder.
Recurrent Cholestasis	Early age of onset and familial incidence. No mechanical biliary obstruction. Normal cholangiogram. Liver morphology shows cholestasis. Cirrhosis does not develop.	Recurrent attacks of pruritus and jaundice, with rise in bilirubin and alkaline phosphatase during attacks.
Recurrent Jaundice of Pregnancy	In 3rd trimester intrahepatic cholestasis. Rise in serum bilirubin usually less than 6 mg/dl. Alkaline phosphatase high. SGOT, SGPT only mildly raised. Benign and self-limiting.	Pruritus and jaundice. Clinical and laboratory abnormalities subside promptly after delivery—normal in 7-14 days. May recur in next pregnancy.

A definitive diagnosis can only be established by liver biopsy; clinical and biochemical criteria cannot make the distinction.

6. *Wilson's Disease*

In adolescents and young adults Wilson's disease may present as acute hepatitis which may mimic viral hepatitis; or it may present as fulminant hepatitis, chronic active hepatitis, or cirrhosis. This diagnosis should be considered in any patient under age 40 with unexplained hepatitis. The diagnostic feature is the Kayser Fleischer ring (green or golden deposit in the cornea) seen on slit lamp examination. The serum ceruloplasmin is less than 200 mg/L and urine copper is more than 100 µg/day.

7. *Ischaemic hepatitis (shock liver)*

Sudden onset of right upper quadrant pain, hepatomegaly and hypotension, with mild jaundice and elevation of SGOT/SGPT may mimic viral or drug-induced hepatitis, but there is clinical evidence of right heart failure, or shock.

8. *Hepatic vein thrombosis*

Sudden onset of severe RUQ pain, gross hepatomegaly and jaundice may mimic viral hepatitis. There is no evidence of right-sided heart failure but there is gross intractable ascites. The diagnosis is established by hepatic venography and radionuclide liver scanning with colloid tracers which will delineate the unaffected caudate lobe of the liver.

Rarer types of jaundice are discussed in **Table 40.7**.

Natural History and Prognosis of Viral Hepatitis

HAV Hepatitis and HEV Hepatitis may rarely be fatal due to fulminant hepatitis but once the patient recovers, there are no chronic sequelae.

On the other hand HBV and HCV and delta virus (which always acts in association with HBV) have chronic sequelae which themselves can be fatal. **Fig. 40.1** shows the worldwide mortality due to viral hepatitis.

Fig. 40.2 depicts the possible outcomes of HBV infection.

Fig. 40.3 depicts the possible outcomes of HCV infection.

Fig. 40.4 gives the differential diagnosis of the controversial clinical entity, 'subacute hepatic failure'. **Fig. 40.5** depicts the determinants of the outcome of HBV infection. **Fig. 40.6** depicts the approach to chronic hepatitis, and the scope of antiviral therapy.

Preventive Measures

All blood banks should have a mandatory screening for HBsAg, Anti HBc, Anti HCV, HIV I and II, and SGOT/SGPT. This will minimize the danger of transfusion-related disease. It is estimated that HCV is responsible for acute hepatitis in 175,000 patients per year in each of the two continents, USA and Europe, and 350,000 per year in Japan. Worldwide there are probably 100 million HCV carriers.

HCV RNA is present in 80 per cent of anti-HCV positive patients (occasionally also in anti-HCV negative patients) hence anti-HCV positivity should be taken as an indicator of infectivity (similar to HIV antibody positivity). Exclusion of high SGOT positive leads to a 40 per cent reduction in transfusion hepatitis and exclusion of anti-HCV positive blood leads to an 80 per cent reduction. The cost of testing could be reduced by pooling ten donor blood samples in each test; only the positive pooled sample can be further tested for individual samples.

Vaccination

The recombinant DNA Pre S$_1$ S$_2$ (Sci-B) HB vaccine is highly immunogenic and well tolerated. In Indian patients the vaccine has a higher seroconversion rate at one month after the second dose injection, compared to the vaccine lacking the pre S components.

Three doses given at 0, 1 and 6 months produce seroconversion (HBs antibody positive) in 100 per cent subjects. Cost considerations are important in developing countries especially for large-scale vaccination. An intradermal injection of 0.1 ml of vaccine is as effective as 1 ml of IM inj. This strategy reduces the cost by a factor of 10.

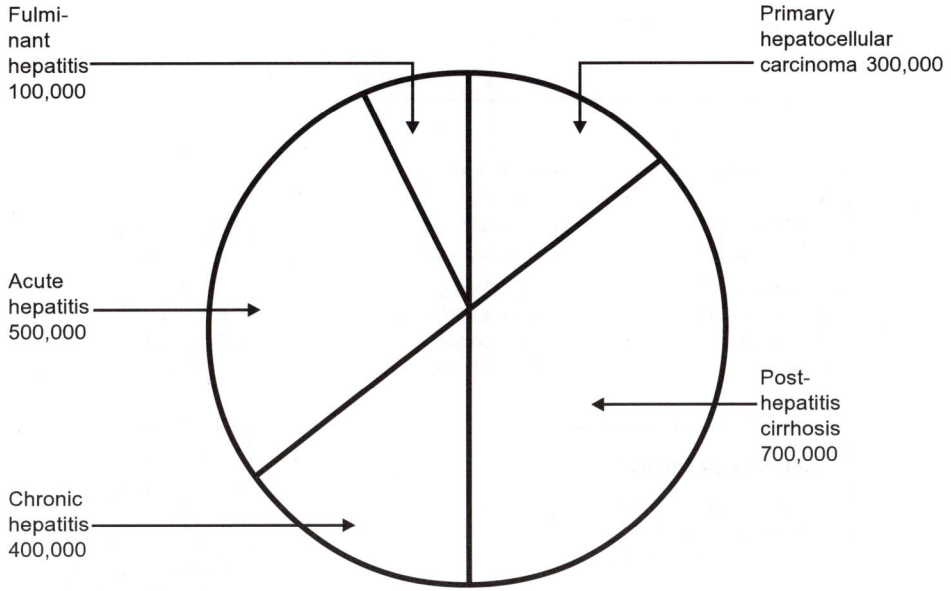

Fig. 40.1: Worldwide mortality due to viral hepatitis

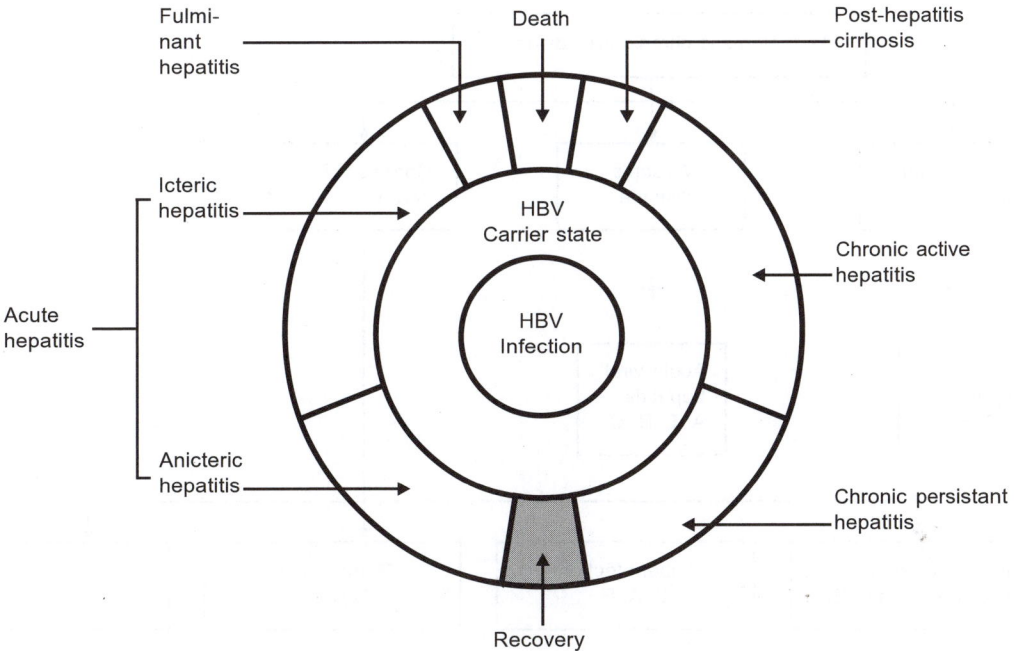

Fig. 40.2: Possible outcomes of HBV infection

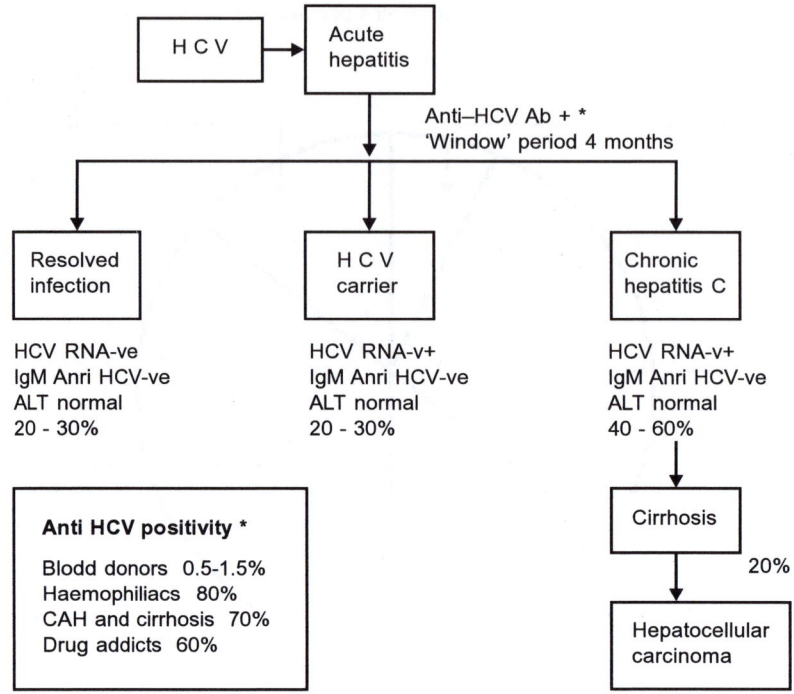

Fig. 40.3: Possible outcome of HCV infection

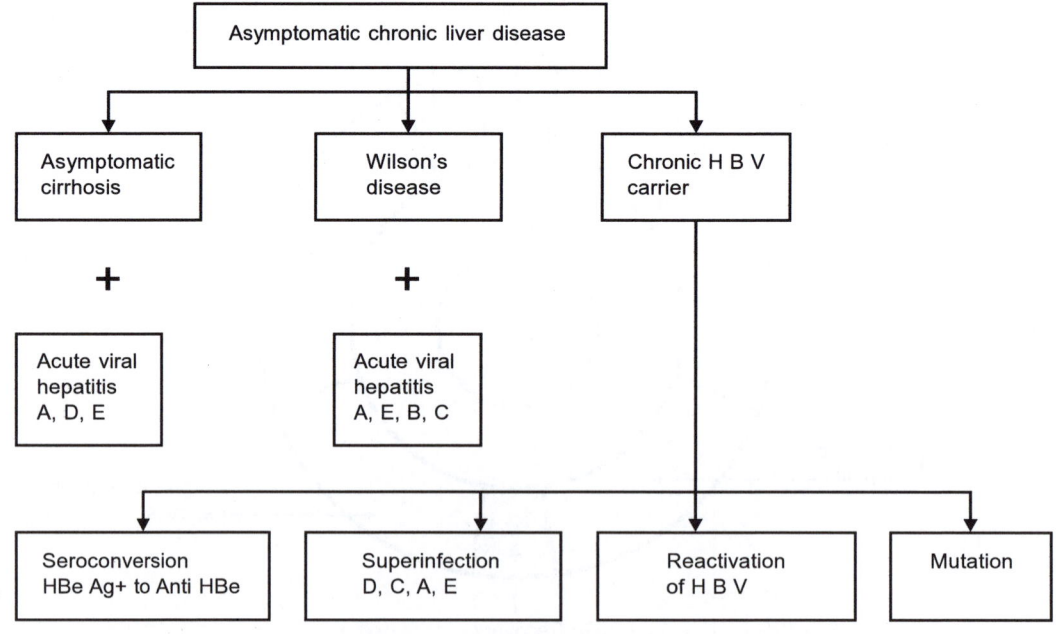

Fig. 40.4: Differential diagnosis of subacute hepatic failure

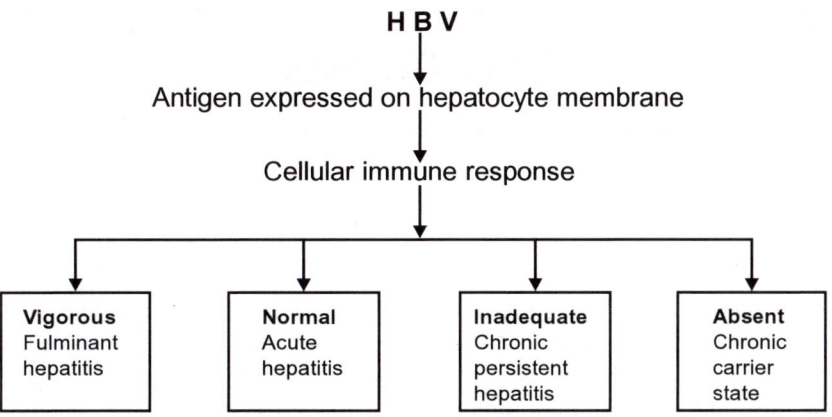

Fig. 40.5: Determinants of the outcome of HBV infection

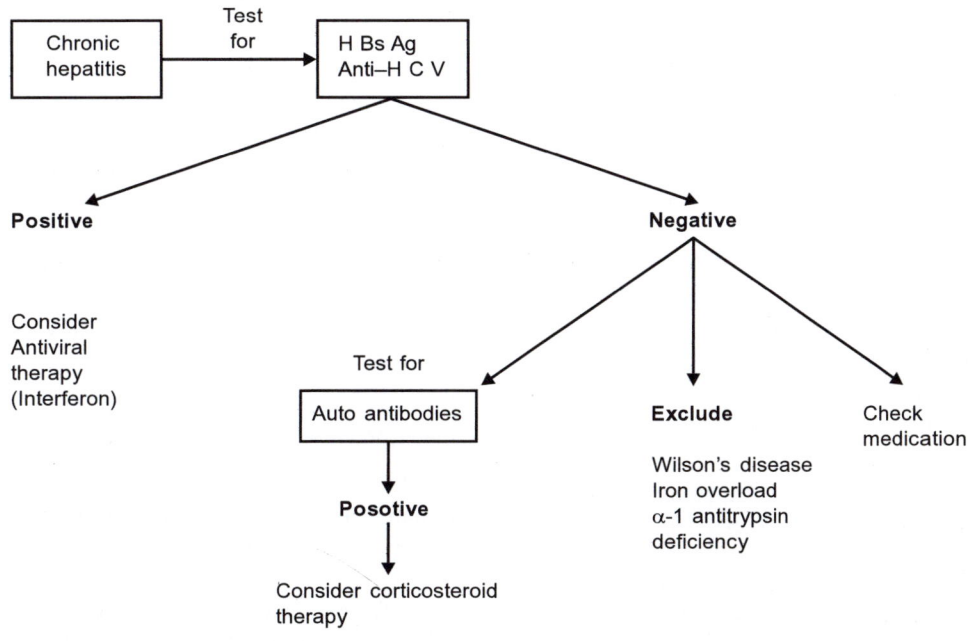

Interferon therapy leads to elimination of circulating H Be Ag and HBV–DNA in 30-40% of cases, and a loss of HBs Ag in less than 5% of cases. In chronic hepatitis C disease, a complete response is seen in 50% of cases, as shown by persistent normal serumtransaminases; a partial response in 25% cases. Unfortunately, after stopping treatment there is a 50-80% relapse.

Fig. 40.6: Approach to chronic hepatits and scope of antiviral therapy

41 Liver Diseases

In normal persons, in the supine position the major part of the liver lies beneath the right rib cage. In some normal persons the liver edge may be palpable 1 to 2 cm below the right costal margin, and a palpable liver edge by itself does not necessarily indicate hepatomegaly.

Normally the upper edge of liver dullness on the right side in the mid-clavicular line is at the level of the 5th rib, but in the asthenic habitus (a tall, thin person) it may be lower. In hyposthenic persons with a very acute costal angle, the liver may lie in the right half of the abdomen, the edge being palpable by as much as 6 to 8 cm below the costal margin. The location of the upper border of liver dullness by percussion is useful to determine whether the liver is displaced downward.

In determining liver enlargement by palpation one has to consider other right upper quadrant masses such as gallbladder, colonic neoplasm, or faecal material in the ascending colon. Hepatic scintigraphy or ultrasonography provide useful means of documenting hepatomegaly for the purpose of prognosis and follow-up.

In many cases of generalized hepatomegaly, the left lobe will be palpable in the epigastrium between the xiphoid and umbilicus. The liver should be carefully palpated during deep inspiration to determine whether the edge is tender, regular or irregular, firm or soft, rounded and thickened, or sharp. The edge is tender and often rounded in hepatic inflammation (e.g. hepatitis) or when the liver is acutely congested as in congestive cardiac failure. Pulsation (expansile) may be found in tricuspid valve incompetence, but this sign disappears when long-standing congestion leads to cardiac cirrhosis. A rock-like hardness of the liver indicates hepatic cancer; the cirrhotic liver is very firm in consistency.

The most massive livers are found in fatty infiltration, Hodgkin's disease and amyloidosis. Rapid decrease in the size of an enlarged liver indicates improvement of congestive heart failure, mobilization of fat from the liver, or massive hepatic necrosis.

Careful percussion is necessary to evaluate the size of a non-palpable liver. A small liver may indicate post-necrotic cirrhosis. A small liver which diminishes further in size suggests massive hepatic necrosis.

Auscultation over the liver sometimes provides useful additional information in a patient with hepatomegaly. A friction rub may be audible (and palpable) in the right upper quadrant; it suggests perihepatitis, hepatoma, or a recent liver biopsy. In portal hypertension, a venous hum may be audible between the umbilicus and the xiphoid. An arterial bruit over the liver may indicate a vascular tumour, usually a hepatocellular cancer.

Causes of a palpable but normal liver are given in **Table 41.1**.

Causes of a palpable and enlarged liver (hepatomegaly) are given in **Table 41.2**.

Jaundice is discussed in Chapter 40.

Hepatosplenomegaly (enlargement of both liver and spleen) with or without lymphadenopathy occurs

TABLE 41.1 CAUSES OF PALPABLE BUT NOT ENLARGED LIVER

1. Low diaphragm: asthma, emphysema.
2. Subdiaphragmatic lesion: abscess.
3. Aberrant lobe of liver: Riedel's lobe.
4. Extremely thin or relaxed abdominal wall.
5. Occasionally present in normal persons.

TABLE 41.2 CAUSES OF PALPABLE AND ENLARGED LIVER

I. Parenchymal
   A. Inflammatory disease
      1. Acute hepatitis: Infectious agents, drug-induced, alcohol.
      2. Chronic hepatitis: Persistent or active.
   B. Cirrhosis
      1. Post-necrotic.
      2. Alcoholic.
      3. Biliary.
      4. Haemochromatosis.
      5. Wilson's Disease.
      6. Alpha$_1$ anti-trypsin deficiency.
      7. Galactosaemia.
   C. Infiltrations
      1. Fatty liver: alcohol, diabetes.
      2. Glycogen.
      3. Amyloidosis.
      4. Leukaemia, lymphoma.
      5. Granuloma: tuberculosis, sarcoidosis.
   D. Space-occupying lesions
      1. Hepatoma, metastases.
      2. Abscess (amoebic, pyogenic).
      3. Cysts (hydatid, polycystic disease).
      4. Gummas.

II. Hepatobiliary
   A. Extrahepatic biliary obstruction
      1. Stones or roundworms in bile duct.
      2. Stricture of bile duct.
      3. Tumour.
   B. Intrahepatic biliary obstruction
      1. Cholangitis.

III. Vascular
   A. Chronic passive congestion & cardiac cirrhosis
   B. Hepatic vein thrombosis (Budd-Chiari syndrome)
   C. Portal pyelophlebitis
   D. Portal vein thrombosis
   E. Arteriovenous malformations

in many infections and immunologically mediated diseases, as well as leukaemias and lymphomas (see also Chapter 53 on Splenomegaly).

The basis of different symptoms and signs produced by liver disease is given in **Table 41.3**.

The liver parenchymal cell (hepatocyte) plays an important role in diverse general metabolic processes that may be deranged as a consequence of liver disease. In addition, this metabolic diversity leads to hepatic involvement in many inborn errors of metabolism, including a wide variety of storage disorders, and less-well-understood disorders of iron metabolism (haemosiderosis and haemochromatosis) and copper metabolism (Wilson's Disease).

The hepatocyte modifies numerous endogenous (e.g. bilirubin) and exogenous (e.g. alcohol, acetaminophen) toxic compounds through oxidation, reduction, and conjugation carried out by several enzymes of the endoplasmic reticulum. Conjugation of substrates generally facilitates their hepatic excretion, converting water-insoluble substances to water-soluble derivatives. Metabolic modifications may significantly alter the pharmacologic activity of drugs through formation of acetaldehyde. These metabolic processes may create intermediaries which are toxic to the liver itself (e.g. carbon tetrachloride, acetaminophen, and alcohol which is converted to acetaldehyde). The principal alterations in hepatic morphology produced by drugs are listed in **Table 41.4**. The hepatocyte produces a variety of soluble proteins for secretion into the circulation (e.g. albumin, prothrombin, fibrinogen, factors V, VII, IX and X). Hepatocyte dysfunction leads to hypoalbuminaemia and bleeding tendency.

The hepatocyte has receptors for various circulating ligands (e.g. LDL receptor). This property is also shared by the Kupffer cells which fulfil their function as constituents of the reticuloendothelial system by clearing a number of serum glycoproteins through asialoglycoprotein receptormediated endocytosis.

The hepatocytes have a capacity for regeneration as shown by complete recovery which usually occurs following fulminant hepatitis (caused by either viral or toxic agents) if the patient can be sustained through the period of actual injury.

Architecturally disordered regeneration in concert with fibrosis is an essential factor in the development of cirrhosis and leads both to disruption of blood flow through the hepatic parenchyma and to uneven hepatocellular function due to distortion of normal lobular structure.

Table 41.3 MECHANISM OF SYMPTOMS AND SIGNS IN LIVER DISEASE

	Pathophysiology	Symptoms and signs
I. Metabolic		
1. Maintenance of blood glucose	Defective glycogenolysis or gluconeogenesis.	Hypoglycaemia.
2. Synthesis of albumin	Reduced albmin production.	Hypoalbuminaemia, oedema, ascites, white nails.
3. Synthesis of clotting proteins (II, V, VII, IX, X)	Reduced production of clotting factors.	Bleeding diathesis.
4. Lipid metabolism	Fatty liver (Multifactorial).	Hepatomegaly.
5. Synthesis and excretion of bile salts	Retention of bile salts in serum.	Pruritus.
6. Conjugation & excretion of bilirubin	Defect of conjugation & glucuronidation of bilirubin.	Jaundice.
7. Conversion of ammonia to urea	Increased blood ammonia.	Encephalopathy.
8. Degradation of hormones	Decreased degradation of aldosterone. Decreased degradation of oestrogens in males.	Aggravation of oedema. Spider naevi, gynaecomastia, palmar erythema, testicular atrophy, loss of body hair.
	Decreased degradation of androgens in females.	Acne, hirsuitism.
9. Processing antigens (dietary, bacterial)		Hyperglolulinaemia.
10. Detoxification of drugs	Failure to metabolize morphine & barbiturates.	Dangerous sensitivity to these drugs.
II. Storage		
1. Fat-soluble vitamins (A, D, E, K)	Deficit of Vit. A. Deficit of Vit. D. Deficit of Vit. K.	Night blindness. Osteomalacia. Clotting defect.
2. Vit. B12	Decreased B12 reserve.	Macrocytic anaemia.
3. Iron	Increased storage of iron.	Haemochromatosis, haemosiderosis.
4. Copper	Increased storage of copper.	Wilson's disease, primary biliary cirrhosis.
III. Disorderly regeneration Following hepatocytic damage, along with fibrosis & scarring	Rise in portal pressure, congestion of splanchnic vessels. Development of portosystemic collaterals. Regenerating nodule more vulnerable to fluctuation in arterial blood pressure than is the normal liver. Porto systemic collaterals, shunting of blood bypassing the liver.	Splenomegaly, anorexia, nausea, flatulence, distension. Oesophageal and gastric variceal bleeding. Hepatic failure following gastrointestinal haemorrhage. Encephalopathy.

TABLE 41.4 DRUG-INDUCED LIVER DISEASE

Major morphologic alteration	Class of drug	Example
Cholestasis	Anabolic steroid	Methyl testosterone
	Antithyroid	Methiamazole
	Antibiotic	Erythromycin estolate
	Oral contraceptive	Norethynodrel with mestranol
	Oral hypoglycaemic	Chlorpropamide
	Tranquillizer	Chlorpromazine
Fatty liver	Antibiotic	Tetracycline
	Anticonvulsant	Sodium valproate
	Antiarrhythmic	Amiodarone
Hepatitis	Anaesthetic	Halothane
	Anticonvulsant	Phenytoin
	Antihypertensive	Methyl dopa
	Chemotherapeutic	Isoniazide
		Rifampicin
	Diuretic	Chlorothiazide
	Laxative	Oxphenisatin
Hepatic necrosis	Hydrocarbon	Carbon tetrachloride
	Metal	Yellow phosphorus
	Mushroom	*Amanita phalloides*
	Analgesic	Acetaminophen
	Solvent	DDimethylforrnamide
Granuloma	Anti-inflammatory	Phenylbutazone
	Chemotherapeutic	Sulfonamides
	Xanthine oxidase inhibitor	Allopurinol

Clinical Approach

In approaching the patient with known or suspected liver disease, the clinician should try to assess if the problem is primarily hepatocellular or cholestatic. Important and reliable clues may often be obtained from a careful history and physical examination. On the other hand significant liver disease can exist without any symptoms or signs.

Clinical History

A number of features In the history may distinguish cholestatic from hepatocellular disease processes. A history of marked right upper quadrant pain or previous indigestion suggest gallstones, cholecystitis or bile duct stones, whereas vague nagging discomfort suggests hepatocellular or infiltrative disease with hepatomegaly causing distension of Glisson's capsule.

Pruritus, jaundice, anorexia, weight loss and fever are important symptoms. Complaints of easy bruising or mental confusion are ominous signs of fulminant acute, or advanced chronic liver disease.

Family history is important in respect of jaundice, anaemia, splenomegaly and cholecystectomy (haemolytic anaemias, congenital or familial hyperbilirubinaemia, gallstones). In Wilson's disease there may be a family history of tremor or neurologic abnormalities (chorea, athetosis). Occupational and environmental factors should be reviewed, including exposure to known or putative toxins such as carbon tetrachloride, beryllium or vinyl chloride. Travel to areas where hepatitis is endemic is important to ascertain. Since alcoholics often deny or underestimate the amounts consumed by them, it is desirable to check this information with relatives or close friends.

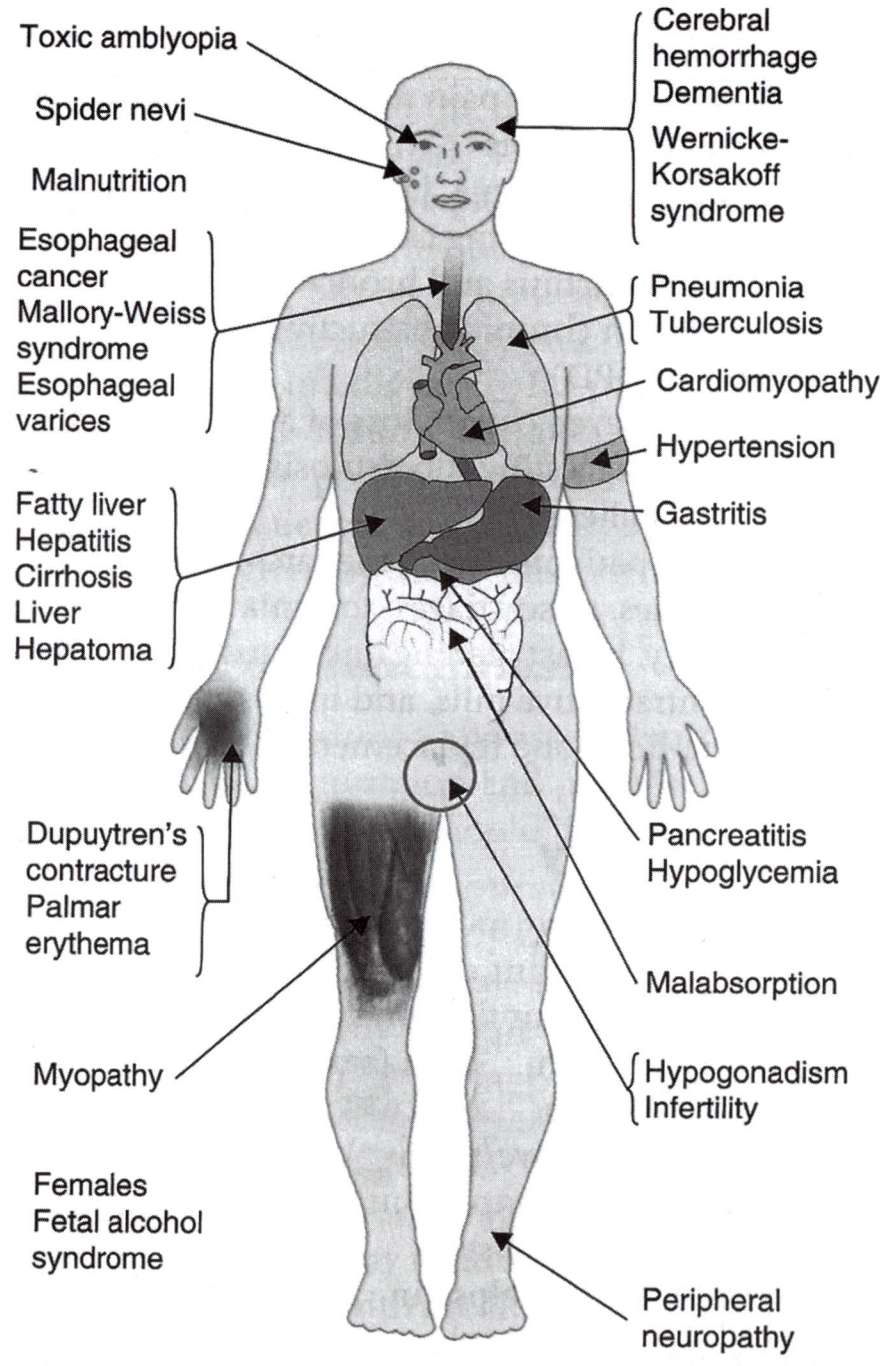

Toxic amblyopia

Spider nevi

Malnutrition

Esophageal
cancer
Mallory-Weiss
syndrome
Esophageal
varices

Fatty liver
Hepatitis
Cirrhosis
Liver
Hepatoma

Dupuytren's
contracture
Palmar
erythema

Myopathy

Females
Fetal alcohol
syndrome

Cerebral
hemorrhage
Dementia
Wernicke-
Korsakoff
syndrome

Pneumonia
Tuberculosis

Cardiomyopathy

Hypertension

Gastritis

Pancreatitis
Hypoglycemia

Malabsorption

Hypogonadism
Infertility

Peripheral
neuropathy

Fig. 41.1

Contact with jaundiced patients (especially intimate kissing or sexual relations) should be noted. History of any injections including blood tests, transfusions, tattooing and dental treatment are important. Post-operative jaundice may be due to the anaesthetic, especially after multiple uses of halothane, or to impaired hepatic excretory function resulting from relative hypoxaemia of liver cells during the operative or post-operative period.

The *onset* of illness is important to note; a relatively abrupt onset of anorexia, nausea and aversion to food or smoking is suggestive of the pre-icteric phase of viral hepatitis.

A gradual development of jaundice associated with pruritus suggests cholestasis.

Intermittent RUQ abdominal pain followed by cholestatic jaundice points to gallstone disease while the gradual onset of painless jaundice with weight loss is suggestive of tumour e.g. carcinoma of the head of the pancreas. Jaundice associated with chills and fever suggest cholangitis and extra-hepatic biliary obstruction, or liver abscess.

The awareness of progressive abdominal distension (tight pants) suggests ascites which may be due to cirrhosis or malignancy. The patient with hepatitis generally feels ill. In cholestatic hepatitis and primary biliary cirrhosis the patient may feel relatively well and may complain only of pruritus.

Physical Examination

Jaundice is looked for in the sclera as well as the skin. Pallor indicative of anaemia suggests a haemolysis, cirrhosis, or neoplasm. Wasting, especially of the extremities, may be associated with cirrhosis and malignancy. In the cirrhotic, parotid and lacrimal gland swelling and Dupuytren's contractures suggest alcohol abuse. Other features of cirrhosis are palmar erythema, gynaecomastia, testicular atrophy and diminished axillary and pubic hair.

The skin may reveal ecchymoses due to prothrombin deficiency, or purpura due to thrombocytopenia. Scratch marks, finger clubbing and xanthoma of the eyelids and extensor tendons of wrists and ankles may be found in chronic obstructive jaundice. A slate colour of the skin due to melanin pigmentation suggests haemochromatosis.

Deterioration of intellectual function and minimal personality changes may suggest hepatocellular disease or portal hypertension.

Abdominal examination may reveal ascites which, together with dilated periumbilical veins, suggest collaterals due to portal hypertension. If additional features of liver disease are lacking, malignancy must be considered more seriously.

Laboratory tests

Serum assays of biochemical markers of liver disease are an integral part of the proper evaluation of liver and biliary tract disease. *It must be remembered that significant liver disease may be present without any symptoms or signs, and may be revealed only by laboratory tests.*

In general, the serum bilirubin is measured to confirm the presence and severity of jaundice and to determine the extent of bilirubin conjugation.

Elevation of aminotransferases (transaminases, SGOT/SGPT) reflects the severity of active hepatocellular damage, while alkaline phosphatase elevations are found with cholestasis and hepatic infiltrates. GGT (gamma glutamyl transpeptidase) is a sensitive indicator of biliary tract disease and also a marker of alcohol-induced hepatic injury.

Serum albumin and prothrombin time are indicators of hepatic synthetic function.

Hepatic mass lesions are identified by ultrasonography, radionuclide scintigraphy, CT and MRI. Peritoneoscopy allows direct visualization of the liver surface and is useful for obtaining a biopsy. ERCP and ascending cholangiography are special tests for obtaining more precise information about the biliary tree.

USG provides non-invasive estimation of liver fibrosis (**Fig. 41.2**)

ARFI (Acoustic Radiation Force Impulse Imaging) scoring is done in an area where the liver tissue is at least 6 cm thick and free of large blood vessels. The tissue is mechanically excited by using short duration (262 sec) acoustic pulses by a curved array of 4 MHz to generate localized tissue displacements resulting in shear wave propagation away from the region of excitation, and are tracked by using ultrasound

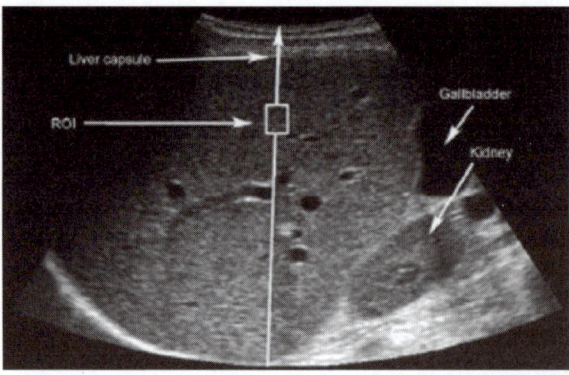

Fig. 41.2 Non-invasive estimation of Liver Fibrosis by UnItrasonography

Dynamic Contrast-enhanced Ultrasound - DCE-US (Fig. 41.3 A to C)

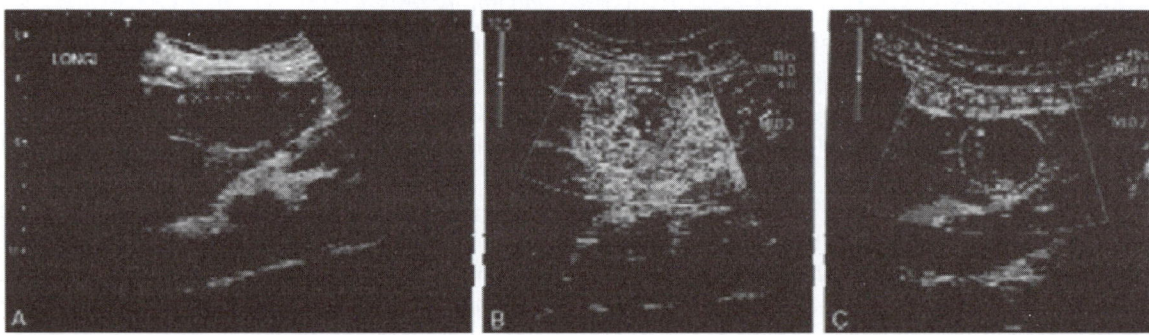

Fig. 41.3 A to C (A) Non-invasive estimation of Liver Fibrosis by UnItrasonography showing 4cm metastasis in the liver from Ca breast, (B) DCE US before treatment showing increased vascularity in the lesion, (C) 2 months after treatment with Bevacizumab (VEGFR Ab), near complete loss of signal, while CT did not show any shrinkage. It would be interesting to know if the lesion if undergoing apotposis as determined by Tc[99] Annexin imaging. (Source D Cosgrove N Lassau Eur J NM Mbl Imaging 2010; 37(5): 5565-85)

correlation based methods. By measuring shear-wave velocity, quantification of stiffness is made possible.

ARFI elastography eliminates the need for invasive liver biopsy for determining the prognosis, surveillance and anti-viral treatment, and evaluate the efficacy of drugs for reversing hepatic fibrosis.

The median shear-wave velocity (m/s) < 1 represents fatty liver; 1-1.5 normal liver, 1.5-2 early fibrosis, 2-2.5 advanced fibrosis, > 2.5 frank cirrhosis.

Inflammation in the liver influences the accuracy of liver fibrosis staging. Higher ARFI values are seen in patients with higher liver enzyme levels and necro inflammatory activity markers (ActiTest).

Microbubble contrast USG demonstrates increased sensitivity and a capability of detection of lesions as small as 2-3 mm. Dynamic contrast enhanced USG helps monitoring tumours response to treatment (**Fig. 41.3**).

42   Lymph Node Enlargement

The lymph nodes and spleen constitute a major portion of the peripheral immune system, and become enlarged in a wide spectrum of infectious, malignant, autoimmune, and metabolic diseases.

The lymph nodes in the human body number over 600 and are important as filters of microbes, producers of antibodies and processors of lymphocytes.

Enlargement of the lymph nodes (lymphadenopathy) and spleen (splenomegaly) are common clinical findings. The clinician should remember the clinical features and the diagnostic evaluation of the important diseases in which lymphadenopathy and splenomegaly occur.

Lymph nodes function as sites of macrophage, T-cell and B-cell contact with antigens with a specialized structure that gives rise to optimal T-cell, B-cell and macrophage interactions. Under normal conditions such interactions result in efficient antigen recognition, activation of the cellular and humoral arms. of the immune response, and ultimate elimination of the antigen.

In a local infection, the regional nodes are involved, but if the barrier is overcome the infection may spread to the blood and to more distant nodes.

When lymph nodes are acutely involved, there is evidence of a cellular infiltration with neutrophils and lymphocytes, and an increase in macrophages, and oedema. In certain illnesses, such as staphylococcal adenitis or plague, fluctuance may be present. Even non-bacterial infections such as LGV (lymphogranuloma venereum) or cat-scratch fever may produce fluctuance.

More chronic inflammation of lymph nodes produces a mononuclear cell inflammation. Usually this inflammatory response is not very specific but in certain illnesses such as toxoplasmosis the architectural findings may in fact be diagnostic. The presence of caseous necrosis, giant cells, and epithelioid cell granulomas, though not diagnostic may point to certain possibilities such as tuberculosis, atypical mycobacterial infection, fungal infection, tularaemia, cat-scratch disease, LGV, or non-infectious processes such as sarcoidosis. In these situations, specific stains such as acid-fast, Gomori silver or PAS may help locate the aetiological agent. With the availability of PCR (polymerese chain reaction) technology it is now possible to make a definitive diagnosis such as tuberculosis, by the demonstration of a specific band such as gp 165.

Causes of lymph node enlargement are listed in **Table 42.1**.

Fig 42.1 shows lymph nodes to be palpated during general examination of every patient.

Lymph node enlargement can be due to the following mechanisms:

1. An increase in the number of benign lymphocytes and macrophages during response to an antigen.

2. Infiltration by inflammatory cells in infections involving the lymph nodes (lymphadenitis).

3. In situ proliferation of malignant lymphocytes and macrophages.

4. Infiltration of nodes by metastatic malignant cells.

5. Infiltration of lymph nodes by metaboliteladen macrophages in lipid storage disease.

Normally in adults the inguinal lymph nodes may be palpable and are generally 0.5-2 cm in size. Elsewhere in the body, smaller lymph nodes due to past infections may be present normally. When a doctor detects one or more new nodes 1 cm or greater

TABLE 42.1 CAUSES OF LYMPHADENOPATHY

I. *Infectious disease*

Viral:	infectious mononucleosis
	infectious hepatitis
	EBV, CMV, rubella, measles
	HIV infection
Bacterial:	streptococcus, staphylococcus
	Pasteurella pestis, Haemophilus
	ducreyi, tularaemia, brucellosis
	catscratch fever, Tuberculosis,
	Atypical mycobacteria
Fungal:	coccidioidomycosis,
	histoplasmosis, sporotrichosis
Chlamydial:	lymphogranuloma venereum
Parasites:	toxoplasmosis
Spirochaetal:	syphilis, yaws, leptospirosis
Mycobacteria:	tuberculosis, leprosy

II. *Immunological*

Serum sickness
Drug reactions: Hydantoin
Rheumatoid arthritis, SLE, dermatomyositis
Angioimmunoblastic lymphadenopathy

III. *Malignant diseases*

Hodgkin's disease
Non-Hodgkin's lymphoma
Leukaemias
Metastases: lung, breast, prostate, kidney, GI tract

IV. *Endocrine*

Hyperthyroidism

V. *Lipid storage disease*

Gaucher's disease.
Niemann-Pick Disease

VI. *Miscellaneous–unclassified*

Sarcoidosis
Amyloidosis
Mucocutaneous lymph node syndrome
(Kawasaki's disease).

in diameter, and which are not known to arise from a previously recognized cause, he should investigate the case. Under certain circumstances new multiple or single smaller lymph nodes also warrant investigation. Important factors in assessing the significance of enlargement of lymph nodes are:

1. *Age of the patient :* Children are more likely to respond to minor stimuli with lymphoid hyperplasia. Lymphadenopathy in patients under 30 years is due to benign causes in about 80 per cent of cases, whereas in patients above 50 years, lymphadenopathy is due to benign causes in only 40 per cent of cases.

2. *Physical characteristics of the lymph node*

- Nodes of lymphoma tend to be rubbery, firm, matted together, and non-tender.

- Nodes involved in metastatic cancer are usually' hard and fixed to the underlying tissue: .

- Nodes in acute infections are tender, matted together, asymmetrically enlarged, and the overlying skin may be erythematous.

- Syphilitic nodes are shotty, painless and discrete.

- Fluctuation in nodes is suggestive of staphylococcal infection, plague, LGV or cat-scratch fever

3. *Location of lymph nodes* (**Table 42.2**) (**Fig. 42.1**).

4. *The clinical setting* is important in assessing lymphadenopathy. A young college student with fever and a recent onset of lymphadenopathy is most likely to be suffering from infectious mononucleosis. High-risk patients for HIV (homosexuals and their heterosexual partners, IV drug abuse and haemophilic patients receiving untested blood transfusions), presenting with generalized lymphadenopathy are likely to be suffering from AIDS or ARC (AIDS-related complex). The commonest lymph nodes affected are cervical, axillary and occipital.

During on outbreak of bubonic plague, every patient with fever and lymphadenopathy (inguinal, axillary, cervical) is suspect until proved otherwise.

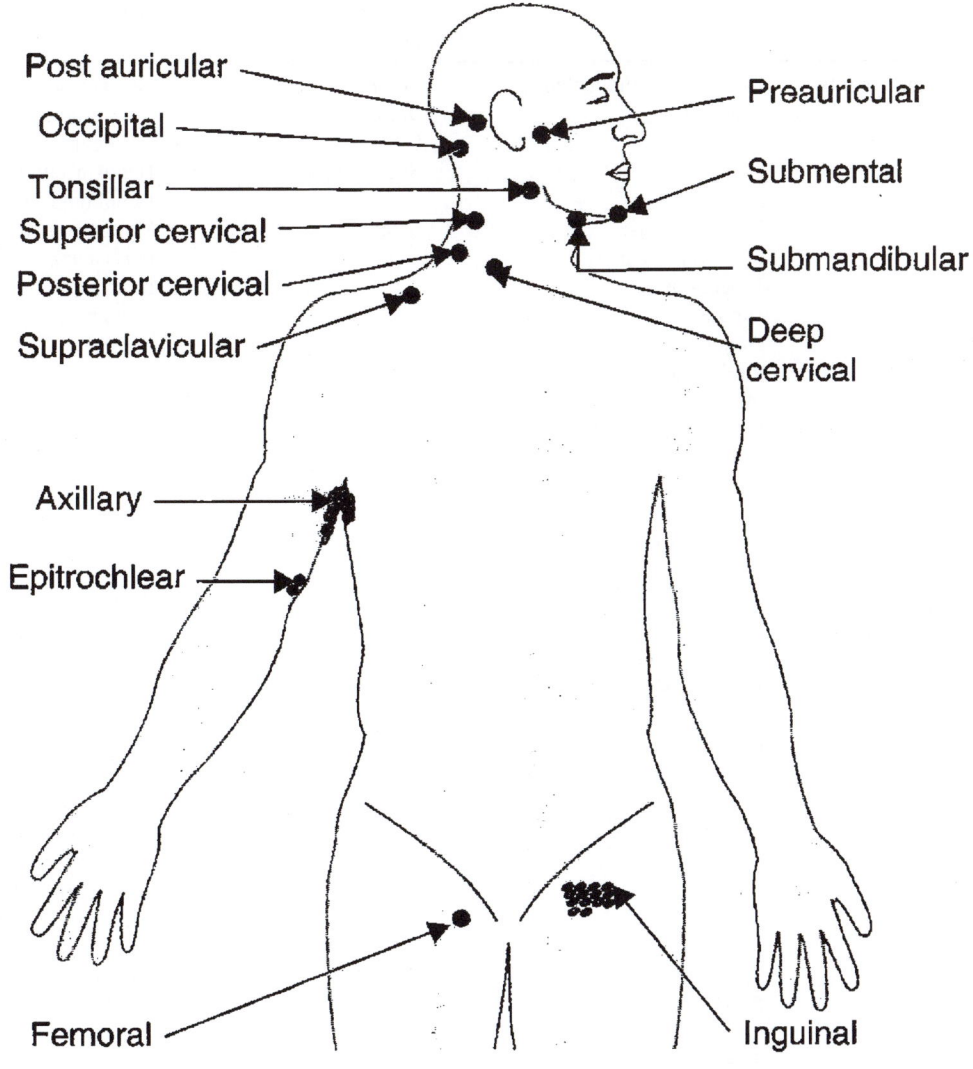

Fig. 42.1 Lymph glands to be palpated in general examination

TABLE 42.2 CAUSES OF LYMPH NODE ENLARGEMENT, ACCORDING TO LOCATION

Anatomic site	Infections	Immune mechanisms and others	Neoplastic
Generalized enlargements	Infectious mononucleosis; Tuberculosis; Syphilis.	Serum sickness; Drug allergy; SLE; Rheumatoid A.	Leukaemia: Chronic lymphatic Acute lymphatic Hodgkin's disease, Lymphoma.
Cervical	Streptococcus; Staphylococcus; Tuberculosis; Fungus; Plague; Viral infections (non-specific).	Sarcoid.	Metastases from: oral cavity, pharynx, nasopharynx, thyroid ca.
Occipital Posterior auricular	Pediculosis capitis. Leprosy; Rubella.		
Anterior auricular	Primary oral chancre; Herpes zoster opthalmicus; Tuberculosis.		Rodent ulcer; Epithelioma.
Supraclavicular & scalene nodes	Tuberculosis.	Sarcoid.	Ca, bronchus, breast, oesoph., stomach, pancreas.
Axillary	Strepto-staphylo; Tuberculosis; Brucellosis; Cat-scratch disease; Plague.		Lympho-reticulosis; Metastases breast.
Mediastinal & hilar	Tuberculosis; Fungal.	Sarcoid.	Hodgkin's lymphoma; Metastases from: bronchogenic ca., breast, stomach, pancreas, colon.
Intra-abdominal and retroperitoneal	Tuberculosis; Salmonella; Filariasis; Plague.		Ca. stomach, pancreas, colon, genitalia; Lymphoma.
Inguinal Unilateral	Strepto-staphylo; Syphilis; Lymphogranuloma venereum; Filariasis; Tuberculosis.		
Bilateral	Tuberculosis; Pasteurella pestis (plague);		Lymphoma. Lymphoma.
Femoral	Tuberculosis.		

Physical Examination

Palpation of the peripheral lymph nodes is one examination the importance of which has not diminished a bit in the modern era of imaging with ultrasonography, scintigraphy, CT and MRI.

Good physical examination techniques for palpation and assessment of lymph nodes are essential for providing useful information on which diagnostic and therapeutic decisions can be based. The size, location, consistency, and mobility (or fixity to the underlying tissue) of the lymph nodes at each examination should be documented for serial evaluation. For cervical node palpation the doctor may stand behind or in front of the seated patient. The sites of various groups of nodes are as follows.

Submental nodes are under the chin in the midline and on either side.

- Submandibular nodes are under the jaw near its angle.
- Jugular nodes are along the anterior border of the sternomastoid muscle.
- Supraclavicular nodes are behind the middle of the clavicle.
- Suboccipital nodes are in the apex of the posterior cervical triangle.
- Pre- and post-auricular glands are in front of and behind the ear.
- Central axillary nodes occur near the middle of the thoracic wall of the axilla.
- Lateral axillary nodes are located near the upper part of the humerus along the axillary vein and are best felt by keeping the patient's arm elevated.
- Subscapular nodes are felt under the anterior edge of the latissimus dorsi muscle.
- Pectoral nodes are beneath the lateral edge of the pectoralis muscle.
- Infraclavicular nodes are felt under the distal end of clavicle.
- Epitrochlear nodes are located about 3 cm proximal to the medial humeral epicondyle.
- Palpation should be done across this area in an anterior to posterior direction.

- Inguinal nodes are felt in the groin and femoral nodes in the region just below the groin.
- Enlarged abdominal lymph nodes can be difficult to palpate and may only be felt if the patient has a shallow abdominal cavity.
- Pelvic nodes are best evaluated with deep palpation of the lower abdomen by rolling the extended fingers over the pelvic brim.

Hilar and mediastinal lymph nodes are not accessible to physical examination but certain symptoms should raise the suspicion that they are enlarged. These are: cough or wheezing due to airway compression; hoarseness due to recurrent laryngeal nerve compression; dysphagia due to oesophageal compression; paralysis of the diaphragm due to phrenic nerve compression; swelling of the neck, face and arm due to superior vena cava or subclavian vein compression. FDGDET/CT, 4MRI and Gallium-67 scintigraphy are extremely valuable for evaluation of mediastinal, abdominal, para-aortic and retroperitoneal nodes.

The investigation of lymphadenopathy can proceed according to the *location* of the enlarged nodes and the *type* of clinical symptoms present.

Enlarged supraclavicular nodes most often result from tuberculosis, lymphoma, gastrointestinal or intrathoracic tumours, and should be biopsied.

Unilateral cervical adenopathy warrants a careful ear, nose and throat examination for malignancy.

In the asymptomatic patient with persistent new axillary and/or inguinal adenopathy, a biopsy specimen should be obtained.

If systemic lymphadenopathy persists without an obvious cause being identified (e.g. serum sickness, drug reactions) lymph node biopsy is warranted. Lymph nodes which have been present for a longer time are preferred for biopsy rather than those which have recently appeared.

Once the decision for lymph node biopsy is made, tissue should be processed for culture of appropriate organisms, frozen in liquid nitrogen for lymphocyte typing or other special diagnostic studies for malignant cell types, and processed for routine pathologic evaluation.

TABLE 42.3 APPROACH TO THE DIAGNOSIS AND THERAPY OF REGIONAL AND GENERALIZED LYMPHADENOPATHY CAUSED BY INFECTIONS

Disease	Diagnostic clues	Treatment
Viral (non-specific)	Exclusion of bacterial causes	Supportive
Infectious mononucleosis	Lymphocytosis with many atypical cell Heterophil antibodies	Supportive corticosteroids for laryngeal obstruction, toxaemia, haematologic and neurologic complications
Streptococci (group A)	Throat culture	Penicillin G for 10 days
Diphtheria	Throat smear and culture	Antitoxin plus erythromycin
Tuberculosis	Biopsy Strongly positive PPD skin test	INAH, rifampicin. pyrazinamide
Plague	Smear and blood culture, aspirate of bubo	Tetracycline. streptomycin, TM/SMZ
Tularaemia	Culture of blood, sputum and exudates	Streptomycin
Cat-scratch disease	Aspiration of node if purulent	Will heal without specific therapy Antibiotics and steroids not indicated
Rat-bite fever	Dark field of bite, rash, or node aspirate VDRL frequently positive	Penicillin G or tetracycline
Sporotrichosis		Oral iodides
LGV		Tetracycline
Chancroid	Smear and culture	Erythromycin
Toxoplasmosis	Serological tests	Most cases self-limited Pyrimethamine and sulfadiazine
Histoplasmosis	Culture of marrow, blood, sputum or lymph nodes	Amphotericin B if disease progressive or severe Ketoconazole
Syphilis	Dark field of moist areas of rash FTA-ABS VDRL	Benzathine Penicillin G
HIV	Lymphopenia Abnormal T_H/T_S ratio	Supportive specific therapy determined by specific opportunistic organism or by presence of Kaposi's sarcoma

Of lymph node biopsies, 50-60 per cent yield firm diagnostic results. About 24 per cent of non-diagnostic biopsies will develop within a year a disease (usually lymphoma) related to the indication of the biopsy. If symptoms or enlarged nodes persist, a repeat biopsy should be done.

Thirty per cent of cases of 'Atypical hyperplasia of lymph nodes' subsequently develop lymphoma, which may be confirmed by repeat biopsy if the nodes persist. In developing countries tuberculosis is equally important.

Imaging Lymph Nodes

Cancer cells (as well as their metastases) take up much more glucose than normal cells, hence a radiotracer Fluorine 18 fluorodexyglucose (FDG) will be avidly taken up and show as "hot" spots even if the lymph node is smaller than 1 cm in diameter. Imaging is done with Positron Emission Tompgraphy (PET). Co-registration of the image with CT gives exact anatomic localization of the lymph nodes as well as the primary site of cancer. PET/CT machines have now become available **Fig. 42.2** shows PET image of a male patient with extensive and non-responding NHL, showing extensive disease (axilla, mediastinum, liver, spleen, abdominal and inguinal nodes) which disappeared after treatment with zevalin.

Activated macrophages and lymphocytes also take up FDG avidly compared to normal cells hence inflammatory and infectious lesions will also show positive FDG uptake. They can be differentiated by another labeled molecule fluoroethyl tyrosine (FET). Cancer cells take up aminoacids avidly similar to glucose, while lymphocytes and macrophages do not. Hence a mismatch between a positive FDG and negative FLT will indicate inflammation / infection such as tuberculosis. This is important in India and developing countries with high prevalence, since tuberculosis can co-exist with a known cancer at some other site.

Therapy

This depends on the cause. **Table 42.3** summarizes the approach to the diagnosis and therapy of regional and generalized lymphadenopathy caused by infections.

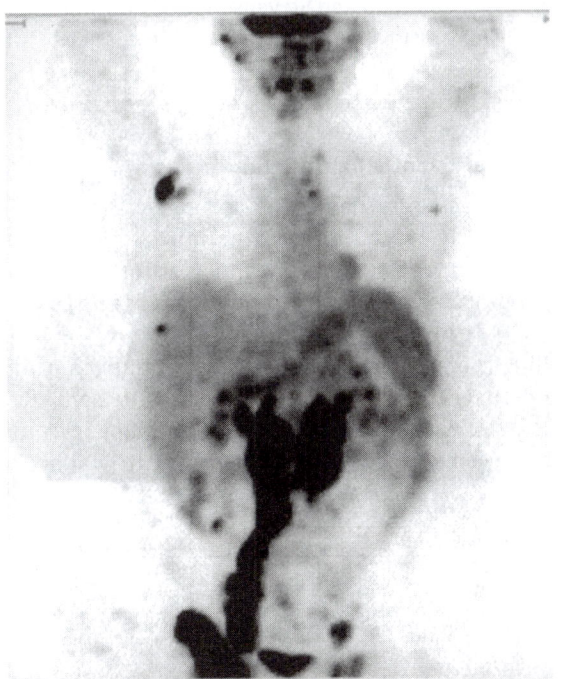 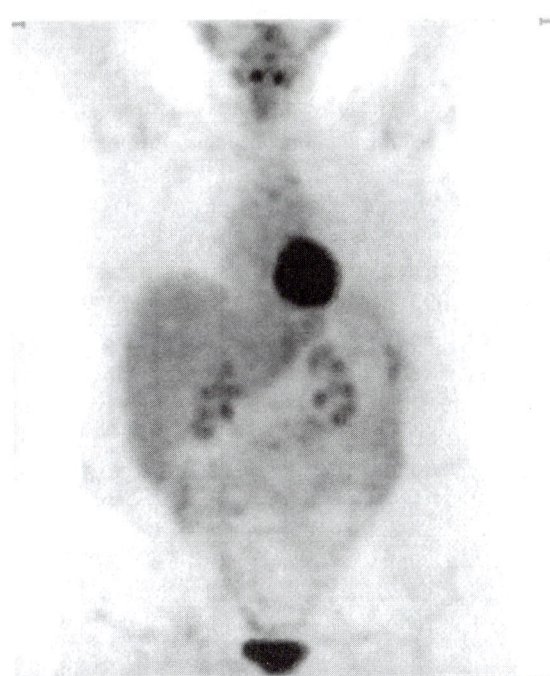

BEFORE   AFTER

Fig. 42.2 Male patient with extensive and nonresponding NHL was treated with Zevalin : Complete disappearance of diseased nodes after therapy

Evolution of the Concept of Insulin Resistance Syndrome/Metabolic Syndrome

In 1973, patients with angina pectoris with angiographically normal coronary arteries were recognized, receiving the label of "Syndrome X". Vascular hyperactivity was plausible explanation of the ischemic pain. Patients with this syndrome were also reported to have hyperinsulinemia. In 1985, hyperinsulinemia was shown as a link between hypertension, obesion and glucose intolerance. In 1988, Reaven postulated the link between insulin resistance, obesion, hypertension and dyslipidemia [high triglyceride (TG) and low high-density lipoprotein (HDL)], and cardiovascular disease (CVD). Again in 1993, Reaven gave an expanded definition of syndrome X.

In 1989, the term "deadly quartet" comprising central OB, hypertension, IGT and hypertriglyceridemia, came to be associated with insulin resistance. In 1991, the multifaceted nature of the insulin resistance

syndrome was established. Subsequent additions to the syndrome were small dense low-density lipoprotein (LDL), increased proinsulin, increased plasminogen activator inhibitor (PAI)-1 and microalbuminuria.

In 1995, Godsland and Stevenson raised the question: Is insulin resistance a syndrome or a tendency? In 1996, the association between insulin resistance and endothelial dysfunction was established.

Normal Endothelial function

Blood vessels are not just passive conduits like water pipes. The vascular endothelium is a dynamic structure that normally maintains vasodilation (via endothelium derived relaxation factors) nitric oxide (NO), prostacyclin and endothelium derived hyperpolarization factor (EDHF), and maintain Coronary blood flow during increased demand. But it is also equipped to cause vasoconstriction instantly if the emergency situation demands it (via locally

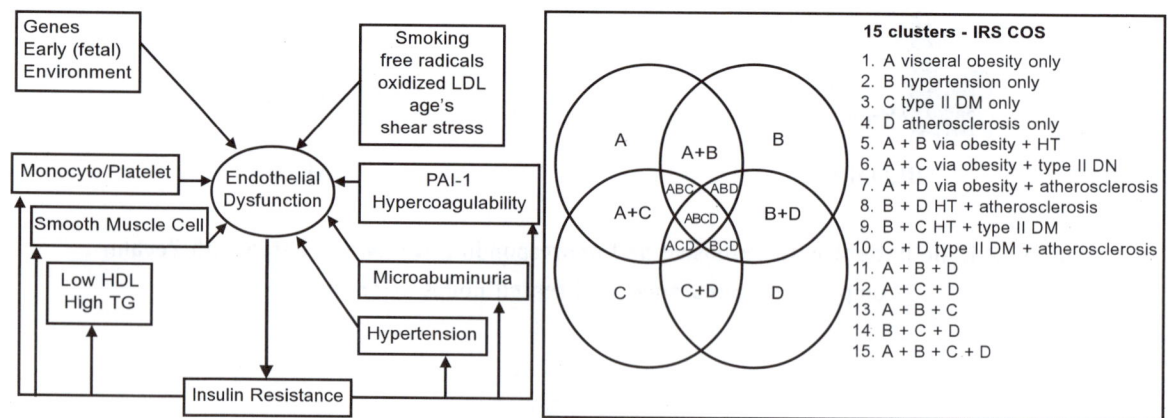

Fig. 43.1

produced endothelin, PGH2 and thromboxane). A healthy endothelium inhibits platelet and leucocyte adhesion to the vascular surface and maintains a balance of pro-fibrinolytic and prothrombotic activity.

eNOS can constitutively produce both NO and superoxide. Tetrahydrobiopterin (BH4) is an essential co-factor for NO synthesis. BH4 deficiency causes deficient NO production. BH4 stabilises NOS dimers which prevents uncoupling of NOS and subsequent superoxide formation. Increased superoxide production has been demonstrated in coronary arteries.

Superoxide dismutase (SOD) normally bound to the outer surface of endothelial cells protects NO from inactivation by superoxide. This protective mechanism is overwhelmed in oxidative stress. The SOD mimetic tempol restores vasodilatation.

Insulin increases NO production via de novo synthetic pathway for BH4 synthesis. Hyperglycaemia-mediated EPC dysfunction is associated with reduced intracellular BH4 concentration, which is reversed by exogenous BH4 treatment.

Nitric oxide inhibits many of the processes that follow endothelial injury such as NFKB activation, monocyte chemotaxis, foam cell formation, leucocyte and platelet adhesion, intimal hyperplasia, vascular smooth muscle cell (SMC) migration and proliferation, expression of adhesion molecules VCAM-1, ICAM-1 and e-selectin, etc.

In patients with coronary atherosclerosis, endothelial vasodilatory dysfunction is not confined only to the epicardial conductance vessels but also extends to the coronary resistance vessels and microcirculation. Excessive inactivation of NO due to increased oxidative stress occurs in smokers, diabetics with increase in advanced glycosylation end products (AGEs) and in hypercholesterolemia. At any level of total and LDL cholesterol the main culprit is the small dense LDL particle which is easily prone to lipid peroxidation and thereby adhere to the proteoglycan of the endothelium. Paraxonase, an antioxidant enzyme located on HDL prevents lipid perioxidation of LDL (hence the protective effect of HDL against the initiation of atherosclerosis). HDL activates eNOS leading to increased production of NO. A variety of stimuli regulate eNOS activity involving Akt kinase and/or mitogen-activated protein kinase.

Diminished production of NO and/or increased inactivation of NO are the basis of endothelial dysfunction, hence increasing the bioavailability of NO and decreasing its inactivation caused by reactive oxygen species (ROS) and reactive nitrogen species (RNS) is the aim of therapy to reverse endothelial dysfunction.

Endothelial Dysfunction as Cause of Insulin Resistance

The endothelium is a dynamic tissue that maintains the integrity of the vasculature. Endothelium produces vasodilators such as NO, BNP, prostacyclins and endothelium-derived hyperpolarization factor. These substances balance the production of vasoconstrictors such as angiotensin II [formed from the enzymatic action of angiotensin-converting enzyme (ACE) located on endothelial cells], endothelin and vasoconstrictive cyclooxygenases (such as thromboxane and prostaglandin H2). These autocrine and paracrine mediators not only direct the behavior of the underlying VSMCs but also mediate interaction of circulating cells such as platelets, neutrophils, monocytes and macrophages with the vascular wall. Damage to endothelium shifts the balance from a vasodilator state to a vasoconstrictor state. Reduced NO activity results in loss of vascular protection (inhibition of platelet and leucocyte aggregation and migration, inhibition of VSMC migration and growth). Thus, an important measure of endothelial health is the ability to produce NO. Defect in NO production or excessive inactivation of NO are seen in subjects with risk factors for atherosclerosis. Endothelial responses are abnormal in the presence of these risk factors even in the absence of angiographically defined disease.

Endothelial injury initiates the process of platelet aggregation releasing platelet-derived growth factors, cytokines, vasoconstrictors and other substances including those that enhance activation of the transcription factor, NFKB an important mediator of inflammation. Enhanced NFKB activity increases monocyte chemotaxis, foam cell formation, white cell adhesion molecule expression, monocyte chemoattractant protein, macrophage colony stimulating factor production and inflammatory cytokine release. These changes not only enhance atherosclerotic lesion formation, but also promote rupture of the atheromatous plaque, the major event leading to myocardial infarction.

Nitric oxide inhibits many of the processes that follow endothelial damage (such as growth and migration of VSMCs, intimal hyperplasia, expression of adhesion molecules such as vascular cell adhesion molecule 1 (VCAM-1), IAM and E-selectin, proinflammatory cytokines such as TNFα and chemokines). NO induces and stabilizes the NF-KB inhibitor IKB? As a result NO attenuates the binding of inflammatory cells to the vascular wall. NO also inhibits the thrombotic process (platelet-adhesion and aggregation) via prostacyclin.

Endothelial Dysfunction as Initial Event

In two epidemiological studies, Von Wille brand factor (VWF) concentrations (as markers of endothelial dysfunction) were correlated with those of insulin, a surrogate marker for IR in nondiabetic subjects. However, no direct association between IR and circulating markers of endothelial dysfunction has been demonstrated.

In a study of 33 subjects (25 men and 8 women) with T2DM, with BMI 29 kg/m^2, glycated hemoglobin (HbA1c) of 10.1% and diabetic duration 5 years, circulating levels of VWF antigen correlated with the metabolic clearance rate of glucose, HDL cholesterol, mean systolic BP (r = -0.35), and marginally with total TGs. These data suggest a relationship between endothelial dysfunction at capillary level and insulin action, as well as providing further evidence for a relationship with other features of the insulin resistance syndrome.

The hypothesis is that peripheral endothelial dysfunction at the arteriolar and capillary level arises through a complex interplay of genetic and environmental factors and leads to a multifaceted metabolic disturbance comprising of insulin resistance and other features of the insulin resistance syndrome. Thus, IRS is a marker for peripheral endothelial dysfunction. In contrast, central large vessel endothelial dysfunction plays a major role in atherogenesis but has little direct metabolic impact. The coexistence of peripheral and central endothelial dysfunction explains the observed association between atherosclerotic vascular disease and IRS.

Endothelial Function in Diabetes

Endothelium dependent vasodilation is impaired in angiographically normal coronary arteries in patients of both T1DM and T2DM. There is increased oxidative stress and raised levels of reactive oxygen species (ROS) in diabetes. Oxygen-derived free radicals impair NO-induced vasodilation in both T1DM and T2DM. There is excessive inactivation of NO by superoxide ions (O2-) to form stable peroxynitrite anion (ONOO).

Sustained hyperglycemia causes nonenzymatic glycation of proteins. There are many adverse effects of AGEs-promotion of auto-oxidation and increased inactivation by quenching of NO. Binding of AGEs to their endothelial receptors causes activation of NF-KB which causes changes in endothelial phenotype expression promoting platelet-aggregation, macrophage migration and cyclooxygenase catalysis.

The oxidative hypothesis of atherosclerosis was proposed by Witztum in 1994. Ting and colleagues found that acute intra-arterial administration of antioxidant vitamin C improved endothelium-dependent vasodilation in both type 1 and type 2 diabetes. Similar benefits have been shown with vitamin E.

Insulin resistance and endothelial dysfunction

Insulin promotes vasodilation by stimulating NO production from endothelial cells. Inhibition of NO-synthase with L-NG-monomethylarginine, acetate salt (L-NMMA) inhibited both insulin-induced blood flow (completely), and muscle glucose uptake (by 30%). L-NMMA infusion significantly increased BP. Scherrer and colleagues suggested that impaired vasodilatory responses to insulin could contribute to the hypertension associated with insulin resistance.

The cause for the common defect in insulin-mediated glucose uptake and insulin-mediated NO production may be the same signaling pathway, the phosphatidyl inositol-3 kinase (PI3K).Chronic exercise and estrogen therapy improve endothelial production of NO and also improve insulin resistance. In IR, the vascular protective effects of insulin, specifically NO production, are blunted while the proatherosclerotic effects proceed normally via stimulation of vascular smooth muscles cells (VSMCs) mediated by the MAPK pathway.

Insulin regulates constitutive NOS gene expression in endothelial cells in vivo. Endothelial dysfunction starts early in life, much before the development of structural coronary atherosclerosis. The multiple risk factors that have been identified for coronary atherosclerosis, can be modified by simple measures such as diet, exercise, and stress control. Patients with risk factors for CAD, normal coronary angiograms and no measurable disease by intravascular ultrasound (IVUS), exhibit selective endothelial dysfunction at both the epicardial and microvascular levels. These findings emphasize the scope and need for life-style management and prevention of "preclinical" coronary atherosclerosis.

With N-13 ammonia PET perfusion studies early detection of abnormal coronary flow reserve (normal: five times the resting flow) due to endothelial dysfunction is now possible in asymptomatic men and women at high risk for CAD. Coronary artery calcium score (CCS) ascertained by high resolution CT provides an indicator of atherosclerotic burden. CCS > 100 provides an indicator for aggressive lifestyle modification.

Demonstration of Endothelial Dysfunction

Endothelial dysfunction may occur in the absence of angiographic or IVUS-detected atherosclerosis in patients with risk factors for atherosclerosis. Animal studies have demonstrated that known risk actors for CAD (hyperlipidemia, hypertension, diabetes) result in impaired endothelium-dependent vascular reactivity before the development of structural atherosclerosis both at the epicardial and icrovascular levels. These findings open the scope for prevention of "preclinical" coronary atherosclerosis.

Coronar y spasm mediated by sympathetic adrenoreceptors can occur in angiographically normal coronary arteries, or it may be superimposed on obstructive coronary vessels. Patients with Prinzmetal's angina, cocaine overdose, and collagen vascular disease like scleroderma are known to have perfusion defects despite normal coronary angiograms. Provocative testing with ergonovine during cardiac catheterization may demonstrate latent coronary artery spasm (as shown by Maseri in 1990).

Syndrome X is defined as stress induced anginal pain with a positive stress test for myocardial ischaemia, with normal coronary angiogram and normal left ventricular function. This represents "small vessel disease" with reduced coronary flow reserve in the coronary microcirculation as shown by N-13 ammonia PET.

FMD (Flow mediated vasodilatation), an indicator of nitric oxide availability is measured by strain gauge plethysmography in forearm resistance vessels or noninvasively using high frequency ultrasound and hyperaemia induced by blood pressure cuff arterial occlusion, a technique described by Correti et al 1995.

Peripheral vascular endothelial function testing by FMD has been shown to correlate well with coronary artery endothelial function. Beneficial effects of l-arginine infusion on myocardial endothelial dysfunction during exercise in patients with angina pectoris and normal coronary angiograms have been demonstrated on myocardial perfusion imaging. Significant improvement in arm FMD is seen during laughter (15%) and reduction (47%) during mental stress.

As inflammation accompanies endothelial dysfunction, markers of inflammation like hsCRP, $TNF\alpha$, IL-6, fibrinogen, sE-selectin, sICAM-1 and sVCAM-1 serve as measures of endothelial dysfunction.

Endothelin, PAI-1, Prostacyclin, TPA, cellular fibronectin and type IV collagen fragments are other markers of endothelial dysfunction.

Microalbuminuria (30-300 mg/day) due to transmembrane leakiness is a marker of generalized endothelial dysfunction. More importantly it represents a stage at which prevention of future cardiovascular and renal deterioration is possible.

EPC Dysf unction

Endothelial progenitor cells (EPCs) are critical for endothelial maintenance and repair. Bone marrow derived EPCs home to sites of ischaemia, incorporate into newly formed capillaries and augment neovascularisation (important for wound healing and tissue repair) under the stimulation provided by erythropoitin (EPO).

In healthy person the number of circulating EPCs serve as a surrogate marker for vascular function and cumulative cardiovascular risk. EPC dysfunction contributes to the pathogenesis of ischaemic vascular disease. EPCs in circulation are depleted in patients with active rheumatoid arthritis (RA). Endothelial inflammation, characterized by permanent over-expression of cellular adhesion molecules and pro-inflammatory cytokine, CRP, matrix metalloproteinase 9 and IL-18 are all elevated in RA and are involved in the development of atherosclerosis.

In patients with cardiovascular risk factors the number and function of EPCs is impaired. EPCs probably secrete angiogenic factors to activate resident endothelial cells. The number of circulating EPCs and circulating angiogenic cells (CACs) are inversely related to the several risk factors for atherosclerosis.

Hyperglycaemia affects EPC proliferation and differentiation. The number of EPCs obtained from T1DM patients in culture was 44% lower compared to age and sex matched healthy controls. EPC dysfunction is a novel concept in the pathogenesis of vascular complications of T1DM. Hyperglycemia causes uncoupling of endothelial NOS, impairing EPC mobilization and function.

Statins are known to increase EPC number, while high TNFα causes decrease in circulating EPCs. The Emory University, USA is currently assessing the role of Mediterranean diet and omega 3 fatty acids on oxidative stress and endothelial progenitor cells.

Caveolin, the structural protein of calveolae plays a central role in EPC mobilization and homing in SDF-1 driven post-ischemic vasculogenesis. It also regulates eNOS turnover and consequently NO release as a result of shear stress.

Anti oxidized LDL Antibodies

Endothelial inflammation is initiated by oxidize LDL, which acts as an immunogen and stimulates the production of auto antibodies by B cells. Anti OX-LDL antibodies are present in healthy individuals as well as in patients with atherosclerosis, Circulating IgG antibodies to OX-LDL are present in cardiovascular risk-free children, and the levels of antibody are significantly higher in children, than adults suggesting that the antibodies may not necessarily be related to atherosclerosis and cardiovascular disease, and indeed may be protective against atherosclerosis by neutralizing and catabolizing the OX-LDL.

It is possible that some infections with phosphorylcholine as a major antigen (e.g., streptococcus pneumoniae) give rise to anti phosphocholine antibodies (IgM) which block the uptake of OX-LDL by macrophages. On the other hand circulating immune complexes (CICs) - OX-LDL and antibodies to OX-LDL may cause damage when deposited in tissues including atheromas.

Only after clearly defining the characteristics of protective anti OX-LDL antibodies and the conditions of their generation will we know whether we can immunize patient with OX-LDL to stimulate protective antibodies especially in patients with accelerated atherosclerosis such as SLE, RA and APS and for the prevention of restenosis.

Adiponectin

Adiponectin, an insulin sensitizing adipocytokine stimulates the production of nitric oxide in endothelial cells using the PI3 kinase dependent pathway. It induces phosphorylation of eNOS at ser 1177 and complex formation of eNOS with heat shock protein HSP90 through activation of AMP-activated protein kinase (AMPK). Adiponectin receptors AdipR1 and Adip R2, expressed on endothelial cells interact with APPL-1, an intracellular protein to mediate the adiponectin-evoked endothelial NO production and vasodilatation. Whether APPL-1 is also involved in other actions of adiponectin such as protection from apoptosis, modulation of cytokine production and alleviation of oxidative stress warrants further studies.

Hypoadiponectinemia is closely linked to the impairment of endothelial function in HT and Type 2 DM as shown by increase in CRP, PAI-1 and tPA (which impair fibrinolysis). On the other hand, transgenic or adenovirus-induced over expression of globular or full length adiponectin results in marked alleviation of atherosclerosis in ApoE deficient mice. The main benefit of PPAR gamma agonist (such asrosiglitazone) is through increased adiponectin production.

Adiponectin activates AMPK in both the liver and skeletal muscle. EPA/DHA induce adiponectin in mice fed a high fat diet.

BH4 oral supplementation (10 mg/kg/day) leads to significant increase in plasma adiponectin and expression of mRNA of adiponectin in adipocytes.

Adiponectin: Adiponectin, a 244 amino acid protein produced exclusively by adipocytes, has an important role in health and disease. Normal levels of adiponectin are 7.9 + 0.5 mg/mL in males and 16.6 + 5 mg/mL in females. Adiponectin circulates in multimeric forms.

Recent reports have focused on high molecular weight (HMW) adiponectin, which is found to be lower in Asian Indian pregnant women compared to Caucasians. Asian Indians with T2DM have low adiponectin levels with higher risk for coronary artery disease (CAD).

PPAR γ agonists such as TZDs stimulate adipocytes to secrete adiponectin. TZDs suppress macrophage-mediated production of proinflammatory cytokines [TNFα, IL-6 IL1b, PAI-1, inducible NOS (iNOS)].

Osmotin, a member of a large pathogenesis-related (PR)-5 protein family is ubiquitous in fruits and vegetables and is a homologue of mammalian adiponectin. The beneficial effects of a diet containing 400 g of fruits and vegetable may partly be due to the osmotin content apart from the antioxidants and high fiber, low fat content. Osmotin activates adenosine monophosphateactivated protein kinase (AMPK) via adipo-R. Further research examining the similarities between osmotin and adiponectin may facilitate development of potential adiponectin agonists.

Hyperhomocysteinemia

Homocysteine > 15 mg % reduces NO bioavailabilty by oxidative stress. Homocysteine may cause ADMA accumulation by inhibition of DDAH. In the Indian population, hyperhomocysteinemia is an indicator of widely prevalent deficiency of Vit B12 and folic acid which must be promptly corrected as emphasised by Yajnik in 2006. Hyperhomocysteinemia as a primary risk factor should be considered in individuals with atherosclerosis at young age, or out of proportion to established risk factors.

How to Improve Endothelial Function?

Dean Ornish set-up a study in 1977 to explore the effect of diet and lifestyle modification on the reversal of coronary atherosclerosis, using the techniques of quantitative coronary arteriography and quantitative myocardial blood flow using N-13 ammonia positron emission tomography (PET) imaging. It became obvious that modification of cardiovascular risk factors that contribute to endothelial dysfunction improves patient outcome disproportionate to the regression in the anatomic atherosclerotic lesions. Patients with "mild" coronary artery lesions can have severe endothelial dysfunction. Long-term follow-up showed more cardiac events in such patients. Myocardial ischemia can occur during exercise in patients without significant epicardial vessel stenosis, due to endothelial dysfunction. Recent insights into vascular biology help us to understand how the benefit occurs in relation to endothelial dysfunction.

High glucose inhibits insulin-stimulated NO production without reducing endothelial NOS Ser 1177 phosphorylation in human aortic endothelial cells. A single high sugar intake may induce heart rate acceleration and BP elevation as a result of sympathetic activation secondary to insulin response and alteration in endothelial function due to activation of oxidative stress. Hyperglycemia activates PKC-b which depresses eNOS expression and increases ET-1 activity. Treatment with vitamin E inhibits PKC, by increasing enzymatic degradation of DAG, the source of PKC, or by activating protein phosphatase-2 which dephosphorylates PKC. This action may be independent of the antioxidant effect of vitamin E.

Endothelial dysfunction caused by vascular PKC-β activation due to hyperglycemia is critical for diabetic microvascular complications. This can be prevented by selective PKC-β inhibitors such as ruboxistaurin. A single high fat meal transiently reduced endothelial function for up to 4 hours in healthy, normocholesterolemic subjects, probably through accumulation of triglyceride-rich proteins. This decrease was blocked by pretreatment with antioxidants, vitamins C and E suggesting an oxidative mechanism which increases superoxide production and deactivates NO.

Lipid lowering agents and antioxidants provide more NO and reduce superoxide, thereby enhance endothelial function, reduce thrombotic potential, reduce inflammatory response thereby preventing rupture of the vulnerable plaque. Clearly mechanisms other than regression of the atherosclerotic stenosis are operating.

Statins, apart from lowering cholesterol also improve nitric oxide production. Patients with low hsCRP do not get significant benefit with statin therapy compared to those with high hsCRP.

Advanced glycosylation end products through their receptors on the endothelium contribute to endothelial dysfunction. Impairment of endothelium-dependent vasodilation in T2DM occurs independent of epicardial coronary atherosclerosis, and cause major cardiac events. Strict control of diabetes reduced the AGEs.

Nitrates (glyceryl trinitrate, isosorbide dinitrate) act as NO donors and thereby improve endothelial function apart from decreasing the preload and after load of the ventricles. Long-term use of nitrates can produce drug tolerance which can be overcome by a combination of nitrate and hydralazine.

Newer selective $\beta 1$ adrenoreceptor antagonists such as nebivolol inhibit ET-1 liberation and increase the availability of NO.

Pioglitazone increases insulin sensitivity by activating insulin receptor kinase and the insulin signaling pathway which are mediated through its binding to the PPARγ receptors.

ACE inhibitors (ACEIs) and angiotensin receptor blockers prevent angiotensin-induced endothelin and superoxide production. ACEIs improve endothelial function in subcutaneous, epicardial, brachial and renal circulation, whereas they are ineffective in potentiating the blunted response to acetylcholine in the forearm of patients with essential hypertension. They can also selectively improve endothelium-dependent vasodilatation to bradykinin, probably related to hyperpolarization. Treatment with an angiotensin I-receptor antagonist can improve basal NO release and decrease the vasoconstrictor effect of endogenous ET-1. Calcium channel blockers can reverse impaired endothelium dependent vasodilatation in subcutaneous, epicardial, renal and forearm circulation.

Nifedipine and lacidipine can improve endothelial dysfunction in the forearm circulation by restoring NO availability probably through an antioxidant mechanism. Tetrahydrobiopterin (BH4) oral tablets are available but are prohibitively expensive; hence no clinical trials have been undertaken. BH4 supplementation prevents endothelial dysfunction and restores adiponectin levels, as described in an earlier section. Administration of sepiapterin (precursor of BH4) restores coronary flow reserve. In healthy adults, oral-glucose induced hyperglycemia and endothelial dysfunction are reversed acutely with BH4 infusion; the same benefit is seen in T2DM.

Normal diet contains 8 g of L-arginine. An additional 8 g/day nutritional supplement on a long-term basis improves endothelial function. Endothelial progenitor cell (EPC) dysfunction is a normal concept in the pathogenesis of vascular complications in diabetes. Endothelial NOS uncoupling impairs EPC mobilization and function in diabetes.

Erythropoietin (EPO) promotes endothelial progenitor cell proliferation and adhesive properties in a PI3 kinase dependent manner. Recombinant human EPO protects the myocardium from ischemia reperfusion injury and promotes beneficial remodeling, a novel protective effect in the infarcted heart.

The vascular action of insulin to stimulate endothelial production of NO leading to vasodilation and increased blood flow is an important component of insulin stimulated whole body glucose utilization.

Exercise training improves coronary flow reserve as a result of improved vasodilation. By increasing shear stress, it induces increase in NO. Regular physical exercise improves insulin resistance in muscles and improves glucose uptake and glycogen synthesis.

The FA composition of skeletal muscle membrane phospholipid is altered by N-3 PUFA, increasing its fluidity, thereby permitting prolonged residence of GLUT4 in the plasma membrane. A daily dietary supplement of essential FAs, EPA and DHA is recommended.

Role of DHA in stress management by modulation of sympathetic activity in the CNS has already been discussed.

Yoga and lifestyle have shown reversal of atherosclerosis. A prospective study done by the Caring Heart Project of International Board Yoga has shown the beneficial effects of Yoga lifestyle on reversibility of ischemic heart disease.

Lifestyle modification is the cornerstone of management of insulin resistance syndrome. Cessation of tobacco smoking decreases oxidative stress and improves endothelial function. Dietary modification, with emphasis on a lactovegetarian diet with at least 400 g green leafy vegetables and fruits will give adequate natural antioxidants (vitamins C, E, carotenoids and flavonoids). Such a diet is low in sodium, high in potassium and fiber.

Need for aggressive revascularization

In Harrison's Principles of Internal Medicine 17th ed. 2005, p. 1304, Eugene Braunwald, eminent cardiologist has stated: "Mechanical revascularization by CABG (Coronary Artery bypass graft) surgery or PTCA (percutaneous trans thoracic coronary angioplasty) with or without drug-eluted stents, is probably being employed too often in USA. The mere presence of angina pectoris and/or the demonstration of severe coronary artery narrowing at angiography should not reflexly evoke a decision to do aggressive revascularization. Instead, this approach should the limited to those patients whose angina has not responseded adequately to medical treatment or in whom revascularization has been shown to improve the natural history of the disease e.g. acute coronary syndrome, or multivessel CAD with left ventricular dysfunction (LVEF < 40%)", and hibernating myocardium.

Unfortunately commercial pressures world-wide have distorted the scientific practice of medicine. Dean Ornish has said in his book "Reversing Heart Disease" "The insurance company will pay at least $ 30,000 for a CABG, at least $ 7500 for a balloon angioplasty, but only $ 150 if a doctor spends the same amount of time and effort educating a heart patient about nutrition, exercise, stress-coping and, life style management. If someone spends the same amount of time and effort teaching a well person how to remain healthy, the insurance company will pay nothing at all. It is not surprising that doctors spend time doing what is reimbursed".

Summary and Conclusions

By the year 2025 half the world's population of type 2 DM will be in India. A polypill strategy (aspirin 75mg, metformin 1gm, ACE inhibitor 10mg and statin 40mg) per day can slash diabetic risks and reduce subsequent events by upto 97 percent over 5 years.

In the larger long-term interest of Indian Society in the next 25 years our emphasis should be on prevention through lifestyle modification beginning from childhood. A vegetarian diet with fat not more than 15%, adequate source of long chain n-3 essential fatty acids EPA and DHA, low sodium, high potassium and high fibre (green vegetables and fruits 400 g/day which also give antioxidants - carotenoids, flavonoids, lycopene, Vit. C, Vit. E) regular physical exercise, avoidance of tobacco and alcohol, and controlling mental stress through Yoga and meditation. Chronic life stressors such as perceived isolation, lack of social support, anxiety, depression, hostility and anger contribute to increased risk of CAD in part by impairing endothelial function. On the other hand positive emotions such as mirthful laughter have the opposite effect. How to keep mental equanimity and how to give and receive love and affection more freely is the key to a happy, healthy life.

44 Nutritional Deficiency

Adequate nutrition is essential for life, but unfortunately it is denied to nearly 800 million people in the world who are desperately poor, most of them in the developing world. The situation is going to remain so in the decades to come. Hence doctors have to deal with a vast population whose primary problem is undernutrition or malnutrition, or where nutritional deficiency compounds the problem of infection, and worm infestation.

On the other hand in the developed world, overnutrition (leading to obesity) is a major problem. Apart from poverty, alcohol, drug addiction, and promiscuous sex (AIDS) will adversely affect the nutritional status of patients, even in the setting of affluence.

The doctor should assess the nutritional status of every patient seen by him (**Table 44.1**). It is a sobering thought that in a hospitalized patient, undernutrition or malnutrition may develop under the very eyes of the caring physicians and surgeons. A significant percentage of patients are undernourished before admission to hospital, and more than 50 per cent of them have signs of malnutrition before they leave it. Clinical manifestations of malnutrition are given in **Table 44.2** and the causes and investigation of malnutrition are given in **Table 44.3**.

Every doctor should learn to assess the *nutritional requirement* of an individual patient, taking into account the age and sex, type of work and recreational activities (**Table 44.2**). The recommended daily caloric intake is given in the 'box' on p. 236. In the hospitalized patient, allowance has to be made to compensate for excessive catabolism (trauma, major sepsis, burns etc). Part of proper management is to ensure a diet adequate in calories, proteins, vitamins, and minerals.

TABLE 44.1 ASSESSMENT OF NUTRITIONAL STATUS

- Dietary assessment
- Weight and Height
  (for optimal weights for heights see 'box' on p. 267)
- Body Mass Index (BMI)

  $$BMI = \frac{Weight\ (kg)}{Height\ (metres)^2}$$

  Normal range = 20-24
  BMI < 18 = marker of malnutrition
  BMI > 24 = marker of obesity
  Grade I obesity : 25-29.9
  Grade II obesity : 30-39.9
  Grade III obesity : > 40
- Skin-fold thickness
  Triceps : < 10 mm-malnutrition
    > 20 mm (males) ⎱ peripheral obesity
    > 28 mm (females) ⎰
  Subscapular ⎱ measure of truncal obesity.
  Supra-iliac crest ⎰
- Mid-arm muscle circumference
  = arm circumference (cm)
    minus triceps skin-fold thickness (mm)
- Waist-hip ratio (WHR) normal : 0.8
  CAUTION: A very muscular man will have a BMI similar to obese patients but his skin-fold thickness is *normal*.

Since most evidence shows that protein energy malnutrition reduces immunological competence, increases the incidence of sepsis, delays wound healing and reduces patient survival, its detection and correction are important. This is particularly so in surgical patients and in those with cancer and gastrointestinal diseases.

Protein and energy providing substances may be given by mouth or by tube feeding (enteral nutrition), or when enteral feeding is impossible, by the intravenous route (parenteral nutrition).

TABLE 44.2 CLINICAL MANIFESTATIONS OF NUTRITIONAL DEFICIENCY

Nutrient	Daily recommended intake	Manifestation of deficiency	Nutrient	Daily recommended intake	Manifestation of deficiency
Calories	30 kcl/kg	Weight loss.	B12 (Cyanoco-balamin)	3 µg	Weakness, Fatigue, Sore tongue, Skin pigmentation, Hair loss, Paraesthesia, Diarrhoea, Anaemia.
Protein	0.6 g/kg	Weakness, Nail & hair change, Oedema.			
Vitamins:					
A (retinol)	5000 IU	Night blindness, Bitot's spots, Xerosis, Keratomalacia.	Minerals:		
			Sodium	92-184 mg	Weakness, Mental confusion, Muscle cramps.
D (calciferol)	200 IU (5mg)	Muscle weakness, Tetany, Rickets, Osteomalacia in adults.	Potassium	2500 mg	Weakness, Paraesthesia, Hyporeflexia, Cramps, Ileus.
			Calcium	800 mg	Rickets in children,
E (tocopherol)	10-20 IU	Areflexia, Gait disturbance, Paresis of gaze.	Phosphorus	1000 mg	Osteomalacia in adults.
			Magnesium	300-350 mg	Tetany
			Iodine	150 µg	Symptoms of hypothyroidism.
K	70-140 µg	Easy bruisability, Bleeding from several sites.	Chromium	30-200 µg	Glucose intolerance, Impaired release of fatty acids.
C (ascorbic acid)	60 mg	Weakness, Irritability, Gingivitis, Joint pain, Loose teeth, Easy bleeding.	Iron	10-18 mg	Anaemia, Koilonychia, Atrophy of tongue papillae, Angular stomatitis.
B1 (thiamine)	1-1.8 mg	Anorexia, Weakness, Paraesthesia, Beriberi, Wernicke's encephalopathy.	Manganese	2.5 mg	Ataxia, Retarded skeletal growth, Decreased reproductive function.
B2 (ribotlavin)	1.2-1.6 mg	Sore lips, Cheilosis, Fissuring of lips and tongue, Angular stomatitis, Skin desquamation, Seborrhoeic dermatitis, Anaemia	Copper	2-3 mg	Neutropenia, Anaemia, Diarrhoea, Scurvy-like bone changes.
			Zinc	15 mg	Facial & extremity rash, Skin ulcers, Alopecia, Apathy, Confusion, Loss of taste, Depression, Dwarfism & hypogonadism.
B3 (niacin)	12-18 mg	Dermatitis on exposed parts, Diarrhoea, Sore tongue, Dementia, Painful tongue, Angular stomatitis.			
B5 (pantothenic acid)	4-7 mg	Fatigue, Paraesthesia, Diarrhoea, Sore tongue Dementia, Painful tongue.	Fluoride	1.5-4 mg	Dental caries.
			Selenium	50-200 µg	Muscle weakness, Cardiac failure.
B6 (pyridoxine)	1-2 mg	Seborrhoea, Cheilosis, Glossitis, Anaemia,	Molybdenum	20-120 µg	Neurologic abnormalities, Hypermethioninaemia, Hypouricaemia, Hyperuricosuria.
B7 (biotin)	100-200 µg	Peripheral neuropathy, Alopecia, Dermatitis.			
B9 (folacin) Folic acid	400 µg	Fatigue, Nausea, Sore tongue, Anaemia, Mouth ulcers.	Fatty acids:		
			Linoleic acid	2-4% of daily calories	Dry scaling dermatitis, Coarse hair, Alopecia, Diarrhoea.
			Linolenic acid	0.5% of daily calories	Numbness, Paraesthesia, Weakness, Blurred vision.

TABLE 44.3 INVESTIGATION OF PATIENT WITH MALNUTRITION

Factor	Disease	Confirmation
Poor intake	Lack of availability; Anorexia due to underlying disease; Anorexia nervosa; Depression; Psychological problems.	Assessment of dietary intake.
Poor absorption	Chr. pancreatitis; Coeliac disease; Tropical sprue; Bacterial colonization; Tuberculosis.	Tests for malabsorption: faecal fat; D-xylose.
Increased catabolism	Tuberculosis; Sepsis; Malignancy; AIDS; GI protein loss.	Screen for infection. Screen for malignancy. Screen for HIV.
Metabolic disease	Uncontrolled diabetes; Addison's disease; Hypopituitarism.	Blood sugar. Plasma ACTH & Cortisol. Absent axillary & pubic hair.
Chronic liver disease	Alcoholic hepatitis; Cirrhosis.	Liver function tests.
Chronic hypoxia	COPD; Interstitial fibrosis.	Lung function tests.
Chronic hypoperfusion	Cardiac cachexia; Chronic renal failure.	Other features of heart disease. Bun, creatinine.
Severe chronic anaemia	Sickle cell disease; Thalassaemia major; Hookworm disease.	Low Hb.

TABLE 44.4 SOME COMPLICATIONS OF TOTAL PARENTERAL NUTRITION

Mechanical	Pneumothorax Catheter embolus, air embolus Thrombophlebitis
Metabolic	Septicaemia Errors in water and electrolyte balance Inappropriate use of energy substrates Excess glucose, excess fat Use of inappropriate substrates— fructose, xylitol, sorbitol, ethanol

Failure to provide individual constituents
Failure to balance constituents
Absolute deficiency syndromes e.g. Zn, Cu, essential fatty acids
Metabolic bone disease

RECOMMENDED DAILY CALORIE INTAKE

Body Weight	Calories
I. Ideal	(30 kcal/kg) 1800 sedentary 2200 heavy manual work
II. Overweight	(20 kcal/kg)
10% overweight	1600
20% overweight	1400
30% overweight	1200
III. Underweight	(40 kcal/kg)
10% underweight	2000
20% underweight	2200-2400

OPTIMAL WEIGHTS (kg) FOR HEIGHTS (cm)		
Height (cm)	Weight (kg)	
	Men	Women
148	52.5	49.0
150	54.0	50.5
152	55.5	52.0
154	57.0	53.5
156	58.5	54.5
158	60.0	56.0
160	61.5	57.5
162	63.0	59.0
164	64.5	60.5
166	66.0	62.0
168	67.5	63.5
170	69.5	65.0
172	71.0	66.5
174	72.5	68.0
176	74.5	69.5
178	76.0	71.0
180	77.5	73.0
182	79.5	74.5
184	81.0	76.0

Prolonged total parenteral nutrition (TPN) has proved its usefulness in many clinical situations (e.g. upper GI fistula, and in patients with cancer, short gut syndrome, and severe granulomatous disease of the bowel). TPN should not be undertaken lightly as it has many complications.

The calculations of TPN are given below:
- Nitrogen: 0.20-0.24g N/kg body weight
- Energy: 40-50 kcal/kg body weight
- Energy-Nitrogen ratio: about 200:1
- Energy source: glucose and fat emulsion equally
- Sodium: 8 mmol/g N
- Potassium: 5 mmol/g N
- Magnesium: 1 mmol/g N
- Calcium: 0.5 mmol/g
- N Phophorus: 0.5-0.75 mmol/kg body weight
- Water soluble vitamins: B 1, B2, B3, B5, B6, B7, B9, Folic acid, B12, C
- Fat soluble vitamins: A, D, E, K
- Tracer elements: Zn, Cu, Mn etc.

Fluid requirements vary widely–usually 2-3 litres are infused daily in most patients.

TPN should be undertaken in specialized units which have the facility to monitor nutrients and trace elements. Some complications of TPN are given in **Table 44.4**.

MEASUREMENT OF RBC MEMBRANE ω3 FATTY ACID STATUS

The RBC membrane ω3 fatty acid content reflects the status of membranes in all cells of the body including neurons, heart muscles and leucocytes. Normal cell membrane contains two types of essential fatty acids in the cell membrane phospholipids; arachidonic acid (ω6) and EPA (eicosa pentanoic acid) which is converted to DHA. While arachidonic acid is the source of pro inflammatory cytokines, EPA is a source of anti inflammatory cytokines-lipoxins, resolvins, protectins, merasins (**Fig. 44.1**)

The normal EPA content of the healthy cell membrane is 6-8%. HS ω3 index is the EPA/DHA content of RBC membrane expressed as a percentage of total RBC membrane fatty acids, assessed by Capillary Column Gas Chromatography (GC).

RBC δ 15 N (ratio of N15 and N14) can be analyzed by a rapid and inexpensive test: mass spectroscopy (MS). There is strong correlation between RBC delta N and EPA/DHA content of the RBC cell membrane.

Intake of 1000 mg/day of EPA/DHA will maintain the targets of 8% in RBC membrane. Women have greater capacity to synthesize EPA/DHA. Breast milk has the ideal ratio of ω6:ω3 of 2:1. High dietary intake such as fish oil leads to high cell membrane EPA/DHA and associated with low level of inflammatory markers even in obese overweight persons (Z Makhout et al Eur J Clin Nutr 2011 65, 808-817). 12 gm/day cow's ghee in daily diet will ensure adequate supply of EPA/DHA. Interestingly our forefathers swore by 'Asli Ghee' and Dara Singh who passed away at age of 82, took 250gms of cow's ghee daily during his wrestling career.

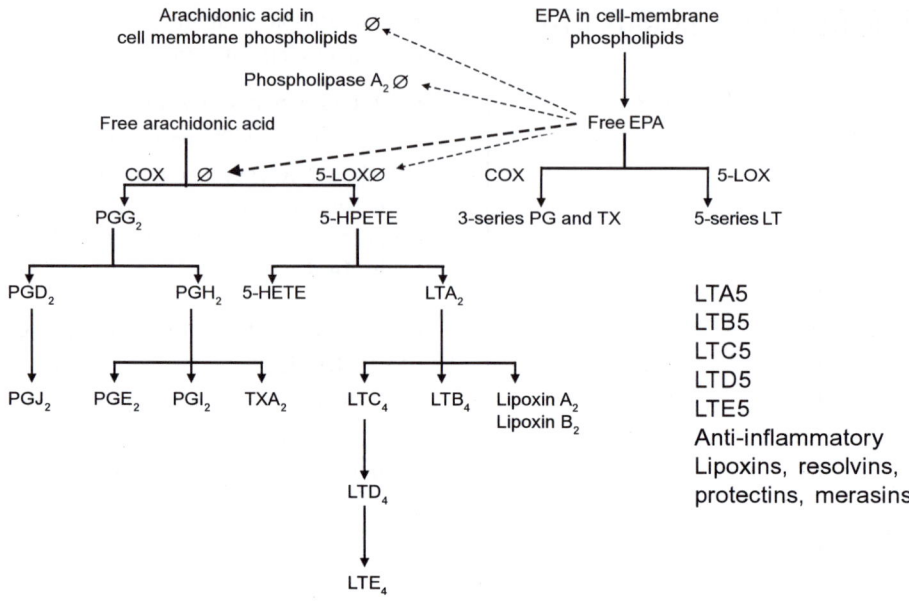

Fig. 44.1: Beneficial effects of EPA/DHA in the cell membrane phosholipids

Low RBC DHA correlates with smaller brain weight and volume even in persons free from clinical dementia. High dietary intake and increased EPA/DHA levels in RBCs have reduced the risk of dementia as assessed by cognitive markers and volumetric imaging by brain MRI (ZS Tan et at Neurology 2912, 78, 659-664). Increasing RBC EPA/DHA level improves GRACE score prediction of 2 year mortality in patients with myocardial infarction (Harris Ws Intl J. Cardiology 2012). It is not generally realized that EPA/DHA deficiency is as rampant as vitamin D deficiency in our Indian population.

Vitamin D and Multiple Health Outcomes

Historically, Vitamin D has been linked to calcium phosphorus and bone metabolism, osteoporosis, fractures, muscle strength and falls. Since 2000 AD observational studies Vitamin D showed deficiency is linked to non-skeletal chronic disease - cancer, cardiovascular, metabolic, infections and autoimmune diseases, Alzheimer's disease as well as mortality (Holick MF. NEJM 2007, 357, 266-81).

Recent data shows the wide-spread prevalence of Vitamin D deficiency in all populations leading an indoors-oriented lifestyle (lack of ultraviolet -

B exposure) several randomised controlled trials have been published regarding the beneficial effects of Vit. D supplementation. Theodaration E. et al (Ref BMJ 1st April 2014, 348, 119).

The Institute of Medicine (10 M) 2011 report states that 50 n mol/L concentrations of 25(OH) D are adequate and 600 IU of Vit. D per day can achieve these concentrations.

Low plasma 25 (OH) D and high BMI are associated with increased risk of diabetes. Genetic variation in DHCR7 (related to endogenous production) and CYP2R1 (related to liver conversion) on plasma 25 (OH) D, are associated with T2DM. Causal relationship between obesity and Vit. D status (PLOS Med 2013, 10, el0013 83).

Vit. D is a negative endocrine regulator of renin angiotensin system and blood pressure. 1,25 $(OH)_2D_3$) suppresses renin gene transcription by blocking the activity of CAMP response element in the renin gene promoter.

The world pandemic of Vit. D deficiency could possibly be explained by cellular inflammatory response activity induced by the renin - angiotensin system (Ferder M et al Am. J Physiol cell Physiol 2013, 304, 1027-39). Potential pathophysiological role of Vit. D deficiency in essential hypertension (Carbone F et al World J cardiol 2014, 6(5) 260-76).

Vit. D could be a powerful weapon in the fight against liver fibrosis (Ronald M. Evans 2013)

The hepatic stellate cells (HSCs) are pericytes formed in the perisinusoidal space (Space of Disse.) are involved in liver fibrosis. Viral infection, alcoholic or drug toxicity or any other factors damaging to hepatocytes elicit and inflammatory response by activation of Kuppter cells which release TGFB, TNFX, PDGF and ROS which activate HSCs to produce large amounts of ECM (exhiacellular matrix protein) fibrotic proteins in an attempt to heal an injury. Under chronic stress, localized fibrosis expands eventually leading to cirrhosis and increased risk of liver cancer.

A synthetic form of Vit. D - Calcipotriol is less susceptible to break down than natural calcitrol, effectively do activates the switch governing the fibrotic response. The synthetic analog produces a strong response without adding calcium to the blood (unlike natural Vit. D which in excess can cause hypercalcemia).

High levels of Vit. D receptor (VDR) on HSCs have been recently discovered calcitral can put a brake on HSCs to prevent fibrosis.

Obesity is defined as a condition in which there is excessive amount of body fat. This is the commonest cause of steady weight gain.

Obesity is a major public health concern in the affluent segment of the world population. It needs medical attention because it is associated with increased mortality, predisposes to the development of important diseases, and diminishes the efficiency and happiness of those affected. Mortality risk is reduced to normal in those who successfully lose weight and maintain it at the desirable level. Obesity can be easily diagnosed by inspection of the patient, and documented by recording the body mass index (BMI), body weight in kilograms divided by the square of body height in metres.

For adults between the ages of 20 and 29, the 85th percentile of BMI is 27.8 for males and 27.3 for females. One snag is that a heavy-muscled individual may be labelled as 'obese' using this index, but the difference can be easily established, simply by inspection, and documented by skinfold thickness measurement (triceps and subscapular), which will be normal in the muscular individual, and high in the obese (above 20 mm in men, 28 mm in women).

The distribution of body fat differs in different obese subjects. The metabolic behaviour of adipose tissue varies as a function of its anatomical sites. Adipocytes isolated from different anatomic sites can vary significantly in terms of cell number and cell size, responsiveness to insulin, glucocorticoids, oestrogen and progesterone, and the rate of catecholamine induced lipolysis (which is opposed by insulin).

Insulin promotes lipogenesis and prevents lipolysis. Hyperinsulinaemia and insulin resistance (more in muscle than in adipose tissue) are common features of obesity.

Adipose tissue is highly sensitive to insulin and obesity is commonly associated with insulin resistance and its consequent hypertension, Type 2 Diabetes mellotous and atherosclerotic coronary artery disease form a part of Insulin Resistance Syndrome – Cardiovascular Dysmetabolic syndrome (IRS/CDS). Insulin promotes leptin production in adipocytes leptin is a measure of adipose mass. Normal females have higher plasma leptin levels. (15-29 ng/ml compared to normal males (3-7 ng/ml). There is a positive correlation between insulin, proinsulin and leptin levels and between these variables and the BMI.

The normal fat content of young adult women is about twice that of young men, and pregnancy is characterized by an increase in body fat.

Obesity commonly begins at puberty, during pregnancy or at menopause. The overwhelming majority of obese patients show no clinical evidence of an endocrine disorder.

TABLE 45.1 Human Genome-Wide Association Study (GWAS) – Obesity Related Genes

		Obesity Related Genes
1.	Thriftness - Low metabolic rate - Low thermogenesis	- ADRB2, ADRB3- beta -adrenoreceptors. - UCP-1, UCP-2, UCP3- uncoupling proteins - ADCY5- Adenyl cyclase 5
2.	Hyperphagia - Abnormal regulation of hunger and satiety	- DRD2- Dopamine D2 receptors - HTR2C- 5hydroxytryptamine - LEP- Leptin - LEPR- Leptin receptor - MC4R- Melanocortin Receptor 4 - NRS3- Nuclear receptor subfamily 3 - NR3C1- Nuclear receptor C member 1
3.	Low rate of lipid oxidation	- ACE- Angiotensin converting enzyme - ADIPOQ- Adiponectin, apelin - GNB3- Guanine nucleotide binding protein 3 - LIPE- Hormone sensitive lipase. - LDLR- Low density lipoprotein receptor.
4.	Adipogenesis - Fat storage	PPARγ - Peroxisome proliferator receptor γ - VDR- Vitamin D receptor - RETN- Resistin - IL-6- Interleukin 6 - TNFα- Tumour necrosis factor α - TIRP Br2 - FTO-fat mass and obesity
5.	Low physical Activity - Modulation of Energy homeostasis - Relation to BMI	- DRD2- Dopamine receptor D2 - MC4R- Melanocortin receptor -4 - TMEM 18- Transmembrane protein 18 - KCTD15- Potassium channel tetramerization domain - GNPDA2- Glucosamine 6 phosphate deaminase 2 - NEGR1- Neuron growth factor regulator gene-1 - FGF21- Fibroblast Growth Factor -21 - TNJK/MSRA- methionine sulfoxide reducing agent. - LYPLAL 1 - PCK1 - PFKP- Phosphofructokinase platelet isoform - PTER- Phosphotriesterase - SEC 16 B- Saccharomyces cerevisae Sec 1 - SH 2 B 1- Scr- homology-2 contatining adapter protein - SDCC AG 8- Serologically defined colon cancer antigen 8.

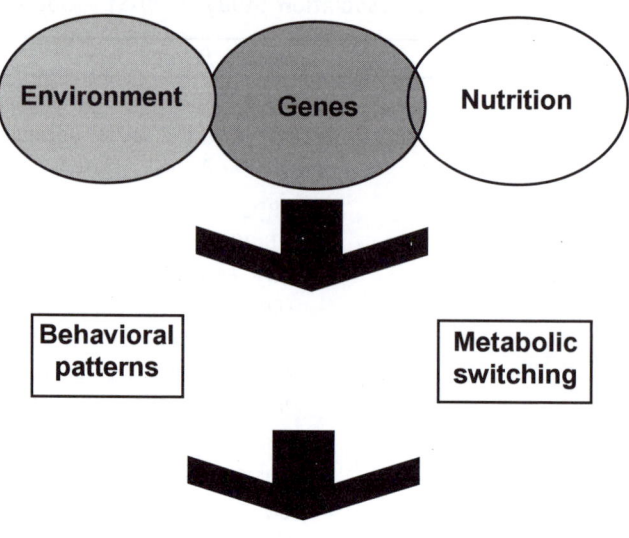

Fig. 45.1

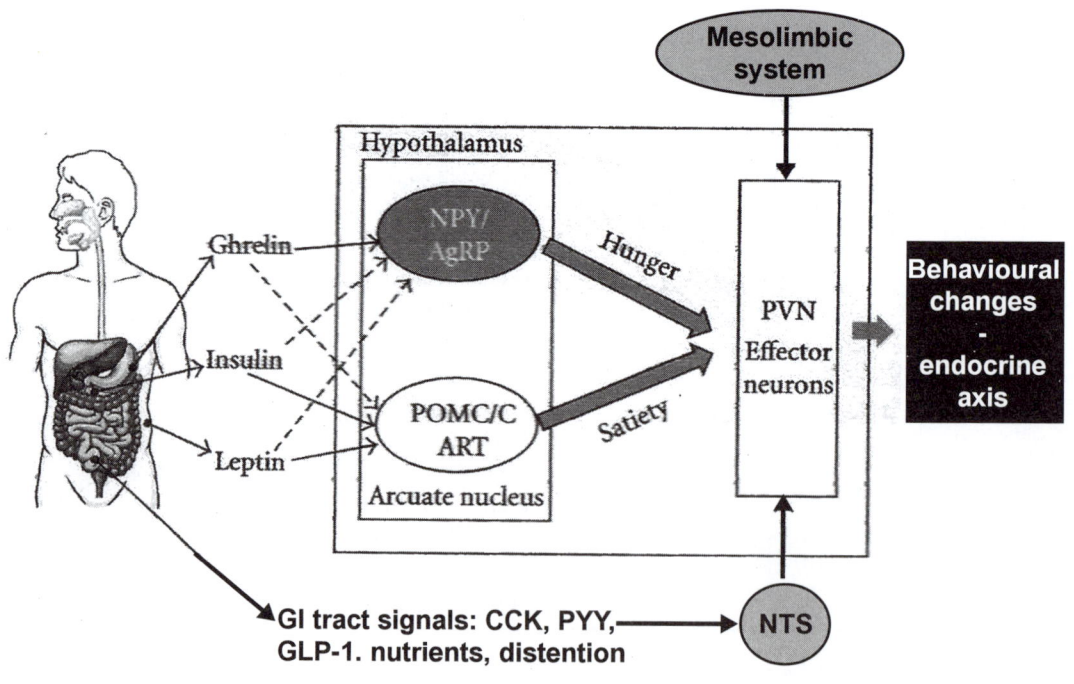

Fig. 45.2

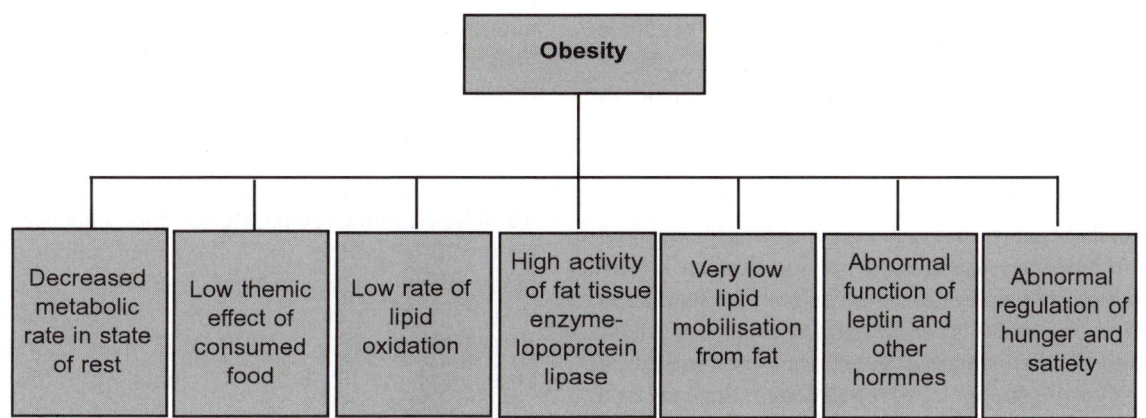

Fig. 45.3. The physiological changes associated with obesity

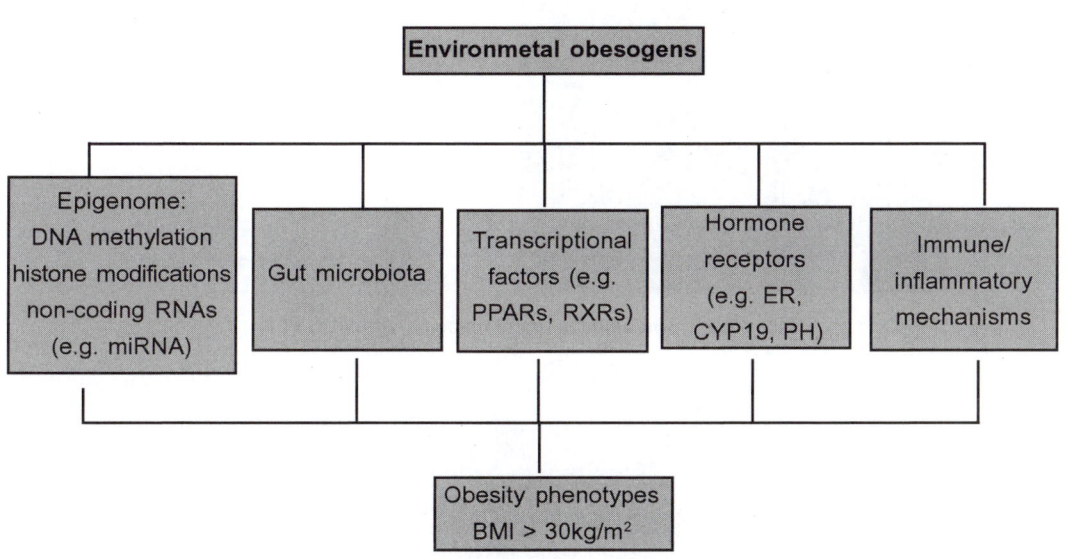

Fig. 45.4 Possible targets of obesogens. Environmental obesogens influence a variety of molecular and/or cellular targets that may act either alone or with each other creating a complex network that affects gene expression and results in obesity phenotypes (abbreviations: miRNA – microRNA, PPARs – peroxisome proliferator–activated receptors, RXRs– retinoid X receptors, ER – oestrogen receptor, CYP19 – Cytochrome aromatase p450, PH – peptidergic hormones, BMI – body mass index).

The causes of obesity are listed in **Table 45.2**. The use of oral contraceptives, phenothiazines, steroids and insulin is commonly followed by obesity mainly because appetite is stimulated.

The complications of obesity are given in **Table 45.3**.

Current Knowledge about Adipose Tissue

Ability to store energy in excess of what is required forimmediate use is essential for survival. White adipose tissueplays a central role in the regulation of energy balance andconservation of body heat through thermogenesis. Functions of adipose tissue include (1) storage of triacylglycerol in thebody, and aromatizaion of sex steroids, storage of fat solublevitamins and (2) protection of vital structures-orbits, palms &soles, vulva, perineal, periarticular, pericalyceal and epiduralregions. It is interesting to note that this supportive function of fat is preserved in lipodystrophy suggesting separate embryonicorigin and genetic regulatory mechanisms of supportive fat. (3)Adipose tissue is an endocrine organ which produces severaladipocytokines. leptin, visfatin, adiponectin, resistin, TNFα, IL-6 PAI-1 etc. (**Fig. 45.4**).Newly formed adipocytes produce adiponectin, an insulin sensitizer while distended adipocytes produce leptin, resistin, TNFα, IL-6. TNFα induces insulin resistance by causing serine phosphorylation of IRS-1in muscle and IRS-2 in liver thereby abrogating the IRS-PI3K-AKT signalling pathway necessary for GLUT4 translocation, glucose transport and glycogen synthesis in muscle.

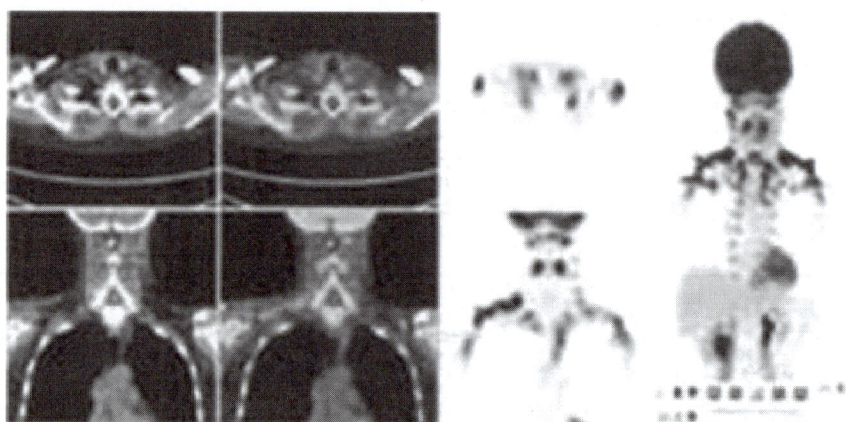

Fig. 45.5 Brown adipose tissue (Imaging with FDG PET)

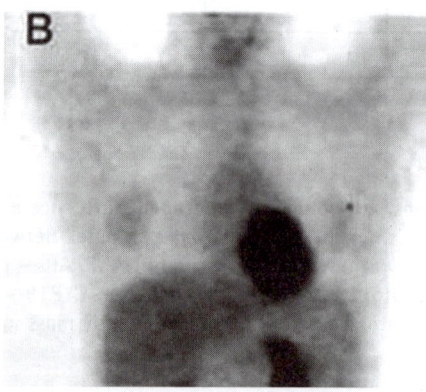

Fig. 45.5B Disappearance of BAT after propranalol

Adipose tissue is a dynamic structure with a good blood supply. The stored fat in adipose tissue is continuously undergoing lipolysis (hydrolysis) and lipogenesis (reesterification). These two processes are not forward and reverse phases of the same reaction but have entirely different pathways in the control of synthesis and hydrolysis. Insulin plays a central role in stimulating lipogenesis and preventing lipolysis. Due to differences in receptors and post-receptor events between human visceral (omental) and subcutaneous adipose tissue, antilipolytic effects of insulin are 3 fold higher in subcutaneous fat than omental. Although the receptor number is similar (~300,000 sites per cell), receptor affinity is higher in subcutaneous fat. I-125 labeled insulin dissociates more rapidly from omental than subcutaneous adipocytes. There is a remarkable heterogeneity in the distribution and metabolic response in adipose tissue in different sites. At any BMI adult females have more body fat than males as reflected in plasma leptin levels. Insulin stimulates adipogenesis and prevents lipolysis at all sites. Growth hormone reduces truncal fat and promotes fat deposition in palms and soles. Estrogen promotes fat deposition in hips, legs, breasts and subcutaneous tissue. Prolactin promotes adipogenesis in femorogluteal & mammary regions. Androgens favour visceral and subsutaneous abdominal fat deposition. Male hypogonadism is associated with increased adipose tissue distribution in female pattern.

Glucocorticoids promote re-distribution of fat from peripheral to central location-truncal and supraclavicular (buffalo hump). Lipodystrophy related to HIV treatment resembles Cushing's syndrome but cortisol levels are not high. adrenoreceptor agonists (isoprenalin) accelerate lipolysis while a2 adrenoreceptor agonists (clonidine) retard lipolysis, more in females. Noradrenaline - induces lipolysis is ten fold more in abdominal than gluteal fat- this difference is 20 fold in females. Regional differences in nor-adrenaline induced lipolysis are not seen when post receptor acting compounds are used such as forskolin (adenylylcyclase & CAMP), enprofyline (phosphodiesterase) or dibutyryl cAMP (protein kinase). (Bolinder J et al) 22. Visceral adipose tissue cells grow slowerin culture than subcutaneous adipose cells Thiazolidine drugs cause proliferation of subcutaneous adipose tissue (but not visceral adipose tissue) and increased UCP2 mRNA expression.

Thermogenesis: Brown fat, muscle and uncoupling enzymes

Brown adipose tissue (BAT) and skeletal muscle are important sites of non-shivering thermogenesis. Non-exercise activity thermogenesis (NEAT) occurs in activities of daily living, fidgetting, spontaneous muscle contractions and maintenance of posture. Till recently there was no information about the presence and distribution of brown fat in adult humans. In new born babies brown fat cells are found in the neck areas helping their tiny bodies generate heat. Brown fat cells largely disappear by adulthood, but their precursors still remain lodged in white adipose tissue (WAT). Brown adipose tissue is characterized by a well developed blood supply, rich sympathetic innervations with high β3 adreno-receptor expression and a high content of mitochondria and cytochromes but low activity of ATP synthase. The proton gradient normally present across the inner mitochondrial membrane of coupled mitochondria is continually dissipated in brown adipose tissue by a thermogenic uncoupling protein thermogenin, which acts as a proton conducting pathway through the membrane. Due to uncoupling of oxidation and phosphorylation much heat is produced but little free energy is trapped in ATP (something similar to thyrotoxicosis) in the mitochondria in BAT, WAT and muscle. UCP1 is exclusively expressed in BAT. UCP2 is expressed in BAT, WAT and muscle. UCP2 locus on human chromosome 11 is linked to obesity and hyperinsulinism. UCP3 is expressed in skeletal muscle, a homologue of UCP1. Diet induced thermogenesis may account for the observation that some lucky individuals "eat a lot but do not get fat‰. It is noteworthy that brown adipose tissue is reduced or absent in obese people. Transgenic mice with reduced BAT are obese indicating the important role of BAT in energy expenditure. Transgenic mice which over express UCP3 have hyperphagia but still do not gain weight. The availability of FDG-PET now enables us to document the presence and distribution of brown adipose tissue in humans. In FDG-PET studies in cancer patients brown fat was located in a very small number in the mediastinum (paratracheal, paraesophagea, prevascular, pericardial) and in the neck, thorax and abdomen. (Fig. 45.5). In thyrotoxicosis there is increased interscapular fat pad weight, its triacylglycerol content and DHA content.

Dysfunction of UCP3 reduces thermogenic capacity, alters energy homeostasis and promotes fat deposition. The C55 promoter polymorphism in UCP3 in South Indian women increases visceral fat deposition. There is inverse relationship between adipose mass and adiponectin production. Expression of UCP-1 in skeletal muscle decreases muscle energy efficiency and affects thermoregulation and substrate oxidation. Uncoupling proteins provide new clues for causation of obesity. Exercising muscle produces a factor "irisin" which converts WAT into BAT ("browning" response) with increased UCP-1 expression.

AMPK: Cellular Energy Sensor and Regulator (Fig. 45.7)

Regulating energy levels is fundamental process in every living organism. At a cellular level ATP must be maintainedat relatively high levels (normally about ten-fold above the concentration of ADP) in order to drive essential metabolic processes. AMPK is activated in response to ATP depletion,which causes a concomitant increase in the AMP : ATP ratio.Activated AMPK causes switching off of ATP- utilizingpathways (eg. Fatty acid synthesis) and switching-on of ATP generating pathways eg. fatty acid oxidation. AMPK is a sensor as well as regulator of cell energy status and plays a key role in maintenance of energy balance at the cellular as well as whole body level. (Towler and Hardie 2007). 40 SIRT1, activated by AMPK, plays an important role inmetabolic function and longevity in mammals. Both act in concert with PGC-1a which interacts with multiple transcription factors to stimulate mitochondrial metabolic capacity. Fibroblast Growth factor-21 regulates energy metabolism by activating AMPK-SIR1-PGC1a pathways. In animal models of obesity FGF21 reduced abdominal fat by 50% (Chau CM et al 2010) Further research is needed to expand our understanding of the diagnostic and therapeutic relevance of FGF21-dependent pathways in humans, and the potential to ameliorate both obesity and diabetes.AMPK activity in the hypothalamus regulates feeding behaviour

Ghrelin activates AMPK and NPY leading to increased food intake and decrease in energy expenditure. Leptin by suppressing AMPK & NPY decreases food intake.

Importance of Physical Exercise

A normal man at rest inhales between 6 and 8 litres of air per minute, from which about 0.3 litre of oxygen is transformed in the lung alveoli to the blood. During maximal physical activity the same man takes in 100 litres of air per minute and extracts five litres of oxygen. Hill studied the effects of breathing pure oxygen during exercise. The immediate effect is to lower considerably the rate of ventilation. Athlets who have breathed oxygen- enriched air during exercise reported a pronounced relief of subjective distress and a decrease in ventilation. Oxygen breathing extended the work capacity of trained athelets. On the other hand the Mexico Olympics showed the adverse effects of high attitude and hypoxia on competitive athletics.

When the body is at rest, the muscles take up no more than about 20 per cent of the total body oxygen consumption (60 to 70 ml of O2 per minute out of 300 ml per minute). During exercise, as in running or swimming the active muscle needs about 3000 ml per minute or about 50 times their resting requirement. Thanks to the presence of myoglobin the special oxygen store, the muscle cell is extraordinarily tolerant to a temporary shortage of oxygen supply. The amount of myoglobin in muscle tissue can be increased by physical training. The increased fuel requirements of exercising muscles (FFAs and glucose) are ensured by the production of 3 hormones noradrenaline, adrenaline and glucagon abetted by growth hormone and cortisol. Physical training results in improved myocardial performance, improved oxygen transport as well as increased oxygen extraction by muscle- the myoglobin levels are elevated, mitochondrial size and numbers increase so also their enzyme content and activity. Exercise increases fibrinolytic activity in plasma which is important in diabetic patients.

Skeletal muscle contains 2 types of fibres: type 1 (slow twitch) fibres are red because they contain myoglobin (a reservoir of oxygen) and high number of mitochondria. They maintain relatively sustained

ADIPOCYTOKINES

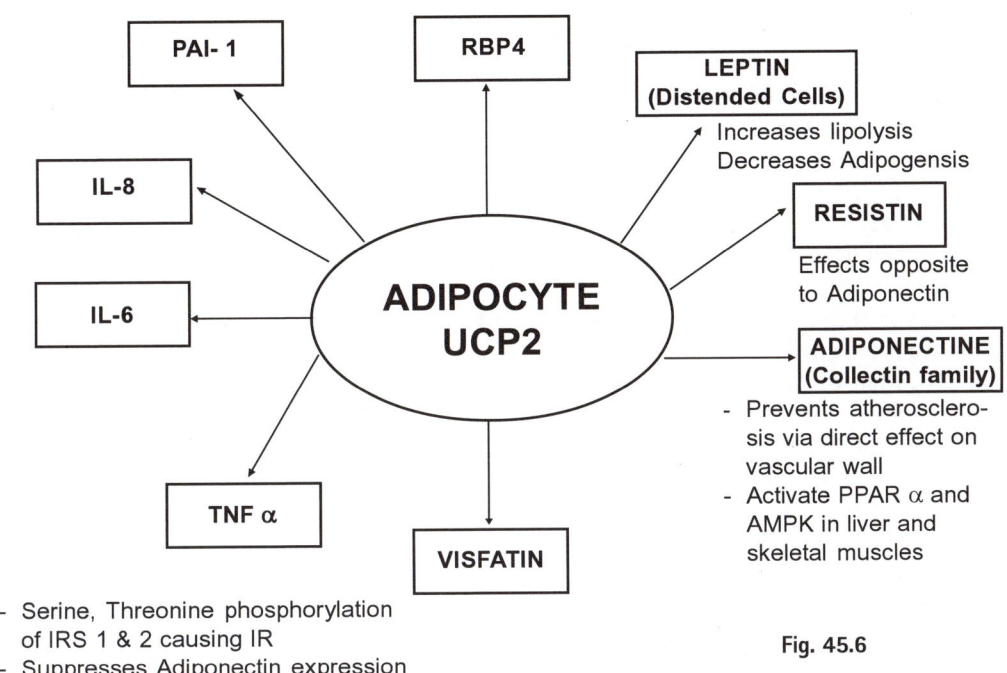

PAI- 1

RBP4

LEPTIN
(Distended Cells)

Increases lipolysis
Decreases Adipogensis

IL-8

RESISTIN

Effects opposite
to Adiponectin

IL-6

ADIPOCYTE
UCP2

ADIPONECTINE
(Collectin family)

- Prevents atherosclero-
  sis via direct effect on
  vascular wall
- Activate PPAR α and
  AMPK in liver and
  skeletal muscles

TNF α

VISFATIN

- Serine, Threonine phosphorylation
  of IRS 1 & 2 causing IR
- Suppresses Adiponectin expression

Fig. 45.6

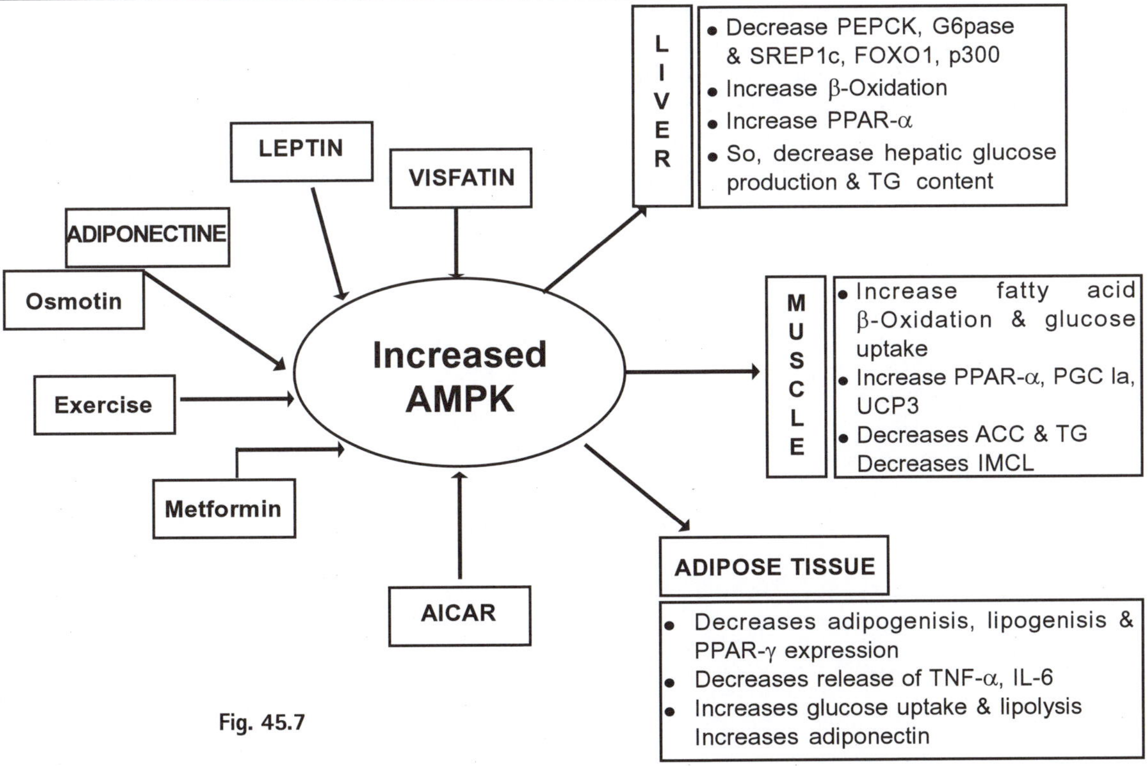

LIVER
- Decrease PEPCK, G6pase
  & SREP1c, FOXO1, p300
- Increase β-Oxidation
- Increase PPAR-α
- So, decrease hepatic glucose
  production & TG content

LEPTIN

VISFATIN

ADIPONECTINE

Osmotin

Increased
AMPK

Exercise

MUSCLE
- Increase fatty acid
  β-Oxidation & glucose
  uptake
- Increase PPAR-α, PGC la,
  UCP3
- Decreases ACC & TG
  Decreases IMCL

Metformin

AICAR

ADIPOSE TISSUE
- Decreases adipogenisis, lipogenisis &
  PPAR-γ expression
- Decreases release of TNF-α, IL-6
- Increases glucose uptake & lipolysis
  Increases adiponectin

Fig. 45.7

---

contraction (such as maintaining of posture) and their metabolism is aerobic.

Type II (fast twitch) and have very few mitochondria, exhibit short duration of contraction and derive their energy from phospho creatine and anaerobic glycolysis of glycogen. Athletes training for marathons have increase in the number of type 1 fibres in certain leg muscles, whereas 100 meter sprinters have a increased in number of type 2 fibres. Exercise increases GLUT-4 and hexokinase II and glycogenin expression in human skeletal muscle. (Kranion Y et al 2000). 45 In human skeletal muscle exercise results in increased mitogenactivated protein kinase (MAPK) activity and activation of down stream targets of MAPK. Impact of exercise training on insulin sensitivity and physical fitness and muscle oxidative capacity has been shown in healthy first degree relatives of T2DM patients (Ostergard T et al 2006). 46 Physical exercise is the most physiological way to overcome insulin resistance in muscle.

Benefits of exercise have not only be shown in metabolic syndrome but also in cancer. Female breast cancer patients who did regular physical exercise lived longer on chemotherapy compared to sedentary patients (Valenti M et al 2008). 47 Immunomodulatory effects of aerobic training in obesity have been demonstrated. Thomas Nickel et al (2011) 48 have analyzed the effects of 10 week intensified exercise training (ET)in obese subjects. There was significant reduction in waist circumference and oxidized LDL levels and increase in serum adiponectin levels, and up-regulation of BDCA-1dendrilic cells and (DCs) TLR-4 and TLR-7, indicating an enhanced immunocompetence with higher antibacterial, antiviral and antitumor activity.

The traditional Indian practice of "Surya Namaskar" is an excellent combination of 12 Yogasanas (which maintain flexibility of all tendons and joints in the body) with dynamic aerobic exercise and deserve to be promoted universally.

The Waist-Hip Ratio (WHR)

Recent data suggest that more than the total body adiposity, it is the central or abdominal obesity which is correlated with risk for diseases like IHD. Central obesity (representing visceral fat mass) is judged by utilizing the waist-hip ratio (WHR). This is better correlated to hyperinsulinism and insulin resistance which may be central to the pathogenesis of hyperlipidaemia, hypertension and atherosclerosis. The visceral fat mass (sensitive to lipolytic stimuli) constitutes around 20 per cent of the total fat mass in centrally obese men. These adipocytes have a very poor density of insulin receptors, and they mobilize free fatty acids (FFA) which in turn contribute to insulin resistance in the liver. This leads to increased secretion of insulin from the islet cells and consequent hyperinsulinaemia. Hence WHR should be assessed along with BMI in the evaluation of obesity (See **Table 45.3**).

Table 45.2 CAUSES OF OBESITY

A. *Primary*
Genetic factors and
environmental factors.

B. *Secondary*
Hypothyroidism
Decreased caloric needs;
only a minority of hypothyroids
are truly obese.

Cushing's disease
Moon face, buffalo hump;
cervical & supraclavicular
fat deposits.

Insulinoma
Increased food intake in
response to hypo glycaemia;
most patients with islet cell
tumour are not obese.

Hypothalamic disorders

Fröhlich's syndrome
Mechanism: overeating
Boys with hypogonadotrophic
hypogonadism, mental retardation;
diabetes insipidus;
visual impairment.

Laurence-Moon-Biedl syndrome
Retinitis pigmentosa;
mental retardation;
skull deformities;
polydactyly, syndactyly;
hypogonadism.

Prader-Willi syndrome
Mental retardation;
hypotonia;
predilection to diabetes;
hypogonadism.

Table 45.3 COMPLICATIONS OF OBESITY

Mechanical disabilities
Flat feet;
Osteoarthritis of knees, hips and lumbar spine;
Venous stasis, varicose veins;
Abdominal hernia;
Diaphragmatic hernia;
Embarrassment of respiratory muscles–
exertional dyspnoea;
Increased susceptibility to respiratory infections.

Metabolic disorders
Insulin resistance;
NIDDM;
Hyperlipidaemia (involving both cholesterol and triglycerides);
Gallstones;
Hyperuricaemia and gout.

Cardiovascular
Waist girth more than hip girth is a risk factor for coronary artery disease (on the other hand triceps skin-fold thickness is not correlated with CAD).

Respiratory
Hypoventilation syndrome
(Pickwickian syndrome);
Snoring and sleep apnoea;
Occasional cardiac arrhythmia due to hypoxia.

Psychological
Cause or effect difficult to assess;
Depression, anxiety.

General
Poor surgical & anaesthetic risks;
More proneness to accidents;
Shortened life span;
30% overweight = 30% increased mortality;
40% overweight = 50% increased mortality.

Cancer
Connection with colon and breast cancer42%

Breast cancer
Obesity associated with breast cancer recurrence and mortality through low physical activities, high calories and fat intake, and changes in hormones (high oestrogen production in adipose tissue)

Prostate cancer
Moreaggressive forms are diagnosed in men with higher BMI (by 15% to 21% higher risk of fatal prostate cancer or biochemical recurrence) 12% to 20% of prostate cancer deaths connected with obesity.

Problems in Weight Reduction

Caloric restriction is the corner-stone of weight reduction irrespective of the cause of obesity. The basic principle in simple: if the food intake is less than the energy expenditure, stored calories (predominantly in the form of fat) will be consumed. In general, a deficit of 7700 kcal (32,000 kilojoules) leads to a loss of about 1 kg of fat. By estimating the patient's daily caloric needs (30 kcal kg body weight) one can calculate the deficit necessary to achieve a given rate of weight loss. Very low caloric diets (500-800 kcal/day) or total starvation for short periods has been tried. These can act as morale boosters to frustrated patients who can then be motivated to comply with long-term weight-reducing programmes. A weekly weight loss of 0.5 to 1 kg should be the general aim, and this can be achieved with a 1500 calorie diet and regular physical exercise. An hour's walk at 5 kilometres per hour will expend about 300 kcal or more for a heavy person. This is equivalent to about 30 g of fat, but if done regularly, it adds up to a weight loss of 9 kg in a year, other factors being equal. The doctor should discuss exercise programmes with the patient and consider which are within the physical capacity of the patient and which can be pursued with religious regularity.

Fenfluramine, a drug which increases release of serotonin in the brain probably acts by stimulating satiety rather than inducing anorexia. It must be given under careful medical supervision since it can cause nausea, diarrhoea, lethargy, breathlessness due to pulmonary hypertension, excessive dreaming, and depression if suddenly withdrawn.

A starting dose of 20 mg bid is gradually increased to a maximum of 120 mg per day, unless adverse effects intervene. Treatment can be continued as long as weight is being lost.

Fibre-rich foods (salads, green vegetables) have an effect on satiety.

The main problem is to maintain the weight loss permanently. This is an area of maximum therapeutic failure.

Newer Treatment Strategies

Cannabinoids and endocannabinoids have CB1 receptors located in CNS, adipocytes and the liver. Their activation in the hypothalamus leads to increased food consumption and their action on the liver leads to increased fatty acid synthesis, hepatic steatosis and obesity via increased fat storage. CB1 antagonists (e.g. SR 141716) have shown therapeutic efficacy and safety in phase III clinical trials in the treatment of obesity. This class of drugs holds considerable therapeutic potential for the future.

Surgical Procedures

For morbidly obese patients (at least 50 kg overweight), surgical procedures have been used, but many of them are accompanied by an unacceptable rate of morbidity and mortality.

Patients on whom jejuno-ileal shunt was performed, lost considerable weight but few returned to ideal weight hence this operation is now rarely performed.

Gastroplasty and gastric bypass result in limited food intake because of a small gastric reservoir and delayed gastric emptying, giving a feeling of fullness after a small meal. The procedures can be reversed if a decision to restore normal anatomy is made at a later date.

Prevention

One of the most useful services that a family doctor could provide for his patient is to record his weight regularly, alert him at the earliest indication of overweight, and give him appropriate advice to correct it. All the health agencies available should be mustered to support a steady campaign of public awareness and education about the need to avoid obesity. It is much easier to prevent obesity than to treat it.

46   Oedema

Oedema is defined as an increase in the extravascular (interstitial) component of the extracellular fluid volume, which may expand by several litres before the abnormality is recognized. A weight gain of several kilograms usually precedes overt manifestation of oedema, and a similar weight loss from diuresis can be induced in a slightly oedematous patient before dry weight is achieved.

Ascites and hydrothorax are to be considered as special forms of oedema. Anasarca refers to gross generalized oedema.

Fig. 46.1 explains the pathogenesis of oedema.

The clinical approach to oedema is on the following lines:

- Is the oedema localized/asymmetrical? (**Table 46.1**).
- Is the oedema generalized? (**Table 46.2**).
- Is the oedema confined to the face and neck, and is not on the legs? (**Table 46.3**).
- 1s the oedema confined to the lower limbs and trunk, and is not on the upper limbs and face? (**Table 46.4**).

As a rule, localized oedema can be readily differentiated from generalized oedema. The vast majority of patients with generalized oedema suffer from advanced cardiac, renal, hepatic, or nutritional disorders. Hence the differential diagnosis of generalized oedema should be directed towards identifying or excluding these conditions.

The *distribution of oedema* is an important guide to the cause.

Oedema of one leg or one or both arms is usually the result of venous and/or lymphatic obstruction.

Oedema resulting from hypoalbuminaemia is typically generalized, but it is especially evident in the very

soft tissues of the eyelids and face, and tends to be most pronounced in the morning because of the recumbent posture assumed during the night.

Oedema associated with heart failure tends to be more extensive in the legs and to be accentuated in the evening (shoes getting tighter in the evening), a feature largely determined by posture.

When patients of heart failure are confined to bed, the oedema may be most prominent in the presacral region.

In constrictive pericarditis, tricuspid stenosis, and endomyocardial fibrosis (seen in Kerala state in India), the lungs are not congested, orthopnoea is absent and the patient actually prefers to lie flat (like the severely anaemic patient); hence the face may be markedly swollen.

The general impression that lymphatic oedema is non-pitting while venous oedema is pitting on pressure, is true in established cases. In early cases of lymphoedema, the oedema is soft and pits easily on pressure.

Similarly classical myxoedema is firm and non-pitting. But patients of hypothyroidism can have pitting oedema as well as pleural and pericardial effusions;

The diagnostic evaluation of lymphoedema should include a search for microfilaria, abdominal and pelvic ultrasound, lymphoscintigraphy, and CT, to detect obstructive lesions such as neoplasms.

Angio-oedema and urticaria may occur in persons with atopy (allergic diathesis) as localized, non-pitting oedema which comes on rapidly and lasts for a few hours.

The most common sites are the face, extremities, and external genitalia. Although self, limiting in duration, angio-oedema of the upper respiratory tract may be

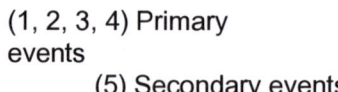

(1, 2, 3, 4) Primary
events
     (5) Secondary events

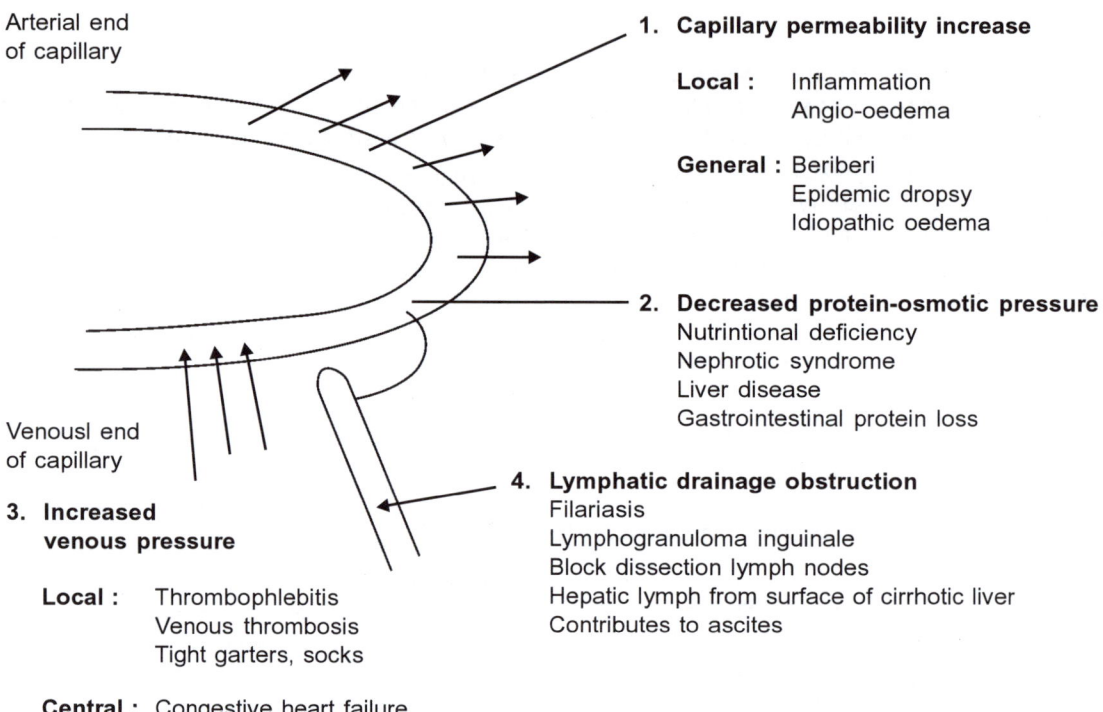

Arterial end
of capillary

1. **Capillary permeability increase**

    Local :   Inflammation
                   Angio-oedema

    General : Beriberi
                   Epidemic dropsy
                   Idiopathic oedema

2. **Decreased protein-osmotic pressure**
Nutrintional deficiency
Nephrotic syndrome
Liver disease
Gastrointestinal protein loss

Venousl end
of capillary

4. **Lymphatic drainage obstruction**
Filariasis
Lymphogranuloma inguinale
Block dissection lymph nodes
Hepatic lymph from surface of cirrhotic liver
Contributes to ascites

3. **Increased
venous pressure**

    Local :   Thrombophlebitis
                   Venous thrombosis
                   Tight garters, socks

    Central : Congestive heart failure
                   Volume overload
                   (e.g. acute glomerulonephritis)

5. **Secondary events**
    - Renin–angiotensin–aldosterone
      response to volume depletion
    - ADH response to volume depletion
    - Renal retention of salt and water

Fig. 46.1: Mechanisms of oedema

Table 46.1 CAUSES OF LOCALIZED/ASYMMETRICAL OEDEMA

1. *Trauma*
   Bruise, sprain, fracture
   haemarthrosis
   Local tenderness & colour changes

2. *Infection*
   Cellulitis, boil, abscess
   Osteomyelitis
   Gas gangrene

3. *Inflammation*
   Insect sting, snakebite
   Inflamed joint
   Trichinosis (facial oedema only)

4. *Venous obstruction*
   Phlebothrombosis & thrombophlebitis
   External pressure (garters, socks)
   Varicose veins & stasis
   Cavernous sinus syndrome (face only)
   Whooping cough (eyelids only)

5. *Lymphatic obstruction*
   A. *Primary*
      i. Presenting at birth (Milroy's Disease)
      ii. Presenting at puberty (Meige's Disease)
      iii. Presenting after age 35

B. *Secondary*
   i. Lymphangitis-bacterial (streptococci)
   ii. Filariasis
   iii. Lymphogranuloma
   iv. Tuberculosis
   v. Neoplasm-prostatic carcinoma, lymphoma
   vi. Surgery-block resection of lymph nodes.
   vii. Radiotherapy (e.g. breast: oedema of upper limb)

6. *CNS lesions*
   (hemiplegia, monoplegia)
   Oedema of paralysed limb due to vasomotor nerve affection (sympathetic dystrophy)
   Also reduced venous & lymphatic flow

7. *Angio-oedema*
   Localized, non-pitting oedema
   Atopic diathesis
   Seasonal occurrence
   Food, drug or physical stimuli (cold, sunrays, exercise)
   Face, extremities, external genitalia
   IgE levels may be high, C_1 esterase may be low.

---

life-threatening due to laryngeal obstruction. Gastrointestinal involvement may present with abdominal colic, with or without nausea and vomiting, and may precipitate unnecessary surgical intervention.

Management of Idiopathic Oedema

The plausible mechanism of idiopathic oedema is increased capillary leak of fluid from the circulation into the extracellular fluid compartment (aggravated by the upright position) with a secondary compensating increase in the renin-angiotensin-aldosterone activity. Diuretics, by further decreasing an already reduced effective plasma volume, stimulate the renin-angiotensin-aldosterone axis, hence they do not provide an effective remedy. The rational approach is to give an angiotensin converting enzyme inhibitor-ACEI like lisinopril, combined with an aldosterone antagonist (spironolactone). Most women have to learn to live with this nuisance if these drugs do not suit them.

Management of Nephrotic Syndrome

Reduced salt intake to 60 mmol/24 hours; in resistant oedema, to 40 mmol/24 hours.

Temporary reduction of water intake.

Diuretics: frusemide 40-80 mg bid plus amiloride 5 mg daily to prevent potassium loss.

In hospitalized patients, up to 500 mg frusemide bid may be given to get rid of the 20-40 litres of accumulated fluid.

In any patient requiring more than 160 mg/day frusemide, an intravenous infusion of albumin is helpful although the benefit may be of short duration. These patients have an increased susceptibility to infection especially pneumococcal peritonitis and septicaemia, also cellulitis from E. coli and other graril-ve organisms: give antibiotics.

Specific treatment: corticosteroids; prednisolone 60 mg/day. High dose *alternate day* treatment (120 mg/alt.days) for 8 weeks is given to reduce steroid-related complications, especially in children.

TABLE 43.2 DIAGNOSTIC FEATURES OF CAUSES OF GENERALIZED OEDEMA

Category	Diagnostic features	Category	Diagnostic features
I. Cardiac		IV. Nutritional	
• Congestive heart failure	History of dyspnoea, orthopnoea; Cardiomegaly, gallop rhythm; Pulmonary basal rates; Raised JVP; Enlarged tender liver; Pedal/sacral oedema.	• Kwashiorkor in children • Famine oedema • Gastrointestinal protein loss	Other stigmata of nutritional deficiency. JVP not raised. No albumin in urine. (Table 43.5)
• Constrictive pericarditis	No orthopnoea.	V. Hypothyroidism	
• Tricuspid stenosis	No pulmonary basal rales.	• Myxoedema	May mimic nephrotic syndrome: Dry coarse skin, hoarse voice;
• Endomyocardial fibrosis	Oedema of face marked since patient can lie flat; Raised JVP.		May have pericardial & pleural effusion; High TSH.
• Beriberi	High output failure; Raised JVP.	VI. Epidemic dropsy	Warm skin; Neovascularization; Oedema of feet; History of ingestion of mustard oil contaminated with Argemone mexicana.
II. Renal			
• Acute glomerulonephritis	Oliguria/anuria.		
• Chronic renal failure	Hypertension; Urine RBCs + albumin + BUN, Creatinine raised.	VII. Drugs causing oedema	Androgens; Carbenoxolone; Corticosteroids in high doses;
• Nephrotic syndrome	Urine albumin more than 3 g/day; Serum albumin less than 3 g/dl; JVP may be raised.		Oral contraceptives (high dose oestrogen); Phenylbutazone and other NSAIDs; Vasodilators;
• Toxaemia of pregnancy	Hypertension; Albuminuria.		Nifedepine (calcium channel blockers).
III. Hepatic		VIII. Idiopathic oedema	Almost exclusively females age 30-40;
• Cirrhosis	Ascites, jaundice; Oedema of lower limbs; Splenomegaly; Spider naevi; White nails; JVP not raised.		Large diurnal variations in weight (more than 1.4 kg/day); Day-to-day weight change as much as 4-5 kg/day, more on ambulation;
• Budd-Chiari syndrome	Sudden onset of tender hepatomegaly & severe intractable ascites; Jaundice; No signs or symptoms of heart failure; JVP not raised.		No evidence of cardiac, renal, hepatic, nutritional, allergic, obstructive venous or lymphatic, or drug-induced oedema.

Table 43.3 OEDEMA OF FACE AND ARMS, NOT OF LEGS

Obstruction of superior vena cava (SVC):	Face, neck and one or both arms swollen and cyanosed (extent depending on anatomical position of lesion in relation to left or right innominate vein or SVC); Collateral veins on front of chest and abdomen; Neck veins *non-pulsatile.*
A. Carcinoma of upper lobe bronchus	Cough, haemoptysis, stridor.
B. Aneurysm of ascending aorta	Chest pain, systolic pulsation, systolic murmur, unequal pulses in both arms.

Table 43.4 OEDEMA OF LOWER LIMBS AND LOWER TRUNK, NOT OF UPPER LIMBS AND FACE

I. *Inferior vena cava obstruction*
Thrombosis;
Extrinsic pressure by tumours, e.g. ovarian;
Invasion by tumour, e.g. hypernephroma.

II. *Cirrhosis of liver*

III. *Pregnancy*

Table 43.5 CAUSES OF PROTEIN–LOSING GASTROENTEROPATHY

	Site	Disease
I.	Stomach	Gastric carcinoma Giant hypertrophy of gastric mucosa Atrophic gastritis Post-gastrectomy syndrome
II.	Small intestine	Intestinal lymphangiectasia Tropical sprue Whipple's disease Lymphoma Intestinal tuberculosis Regional enteritis Acute infectious enteritis Scleroderma Jejunal diverticulosis Allergic gastroenteropathy
III.	Colon	Colonic neoplasm Ulcerative colitis Crohn's disease Megacolon
IV.	Heart	Chronic congestive heart failure Constrictive pericarditis Primary cardiomyopathy Inter-atrial septal defect
V.	Misce-llaneous	Oesophageal carcinoma Gastro-colic fistula Agammaglobulinaemia Nephrosis

Management of Ascites in Cirrhosis

Bed rest.

Salt restriction (2 g NaCl/day).

Fluid restriction 1500 ml/day.

Spironolactone 25 mg qid; increase gradually to 100 mg qid (upto maximum 400 mg/day).

Frusemide 40-80 mg daily.

For refractory ascites: IV infusion of salt-poor albumin.

Peritoneovenous shunt.

Doctors should always remember that in the majority of patients suffering from renal disease, symptoms and signs are not referred to the anatomic site of the kidneys. Clinical features of renal disease most frequently arise from:

(1) Abnormalities in the chemical composition of the blood (hence the importance of a routine measurement of BUN and Creatinine).

(2) Hypertension (hence the importance of checking BP in every patient).

(3) Anaemia (hence the importance of estimating Hb and CBC).

(4) Metabolic bone disease (indicated by alterations in serum calcium, phosphorus and alkaline phosphatase).

Their true origin may be suggested only after the detection of urinary abnormalities (provided of course that the clinician is in the habit of including *urine examination as a part of routine physical examination*. The importance of this (often neglected) procedure cannot be emphasized too much.

There are ten clinical syndromes (**Table 47.1**) that, singly or in combination, call attention to the possibility of renal disease, and thereby become useful starting points for patient evaluation. Their detection depends upon a small range of clinical and laboratory data (**Table 47.2**) that are usually collected in the course of routine health evaluation. Once the syndromes are recognized, they must be analysed to determine which prognostically or therapeutically significant causes are present, to evaluate the extent and severity of the causal disorder, and to institute proper treatment.

Drug history is important because drugs cause a variety of renal manifestations (**Table 47.3**).

TABLE 47.1 TEN SYNDROMES IN NEPHRO–UROLOGY WITH OPERATIONAL EFINITIONS

Syndrome	Operational definitions
1. Acute nephritis (AN)	Haematuria, oliguria Oedema Transient hypertension $\uparrow$ BUN, Creatinine
2. Nephrotic syndrome (NS)	Oedema Urine protein > 3.5 g/day $\uparrow$ Serum cholesterol
3. Asymptomatic urinary abnormality (AUA)	Urine showing RBCs, protein
4. Acute renal failure (ARF)	Oliguria, anuria $\uparrow$ BUN, Creatinine No anaemia
5. Chronic renal failure (CRF)	Anaemia $\uparrow$ Serum P J, serum Ca Small kidneys on US
6. Urinary tract infection (UTI)	Urine pus cells Culture: bacteria > 10^5 col/ml
7. Urinary tract-obstruction (UO)	Residual urine Obstruction seen on IVU/US
8. Renal tubular defect (RTD)	Glycosuria, aminoaciduria renal tubular acidosis etc.
9. Hypertension (HT)	High BP
10. Nephrolithiasis (NL)	Stone passed or seen on X-ray, or stone removed surgically

Routine urinalysis, Hb and CBC, BUN and creatinine are sufficient for syndrome detection. Currently available enzyme-coated dip-sticks make it very simple to detect urine albumin and glucose. Glycosuria without hyperglycaemia is a useful clue to defective renal tubular dysfunction.

TABLE 47.2 INITIAL CLINICAL DATABASE IN RENAL DISEASES

Findings	AN	NS	AUA	ARF	CRF	UTI	UO	RTD	HT	NL
Haematuria	N	O	●	O		O		O		●
Oliguria	●	O		●	O		●			
Anuria	●			●	O		●			
Polyuria							●			
Nocturia		O				O	O	O		
Urine retention								S		
Slow stream							●			
Oedema	O	●		O	O					
Azotaemia symptoms				●	●					
Renal colic										●
Stone passed										S
Hypertension	●			●	●				NS	
Tender bladder or flank						●	●			
Full bladder after voiding						S				
Large prostate							●			
Large kidney							●	●		
Bone pain/s fractures					●			●		

O = occurs in syndrome
● = important clue to syndrome
N = necessary for diagnosis
S = sufficient for diagnosis

Urine Examination

The tests which may be of value include:

1. Determination of 24-hour urine volume.
2. Determination of specific gravity of morning sample of urine after 12-hour water restriction (8 p.m.-8 a.m.).
3. Detection of the presence of abnormal urinary constitutents–protein, RBCs, WBCs, casts.
4. Bacteriological examination.
5. In certain circumstances the urine pH and osmolality.

Urine volume:

Normal range: 800-2500 ml per day. A minimum volume of 500 ml per day is required to excrete the solid urinary constituents (mainly urea and electrolytes). A diet rich in carbohydrate and fat and low in protein and salt, may require as little as 250 ml of urine per day to do the same.

Oliguria is the production of insufficient urine. Oliguria develops in conditions associated with a reduction in renal blood flow and rate of glomerular filtration, e.g. diseases giving rise to water and salt depletion, hypotension, cardiac failure, acute glomerulonephritis and other organic diseases of the kidney like acute tubular necrosis.

Anuria is complete cessation of urine flow. It should be distinguished from urinary retention (full bladder relieved by catheterization).

Polyuria denotes a persistent increase in urine output. It must be distinguished from frequency of micturition (small quantities passed frequently without an increase in the total volume. Polyuria may be due to:

(a) Need to excrete an abnormally large amount of solute which prevents reabsorption of water in the tubules (osmotic diuresis), and in uncontrolled diabetes mellitus (sugar) and uraemia (urea) urine specific gravity is high > 1024.

Table 47.3 DRUGS CAUSING NEPHROUROTOXICITY

Nephrotic syndrome	Captopril Gold salts Penicillamine Phenindione Probenecid
Interstitial nephritis	Allopurinol Diuretics: thiazides, frusemide Penicillins, esp. methicillin Phenindione Sulphonamides
Concentrating defects with polyuria	Democycline Lithium Methoxyflurane Vitamin D
Acute tubular necrosis	Aminoglycosides Amphotericin B Polymyxins, colistin Cyclosporine Sulphonamides Tetracyclines
Renal tubular acidosis	Acetazolamide Amphotericin B Degraded tetracyclines
Renal dysfunction	NSAIDs Cyclosporine Triamterene
Analgesic nephropathy	Phenacetin
Calculi	Acetazolamide Vitamin D
Obstructive uropathy:	
intrarenal	Cytotoxic drugs
extrarenal	Methysergide
Haemorrhagic cystitis	Cyclophosphamide
Bladder dysfunction	Anticholinergics Disopyramide Monoamine oxidase (MAO) inhibitors Tricyclic antidepressants
Prostate	Ephedrine

(b) Reduction in the ability of the kidney to concentrate urine so that an increased volume of water is needed to eliminate a given amount of solute. The second defect may arise because of a lack of circulating vasopressin or insensitivity of the renal tubular concentrating mechanism to its presence (e.g. chronic pyelonephritis, chronic obstructive nephropathy, recovery phase of acute tubular necrosis, hypercalcaemia, potassium depletion, and nephrogenic diabetes insipidus).

Drugs like lithium and amphotericin can cause unresponsiveness to vasopressin.

In all conditions mentioned in (b) urine specific gravity is *low*.

Urine reaction:

In health the urine pH is acid (below 6) over a wide range depending upon the dietary intake and time of the day. In the presence of systemic acidosis, a urine pH above 6.0 in the absence of urinary tract infection indicates renal tubular acidosis. Urine infected with organisms capable of splitting urea may give false high pH values.

Abnormal urine constituents:

Protein in the urine almost invariably indicates the presence of disease of the kidneys (**Table 47.4**). Its magnitude bears little relation to the overall level of renal function. Significant proteinuria does not occur in disease of the lower urinary tract, though a small amount can be detected in severe urinary tract infection or in obvious haematuria. Small amounts of protein are usually found in the urine in chronic renal disease, in the course of febrile illness, and in heart failure. Large amounts of protein (e.g. 3 g/day or more) are found in the nephrotic syndrome and invariably indicate glomerular disease.

The great bulk of urinary protein is albumin. The pattern of proteinuria can be determined and an index of selectivity assessed. A highly selective is one in which the larger proteins are found in significant amounts. The degree of selectivity is an indication of the amount of glomerular damage, and helps in predicting the response to be expected to the administration of corticosteroids. Postural (orthostatic) proteinuria is seen in a number of apparently healthy children and adolescents, less commonly in adults. This is a harmless abnormality and does not warrant further investigation. It should be remembered that postural proteinuria sometimes occurs in the presence of organic renal disease.

TABLE 47.4 APPROACH TO PROTEINURIA

Mild	Moderate	Marked	Massive
(50-100 mg/d)	150-1000 mg/d	1-3 g/d	3-20 g/d
Exclude benign causes: Fever Mucus contamination from genital tract	When benign causes are excluded, persistent proteinuria in excess of 0.5 g/d is unequivocal evidence of renal disease		'Nephrotic syndrome' A. Primary renal disorders B. Nephrotoxins and allergens C. Systemic illness (See **Table 47.1** for details)
Vigorous exercise Postural orthostatic proteinuria	Consider diagnostic renal biopsy		

Blood in the urine is seen in a wide variety of clinical conditions. Haematuria commonly indicates serious disease of the urinary tract and the aetiology should always be sought without delay-important causes being tuberculosis, benign and malignant neoplasms, or unsuspected stone. Haematuria alone may also arise in severe urinary tract infection and haemorrhagic cystitis due to cyclophosphamide therapy. RBCs in the urine (microscopic haematuria) occur in glomerulonephritis, malignant hypertension, renal infarcts due to infective endocarditis, polyarteritis nodosa and SLE affecting the kidneys, renal tuberculosis, congenital cystic disease, renal calculi, benign hyperplasia and carcinoma of the prostate.

Many of these conditions can be diagnosed by the presence of characteristic symptoms and signs in addition to haematuria. When haematuria is the sole or presenting symptom, the cause is most likely to be renal carcinoma, papilloma of the bladder, benign prostatic hypertrophy, or in some geographic regions, schistosomiasis.

When blood appears only at the beginning of micturition, the rest of the urine voided being clear, the source of bleeding is distal to the bladder.

When blood is uniformly mixed with the urine it may have come from any part of the urinary tract other than the urethra. Renal colic accompanying haematuria indicates that the bleeding is renal or ureteric in origin.

Haematuria can be mimicked by other rare causes of discoloration of the urine.

Haemoglobinuria occurs in various disorders characterized by intravascular haemolysis, and occasionally in normal people. The urine gives the chemical test for haemoglobin, but no RBCs are present on microscopic examination of the centrifuged deposit of a fresh sample of urine.

Myoglobinuria
Acute intermittent porphyria produces dark red 'port wine' coloured urine.

Beetroot, senna, dyes used to colour sweets, phenolphthalein and rifampicin produce red coloured urine mimicking haematuria.

Pus cells may be found in the urine in inflammation of any part of the urinary tract. A *mid-stream* urine sample should be obtained and a culture should be set up within 2 hours.

WBC casts and *RBC casts* are important clues of a renal source of pyuria and haematuria. In a patient with urinary tract infection their presence strongly suggests *renal infection*.

Cellular casts indicate renal inflammation and bleeding.

Table 47.5 lists the syndromes of urinary tract infection.

Bladder and urethral infection decrease the tolerance to bladder distension, so a desire to void urine occurs even when a small amount of urine is present. Dysuria and urgency about voiding are also common, especially when the urethra or bladder trigone is involved. All these symptoms can be mimicked by a stone at the ureterovesical junction, so that they are not specific for infection.

Kidney infection usually but not always causes painful tender flanks, fever and chills. During severe infections, the renal papillae occasionally become necrotic, slough into the renal pelvis and, like stones, obstruct the kidney or pass through the urinary tract causing renal colic.

While most symptoms enumerated in **Tables 47.1** and **47.4** point to the kidneys as the site of trouble, it must be remembered that symptoms of renal failure are *non-specific* and *systemic*. Lassitude, drowsiness, itching, anorexia, nausea, vomiting, bad taste in the mouth and singultus, are examples of symptoms whose significance can be totally missed unless the clinician thinks of renal failure and uraemia as a possible mechanism. Other presenting features are *neuropathy* with numbness and paraesthesia, pericarditis with chest pain and dyspnoea, hyperventilation due to uraemic acidosis, and coma.

In chronic renal failure osteomalacia (because of vitamin D resistance) and osteitis fibrosa cystica (because of secondary parathyroid overactivity) may coexist in the same patient. Both can cause bone pain and pathologic fractures. Osteomalacia produces pelvic girdle muscle weakness and waddling gait, and inability to rise easily from the squatting position or from a chair. Several renal tubular defects including renal tubular acidosis and primary or acquired renal phosphate wasting can present as osteomalacia.

Investigations of Nephro–urological Problems

Radiology

1. *A plain radiograph* of the abdomen reveals radio-opaque calculi, or other areas of calcification such as nephrocalcinosis. Calculi are easily missed especially if they are less than 1 cm in diameter as they are easily obscured by bowel shadows or overlying bone. The plain film may also demonstrate the renal outline and so give an indication of renal size.

2. *Excretory urography* shows the size of the kidneys (normal adult kidneys are 11-14 cm in length, and differ from each other by less than 2 cm). The nephrogram phase may reveal scars of pyelonephritis, often associated with a calyceal abnormality, or reveal localized masses or tumours. Foetal lobulation is a normal variation. Clubbed calyces and slow excretion are

TABLE 47.5 SYNDROMES OF URINARY TRACT INFECTION

Condition	Symptoms	Signs	Urine tests
Acute cystitis	Dysuria, frequency, back' pain, lower abd. pain.	Low grade fever, suprapubic tenderness.	Pus cells, Red blood cells, proteins, bacteria.
Acute pyelonephritis	Chills, flank pain, malaise, dysuria, frequency.	Fever, tenderness of costovertebral angle, splenomegaly.	± Pus cells, RBCs, proteins, hyaline & WBC casts.
Asymptomatic bacteriuria	Usually none, occasionally nocturia.	Usually none, occasionally flank tenderness.	Bacteria, ± cells
Chronic pyelonephritis	May be asymptomatic, may present as uraemia, may come with acute exacerbations: malaise, back pain, nocturia, polyuria.	May be none, ± tenderness over kidneys.	

Common setting of urinary infection in females

'Honeymoon cystitis'

Pregnancy

Catheterization during delivery

Urethrocoeles & rectocoeles

commonly found in chronic urinary obstruction. Calyceal abnormalities may also suggest papillary necrosis, renal tuberculosis or atrophic pyelonephritis. In renal tuberculosis calcification and cavitation are common. Polycystic kidney disease causes bilateral renal enlargement and the calyceal structure is stretched and spidery.

3. *Retrograde urography* is mainly used to investigate lesions of the ureter and to define the cause of obstruction.

4. *Micturating cystogram* is useful in the investigation of urinary infection in childhood often associated with ureteric reflux.

5. *Renal arteriography* is helpful to demonstrate renal artery stenosis or fibromuscular hyperplasia, and intra-renal microaneurysms typical of polyarteritis nodosa.

6. A finding of both kidneys of small size indicates end-stage renal disease (which requires dialysis). Kidney size may be normal or large in CRF due to polycystic kidneys, diabetes, amyloidosis and collagen disease (e.g. SLE).

Ultrasonography (US)
This is most useful in assessing kidney size and in distinguishing solid from cystic lesions, and hydronephrosis.

When a patient with oliguria or anuria presents for the first time, ultrasound will distinguish obstructive causes (which need surgical relief) from other causes of ARF.

Laboratory values alone do not distinguish between ARF and CRF, although low serum calcium and high serum phosphorus favour CRF.

Computed tomography
This is particularly helpful in the diagnosis of masses in the kidneys and retroperitoneal tissues, and in defining the spread of bladder and prostatic tumours.

Radionuclide studies
These give a quantitative idea of individual kidney function (GFR, tubular function). renal blood flow, and urine flow. Diuretic renography helps to differentiate obstructive uropathy (which needs surgical relief) from passive dilatation of the pelvis (which can be left alone). Captopril renography is valuable in predicting *reversible* renovascular hypertension by surgery or renal angioplasty. It is useful in monitoring renal transplant for all possible complications.

Renal biopsy
This is especially useful in unexplained renal failure when the kidneys are of normal size, in suspected systemic disease associated with abnormal urinary constituents, and in haematuria in which lesions of the lower urinary tract have been excluded.

Drugs and the Kidneys
The susceptibility of the kidney to damage by drugs stems from the fact that it is the route of excretion for many water soluble compounds including drugs and their metabolites. Damage to the kidney may arise in the course of treatment with a large number of drugs and may be severe enough to result in acute renal failure (**Table 47.3**).

Drugs should never be given to patients with impaired renal function unless specific indications for their use exist. Commonly used drugs the dose of which needs to be reduced in renal failure include cephalosporins, cimetidine, hydralazine, digoxin, cotrimoxazole, aminoglycosides, narcotics, analgesics, aspirin, and phenylbutazone. **Table 47.6** lists the use of antimicrobial drugs in the face of renal failure.

Management of Acute Renal Failure (ARF)
Conservative measures
These usually suffice for pre-renal and post-renal causes of ARF.

1. Fluid management: Correct fluid deficit by 5 per cent dextrose in N saline; avoid volume overload.

2. Dietary modification: Protein intake restricted to 0.5 g/kg/day. Restrict potassium. Salt restriction 2-4 g /day.

3. Hypotension corrected with volume expansion or vasopressors.

Dialysis is indicated for the following conditions, where conservative management fails to control.

1. Fluid overload;

2. Hyperkalaemia (K more than 6 meq/L)

3. Acidosis (HCO_3 less than 10 meq/L)

4. Azotaemia (creatinine more than 10 mg/dl)

5. Pericarditis

6. Bleeding diathesis

TABLE 47.6 ANTIMICROBIAL DRUGS IN RENAL FAILURE

Group I: Major extra-renal pathway of elimination.

Methicillin	Sulphadimidine
Cloxacillin	Chloramphenicol
Ampicillin	Fusidic acid
Erythromycin	Novobiocin

Group II: Minor adjustment sufficient. Wider spacing of dose than normal.

Penicillin G	Sulfamethoxazole
Cephalothin	Trimethoprim
Cephaloridine	Nalidixic acid
Lincomycin	INAH

Group III: Major adjustment necessary. Doses 24 hours apart.

Tetracycline	Kanamycin
Oxytetracycline	Gentamycin
Streptomycin	Vancomycin
Polymyxin B	
Colistin	
Amphotericin B	
PAS	
Cycloserine	

Group IV: Avoid altogether.

Chlortetracycline
Nitrofurantoin

However, the choice between haemodialysis and peritoneal dialysis depends upon the *hypercatabolic state* (rate of rise of blood urea more than 60 mg/dl/day) which needs haemodialysis. Patients who have undiagnosed intra-abdominal disease or who have had recent abdominal surgery (where peritoneal dialysis is contraindicated) are subjected to haemodialysis; the patient has to be haemodynamically stable for it.

For the non-hypercatabolic, haemodynamically unstable person with poor vascular access, or with active bleeding, peritoneal dialysis is indicated.

The recent introduction of continuous arteriovenous haemodialysis (CAVHD) provides one more option which is technically simple, able to correct volume overload quickly In haemodynamically unstable patients, and is applicable where peritoneal dialysis is contraindicated.

With the onset of the diuretic phase, dialysis may not be required once the serum creatinine falls to less than 8 mg/dl.

Management of Chronic Renal Failure (CRF)

Conservative management: Dietary modification. Restriction of protein to 0.5 g/kg/day; restriction of potassium and phosphorus; ACE inhibitors for control of hypertension; oral $NaHCO_3$ 300-600 mg/day for acidosis; inj. erythropoietin for anaemia to maintain Hb above 7 g per cent. Treatment of urinary infection with antibiotics.

When the progression of CRF can no longer be controlled with conservative measures, renal dialysis/transplant is indicated. Emergency indication for dialysis' is based on:

Hyperkalaemia (K more than 5.5 mEq/L)
Acidosis (HCO_3 less than 12 mEq/L)
Azotaemia (BUN more than 100 mg per cent)
   (serum creatinine more than 10 mg per cent)
Bleeding diathesis
Pericarditis
Polyneuropathy
Volume overload (pulmonary oedema)
Coma

Haemodialysis is administered 2-3 times per week as a long-term measure if transplant is not feasible. Continuous ambulatory peritoneal dialysis is an option, but there is the problem of infection.

Cadaver kidney transplant is preferable to living related donor transplant with improved recipient selection (HLA DR matching) and cyclosporine. The one-year graft survival is 87 per cent for cadaver grafts and 92 per cent for related donor grafts. Life-long monitoring of renal function and close follow-up form the key to success.

Detection of sexual problems depends upon asking appropriate questions specifically about sexual function, because patients are usually reluctant to raise the topic themselves. The doctor may also feel uncomfortable or embarrassed about discussing sexual problems hence this aspect of history taking is often neglected. When the patient is accompanied by the spouse or relatives, it is not discreet to ask questions about sexual function in their presence since this is not likely to evoke authentic answers.

A good strategy is to keep interrogation on this aspect until the physical examination has been started. Often the sudden change from the armchair interview across the table to the greater intimacy of the examination couch encourages the patient to mention spontaneously problems not previously aired. Uncovering of the body often makes uncovering of the mind much easier.

The general practitioner should be aware of the types of dysfunction that may occur so that he may reassure the couple and refer them to a specialist for appropriate treatment and counseling.

Elements of Sexual Dysfunction

The following four cardinal elements of the normal sexual function have to be probed into for detecting any abnormality of function.

Male	Female
Desire (libido)	Desire (libido)
Erection	Lubrication
Intromission	Intromission
Ejaculation & orgasm	Orgasm

Libido

Loss of libido can be due to psychogenic and/or organic causes. Common psychogenic causes are:

- Dislike of the partner
- Disturbed interpersonal relationship
- Depression
- Schizophrenia

Sexual interest is temporarily diminished in any debilitating illness. Libido returns to normal after resolution of the physical illness. More specifically, it may be due to particular diseases such as diabetes mellitus, or liver disease causing suppressed androgenic activity. Hyperprolactinaemia is worth remembering as a cause since it provides no particular clues in the history or physical examination.

Drug history is important since many commonly used drugs can decrease libido (**Table 48.1**).

Increased libido is seen in manic and schizophrenic patients, as also in frontal and temporal lobe lesions. The anti-Parkinsonism drug L-dopa and the Ayurvedic drug for Parkinsonism, Mucona pruriens, do increase the libido. Alcohol 'stimulates the desire but takes away the performance'.

Erection

Previously it was thought that the great majority of cases of men with failure to have an erection have a psychologic aetiology. It is now believed that a majority of cases of erectile impotence have a component of organic disease, which may be amenable to treatment.

The crucial single question is about the occurrence of spontaneous nocturnal or early morning erection with which the patient may wake up. Nocturnal penile tumescence (NPT) occurs during rapid eye movement (REM) sleep, lasting about 100 minutes per night. NPT indicates that the afferent neurologic and circulatory apparatus that mediate erection are intact. An occasional patient with early sensory neuropathy may have NPT. With this single

Table 48.1 ORGANIC CAUSES OF IMPOTENCE

I. *Endocrine causes*
   A. Testicular failure
      Primary
      Secondary to gonadotrophin deficiency
   B. Hyperprolactinaemia

II. *Penile diseases*
   A. Peyronie's disease
   B. Previous priapism
   C. Penile trauma

III. *Neurologic diseases*
   A. Anterior temporal lobe lesions
   B. Diseases of the spinal cord
   C. Loss of sensory input
      Tabes dorsalis
      Dorsal root ganglia lesion
   D. Nervi erigentes
      Radical prostatectomy and cystectomy
      Rectosigmoid operations
   E. Diabetic autonomic neuropathy
      Various polyneuropathies.

IV. *Vascular disease*
   A. Aortic occlusion (Leriche's syndrome)
   B. Atherosclerotic occlusion or stenosis of pudendal and/or cavernosal arteries
   C. Venous leak
   D. Disease of the sinusoidal space.

V. *Drugs* (**Table 48.2**)

exception, NPT excludes organic disease and points to psychological causes of dysfunction.

As noted about libido, a large number of drugs taken for hypertension or other diseases can produce erectile impotence. It is useful to remember the three groups of anti-hypertensive drugs that *do not* cause erectile impotence: ACE inhibitors, calcium channel blockers and peripheral vasodilators.

Diabetes mellitus is the commonest organic disease that can lead to erectile failure. About 50 per cent of diabetic patients develop this complaint within 6 years after onset, as a manifestation of diabetic autonomic neuropathy. Other features of autonomic neuropathy may be present e.g. postural hypotension and bladder disturbance.

Vascular insufficiency due to atherosclerosis is also an important contributing factor.

Failure of ejaculation, more commonly retrograde ejaculation, is also seen in diabetic impotence. Difficulty of vaginal lubrication during sexual stimulation has been observed in female diabetics.

Spinal cord injuries, pelvic fractures, surgery involving the pelvis such as radical prostatectomy, surgery of the bladder or rectum may result in erectile impotence.

Psychogenic erectile dysfunction is sudden in onset, and may be intermittent, erections occurring occasionally.

Intromission

In some patients intromission is accomplished but the penis loses its stiffness in the vagina during the sex act. This may be due to performance anxiety, or a venous leak, or external iliac steal syndrome.

Orgasm

Early orgasmic response (EOR) or premature ejaculation is a common complaint, often frustrating to the partner. It may be due to performance anxiety, over excitement, or long periods of abstinence. There is seldom any organic cause.

Delayed orgasmic response (DOR), impaired orgasmic response (IOR) or absent orgasmic response (AOR), failure of ejaculation, and retrograde ejaculation, are problems encountered in the sex act.

Drugs such as guanethidine, phenoxy benzamine and phentolamine primarily impair ejaculation rather than libido or erection.

Physical Examination

Examination of the penis: for presence of fibrosis/plaques on the dorsum of the penis (Peyronie's disease).

Examination of testicles: length less than 3.5 cm indicates testicular atrophy.

Look for gynaecomastia as evidence of androgenic deficit or oestrogenic overactivity as in hepatic disease.

Palpate all peripheral pulses, including the dorsal penile pulse for evidence of vascular disease. However, it must be remembered that significant disease of the pudendal and cavernosal arteries can occur in the absence of other clinical manifestations of peripheral vascular disease.

TABLE 48.2 DRUGS WHICH CAN AFFECT SEXUAL FUNCTION

Class	Drugs	Effect on sexual function		
		Libido	Arousal	Orgasm
Anticholinergic:	Pro-Banthine		Erectile impotence	
Antidepressants:	Tricyclics		Erectile impotence	Delayed ejaculation
	MAOIs		Erectile impotence	Delayed ejaculation
Antihypertensives:				
Centrally acting:	Methyldopa	Reduced	Erectile impotence	Delayed ejaculation
Alpha blockers:	Clonidine			Retrograde ejaculation
	Guanethidine,			Impaired ejaculation
	Phenoxybenzamine,			
	Phentolamine			
Beta blockers:	Propranolol	Reduced	Erectile impotence	Failure of or retrograde ejaculation
Anti-inflammatory:	Indomethacin	Reduced		
Anti-Parkinsonian:	L-Dopa	Increased		
Diuretics:	Thiazides	Reduced	Erectile impotence	
	Spironolactone	Gynaecomastia	Erectile impotence	
Hormones:	Androgen	Increased in females	Erectile impotence	
	Corticosteroids	Reduced	Erectile impotence	Delayed ejaculation
	Oestrogen	Reduced (male)	Erectile impotence	Delayed ejaculation
Major tranquillizers:	Chlorpromazine	Reduced	Erectile impotence	Delayed retrograde ejaculation
	Thioridazine	Reduced	Erectile impotence	
CNS depressants:	Barbiturates	Reduced		
	Diazepam			
	Alcohol	Increased		
	Marijuana	Increased		
	Heroin	Increased		
	Methadone			

Neurological examination
Relevant examination includes tendon reflexes, touch, pain and vibration sense, perineal sensation, anal sphincter tone, and bulbocavernous reflex (squeeze glans penis and note the degree of anal sphincter contraction).

Assessment of penile blood flow
Penile-brachial index is derived by dividing the penile systolic blood pressure (as derived by Doppler) by supine brachial systolic pressure. An index less than 0.6 indicates decreased flow through the dorsal penile artery. It is possible, however, that flow may' be normal in the dorsal penile artery (which is not directly involved in the erectile process) while that in the cavernosal arteries is deficient.

Cavernosal arterial blood flow can be assessed by pulsed Doppler and high resolution ultrasonography in conjunction with intra-cavernosal injection of papaverine. Venous leak is also diagnosed by this method.

Pudendal arteriogram is an invasive but definitive procedure to establish vascular insufficiency as a cause of erectile impotence. In order not to miss distal arterial lesions, this procedure may also be done after papaverine injection. Abnormalities in the venous occlusive mechanism of the penis can cause impotence due to venous leak and can be diagnosed with the use of papaverine induced erection in combination with ultrasonography. Venous leak may be secondary to arterial inflow and sinusoidal disease.

Nevertheless, in carefully selected patients, surgical ligation or clinical obliteration of the incompetent veins can improve erectile function.

Laboratory Studies

Hormonal blood tests

Clinicians should make decisions to measure hormone levels on a case-by-case basis, in accordance with the patient's clinical presentation.

Patients who express a loss of libido, depression, or any signs of diminished secondary sexual characteristics should undergo an endocrine evaluation. At a minimum, this should consist of measuring morning serum testosterone levels.

The relative merits of measuring total, free, and bioavailable testosterone levels and serum hormone-binding globulin are controversial. In screening for hypogonadism, total and free testosterone levels should be measured to investigate the hypothalamic-pituitary-gonadal axis. Testosterone levels peak at about 8:00 AM; thus, a morning level should be checked whenever possible. Free or bioavailable testosterone is important because it is the testosterone that is usable; the rest is attached mainly to serum hormone-binding globulin.

Measurement of luteinizing hormone (LH) may be helpful. LH levels vary according to the body's need for testosterone. The hypothalamus regulates testosterone levels by releasing or inhibiting LH-releasing hormone (LHRH), which acts in the pituitary to produce LH. A high LH level associated with a low testosterone level implies primary testicular (Leydig cell) failure. Conversely, a low LH level associated with a low testosterone level suggests a central defect.

In some instances, prolactin levels may be helpful as well. A serum prolactin level is obtained if the patient has evidence of pituitary hyperfunction (e.g. from a pituitary tumor) or if low serum testosterone levels have been documented.

A serum thyroid-stimulating hormone (TSH) evaluation is appropriate in selected patients.

Other blood tests

Additional useful screening studies include the following:

- Hemoglobin A1C
- Serum chemistry panel
- Lipid profile

These studies should be considered unless the patient has had them performed recently and the results are available.

Measurement of prostate-specific antigen (PSA) levels may be appropriate if the patient is a candidate for prostate cancer screening. Such screening is controversial, however, and should be performed only after its risks and benefits have been reviewed with the patient (see Prostate Cancer).

Urinalysis

Performing a urinalysis is recommended. The presence of red blood cells (RBCs), white blood cells (WBCs), protein, or glucose can be important clues to a genitourinary disorder.

Injection of Prostaglandin E1

A test used to evaluate penile function is the direct injection of prostaglandin E1 (PGE1; alprostadil) into one of the corpora cavernosa (see the images below). If the penile vasculature is normal or at least adequate, an erection should develop within several minutes. The patient and the clinician can judge the quality of the erection. If successful, this test also establishes penile injections as a possible therapy.

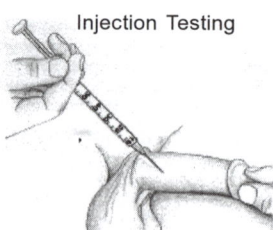

Injection Testing

A vasodilator such as prostaglandin E1 can be injected into one of the corpora cavernosa. If the blood vessels are capable of dilating, a strong erection should develop within 5 minutes

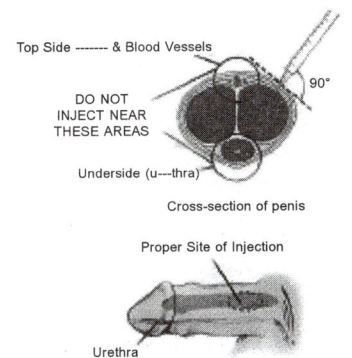

Top Side ------- & Blood Vessels

DO NOT
INJECT NEAR
THESE AREAS

90°

Underside (u---thra)

Cross-section of penis

Proper Site of Injection

Urethra

Erctile dysfunction. This diagram depicts a cross-section of penile anatomy and is used to instruct patients in the technique of administering intracorporeal medications

Biothesiometry

The sensitivity of the skin of the penis to detect vibrational stimuli (i.e. biothesiometry) can be employed as a simple nerve function office screening test, but it is infrequently indicated. In this test, a small electromagnetic test probe is placed on the right and left sides of the penile shaft and on the glans. The vibrational amplitude is adjusted until the subjective sensory threshold is reached, which is determined by questioning the patient (see the image below).

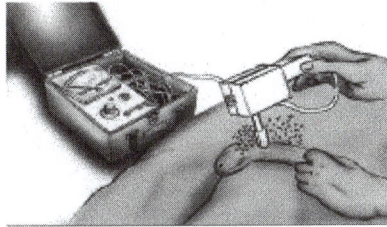

Skin Vibration Testing (Biothesiometry)

The presence of normal skin sensation adequate to produce an erection is measured with this device.

A series of these tests determines the average vibrational sensory threshold in each location; these thresholds are then compared with reference range standards for the patient's age group. Although this test does not directly measure erectile nerve function, it serves as a reasonable means of screening for possible sensory deficit and is simple to perform. Formal nerve conduction studies (e.g. bulbocavernosus reflex latency time) are reserved for very specific situations.

Ultrasonography

Vascular function within the penis can be evaluated by means of duplex ultrasonography. In this procedure, blood flow in the cavernosal arteries within the corpora cavernosa is measured before and after the intracavernosal injection of a test dose of a standard vasodilator (e.g. 20 µg of PGE1).

Criteria for evaluating the study results vary to some degree. A peak systolic velocity lower than 25 cm/sec is generally agreed to indicate arterial insufficiency. The proposed value for the lower limit of normal ranges from 25-35 cm/sec, but a peak systolic velocity of 35 cm/sec or higher clearly rules out arterial insufficiency. End-diastolic velocity serves as a proxy for venous outflow; a velocity of 5 cm/sec or lower when the penis is at full rigidity indicates the absence of abnormal venous leakage.

Nocturnal Penile Tumescence Testing

Nocturnal penile tumescence testing involves placing several bands around the penis, connected to a device such as the Rigiscan monitor, and instructing the patient to wear the assembly for 2 or 3 successive nights. If an erection occurs, which is expected during rapid eye movement sleep, its force and duration are measured on a graph (see the image below). Inadequate or absent nocturnal erections suggest organic dysfunction, whereas a normal result indicates a high likelihood of a psychogenic etiology.

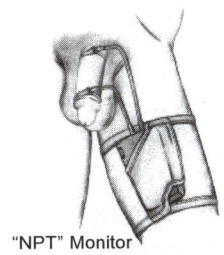

"NPT" Monitor

This penile tumescence monitor is placed at the base and near the corona of the penis. It is connected to a monitor that records a continuous graph depicting the force and duration of erections that occur during sleep. The monitor is strapped to the leg. The nocturnal penile tumescence test is conducted on several nights to obtain an accurate indication of erections that normally occur during the alpha phase of sleep

Nocturnal penile tumescence testing was once frequently performed; it was thought to be useful in distinguishing psychogenic from organic impotence. Currently, other devices are available that provide similar information. Some are also able to measure rigidity (resistance to mild compression) and tumescence (size). Nocturnal penile tumescence testing is rarely used in current practice, but it can be helpful in situations where the diagnosis is in doubt.

Other Studies

Angiography is useful if the patient is a potential candidate for some type of vascular surgery. Young men with traumatic vascular injuries resulting in ED are candidates for this angiography because they may qualify for a vascular reconstruction.

In the vast majority of patients with ED, formal neurologic testing is unnecessary. However, those with a history of central nervous system (CNS) problems, peripheral neuropathy, diabetes, or penile sensory deficit may benefit from some level of neurologic testing.

Treatment of Impotence

Sildenafil (Viagra) 25 to 100 mg. taken about an hour before sexual act helps to sustain erection in an aroused person. Patients who are using vasodilator nitrates for CAD or recently recovered from myocardial infarct should not take the drug for fear of vascular collapse.

Except for hypogonadal males (low serum level of testosterone with high LH) androgen therapy offers little more than a placebo effect.

In a prolactin-producing pituitary tumour treatment with dopamine agonist bromocriptine usually results in return of potency.

The efficacy of penile revascularization and balloon embolization for vasculogenic impotence remains uncertain.

Men with primary venous leak impotence without associated arterial or sinusoidal disease may benefit from venous ligation.

Self-injection with vasoactive drugs like papaverine, with or without phentolamine produces erection in patients with psychogenic, neurogenic and mild vasculogenic impotence.

Possible complications are priapism and penile fibrosis.

Vacuum devices to produce an erection and a rubber band to restrict venous return at the base of the penis provide a successful non-surgical alternative in many patients, including diabetics.

Side effects of vacuum devices

Bruising, skin breakdown, and penile pain associated with the application of the constriction band have already been discussed. The tightness of the band may also result in failure to achieve an ejaculation (although no interference with orgasm should occur) and the development of a temporary penile numbness. One of the other problems with the erection achieved with the vacuum device is that it may hinge at the point of application of the constriction ring. That is, the penis behind the ring is soft and only that portion of the shaft that is beyond the ring has any degree of hardness. Therefore, the ring must be applied as far towards the base of the penis as possible.

Penile protheses of various types are currently in use.

Painful intercourse (dyspareunia)

Dyspareunia is manifested by sharp, burning, stinging or stabbing pain in the vaginal or pelvic area, with or without lingering post-coital soreness or aching. The longer the duration of painful experience the more likely is the patient to become fearful and averse to coitus. There may be complaints of dryness (lack of lubrication).

The diagnostic possibilities are

Vaginismus	Pain reproduced on pelvic examination
Vulvitis	Tender mass at left or right lateral introitus
Bartholin cyst or abscess	
Vaginitis: bacterial allergic atrophic	
Endometriosis	
Pelvic infection	PV: pain on moving cervix
Prolapsed ovary syndrome	Palpation of tender ovary in cul-de-sac

TABLE 48.3 Advantages and Disadvantages of Different Types of Penile Implants for Erectile Dysfunction

Treatment	Advantages	Disadvantage
Semirigid or malleable rod implants	Simple surgery Relatively few complications No moving parts Least expensive implant Success rate of 70-80% Highly effective	Constant erection at all times May be difficult to conceal Does not increase width of penis Risk of infection Permanently alters or may injure erection bodies Most likely implant to cause pain or erode through skin If unsuccessful, interferes with other treatments
Fully inflatable implants	Mimics natural process of rigidity-flaccidity Patient controls state of erection Natural appearance No concealment problems Increases width of penis when activated Success rate of 70-80% Highly effective	Relatively high rate of mechanical failure Risk of infection Most expensive implant Permanently alters or may injure erection bodies If unsuccessful, interferes with other treatments
Self-contained inflatable unitary implants	Mimics natural process of rigidity-flaccidity Patient controls state of erection Natural appearance No concealment problems Simpler surgical procedure than that required for fully inflatable prosthesis Success rate of 70-80% Highly effective	Sometimes difficult to activate the inflatable device Does not increase width of penis Mechanical breakdowns possible Long-term results not available Risk of infection Relatively expensive Permanently alters or may injure erection bodies If unsuccessful, interferes with other treatments

Side effects of Vacuum Devices

Brusing, skin breakdown and penile pain associated with the application of the constriction band have already been discussed. The tightness of the band may also result in failure to achieve an ejaculation (although no interference with orgasm should occur) and the development of a temporary penile numbness.

One of the other problems with the erection achieved with the vacuum device is that it may hinge at the point of application of the constriction ring. That is, the penis behind the ring is soft and only that portion of the shaft that is beyond the ring has any degree of hardness. Therefore, the ring must be applied as far towards the base of the penis as possible.

49   Sexually Transmitted Diseases

Sexually transmitted diseases (STD) are a major and growing public health problem. Many of these infections are associated with a wide range of clinical complications that extend beyond the traditional sphere of venereology. It is therefore important that the general practitioner is fully aware of the entire spectrum of STD.

Table 49.1 lists all the STD, giving the names of the pathogens, the clinical picture and complications of each disease entity, diagnosis, and treatment. Individuals at risk for STD are listed in Table 49.2 and social factors which promote STD are listed in Table 49.3.

The list of STD contains bacterial, treponemal, fungal, viral and protozoal pathogens. Nevertheless, common principles should be applied when caring for any patient presumed to have STD.

The history should include the patient's sexual practices to identify risk factors for particular infections.

The physical examination and microbiological studies should be directed towards the urogenital, rectal and oropharyngeal areas. Since infection with multiple pathogens is common, studies for gonorrhoea and syphilis should be routinely included when evaluating patients of STD. In view of the rising tide of HIV infection, routine HIV testing and counselling for those found positive is a sound public health practice.

Efforts should be made to obtain cultures from sexual contacts, as treatment of asymptomatic carriers may prevent the spread of infection.

Follow-up cultures or serological studies should be done after completion of therapy to document cure. An STD apparently refractory to treatment may represent reinfection, a concomitant previously undiagnosed STD, or antimicrobial drug resistance (e.g. gonococci with plasmid-mediated penicillinase production, or plasmid-mediated high level tetracycline resistance, or chromosomally-mediated antibiotic resistance to penicillin and other commonly used antibiotics). All Neisseria gonorrhoeae isolates should be tested for penicillinase production. In addition, all post-treatment isolates and isolates from patients with disseminated gonococcal infections or gonococcal ophthalmia should be tested for resistance.

Pelvic Inflammatory Disease (PID)

The term PID refers to the ascending spread of micro-organisms from the vagina and cervix to the endometrium, fallopian tubes and/or contiguous structures. PID is one of the most significant complications of STD in women, and is probably the most common serious infection in women of childbearing age. PID is the major cause of female infertility and ectopic pregnancy. Chronic abdominal pain with dyspareunia can be particularly distressing.

A clinical diagnosis of PID is suggested by:

1. Abdominal tenderness
2. PV: cervical motion causing tenderness
3. Bimanual examination: adnexal tenderness

In addition, at least one of the following 5 should be present:

4. Temperature higher than 38°C
5. Pelvic mass on examination or sonography
6. Intracellular gram negative diplococci or gram stain of cervical smear
7. WBC count 10,000 or more per μl
8. Purulent material obtained by culdocentesis or laparoscopy

TABLE 49.1 SEXUALLY TRANSMITTED DISEASES

Pathogen	Disease	Complications	Diagnosis	Treatment
I. Neisseria gonorrhoeae	Urethritis, cervicitis, proctitis, vaginitis, pharyngitis, conjunctivitis.	Pelvic inflamm. disease (PID), urethral stricture, septic arthritis, endocarditis, epididymitis, prostatitis, infertility.	Gram stain intracellular gram negative diplococci. Growth on Thayer-Martin media under 5% CO_2.	See under 'Treatment of Gonorrhoea'.
II. Non-gonoccocal urethritis (NGU)	Urethritis.			
i. Chlamydia trachomatis		Ectopic pregnancy, prematurity, blindness.		
ii. Ureaplasma urealyticum	Urethritis.	PID, prostatitis, infertility.		
III. Treponema pallidum	Syphilis Primary: chancre. Secondary: rash, snail-track ulcers. Tertiary; neurological cardiovascular, skeletal.	Tabes dorsalis, Charcot's joints, meningovascular syphilis, dementia, aortitis, gummas congenital syphilis.	Dark field examination of chancre, condyloma lata, or lymph node aspirate. Serological tests for syphilis.	*Early* Benzathine penicillin G, 2.4 megaU IM inj. *Late* As above once weekly for 3 weeks. *Neurosyphilis* aqueous crystalline penicillin G, 3 megaU 4 hrly x 10 days.
IV. Chlamydia trachomatis (antigenically different from that causing NGU)	Urethritis, cervicitis, proctitis, lymphogranuloma venereum (LGV).	PID, epididymitis, infertility, ectopic pregnancy, prematurity, neonatal pneumonia.	Isolation in tissue culture.	Tetracycline 500 mg PO qid x 7 days. For LGV as above for at least 2 weeks or till lesions are healed.
V. Haemophilus ducreyi	Chancroid, painful non-indurated ulceration, tender inguinal lymphadenitis.	Spontaneous rupture of fluctuant nodes.	Isolation on supplemented agar.	Erythromycin 500 mg PO qid x 10 days *or* TMP/SMX 80/400 mg PO bid x 10 days. Aspiration of fluctuant nodes.

(Contd)

TABLE **49.1** (Contd)

	Pathogen	Disease	Complications	Diagnosis	Treatment
VI.	Calymmatobacterium granulomatis (Donovan bodies)	Granuloma inguinale.	Squamous cell carcinoma.	Giemsa or Wright's stain of scraping or biopsy; coccobacilli in cytoplasm.	Tetracycline 500 mg PO qid until lesion is healed.
VII.	Candida albicans	Vaginitis.	None.	Fungal elements or KOH 10% preparation.	Miconazole 7 g daily intravaginally x 7 days.
VIII.	Herpes simplex virus	Genital herpes, proctitis, pharyngitis.	Recurrent attacks, disseminated disease, meningitis, encephalitis, cervical cancer.	Tzane smear; multinucleated giant cells. Tissue culture: Four-fold rise. Complement fixing antibodies.	Symptomatic topical anaesthetic benzocaine spray. Acyclovir 200 mg PO x 5/d for 7-10 days 5 mg/kg IV 8 hrly.
IX.	Trichomonas vaginalis	Vaginitis.	None.	Motile organisms on wet mount.	Metronidazole 2 g PO single dose.
X.	Cytomegalovirus (CMV)	Infectious mononucleosis syndrome.	Congenital birth defects, prematurity.	Tissue culture serology.	
XI.	Gardnerella vaginalis	Non-specific vaginitis.	Postpartum endometritis.		Metronidazole 7g intra-vaginally daily for 7 days.
XII.	HIV	Acquired immuno-deficiency syndrome (AIDS).	Kaposi's sarcoma, PCP & other opportunistic infections.	ELISA Western blot.	Treatment of infectious complications.

TABLE **49.2** INDIVIDUALS AT RISK FOR STD

Men aged 18-35 years

Women aged 16-25 years

Frequent travellers

Prostitutes (sex workers)

Armed services personnel

Merchant navy seamen

Entertainers

TABLE **49.3** SOCIAL FACTORS WHICH PROMOTE STD

Affluence

Increased leisure

Permissive society, personal freedom, promiscuity large number of sexual partners

Alcohol consumption

Drug addiction

Prostitution–professional & clandestine

Ignorance about safe sex

Patients of PID who fulfil the following criteria should be hospitalized:

1. Patients with diffuse rebound tenderness
2. Patients with a mass (palpable or ultrasonographic)
3. Patients who are pregnant
4. Patients who cannot take oral therapy due to nausea or vomiting
5. Patients in whom diagnosis is uncertain or surgical emergencies need to be excluded (See Chapter 3 on Acute Abdominal Pain)
6. Patients who fail outpatient therapy
7. Patients for whom outpatient follow-up cannot be arranged Examination and treatment of sexual partners is important.

Treatment of Gonorrhoea

1. *Uncomplicated urethral and endocervical infection*
   Co-existent non-gonococcal urethritis occurs In upto 40 per cent women and 23 per cent heterosexual men with gonorrhoea. Hence both infections should be treated.
   i. Ceftriaxone 125-250 mg IM inj. is the therapy of choice for all patients.
   ii. Penicillin-sensitive isolates may be treated with:
      amoxycllin 3 g PO single dose or
      ampicillin 3.5 g PO single dose or
      procaine penicillin G 4.8 megaunits IM distributed in two injection sites.

With all penicillins probenecid 1 g PO should follow.
   iii. Patients allergic to beta lactam antibiotics may be given:
      spectinomycin 2 g IM single dose *or*
      ciprofloxacine 500 mg PO
      followed by doxycycline 100 mg PO bid for 7 days.
   iv. Pregnant women or those unable to tolerate tetracycline may be given:
      erythromycin 500 mg PO qid for 7 days.

2. *Acute salpingitis*
   Hospitalized patient:
   doxycycline 100 mg IV of 12 hrs for 4 days.
   cefoxitin 2 g IV of 6 hrs

3. *Disseminated gonococcal infection*
   IV therapy for at least 3 days or until improvement occurs followed by oral antibiotic to complete a minimum of 7 days of treatment. Ceftriaxone 1 g IV qid for 7 days is the drug of choice.
   For penicillin-sensitive strains:

      acquem penicillin G 2 megaunits IV of 4 hrs
      followed by amoxycillin (or ampicillin) PO 500 mg qid to complete 7 days of treatment.

Meningitis or endocarditis :
Ceftriaxone 2 g IV per day for 10 days (meningitis) or 4 weeks (endocarditis).
For penicillin-sensitive isolates:
Penicillin G 10 megaunits/day for same duration as specified above.

The control of STD is based on the effective treatment of established disease, contact tracing, community education, and screening.

The skin, the largest organ in the body, lends itself totally for inspection and palpation by the doctor who can thereby gain a lot of valuable information. It is unfortunate that many doctors show little enthusiasm about learning more about skin disorders, leaving them entirely to the specialists. In fact only a minority of skin lesions are of purely dermatological interest, and of no concern to the general physician. Many common and important diseases have cutaneous manifestations, and all that is needed to recognize them is adequate natural light and trained observant eyes. A good example is leprosy which afflicts 20 million people worldwide. It is a good practice to examine the entire skin even though the patient may complain of only a localized lesion.

Dermatology is mainly descriptive, with more than 1000 named entities. Fortunately, fewer than a dozen diseases represent 70 per cent of dermatological practice–acne; bacterial, viral, parasitic and fungal infections; dermatitis, psoriasis; leg ulcers; warts; and tumours.

Every good physician looks at the skin all the time while he is listening to the patient or eliciting physical signs.

A doctor should know enough to recognize a skin lesion which is a threat to life such as the malignant pustule of anthrax, melanoma, or the eroded blisters in the mouth in pemphigus vulgaris. He should also know how to recognize skin lesions which are significant indicators of systemic disease such as erythema nodosum, splinter haemorrhages, xanthomas, and the white macules of tuberous sclerosis.

The physician should also look at the skin lesions from the patient's perspective.
The greatest handicap of all is to be unwelcome. Acne vulgaris is a cosmetic disability which makes a teenager feel unwelcome and contributes to delinquency. The white patches of vitiligo and albinism are a social embarrassment. The severe psoriatic lesions which leave blood on the sheets and scales on clothing and furniture, are a huge disadvantage in social life. The unfortunate social stigma attached to leprosy has not yet disappeared from society. The patient with skin disease is unemployable in any job in which he or she is in the public eye or involved in food preparation or serving.

It is also important to recognize the role of psychological factors in producing skin lesions.

Important Questions in History

1. How long have you had the lesion? Exactly when did it start? Have you had it before?

2. Which part of the skin was first affected? Where were you when it started? What were you doing?

3. How did it progress? To what sites?

4. Does it come and go? How long does each lesion last?

5. Does it itch? Is it painful, tender, anaesthetic?

6. Does it develop blisters or clear fluid?

7. Does anything make it better?

8. Does anything make it worse?

9. What ointments, creams, lotions or bath oils have you used?

10. Have you had any medicines or injections prior to the onset? Any blood transfusion?

11. Has anyone else you know got it? Does it run in your family? Do other diseases like asthma, eczema or hay fever run in your family?

12. Have you had any previous illness? Have you had exposure to sexually transmitted disease?

Physical Examination

A full examination includes looking at the skin of the entire body including the mucosa of the mouth, and the genitalia. One should look at (1) the type of skin lesion; (2) the configuration (single, linear, annular, grouped etc); (3) the distribution of the lesion.

Touching the lesion differentiates a papule (palpable) from a macule (non-palpable). For instance, palpable purpura is a useful clue for vasculitis. Compression distinguishes between erythema or telangiectasia (which blanch on pressure) and purpura (which does not blanch on pressure).

General examination of the skin reveals many useful clues-pallor, cyanosis, jaundice, pigmentation, erythematous or purpuric rash etc.

Types of skin lesions

(a) *Primary lesions*

These should be characterized by local examination.

Macules: circumscribed alterations in colour of the skin, without any elevation or depression of the skin; for example erythema. Diseases causing macular lesions are listed in **Table 50.1**. Causes of erythematous rashes are given in **Table 50.2**.

Papules: are solid lesions raised above the surface of skin, both visible and palpable, usual size 1 cm. Large papules are called nodules. Large nodules are called tumours. Large papules coalescing are called plaques. Sometimes lesions depressed below the skin are also called plaques. Comments on important papular lesions are given in **Table 50.3**. The significance of nodules is given in **Tables 50.4** and **50.5**.

Wheals and urticaria: These are evanescent papules or plaques that are pale and oedematous, generally with an erythematous halo around them. Comments on wheals and urticaria are given in **Table 50.6**. One unique cutaneous symptom is pruritus. Its causes are listed in **Table 50.7**.

Vesicles: are circumscribed small lesions filled with fluid. Large vesicles are called bullae. Comments on bullous lesions are given in **Table 50.8**.

Pustules: are elevated lesions filled with pus.

Purpura: is the appearance of haemorrhages under the skin. The significance of purpura is given in **Table 50.9**.

Alopecia or loss of hair may be patchy or diffuse and with or without scarring (**Table 50.10**).

(b) *Secondary lesions*

Scales: These are sheets of adherent epidermal cells, which may be white or silvery as in psoriasis, greasy as in seborrhoeic dermatitis, or fish-like as in ichthyosis. Comments on scaly lesions are given in **Table 50.11**.

Crusts or scabs are formed by dried secretions, whether serum, pus or blood. Crusts from serous fluid are golden or honey coloured, those from pus are dirty grey, and those caused by blood are chocolate brown in colour.

Ulcers: An ulcer is a breach in the continuity of the skin or mucosa. An ulcer may be superficial and confined to the epidermis, or deep, involving the whole skin or the underlying tissue (fascia, muscle) and may even expose the bone. Ulcers caused by scratching are linear and are called excoriations. Comments on ulcers are given in **Table 50.12**.

Scars: are formed by replacement of dermis or even subcutaneous tissue by newly formed connective tissue. Scars maybe hypertrophic or keloidal.

Lichenification: This is a distinctive thickening of the skin with accentuated skin-fold markings; it is thick and firm on palpation.

Configuration of skin lesions

This is diagnostically important. For instance,

Annular lesions occur in ringworm, pityriasis annulare, leprosy, secondary syphilis, and granuloma annulare.

Linear lesions occur in lichen planus, sporotrichosis, warts and morphea.

Grouped lesions occur in herpes simplex, herpes zoster and dermatitis herpetiformis.

Distribution of skin lesions

This is suggestive but not necessarily diagnostic of specific diseases. Some illustrative examples are:

Acne occurs on the face, upper trunk, and back.

Contact dermatitis is determined by the sites of contact e.g. footwear, necklace, ear-rings, bra hook, wristwatch band etc.

Seborrhoeic dermatitis is localized preferentially to the scalp, nasolabial and retroauricular folds, front of chest, axillae, pubic region and interscapular areas.

Photosensitivity dermatitis is localized to areas exposed to sunlight, particularly the face and dorsum of the hands; it usually spares the covered regions such as the undersurface of the chin, and areas covered by hair.

Lichen planus usually involves the flexors of the wrists and legs; the genital and buccal mucosa may also be involved.

Psoriasis affects the knees, elbows, lumbosacral region, back, scalp, extensors of the extremities, and nails.

Scabies occurs in the interdigital clefts of the hands and creases of the wrists, axillary fold, male genitalia, and areola of the female breast; it affects the palms and soles in infants and children. The face is never involved.

Fig. 50.1 illustrates the distribution of various types of skin rashes.

The cutaneous manifestations of systemic diseases are listed in **Table 50.13**.

TABLE **50.1** DISEASES CAUSING HYPER PIGMENTATION

A.	*Circumscribed*	
	Fungus infection	Pityriasis versicolor-axillae.
	Café-au-lait spots	Associated with neurofibromatosis, Albright's syndrome.
	Acanthosis nigricans	Malignancy associated; hormone-associated; insulin resistance; idiopathic.
B.	*Generalized*	
	Metabolic	Haemochromatosis; Porphyria cutanea tarda; Chronic liver disease; Uraemia.
	Endocrine	Pregnancy; Addison's disease; Cushing's syndrome; Pernicious anaemia; Scleroderma; Thyrotoxicosis; Myxoedema; Ectopic ACTH production in malignancy.
	Nutritional	Vit. B12 deficiency; Pellagra; Malabsorption; Whipple's disease.
	Drugs	Arsenic Busulphan (Myleran) Vinca alkaloids Chlorpromazine Phenothiazines.
•	Slate-gray or yellowish	Antimalarials.
•	(Blue-grey to blue-black)	Industrial exposure— Silver, gold, mercury, bismuth (heavy metals).
•	Chloasma-like pigmentation in women	Long-term phenytoin Oral contraceptives.
•	Red skin	Clofazimine Methysergide.
	Brown pigmentation	Nicotinic acid in large doses; Cigarette stains on fingers.

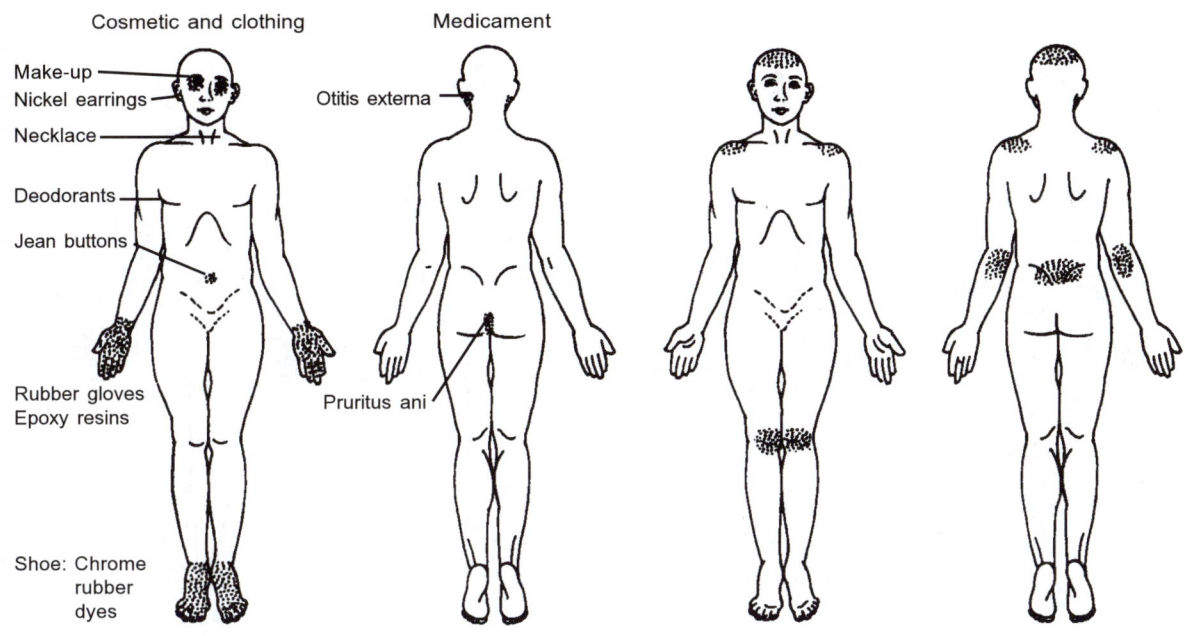

Cosmetic and clothing

Make-up
Nickel earrings
Necklace

Deodorants

Jean buttons

Rubber gloves
Epoxy resins

Shoe: Chrome
rubber
dyes

Medicament

Otitis externa

Pruritus ani

1. Contact dermatitis

2. Dermatitis herpetiformis

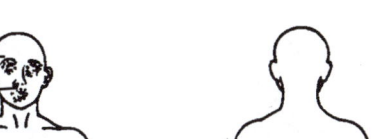

Eyes
Mouth

Hands

Feet

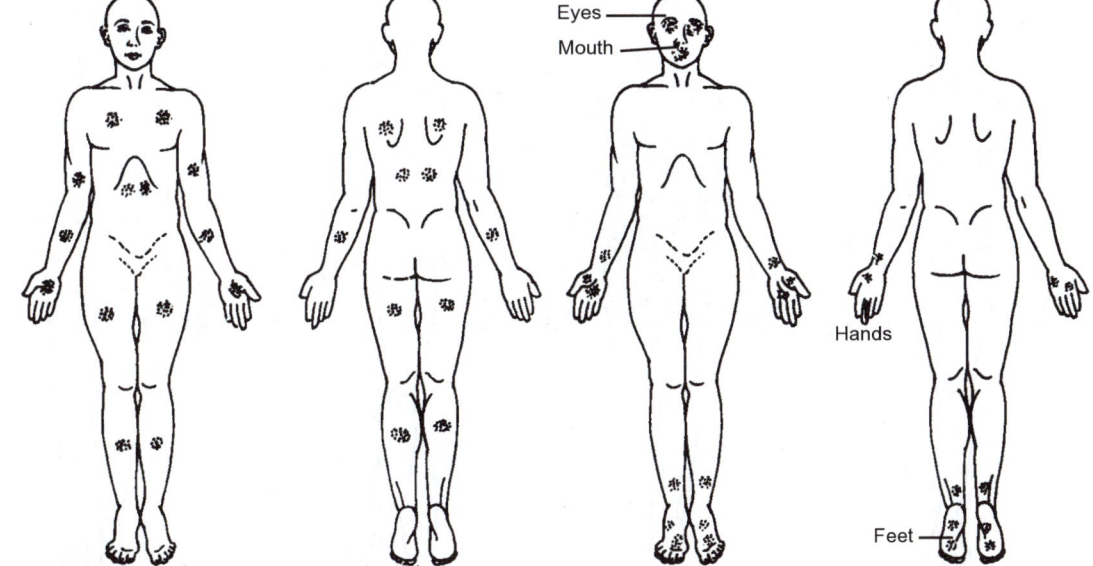

Discoid lesions can be in any distribution but they tend to
be symmetrical and coin-sized

3. Discoid lesions

4. Erythema multiforme

Fig. 50.1: Distribution of skin rashes (contd)

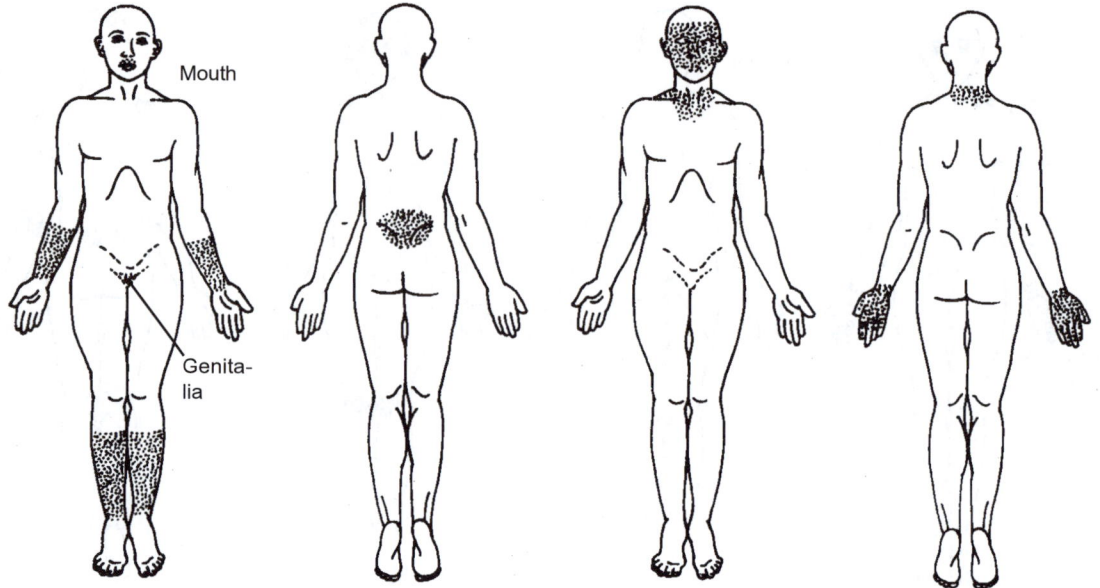

5. Lichen planus

6. Photosensitivity dermatitis

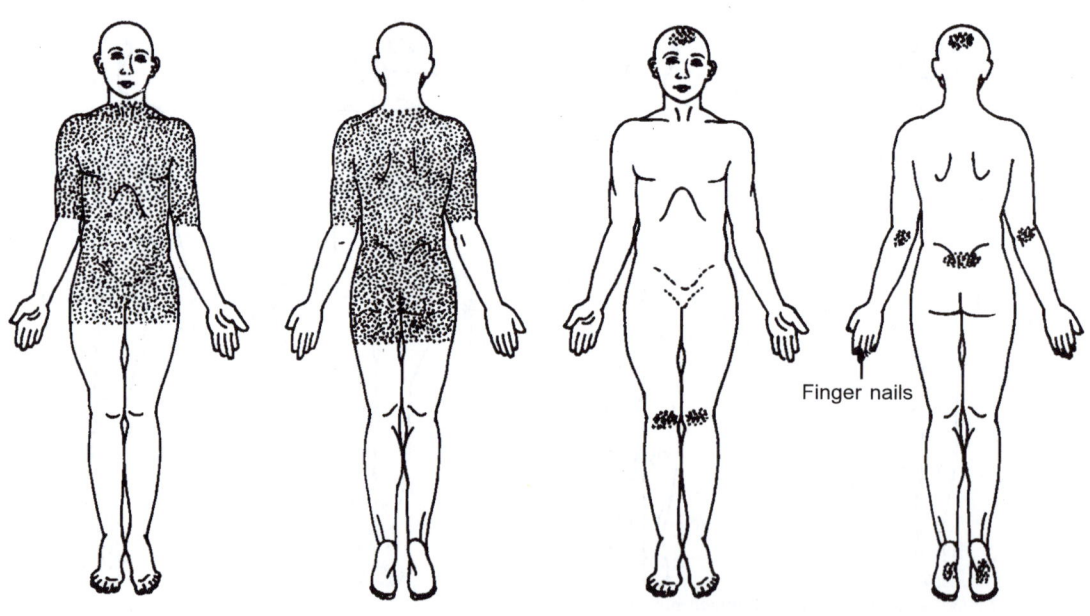

7. Pityriasis rosea

8. Psoriasis

Fig. 50.1: Distribution of skin rashes (contd)

Skin Lesions

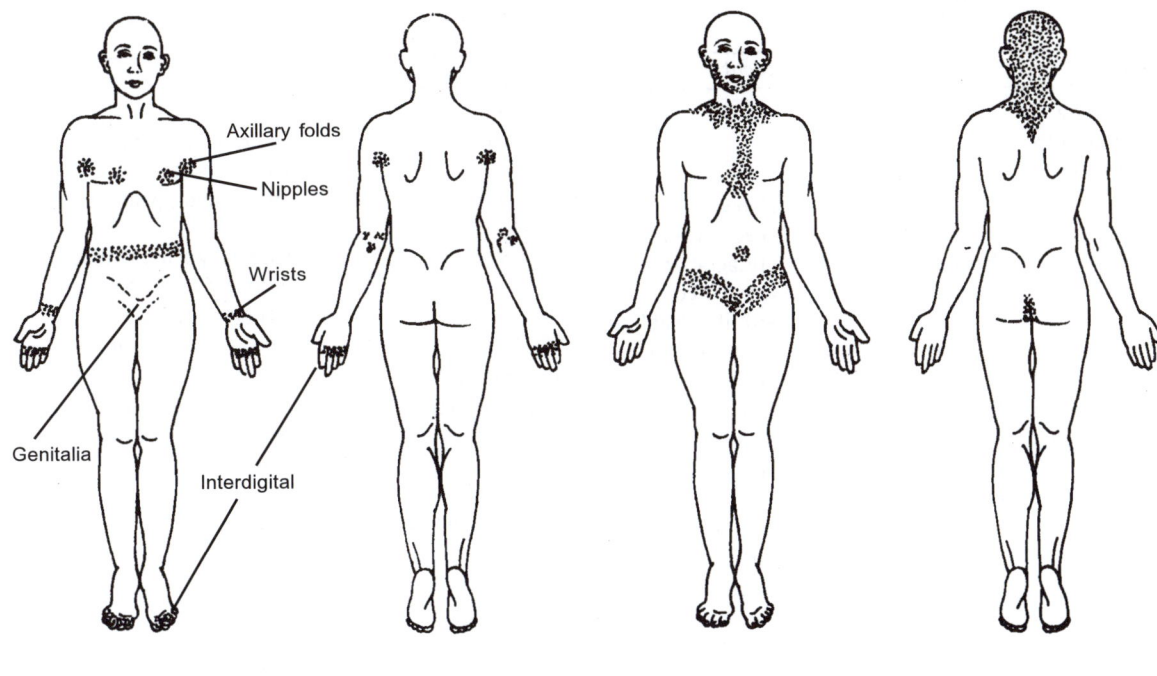

9. Scabies   10. Seborrhoeic dermatitis

Fig. 50.1: Distribution of skin rashes

TABLE 50.2 ERYTHEMATOUS LESIONS

Generalized

- Exanthemata or eruptive fevers:
  Measles
  German measles
  Erythema infectiosum
- Early HIV
- EBV, coxsackie, adenovirus
- Secondary syphilis
- Pellagra
- Drug-induced:
  Penicillin, especially ampicillin

Sulphonamides
Captopril
Phenytoin
Gold

Localized

- Sunburn: face, exposed parts
- Rosacea
- Systemic lupus erythematosus
  face 'butterfly rash'
- Fixed drug eruptions

Table 50.3 PAPULO-SQUAMOUS SKIN DISEASES

Disease	Characteristics	Location
A. Primary cutaneous disease		
Psoriasis	Pink-red silvery scales. sharply demarcated. Nails: dystrophy, pitting, onycholysis, yellow discoloration.	Elbow, knees. scalp, presacral area. Associated arthritis distal interphalangeal joints.
Pityriasis rosea	Salmon-pink, oval shape. Herald patch initial & largest lesion.	Trunk, proximal limbs.
Lichen planus	Violet coloured, polygonal, flat-topped pruritus Oral mucosa: lacelike white plaques.	Flexors of forearms, wrists, ankles, genitals, front of legs.
Tinea	Pink-red, central clearing common, active, scaling border.	Inner thigh, palms, soles, any area of body.
B. Secondary to systemic disease		
Systemic lupus erythematosus	Erythematous papular lesions, loss of hair.	Nose, cheeks, back of hands, feet, trunk.
Secondary syphilis	Red brown papules.	Palms, soles.
Reiter's disease	Heaped up scaly lesions, accompanied by urethritis.	Palms, soles.
Cutaneous T cell lymphoma	Psoriasiform lesions. thickening of skin.	No specific location.
Bazex' syndrome.	Psoriasiform lesions.	Hands, feet, nose, ears, fingers and toes.
C. Drugs		Trunk more than limbs.

Table 50.4 SIGNIFICANCE OF SKIN NODULES

	Distribution
Chronic inflammatory lesions	
Tuberculosis	Lupus vulgaris: face, cheeks, nose
Syphilis } Yaws }	Trunk, limbs, palms, soles
Leprosy	Especially lepromatous variety: face, ears, 'Leonine facies'.
Sarcoidosis	Nose, face, ears, neck.
Reticulosis	
Hodgkin's disease	Itchy nodules, pruritus may precede the skin involvement.
Leukaemia	
Mycosis fungoides	
Malignancy	
Secondaries from bronchogenic Ca.	No particular site.
Melanoma	Slate colour, dark brown, black.
Basal cell epithelioma:	Face, trunk, scalp. Itching, rapid increase in size, new satellite lesions, enlargement of local lymph nodes.
Metabolic	
Xanthoma tuberosum	Buttocks. thighs, arms, back, chest.
Amyloid	Central area of face: glistening waxy papules.
Gout	Olecranon, pinna of external ear.
Genetically determined diseases	
Neurofibromatosis	Look for associated pheochromocytoma and acoustic neuroma.
Adenoma sebaceum (epiloia)	Widespread benign tumours in various organs, including brain, epilepsy, mental retardation.
Autoimmune disorders	
Rheumatoid nodules	Extensor surface of forearms, patellae, bony prominences.
Polyarteritis nodosa	
Erythema nodosum **(Table 50.5)**	

Table 50.5 CAUSES OF ERYTHEMA NODOSUM

Cause	Comfirmation
Infection	
Streptococcus	Throat swab
Tuberculosis	Chest X-ray, Mantoux
Leprosy (lepromatous)	Hypopigmented anaesthetic patches
Lymphogranuloma venereum	Genital & inguinal lesions
Psittacosis	Serological tests
Yersinia	
Tularaemia	Skin tests with appropriate fungal antigen
Cat-Scratch fever	
Histoplasmosis	
Coccidiodidomycosis	
Blastomycosis	
Systemic Diseases	
Sarcoidosis	X-ray chest (BHL), ↑ ACE in blood
Inflammatory bowel disease	Sigmoidoscopy Oral & genital ulcers
Behiet's disease	
Drugs	Drug history
Sulfonamides	
Penicillin	
Bromides and riodides	
Oral contraceptives	
Pregnancy	

Abnormalities of Nails

Observation of the nails can often lead the physician to suspect the presence of certain diseases. Table 50.14 lists the abnormalities in nails which occur in various conditions.

Cutaneous Drug Reactions

Cutaneous reactions are among the most frequent adverse reactions to drugs. Penicillins, sulphonamides and blood products account for two-thirds of cutaneous reactions, most of which occur *within* one week of exposure to the drug. With semisynthetic penicillins and ampicillin, about half the reactions occur more than a week after initial administration. Skin reactions are more frequent among women.

Table 50.6 URICARIA

Causes	Examples	Diagnostic clues
Drugs	penicillins Sulfonamides Aspirin Anti-TB drugs Vit. B complex	Soon after intake; Occasionally may occur/persist for long even after drug is stopped; Scratch, prick & intradermal tests.
Food and food additives	Eggs, meat, fish, milk, cheese, pulses, wheat, rice	After a variable period following ingestion; Diet elimination and provocation test.
Inhalants	Pollen, fungi, house dust, paper dust in libraries	Scratch, prick or intradermal tests.
Infection and parasite infestation	Bacterial, viral, intestinal worms	Stool for cysts and ova.
Systemic disease	Hepatitis B infection, SLE, vasculitis, Hodgkin's D, lymphoma Hyperthyroidism hypothyroidism	Underlying disease features obvious.
Physical: = Dermato- graphism		Mastocytosis Urticariapigmentosa Hepatosplenomegaly High IgE.
= Cold	Cold water bath, rain	Ice cube test.
= Cholinergic stimuli	Physical exertions exposure to sun, heat	Intradermal carbachol test.
Psychogenic stimuli	Emotional stress esp. anxiety	No laboratory tests.
Hereditary angio- oedema	Serum complement C_4 and C_1 esterase inhibitor low	Serum complement C_4 level and C_1 esterase inhibitor level persistently low.
Acquired angio- oedema	Contact with benzoic & other acids, antibiotics	Patch test.

TABLE 50.7 CAUSES OF PRURITUS

A. *Pruritus secondary to visible skin disease*

Scabies

Dermatitis herpetiformis

Eczema

Urticaria

Lichen planus (usually seen in middle life)

B. *Localized pruritus without visible skin lesions*

Pediculosis capitis & pediculosis pubis (e.g. flea, bedbug)

Insect bites

Localized neurodermatitis

Onchocerciasis (in Africa)

C. *Generalized pruritus without visible skin lesions*

Diabetes mellitus

Pregnancy during the last month

Reticulosis-Hodgkin's disease

Leukaemia, polycythaemia

Obstructive jaundice esp. primary biliary cirrhosis

Hypothyroidism, hyperthyroidism

Renal failure-uraemia

Old age, especially in winter: dry skin

Psychogenic; nervous tension, anxiety

D. *Drug-induced*

Aspirin

Barbiturates, opiates

Captopril, enalepril

Penicillin, sulphonamides

The most common morphological pattern of drug reactions are exanthematous (46 per cent), urticaria and/or angio-oedema (23 per cent), fixed drug eruption, (19 per cent), erythema multiforme (5.4 per cent), Steven Johnson syndrome (4 per cent), exfoliative dermatitis (4 per cent), photosensitivity reactions (3 per cent), anaphylaxis (1.5 per cent), toxic epidermal necrolysis (1.5 per cent).

Cutaneous drug reactions can arise out of immunological or non-immunological mechanisms, the latter being responsible for the majority of drug reactions.

TABLE 50.8 BULLOUS ERUPTIONS

Disease	Characteristics	Treatment
Staphylococcal scalded skin syndrome	Proteolytic enzymes split granular layer of skin.	Antibiotics.
Pemphigus vulgaris	IgG directed at epidermal intercellular layer. Split at basal layer. Flaccid bullae: oral mucosa.	Corticosteroids Immunosuppressives. Gold.
Bullous pemphigoid	IgG and complement directed at basal lamina. Split sub-epidermal. Older age group (60-70 yrs).	Corticosteroids. Immunosuppressives.
Dermatitis herpetiformis	IgA in dermal papillae. Split subepidermal. Back, buttocks, extensor surface of limbs.	Sulphones.
Epidermolysis bullosa	Genetic defect: localized to areas of trauma. Split sub-dermal. Excessive collagenase activity.	Protection against skin friction. Dilantin blocks collagenase.
Erythema multiforme	Iris target lesions. Split subepidermal.	Corticosteroids.
Toxic epidermal necrolysis	Drug-induced (e.g. INAH) or idiopathic split at basal layer.	Corticosteroids.

Special Diagnostic Procedures

Skin scrapings for fungus for direct microscopic examination in a 10-20 per cent KOH solution.

Cytologic examination of fluid or scrapings from the base of a vesicle, both for acantholytic cells or inflammatory cells in pemphigus and other bullous lesions.

Bacterial culture to determine the causative or complicating microbes and their sensitivity to antibiotics.

Biopsy of lesions e.g. for Hansen's disease, SLE.

TABLE 50.9 SIGNIFICANCE OF PURPURA

Drug-induced

Sulphonamides
Thiouracil

Primary cutaneous disorders (Non-palpable)
Trauma
Solar purpura
Steroid purpura
Capillaritis

Systemic diseases

A. *Non-palpable*	B. *Palpable*
1. Clotting disturbances Thrombocytopenia Abnormal platelet function (uraemia) Clotting factor defects	1. Vasculitis Leucocytoclastic (allergic) (circular or oval outline) e.g. Henoch-Schönlein purpura Polyarteritis nodosa (irregular outline)
2. Vascular fragility Scurvy Ehlers-Danlos syndrome Amyloidosis	2. Emboli Acute meningococcaemia Disseminated gonococcal infection Ecthyma gangrenosum
3. Thrombi Disseminated intravascular coagulation (DIC) Monoclonal cryoglobulinuria Multiple myeloma Thrombotic thrombocytopenic purpura Warfarin reactions	(Pseudomonas, Klebsiella) Typhus
4. Emboli Cholesterol (following arteriography) Fat	
5. Waldenstrom's hypergamma-globinaemic purpura	

TABLE 50.10 ALOPECIA

1. *Patchy hairless:*

Without scarring	*With scarring*
Alopecia areata Ringworm (common type) Secondary syphilis Use of curlers	Ringworm (less common type) Lichen planus SLE and discoid lupus erythematosis Lupus vulgaris

2. *Diffuse hairless:*

Without scarring	*With scarring*
Male pattern baldness Ectodermal defects. Alopecia totalis SLE Fevers e.g. typhoid Drugs e.g. cyclophosphamide Myxoedema	X-ray atrophy Associated telangiectasia and pigmentation

TABLE 50.11: ERUPTIONS IN WHICH SCALES ARE A CONSPICUOUS FEATURE

- Psoriasis: Knees & elbows, scalp, trunk, nails.
- Seborrhoeic dermatitis: Scalp, face, midline of chest & back, flexures.
- Pityriasis rosea: Trunk, thighs, upper arms.
- Tinea circinata: Non-shaving skin-tine scaling.
- Ichthyosis: Extensor surfaces of upper arms, hands & legs.
- Exfoliative dermatitis: Trunk more than the extremities.

Immunofluorescence in differentiating various types of bullous dermatoses, systemic lupus erythematosus, and discoid lupus and lichenoid dermatoses.

Table 50.12 CAUSES OF LEG ULCERS

Trauma	External injuries: bums, scalds, chemicals, self-inflicted, artefacts, contact dermatitis	Neuropathic (trophic)	Painless ulcers Leprosy Diabetic neuropathy Tabes dorsalis Syringomyelia
Infection	Acute– 'desert sore', gas gangrene Chronic–tuberculosis, leprosy Swimming pool granuloma Syphilis, yaws Tropical ulcer Mycotic	Blood disorders	Chronic haemolytic anaemias, sickle cell, spherocytosis Polycythaemia Thrombocythaemia Dysglobulinaemia
Metabolic	Diabetes mellitus		
Vasculitis	SLE, PAN, immune complex disease	Malignancy	Basal cell carcinoma
Pyoderma gangrenosum	Associated with ulcerative colitis and Crohn's disease or blood dyscrasias		Squamous cell carcinoma Melanoma
Venous stasis	Post-thrombotic, varicose veins		Kaposi's sarcoma

Table 50.13 CUTANEOUS MANIFESTATIONS OF SYSTEMIC DISEASES

Disease	Features in skin
Endocrine	
Hyperthyroidism	Smooth, moist, soft skin; Hyperpigmentation or vitiligo; Pretibial myxoedema.
Hypothyroidism	Dry, cold, yellowish skin, thickening.
Hypoparathyroidism	Dry, scaly, sparse hair, patchy alopecia; Extensive candidiasis of skin.
Diabetes mellitus	Dermopathy: round or oval red papules (I cm diameter) on shins, heal with a pigmented scar; Necrobiosis lipoidica: oval indurated reddish yellow plaques with central atrophy, on shins, thighs.
Acromegaly	Diffusely thickened & furrowed skin; Greasy due to excessive sebaceous glands.
Cushing's syndrome	Striae atrophicans on trunk and limbs; Moon face and buffalo hump.
Addison's disease	Pigmentation of skin and mucosa.
Insulin resistance	Acanthosis nigricans; Lesions on nape of neck.
Glucagonoma	Necrolytic migratory erythema on lower abdomen, perineum, groin.
Gastrointestinal	
Ulcerative colitis	Pyoderma gangrenosum.
Peutz-Jeghers syndrome	Pigmentation of skin and oral mucosa.
Zinc malabsorption	Acrodermatitis.
Pancreatitis	Nodular fat necrosis: lower limbs and trunk.
Autoimmune disease	
Dermatomyositis	Erythematous patches on upper anterior chest, face (butterfly), extensor surface, arms, legs, hands; Periungual telangiectasis.
SLE	'Butterfly' erythema of face, upper chest; Papulo-squamous lesions resemble psoriasis.

(Contd)

TABLE 50.13 (Contd)

Disease	Features in skin
Scleroderma and morphea	Face, hands, feet, sclerodactyly; calcinosis cutis.
Sarcoidosis	Blue-red subcutaneous nodules; Lupus pernio.
Internal malignancy	
Any site	Dematomyositis in 10-15% adults.
GI malignancy	Acanthosis nigricans (hyperpigmented hyperkeratotic lesions in body flexures).
Lymphoma/solid tumours	May be heralded by acquired ichthyosis.
Hodgkin's disease	Herpes zoster, pruritus.
Breast/thyroid ca	Multiple papules and papillomata on the face, hands & forearms– cobblestone appearance of mucous membranes.
Immunosuppression	
AIDS	Kaposi's sarcoma; Atypical seborrhoeic dermatitis; Herpes simplex, Herpes zoster (multiple sites simultaneously); Folliculitis; Psoriasis; Warts (Molluscum contagiosum).
Metabolic	
Porphyria cutanea tarda	Photosensitivity, blister formation, hyperpigmentation, hypertrichosis.
Hyperlipidaemias	Xanthelasma (white or yellow plaques of lipid deposited in the periorbital skin); Xanthomata on tendons and dorsum of hands.

NOTE: See also Chapter 44 on Nutritional Deficiency for skin lesions in nutritional diseases.

TABLE 50.14 ABNORMALITIES OF NAILS

Appearance of nail	Likely cause	Appearance of nail	Likely cause
Absence or atrophy	Congenital ectodermal defect Nail-patella syndrome Radiation exposure	Brown Grey	Hydroquinone Argyria Phenolphthalein Mercuric chloride
Hypertrophy	Fungal (trichophyton) infection Chronic mucocutaneous candidiasis	Green Yellow	Pseudomonas infection Chronic oedema
Pits Psoriasis		Nail plate separation (onycholysis)	Fungus infection (KOH positive) Psoriasis Graves' disease
Lines	Single line of pits: major metabolic disturbance		
White bands	Hypoalbuminaemia Arsenic	Sub-ungual haemorrhage	Subacute bacterial endocarditis Vasculitis Trauma
Clubbing	Familial Pulmonary infection/neoplasm Cyanotic heart disease Cirrhosis	Peri-ungual inflammation	Paronychia: factorial or fungal infection
Spooning	Iron deficiency anaemia	Peri-ungual neoplasm	Myxoid cysts (clear jelly on puncture)
Colour: Black	Hair dyes Vit. B12 deficiency Peutz-Jeghers syndrome		Glomus (bluish colour) Enchondroma (firm papule) Warts
Grey-black	Melanoma		Squamous cell carcinoma

Management of Common Skin Lesions

I. *Fungal skin infection*
1. Candidiasis
   (a) Intertriginous — Nystatin cream 100,000 units/g topical application. Miconazole cream *or* lotion 2%. Clotrimazole cream *or* solution 1% twice daily. Ketoconazole cream once daily.

   (b) Periungual — Thymol 2-4% in absolute alcohol applied bid or tid.
2. *Dermatophyte infection*
   (a) small areas of glabrous skin and feet — Miconazole bid *or* Clotrimazole bid *or* Ketoconazole once daily.

   (b) widespread infection, tinea capitis, onychomycosis — Griseofulvin 500 mg PO twice daily for 4 weeks; 6-8 months for nail infection. Oral Ketoconazole in patients not tolerating Griseofulvin.

   (c) tinea versicolor (often recurs regardless of mode of therapy) — Selenium sulfide 2.5% suspension applied with scrubbing for 15 minutes daily for 1-2 weeks. Clotrimazole and other drugs also effective but more expensive.

II. *Bacterial infections of skin*
1. *Impetigo* (usually streptococcal) more common in children rarely in adults — Penicillin VK 250 mg PO qid *or* Erythromycin stearate 250 mg PO qid (1 g per day). Dicloxacillin 250 mg PO qid (for bullous staphylococcal lesions). Topical mupirocin ointment for resistant staph.

2. *Cellulitis & erysipelas* (Staphylococcal or streptococcal) — Dicloxacillin 1 g/day *or* Cephalexin *or* Erythromycin.

3. *Boils or Carbuncles* — Dicloxacillin g/day *or* Cephalexin *or* Erythromycin.

III. *Scabies* (groin, axillae, between fingers & toes, below breasts) — 1 % gamma benzene hexachloride (Lindane*) cream or lotion applied to the entire body chin downwards, esp. intertriginous areas, skin folds and finger webs at bedtime; left overnight; repeat procedure the next evening.

IV. *Warts*
1. *Common warts* — Liquid nitrogen cryotherapy or local flexible collodion containing 16.7% salicylic acid and 16.7% lactic acid daily for several days.

2. *Plantar warts* — Salicyclic acid 40% plaster cut to fit the lesion applied daily under adhesive tape occlusion.

3. *Condyloma acltminata* — Podophyllin 20-25% in tincture of benzoin should be applied by the doctor, avoiding normal skin and washed off thoroughly 4 hours later. Repeat application weekly. Liquid nitrogen cryotherapy is also helpful.

*Note: Lindane is contraindicated in pregnancy and infancy. Crotamiton (Eurax) 10% every night for 4-5 nights is ideal for children.

V.	*Dermatitis (eczema)*	
	Face, neck, extensor surface, groin	Topical corticosteroids (1% hydrocortisone) as lotion, creams or ointment for control of inflammation.
	For acute, weeping lesions	Cream or lotion preferable
	For chronic dry eczema	A lubricating ointment
	Low strength:	for facial use, and for infants and children,
	Medium strength:	for most dermatoses of average severity, and
	High strength:	for severe or resistant lesions and for hand and foot involvement.
	Sun screens (for protection of patients prone to solar dermatitis)	
	To protect from UVB (280–320 nm) causing sunburn	PABA (para-amino benzoic acid) and its esters padimate A, padimate O for routine prophylaxis in sunbathing and outdoor sports.
	To protect from UVA (320–400 nm)	Oxybenzone and dioxybenzone for patients with porphyria, photodermatitis (SLE), drug sensitivity (Sulphonamides, tetracycline, thiazides).
	To protect from both	Titanium dioxide and zinc oxide.
VI.	*Acne* (face, upper back)	(1) Topical benzoyl peroxide 5–10% bid. (2) Topical retinoic acid 0.05–0.1%. (3) Topical antibiotic-clindamycin, erythromycin tetracycline. (4) Systemic antibiotic tetracycline 500 mg PO bid. (5) Isotretinoin 1 mg/kg/day: 2 oral doses, given with meals for 15–20 weeks.
VII.	*Eczematous dermatitis*	
	Acute	Wet compresses. Topical steroids. Oral steroids.
	ChronicTopical corticosteroid cream.	Topical antipruritic. Systemic antipruritic.
VIII.	*Psoriasis* (elbows, knees, scalp, lower back, fingernails)	
	Mild	Topical cortocosteroid cream and ointment. Sunlight or UVL. Tar compound e.g. Target. Keratolytic agent. Salicylic acid 6% gel: overnight occlusion. Corticosteroid solutions and tar shampoo.
	Severe (To be treated only by an expert dermatologist)	Chemotherapeutic agents. Large wave length UVL. Etretinate

IX.	*Seborrhoeic dermatitis* (scalp and face, eyebrows, perinasal)	2.5% selenium sulfide shampoo for 5-10 minutes, upto 3 times/week. For more inflammatory scalp lesions: steroid lotion or solution. For face: hydrocortisone 1% cream applied twice daily.
X.	*Urticaria and angio-oedema*	Oral antihistaminics (HI antagonists) e.g. terfenadine. Topical antipruritic adjuncts. Inj. adrenaline for laryngeal oedema / anaphylaxis. Danazol or stanazol to prevent attacks in hereditary angio-oedema.
XI.	*Pruritus*1.	*Topical agents:*

XI. *Pruritus*1.

Topical agents:

    (a) Camphor 1-3% and menthol 0.25-2%.

    (b) Phenol 0.25-2% causes local hypoaesthesia and should not be used on a raw or ulcerated skin.

    (c) Calamine lotion can be helpful.

2. Systemic agents: Anti-histamines (HI receptor antagonists)
Diphenehydramine 25-50 mg PO of 4-8 hrs.
Hydroxyzine hydrochloride.
Hydroxyzine palmoate 10-50 mg PO of 4-8 hrs.
Cyproheptadine.
Drimeprazine.

COMMONLY USED TOPICAL CORTICOSTEROIDS (CREAM/OINTMENT)

Low strength
Hydrocortisone
    0.1%, 1%, 2.5%
Fluocinolone acetonide
    0.01%
Bec1omethasone diproprionate
    0.025%

} Suitable for face and flexures.

Medium strength
Hydrocortisone 17 butyrate
    0.1%
Flurandrenolone
    0.0125%
Betamethasone valerate
    0.1%

} Can produce unchecked growth of fungal infection 'tinea incognito'. Perioral dermatitis if used on face.

High strength
Betamethasone 17 valerate
    0.1%
Ditlucortolone valerate
    0.1%
Bec1omethasone diproprionate
    0.25%

} Chronic use can produce atrophy of the skin, especially axilla.

Very strong
Bec1omethasone diproprionate
    0.5%
Clobetasol proprionate
    0.05%

} Avoid in children. Can produce adrenal suppression. Not to exceed 50 g/week.

51 — Sleep Disorders

Introduction

Sleep plays an important role in the preservation of health and well-being of the individual, for memory consolidation, restorative and recovery function and neurogenesis. Good sleep and exercise are related to longer telomeres and telomerase activity. Quality of sleep as well as duration is important. The average sleep duration is 7 to 8 hours. Some persons may do with 3-4 hours of sleep while some others may need 9 hours. Babies may sleep for as long as 16 hours in a day. Partial sleep dept - occurs when a person sleeps too little for many days. Total sleep dept leads to physical and mental fatigue.

There are approximately 85 different types of sleep disorders known today.

Sleep Architecture

Each night a person goes through two types of sleep that alternate with each other.

- Slow wave or non-rapid eye movement (NREM) sleep.
- Rapid eye movement (REM) Sleep.

Non-REM sleep occupies 75-80% of total sleep. REM sleep occupies the remaining 20-25% total sleep. REM sleep tends to occur more during early hours of the morning, during the later part of a person's sleep. It is accompanied by an aroused EEG pattern, and lower muscle tone.

Non-REM sleep is divided into 3 stages - 1, 2, 3 accompanied by slowing of EEG waves, higher muscle tone and absence of thought - like activity.

Although dreams occur in both types, only dreams occurring during REM are remembered.

Sleep Laboratories have the facility of Polysomnography - EEG, EMG, EOG, ECG and Oxygen saturation.

Classification of Sleep Disorders

Dyssomnia - Difficulty in falling asleep or maintaining sleep.

Insomnia - Difficulty in falling asleep or difficulty in maintaining sleep. Primary insomnia is not associated with any underlying medical or Psychiatric condition. It is most common in the elderly population. Secondary insomnia is associated with anxiety, depression, congestive heart failure, GERD, asthma, arthritis, irritable bowel syndrome and cancer.

Insomnia is more common in females compared to males. Insomnia is associated with several undesirable effects - fatigue, irritability, poor memory, poor concentration, headaches, day time sleepiness.

Sleep Hygiene - Consists of going to bed only when feeling sleepy, getting up at the same time each day, to reinforce the body's biological clock; keeping the bedroom dark; avoid spicy and fatty food before sleep, avoid strenuous exercise 4 hours before sleep, avoid tea or coffee 4 hours before sleep.

Conventional sleeping pills contain benzodiazepines (Triazolam, Estazolam, Temazepam etc.) prescribed for less than 4-6 weeks. Alcohol should be avoided while using these drugs. Abrupt withdrawal of these drugs can lead to rebound insomnia which may be more problematic than the primary sleep disorder itself.

Newer benzodiazepine compound - Zolpidem, Zaleplon and Eszopielone, can be prescribed for periods as long as 6 months.

Zolpidem (1.75 mg) in females, (3.5 mg) in males through sub-lingual route for patients who have difficulty in falling asleep after waking up in the middle of the night.

Ramelteon, a melatonin receptor agonist 8 mg at bed time is a new FDA - approved drug for sleep onset insomnia.

Mirtazapine a newer antidepressant is used in insomnia associated with depression (7.5 to 30 mg at bed time). Unwanted effects include weight gain, drowsiness and rebound insomnia on its withdrawal.

Narcolepsy

Narcolepsy is a sleep disorder characterized by extreme day-time sleepiness. Patients may fall asleep suddenly even in the middle of a conversation or any other activity.

Cataplexy involves a sudden loss of muscle tone in the limbs, neck and face. These episodes of muscle weakness are usually provoked by strong emotions such as anger, laughter or surprise.

Onset between age 15-25, with a predilection for males, these episodes last for a few seconds to minutes, followed by immediate and complete recovery.

Diagnosis is made by Polysomnography and Multiple Sleep Latency Test (MSLT). An opportunity to sleep at two hours intervals over a day is given to the patient. A Mean sleep latency less than 8 minutes forms the diagnosis of narcolepsy.

Hypocretin-1 levels in CSF help to establish the diagnosis of narcolepsy. Levels lower than 110 pg/ml are confirmatory.

The absence of HLA DQ B1 0602 or HLA DQAI 0602 virtually exclude the diagnosis of narcolepsy.

Modafinil (200 mg once daily) is the drug of choice for promoting wakefulness.

Armodafinil, an enantiomer of modafinil produces less adverse effects than modafinil.

Obstructive Sleep Apnoea (OSA)

Extreme obesity associated with alveolar hypoventilation (Pickwickian syndrome) was described by Burwell C. S. et al in 1956. Obstructive Sleep Apnoea is characterized by an obstruction of the upper airway during sleep leading to a decrease or cessation of air flow and hypoxia leading to

disturbed sleep followed by excessive daytime sleepiness (EDS). EDS is assessed using the Epworth Sleepiness Scale (ESS). This involves the patients response to 8 questions regarding the probability of dozing under specific situations with a 4 point scale. A score of > 10 is suggestive by EDS.

Sleep Laboratories are now functioning in many parts of India where the diagnosis of OSAs is established by Polysomnography (PSG) which includes EEG, EMG and EOG recordings to differentiate between REM and NREM sleep.

PSG yields an important parameter known as Apnoea Hypopnea Index (AHI) defined as the total number of apnoeas and hypopnes that occur per hour of sleep.

Apnoea is defined as complete cessation of airflow for 10 or more seconds.

Hypopnea is defined as > 30% airflow reduction and > 4% oxygen desaturation.

Based on AHI, patients are classified as having mild (5-15), moderate (15-30) or severe (> 30) OSAS.

The major consequences of OSAS are: neuro cognitive dysfunction; poor quality of life; hypertension and endothelial dysfunction, sympathetic surges in early morning, and hypercoagulability.

Presence of OSA with Metabolic syndrome is known as Syndrome Z.

Treatment options in OSAS are.

- Sleeping in upright position; avoidance of smoking and alcohol.
- CPAP- Continuous positive air pressure maintenance via nasal catheter is therapy for moderate to severe OSAS.
- Oral appliances to stabilize lower jaw.
- Surgery involving soft palate, uvula, tonsils, tongue or adenoids

Central Sleep Apnoea Syndrome

Central sleep apnoea is an intermittent reduction or absence of respiratory efforts leading to a fall in Oxygen saturation levels. This is usually associated with OSA.

Restless Legs Syndrome (RLS)

RLS is characterized by discomfort and irritable sensations in the legs, leading to a desire to move them constantly. Symptoms may even include pain and occur mostly during evening or night.

Periodic Limb movement of sleep (PLMS) is characterized by involuntary twitching or jerking movements of the legs during sleep is recurring every 15 to 40 seconds leading to disturbed sleep.

Useful medications in RLS include Dopaminergic agents, benzodiazepines, opioids and anti convulsants, Gabapentin enacarbil is recently approved for RLS.

Circadian Rhythm Sleep Disorder (CRSDs)

Delayed Sleep Phase Disorders (DSPDs) sleep times that are delayed as compared to usual sleep times. Patients usually have a problem in falling asleep before 2-6 am and find it difficult to wake up in the morning.

Chrono Therapy involves a progressive slide of the sleep time in the same direction as the patients tendency to sleep.

Patients with DSPD will benefit by Melatonin 3-5 mg, 3-4 hours before bed time.

Advanced Sleep Phase Disorders (ASPDS)

These patients have sleep and wake times that are a few hours earlier than usual. Patients wake up early in the morning and have a compensatory early sleepiness in the evenings. Bright light may be used in the evening as a therapeutic modality.

Free Running Type Sleep Disorders

A daily drift of sleep and waking times. Blind persons have a non-entrained circadian rhythm in the absence of light stimulation (light - being the most important zeitgeber).

Despite the absence of photic stimulation the circadian rhythm of blind persons may respond to bring light

Shift Worker Sleep Disturbances

Shift workers frequently complain of sleep disturbances. Either sleepiness or insomnia may occur depending on the work schedule. Patients complain of an unrefreshing sleep. Symptoms may last even after restoration of usual sleep times. Melatonin 0.5-5 mg at bed time is useful.

Jet Lag Syndrome

Jet Leg occurs due to an ansynchrony between environmental and endogenous factors due to air travel across time zones. The body's circadian rhythm which dictates when to sleep and when to get awake in the old time zone, is out of sync with cues from the new time zone such as light exposure and dining times. Jet lag is temporary but it can significantly affect your vacation or business travel comfort, difficulty in concentrating and functioning at your usual level. Pilots, flight attendants and business travelers are most likely to experience jet lag. Older adults need more time to recover from jet lag.

Features include excessive sleepiness, insomnia, day time fatigue, mood changes, difficulty in concentration etc. Jet Lag is more pronounced in eastward travel when you "lose" time as compared to westward travel, where you gain time. No jet lag is experienced in north-south flying.

Melatonin 0.5-5 mg at bet time is useful short term use of short acting non- benzodiazepines such as zolpidem, eszopiclone, Zaleplon or Benzodiazepines such as triazolam. Exposure to sunlight combined with exercise such as walking or jogging help to restore the sleep- wake cycle.

Parasomnias

There are episodic behaviors that intrude into sleep.

Common parasomnias include night terrors (during NREM sleep), night mares (during REM sleep), sleep enuresis, bruxism etc.

REM sleep behavioral disorders (RSBDs) are specific types of parasomnias characterized by dream enacting behaviors which occur during REM sleep. Polysomnographic video recording is the test of choice for RSBDs. Clonazepan is the drug of choice. Providing a safe environment in the bed room and removing of dangerous objects is important. RSBDs may be an early feature of neuro degenerative disorders.

Sleep Disorders in Children

Sleep enuresis

Sleep bruxism

Infant - Sleep apnoea

Sudden infant death syndrome

Attention - Deficit hyperactivity disorder may in particular be associated with sleep apnoea snoring, RLS etc.

Sleep disorders may be associated with mental, neurological or other disorders.

Psychiatric disorders are closely related to sleep disorders, particulars depression. Therefore the importance of a thorough psychiatric evaluation cannot be over emphasized in patients with sleep disorders to rule out an underlying psychiatric illness.

References

International classification of Sleep Disorders ICS D-2 2005. American Academy of Sleep Medicine.

TABLE 51.1: Demographic details of patients seen in sleep disorders clinic over an 8 year period

	Group 1	Group 2
Total no. of patients studied	222	247
Mean age at presentation	43.1± 17.6 years	41.7 ± 15.0 years
Male:Female ratio	2.48:1	2.1:1
BMI	26.56	28.24
Occupation		
housewives	18.64%	12.05%
students	9.09%	3.61%
retired from service	12.73%	12.05%
under government employment	22.27%	39.76%
working in private enterprise/self employed	33.64%	32.53%

TABLE 51.2: Distribution of sleep disorders seen over the first 4 years versus the next 4 years

ICSD-R category of sleep disorder	Group 1	Group 2	P value
Insomnias	38	29	0.000
Sleep-related breathing disorders	67	117	0.000
Hypersomnias	28	43	0.012
Circadian rhythm sleep disorders	5	4	0.776
Parasomnias	44	28	0.011
Sleep-related movement disorder	69	86	0.000
Isolated symptoms, unresolved	6	3	–

52 Sore Throat

Sore throat is a common complaint. Most cases of sore throat or pharyngitis are viral in origin, self-limiting in course, and do not need any specific antimicrobial therapy. The causes of sore throat are given in **Table 52.1**. The important consideration for the doctor is not to miss a serious or life-threatening infection like *diphtheria* (which has fortunately become extremely rare due to the universal practice of immunization), or an underlying serious haematologic condition like *agranulocytosis, aplastic anaemia or leukaemia*. In the immunosuppressed patient candida infection may present as sore throat. An unusual cause of sore throat is gonococcal infection in those practising oral sex. Oral ampicillin or amoxicillin are not effective for gonococcal pharyngitis, and the bacteriologist will probably not examine the swab for gonococci unless alerted to this possibility in appropriate adult cases.

The importance of making a specific diagnosis of sore throat by throat culture is to permit identification of group A haemolytic streptococcus infection and thus prevent acute rheumatic fever by prompt treatment with penicillin. By prophylactic use of penicillin, rheumatic fever and its consequent rheumatic valvular disease have been stamped out from developed countries like Sweden long back. There is no reason why the same cannot be achieved in developing countries by a determined effort.

The treatment of streptococcal throat infection is oral penicillin VK 250 mg qid for 10 days, or IM inj. benzathine penicillin 1.2 megaunits.

The treatment of gonococcal pharyngitis is ceftriaxone 125-250 mg IM inj. or procaine penicillin G 4.8 megaunits distributed over two injection sites. The treatment of Vincent's angina IS with penicillin.

Thrush (candida) is treated with ketaconazole.

Agranulocytosis: Stop the drug which precipitated it. Give oral penicillin cover to prevent superadded infection. Avoid 1M injection to avoid infection at injection sites. Give fresh leucocyte transfusion or granulocyte colony-stimulating factor if affordable.

Ampicillin should not be given to patients with suspected infectious mononucleosis, because of the higher incidence of erythematous rash.

Treatment of Diphtheria

This is one condition where prompt early diagnosis is important. Every moment of delay increases the danger to the patient's life because the exotoxin, once fixed to the tissues, can no longer be neutralized by antitoxin. The complications of untreated diphtheria are given in **Table 52.2**. Hence if the doctor suspects diphtheria, he will have to initiate therapy without waiting for the bacteriological report on the throat swab. Before giving anti-diphtheritic serum, the following three questions have to be answered:

1. Has the patient received horse serum before?
2. Has he suffered from asthma, eczema or allergy?
3. Is there a family history of asthma, eczema or allergy?

If the answer is affirmative, a small test dose of antiserum is given keeping an adrenaline syringe ready. If a reaction does occur, rapid desensitization must be undertaken with the adrenaline syringe at hand, to deal with any anaphylactic reaction.

TABLE 52.1 DIFFERENTIAL DIAGNOSIS OF SORE THROAT

	Disease	Clinical features	Throat appearance	Confirmation
1.	Streptococcal tonsillitis	Abrupt onset, high fever 104°F, cervical lymph nodes enlarged & tender.	Widespread inflammation of throat with purulent yellowish-white exudate on tonsil which can be swabbed off easily.	Throat-swab culture.
2.	Diphtheria,	Onset insidious, fever not high (99-100°F), cervical lymph nodes enlarged & tender.	Pearl-grey membrane, elevated with well-defined edge & surrounding inflamed area, firm and adherent–cannot be swabbed off. In mild infections no membrane, only injected throat; clinical diagnosis can be missed.	Microscope examination of throat-swab culture for virulence.
3.	Thrush (candida)	No constitutional symptoms, no enlarged or tender regional lymph nodes.	White deposits adherent to buccal mucosa, palate & tonsils, very little surrounding inflammation.	Microscopic exam. of throat swab: budding yeas Hike growths with mycelial threads.
4.	Infectious mononucleosis	Fever with generalized lymph-adenopathy, ± skin rash & splenomegaly.	Inflamed throat accompanied by exudate.	Microscopic exam. of throat swab negative for bacteria. Peripheral smear shows increased mononuclear cells. Paul-Bunnell test positive.
5.	Other viruses- adenovirus, herpes simplex, Epstein-Barr, CMV	Similar to infectious mononucleosis.	Similar to infectious mononucleosis.	Peripheral smear; monocytosis. Paul-Bunnell negative. Throat swab negative.
6.	Vincent's angina	No fever and constitutional disturbances.	Ulcero-membranous lesions on gums, spreading to buccal mucosa & tonsils.	Stained smear: spirochaetes and fusiform bacilli.
7.	Agranulocytosis, Aplastic anaemia, Acute leukaemia	Fever, pallor, bleeding manifestations.	Necrotic ulcers in mouth and throat.	Peripheral blood smear. Bone marrow.

Table 52.2 COMPLICATIONS OF DIPHTHERIA

Time	Complication	Management
1st week	Nasal bleeding. Hoarse voice, stridor (watch for laryngeal obstruction). Disproportionate tachycardia, fall of blood pressure (myocarditis), peripheral circulatory failure.	Be in readiness for tracheostomy.
2nd week	Arrhythmia (atrial tibrillation), congestive heart failure. Paralysis of palate, nasal regurgitation, usually at 10 days. Paralysis of accommodation, difficulty in reading small print.	Digitalis. Feeding via nasogastric tube and reassurance about complete recovery.
3rd week	Multiple neuritis, watch for paralysis of diaphragm and respiratory muscles (counting ten aloud).	Reassurance about complete recovery. Be ready with mechanical ventilator.

If there is no contraindication as above,

4000–8000 units IM inj. are given in a mild case

16,000–32,000 units IM inj. are given to a moderately severe case.

100,000 units IV are given to a severe case.

In addition to antiserum, phenoxymethyl penicillin should be given for one week to eliminate the organisms from the throat. Erythromycin is given to those patients who are allergic to penicillin.

If the patient has not already received immunization against tetanus, tetanus toxoid should be given now.

53 Splenomegaly

The spleen is a lympho-reticular organ that serves at least four major physiological functions:

1. *Immune system:* major site of clearance of micro-organisms and particulate antigens from blood stream, and generation of humoral and cellular immune response to foreign antigens. The importance of this function is seen in the proneness of splenectomized patients to life-threatening infections.

2. Sequestration: removal of normal senescent and abnormal blood cells.

3. Regulation of portal blood flow.

4. Extramedullary erythropoiesis when bone marrow is replaced or overstimulated to respond.

There are six basic pathophysiological mechanisms of splenic enlargement:

1. Immune system hyperplasia:
   (a) infections e.g. bacterial endocarditis.
   (b) autoimmune diseases e.g. Felty syndrome.
   (c) destruction of abnormal red cells: hereditary spherocytosis, thalassaemia, sickle cell disease.

2. Disordered splenic blood flow e.g. cirrhosis.

3. Malignant neoplasms: lymphoma, angiosarcoma, leukaemia.

4. Extramedullary erythropoiesis: myeloid metaplasia.

5. Infiltration with abnormal material: amyloidosis, Gaucher's Disease.

6. Space-occupying lesions e.g. haemangiomas, cysts.

Approach to a Patient with Enlarged Spleen

A normal-sized spleen is about 12 cm long and 7 cm wide. Because of its oblique orientation in the abdominal cavity, its long axis lies behind and parallel to the 10th rib in the mid-axillary line, with the splenic width located between the 9th and 11th ribs; therefore to percuss for splenic dullness, the patient lies on his right side and the left 9th intercostal space is located by finding the tip of the scapula lying in the 7th intercostal space and counting down to the 9th intercostal space. Dullness outside the 9th and 11th intercostal spaces suggests splenomegaly, although fluid in the stomach or faeces in the colon can cause dullness in the splenic area.

Palpation of the left upper quadrant for splenic enlargement is done with the patient supine or lying on his right side. The examiner's left hand is placed under the lower thorax grasping the lower rib posteriorly. The examiner's right hand is kept steady with the patient taking deep breaths to permit the examiner to feel the inferior tip of an enlarged spleen. To avoid missing a massively enlarged spleen, palpation of the left upper quadrant should begin in the lower abdominal cavity with gradual movement up to the left upper quadrant.

Physical examination may miss mild to moderate splenomegaly especially in obese patients. Radionuclide colloid liver-spleen scan or ultrasound of the left upper quadrant are more reliable methods for documenting splenomegaly in such situations. Imaging techniques provide additional information such as the presence of cysts, infarct or tumours, or in defining accessory splenic tissue or residual splenic tissue following splenic rupture (splenosis). It is useful to consider splenomegaly in (a) an acute setting; (b) a chronic setting.

Acute left upper quadrant pain with an enlarged tender spleen suggests subcapsular haematoma, splenic infarct, or splenic rupture. This can occur from direct or remote trauma, infectious mononucleosis, malaria, or typhoid fever. Splenic infarcts can occur due to sickle cell disease, or emboli from bacterial endocarditis, or atrial myxoma.

Acute febrile illness with splenomegaly suggest bacterial endocarditis, infectious mononucleosis, typhoid or tuberculosis.

Fever, lymphadenopathy and splenomegaly with or without a rash or arthralgia suggest infectious mononucleosis, sarcoidosis, SLE, serum sickness or lymphoma.

An acute illness with splenomegaly associated with signs and symptoms of anaemia, with or without bleeding, suggests leukaemia, autoimmune haemolytic anaemia, or myeloproliferative syndrome.

Splenomegaly in a chronic setting suggests a wide range of disorders, many of which are listed in **Table 53.1**. Liver disease with portal hypertension is a common cause. The patient may be asymptomatic and the condition may be discovered during a routine physical examination.

With the clinical features of rheumatoid arthritis and leucopenia, Felty's syndrome should be considered.

The presence of lymphadenopathy along with splenomegaly suggests chronic lymphocytic leukaemia or lymphoma. Plethora and an elevated haematocrit suggest polycythaemia vera or chronic lung disease with right-sided heart failure and congestive splenomegaly.

Weight loss or other signs of chronic illness suggest myeloproliferative syndromes, or leukaemia, or haemoglobinopathies.

Hypersplenism

This refers to any clinical situation in which an enlarged spleen removes excessive numbers of RBCs (anaemia), granulocytes (neutropenia) or platelets (thrombocytopenia). The bone marrow tries to compensate for the excessive destruction

TABLE 53.1 CAUSES OF SPLENOMEGALY

Disease	Mechanism	Important examples
I. Infection	Reticulo-endothelial or immune system hyperplasia in response to a variety of micro-organisms, macrophage, T & B cell proliferation.	Infectious mononucleosis, bacterial endocarditis, septicaemia, malaria, tuberculosis, leishmaniasis (kala azar), viral hepatitis, AIDS.
II. Immunological injury and autoimmune diseases	Lymphoid hyperplasia.	Felty's syndrome (variant of RA), SLE, immune haemolytic anaemias, serum sickness & drug reactions.
III. Diseases with abnormal RBCs	Hypersequestration and destruction of abnormal red cells, Pooling in sinuses, pulp cords.	Hereditary spherocytosis, ovalocytosis, thalassaemia, sickle cell disease.
IV. Diseases with disordered splenic blood flow	Chronic passive venous congestion of increased portal venous pressure or portal venous obstruction.	Cirrhosis liver with portal hypertension, hepatic vein obstruction, hepatic schistosomiasis, portal vein obstruction, splenic vein obstruction, chronic congestive heart failure.
V. Infiltrative disorders	Focal or generalized increase in white pulp.	Benign.
VI. Miscellaneous	Unknown mechanism of lymphoid hyperplasia.	Iron deficiency anaemia, sarcoidosis, berylliosis, thyrotoxicosis.

by undergoing hyperplasia with normal representation of the cell-line deficient in the circulation, and showing increased turnover of the cell-line affected Le. reticulocytosis, increased band forms of neutrophils, or circulating immature platelet forms.

If the underlying disorder responsible for hypersplenism cannot be corrected, splenectomy is an option.

Indications for Splenectomy

1. Splenic trauma.

2. Haemolytic anaemias:
   Hereditary spherocytosis and elliptocytosis;
   Thalassaemia with increased transfusion requirements;
   Thrombocytopenia;
   Immune haemolytic A with warm IgG antibody;
   Pyruvate kinase deficiency.

3. Staging laparotomy for Hodgkin's disease with splenectomy.

4. Hypersplenism (lymphoma, B cell hairy leukaemia, Felty's syndrome) (CLL, CML, myeloid metaplasia).

Hyposplenism

Sickle cell anaemia patients may undergo repeated splenic infarcts leading to autosplenectomy. Persistence of a palpable spleen after the age of 5 years in a patient with sickle cell disease suggests associated thalassaemia.

Findings in the peripheral blood that indicate hyposplenism include the presence of nucleated red cells, Heinz bodies and Howell Jolly bodies, target cells, and burr cells.

These patients, as well as the splenectomized patients are prone to frequent, overwhelming, and life-threatening bacterial infections (pneumococcus, meningococcus, E. coli, H. influenzae). Immunization with pneumococcal vaccine is recommended in hyposplenie patients older than two years and prior to elective splenectomy.

Thyroid Diseases

A patient may present to the doctor with the complaint of a swelling in the front of the neck, or the doctor may notice a thyroid swelling while he is examining a patient for some other complaint; the patient may not be aware of it, and on checking, has no accompanying complaints suggestive of thyroid dysfunction.

That the swelling in the neck is related to the thyroid is established by giving the patient a sip of water to swallow, and noticing whether the swelling moves with deglutition.

The next step is to assess whether the thyroid swelling is associated with (a) deficient hormonal activity (hypothyroid); or (b) excessive hormonal activity (hyperthyroid); or (c) normal hormonal activity (euthyroid). This is done by asking the patient certain key questions and looking for certain crucial signs in the physical examination. These are given in **Table 54.1** and **Table 54.2**. **Table 54.3** lists causes of hypothyroidism and **Table 54.4** lists causes of thyrotoxicosis which can occur with or without associated hyperthyroidism.

Euthyroid goitre is a common condition, particularly during puberty and adolescence, and during pregnancy especially in regions of iodine deficiency.

Examination of the Thyroid Gland

Movement on swallowing is characteristic of the thyroid gland. but this movement may be lost if the goitre is very large occupying the whole space in the neck, or is fixed to underlying tissues as in malignancy or Riedel's thyroiditis.

A swelling in the mid-line of the neck in front, which moves up on protrusion of the tongue is indicative of a thyroglossal cyst.

TABLE **54.1 SYMPTOMS AND SIGNS OF HYPOTHYROIDISM**

(Arranged in the order of frequency of occurrence)

Symptoms

Weakness	99%
Lethargy	91%
Sensation of cold	89%
Decreased sweating	89%
Memory impairment	66%
Constipation	66%
Weight gain	59%
Loss of hair	57%
Dyspnoea	55%
Anorexia	45%
Nervousness	35%
Menorrhagia	32%
Palpitations	31%
Precordial pain	25%

Signs

Dry skin	97%
Coarse skin	97%
Slow speech	91%
Oedema of eyelids	90%
Cold skin	83%
Thick tongue	82%
Oedema of face	79%
Coarse hair	76%
Pallor of skin	67%
Pallor of lips	57%
Peripheral oedema	55%
Hoarseness	52%
Deafness	30%
Stiff and painful muscles	25%

TABLE 54.2 SYMPTOMS AND SIGNS OF HYPERTHYROIDISM

(Arranged in the order of frequency of occurrence)

Symptoms	%
Nervousness	99
Increased sweating	91
Heat intolerance	89
Palpitations	89
Fatigue	88
Weight loss	85
Dyspnoea	75
Weakness	70
Increased appetite	65
Frequency of stools	33
Diarrhoea	23
Anorexia	9
Constipation	4
Weight gain	2

Signs	
Tachycardia	100
Fine tremors	97
Bruit over gland	77
Eye signs	71
Swelling of legs	35
Atrial fibrillation	10
Gynaecomastia	10
Splenomegaly	10
Liver palms (erythema)	8

Palpation of the thyroid is best undertaken standing behind the seated patient and palpating with the fingertips of both hands. The feel of the normal gland, diffuse colloid goitre, and Graves' disease is smooth and soft, while the Hashimoto gland is firm; Riedel's thyroiditis and cancer may feel stony hard. Irregularities of the surface, variations in consistency (solid, cystic) and tender areas should be noted. If nodules are palpable, their shape, size, position and consistency in comparison with the surrounding tissue should be noted. Palpation should always include the regional lymph nodes.

TABLE 54.3 CAUSES OF HYPOTHYROIDISM

Thyroprivic	Post-ablative
	Primary idiopathic
	Sporadic athyreotic cretinism
	(Thyroid aplasia/dysplasia)
Trophoprivic	Sheehan's syndrome
	Infiltrative disorders of pituitary or hypothalamus
Goitrous	Hashimoto thyroiditis
	Endemic iodine deficiency
	Antithyroid agents
	PAS, phenylbutazone, resorcinol lithium, cassava cruciferous plants
	Iodide goitre and hypothyroidism
	Heritable defects of hormone synthesis
	Peripheral resistance to thyroid hormones (may be nongoitrous)

TABLE 54.4 VARIETIES OF THYROTOXICOSIS

A. *Hyperthyroidism (RAIU high)*
   1. Graves' Disease
   2. Toxic multinodular goitre
   3. Toxic adenoma
   4. Iodine-induced (Jed Basedow)
   5. Trophoblastic tumour: Choriocarcinoma
                             Hydatidiform mole
   6. Increased TSH secretion: hypothalamic/pituitary 'Graves' disease'.

B. *Not associated with hyperthyroidism (RAIU low)*
   1. Subacute thyroiditis.
   2. Chronic thyroiditis with transient thyrotoxicosis (painless thyroiditis).
   3. Ectopic thyroid tissue (struma ovarii, functioning metastases).
   4. Factitious thyrotoxicosis: Exogenous administration of thyroxine.

During palpation a vascular thrill may be felt. Auscultation of the neck should be performed because it gives some indication of the vascularity of the gland. A systolic or continuous bruit is commonly heard over the hyperplastic gland of Graves' disease or the rare dyshormonogenesis syndromes. Care should be taken to distinguish a thyroid bruit from a carotid artery murmur transmitted from the aortic valve, and from a venous *hum* (that can be obliterated by compression of the external jugular veins, or by turning the head). Bruits and thrills do not occur in simple goitre.

Transillumination of the gland is readily performed with a pen light and serves to distinguish between a cystic and solid mass in the thyroid. The transillumination in the lesion should be compared with that in an indifferent area.

The arm-raising test is useful when retrosternal extension of a goitre is suspected. Raising both the arms until they touch the sides of the head will further narrow the thoracic inlet and cause congestion of the face and respiratory distress (Pemberton sign).

Position of the trachea and evidence of compression of adjacent structures should be sought. Hoarseness of voice may indicate compression of the recurrent laryngeal nerve, usually by a malignant thyroid neoplasm, and this should be confirmed by laryngoscopy. Inspiratory stridor may indicate compression of the trachea.

Eye signs in Graves' disease are described in **Table 54.5**. Occasionally unilateral or bilateral exophthalmos may be a *presenting feature* of Graves' disease before the thyroid signs are manifest. Or the eye signs may appear following the therapy of Graves' disease. The natural course of Graves' ophthalmopathy is independent of the clinical course of Graves' disease itself.

TABLE 54.5 EYE CHANGES IN GRAVES' DISEASE

Class	Definition
0	No physical signs or symptoms
1	Only signs: upper lid retraction, lid lag, proptosis to 22 mm
2	Soft tissue involvement
3	Proptosis more than 22 mm
4	Extra-ocular muscle involvement
5	Corneal involvement
6	Sight loss (optic nerve involvement)

SOURCE: American Thyroid Association

Clinical Evaluation

It is worth emphasizing that clinical evaluation based on history and physical examination alone, has a high degree of sensitivity, specificity, and predictive value in the diagnosis of thyroid dysfunction. However, one must beware of the tricky situations in hyperthyroidism.

1. 'Apathetic' rather than 'hyperactive' Graves' disease.
2. No thyromegaly, no eye signs.
3. Presentation with atrial fibrillation alone.
4. Presentation with congestive heart failure alone.
5. Presentation with muscular weakness alone.
6. Presentation with diarrhoea alone.
7. Presentation with weight loss alone.

A useful common clue is resting or sleeping tachycardia for which there is no other explanation (fever, anaemia etc).

Hypothyroidism often begins so insidiously that it can be easily missed by persons who see the patient daily (including the family doctor), while it strikes someone seeing the patient for the first time, as very abnormal. Hypothyroidism is the commonest endocrine disorder which is missed by doctors. Hypothyroidism is also the commonest mis-diagnosis for a middle-aged female who is putting on weight and feeling tired. If she says she loves winter and hates summer, and if she is comfortable in an air conditioned room for half an hour, hypothyroidism is out of consideration.

Slow relaxation of the Achilles tendon reflex is a very useful (but not pathognomonic) physical sign in hypothyroidism. Other causes of slow relaxation are given in **Table 54.6**.

In the evaluation of a goitre, it is useful to have a plain X-ray of the thoracic inlet which may reveal displacement or narrowing of the trachea due to retrosternal extension of the goitre. During a barium swallow displacement of the oesophagus may be seen. Calcification of the thyroid gland may be seen on the plain X-ray and, by its nature, aids in distinguishing between benign and malignant lesions. Cyst walls are often calcified in a linear fashion.

TABLE 54.6 CAUSES OF DELAYED ACHILLES REFLEX TIME

Hypothyroidism: 90% with moderate or severe disease

Diabetes mellitus

Pernicious anaemia

Anorexia nervosa

Oedematous states

Peripheral vascular disease

Hypothermia of any cause

Drugs:	Morphine
	Propranolol
	Quinidine
	Procainamide

The differential diagnosis of a single nodule is given in **Table 54.7** and the evaluation of a solitary nodule is given in **Table 54.8**. A rapidly growing non-tender nodule should be highly suspect for malignancy.

Investigation of Thyroid Disease

The doctor seeks two types of information from the thyroid tests of which there are a large number available.

A. *Tests that document function:* hyperfunction, hypofunction, or normal function

    I. Measurement of T_3, T_4, TSH

    II. Radioactive iodine uptake (RAIU)

  *III. Technetium-99m TcO_4 uptake and scan

    IV. Stimulation by exogenous TSH

B. *Tests that help to determine specific aetiopathology*

    V. Tests for antibodies

    VI. Tests for thyroglobulin

    VII. PBI and BEI

    VIII. Fluorescent scanning

    IX. Ultrasound

    X. Fine needle aspiration cytology (FNAC)

*Technetium uptake and scanning gives both A & B types of information.

TABLE 54.7 DIFFERENTIAL DIAGNOSIS OF A SOLITARY THYROID NODULE

Primary thyroid lesion	*Non-thyroid lesion*
Adenoma	Lymphadenopathy
Carcinoma	Parathyroid adenoma
Cyst	Cystic hygroma
Focal Hashimoto	Bronchocoele
Thyroglossal duct cyst	Laryngocoele
Thyroid hemiagenesis	Carotid aneurysm
Prior hemithyroidectomy	Metastases
Lymphoma	

TABLE 54.8 INITIAL EVALUATION OF A SOLITARY THYROID NODULE

History	Radiation to face or neck during childhood
	Family history of tumour
	Recent change in size
	Hypothyroidism or Hashimoto thyroiditis
	Thyrotoxicosis
Physical examination	Thyroid status
	Tracheal deviation
	Hoarseness
	Single vs multiple nodules
	Fixation, consistency, tenderness
	Lymphadenopathy
Laboratory tests	T_3 T_4 TSH
	Thyroid microsomal antibodies
	Serum calcitonin (medullary carcinoma)
	Needle aspiration

I. *Measurement of Hormones in the Blood*

Normal range: Tri-iodothyronine (T_3): 88-193 ng/dl
                Thyroxine (T_4): 5.4-13.4 µg/dl
                Thyroid stimulating hormone
                (TSH): 0.5-5 mIU/ml

i. The normal range of T_3 and T_4 is wide, hence it is possible for an individual patient's level to rise two-fold or fall to half the original level, and yet be 'within the normal range'.

ii. The blood level of hormones is determined by the amount of binding proteins. **Table 54.9** lists conditions of increased and decreased T_4 binding, which may give the erroneous impression of 'hyper' or 'hypo' thyroidism looking at the T_4

TABLE 54.9 CAUSES OF ALTERATION IN BINDING OF T$_4$ BY TBG	
Increased binding	*Decreased binding*
Pregnancy	Androgens
Oral contraceptives	Anabolic steroids
Oestrogens	Large dose glucocorticoids
Tamoxifen	Acute acromegaly
Acute intermittent	Nephrotic syndrome
porphyria	Major systemic illness
Infectious hepatitis	Asparaginase
Chronic active hepatitis	Genetic defect
HIV infection	
Perphenazine	
Neonatal state	
Genetic defect	
Significance	*Significance*
RIA of T$_4$: *high level*	RIA of T$_4$: *low level*
may be misinterpreted as	may be misinterpreted as
'Thyrotoxicosis'	'Hypothyroidism'
(but *free* T4 normal);	(but *free* T4 normal);
TSH normal	TSH normal

figures alone, but the 'free' hormones–'free T$_4$' and 'free T$_3$' are normal (i.e. are not affected by changes in binding proteins).

iii. T$_3$ is mostly derived from peripheral conversion of T$_4$. **Table 54.10** lists the physiological, pathological and pharmacological factors which impair peripheral conversion of T$_4$ to T$_3$. The resultant low T$_3$ level in the blood may give an erroneous impression of hypothyroidism.

For all these reasons it is good strategy always to combine the estimation of T$_3$ and T$_4$ with TSH, which together are more informative than doing each one alone.

(a) TSH is very sensitive to the rise and fall of free T$_4$ and free T$_3$. Thus T$_3$ and T$_4$ levels at lower limits of the normal, combined with higher than normal TSH indicate diminished thyroid reserve or subclinical hypothyroidism. The same T$_3$ and T$_4$ values with a normal TSH indicate the euthyroid state.

(b) TSH is not affected by changes in thyroxine binding proteins, thus a high T$_4$ with normal TSH would indicate probable increased binding, while a low T$_4$ with normal TSH indicates decreased binding.

TABLE 54.10 FACTORS THAT IMPAIR PERIPHERAL CONVERSION OF T$_4$ TO T$_3$	
Physiological	Foetal and early neonatal life
	Old age
Pathological	Fasting, malnutrition
	Hepatic or renal dysfunction
	Systemic illness
	Trauma
	Post-operative state
Pharmacological	Drugs:
	Propylthiouracil
	Glucocorticoids
	Propranolol
	Amiodarone
	Oral cholecystographic agents

(c) Low T$_3$ with normal TSH would indicate 'euthyroid sickness' due to non-thyroid illness. If a reverse T$_3$ (r T$_3$) is estimated in these conditions it would be found to be high but this estimation is not clinically necessary.

Table 54.11 summarizes the various disease states indicated by routinely combining T$_3$ and T$_4$ with a super-sensitive TSH assay.

Patients with primary hypothyroidism have elevated TSH that can range from 15 to 100 mIU/L. In general there is a correlation between the degree of TSH elevation and the clinical symptoms. Patients with values in the range of 6–15 mIU/L have few if any symptoms since their T$_3$ level is normal, T$_4$ level may be low normal or even slightly reduced.

Patients with hypopituitary or hypothalamic hypothyroidism generally have normal or slightly elevated TSH. In thyrotoxic patients TSH levels are often unmeasurable (less than 0.1 mIU/L).

Accurate measurement of both elevated and suppressed TSH have led to the suggestion that TSH by IRMA (immunoradiometric assay) could be used as a *single* screening test for *all* thyroid cases. There are two limitations to this approach. (i) a number of significantly ill individuals who do not have primary hypothyroidism have elevated TSH; (ii) hospitalized patients receiving dopamine and glucosteroids may have suppressed TSH in the absence of hyperthyroidism.

TABLE 54.11 USEFULNESS OF RIA OF T_3 T_4 & TSH IN 5780 PATIENTS

Group	T_3	T_4	TSH	Comments
1.	Normal	Normal	Normal	Euthyroid
2.	High	High	Low	Classical Graves' disease
3.	High	High	High	'Hypothalamic' Graves' End-organ insensitivity
4.	High	Normal	Low	T_3 toxicosis
5.	High	Normal	Normal	Euthyroid goitre
6.	Normal	High	Low	T_4 toxicosis or exogenous thyroxine
7.	Low	Normal	Normal	Euthyroid sick
8.	Normal	Low	High	Subclinical hypothyroid
9.	Low	Low	High	Primary hypothyroidism
10.	Low	Low	Low	Hypopituitarism*
11.	Normal	Normal ±	High ±	Monitoring thyroxine therapy
				* Ca. breast on androgen.

II. RAIU (Radioactive Iodine Uptake)

The rate of uptake of radioiodine by the thyroid gland is a direct measure of thyroid function. With the routine availability of RIA of T_3 T_4 and TSH, RAIU today is indicated in only certain special situations. In a patient with clinical thyrotoxicosis the RAIU is expected to be very high.

A *low RAIU* in that context indicates:

1. Exogenous thyroid administration.
2. Iodine-induced hyperthyroidism.
3. Subacute thyroiditis with transient thyrotoxicosis.
4. Struma ovarii: extrathyroidal source of hormone.

RAIU can also be used to demonstrate a defect in organification of the trapped iodine. Normally when radioiodine enters the thyroid gland it does not come out, hence there is no fall in the neck counts after administration of perchlorate. A drop in the neck counts ('perchlorate washout') indicates on organification defect typically seen in Hashimoto's disease and in one variety of dyshormonogenesis.

III. Tc-99m uptake test

Technetium-99m is a pure gamma emitting radionuclide with a short half life of 6 hours; hence it gives very little radiation dose to the thyroid (unlike I-131 which has undesirable B emissions). The Technetium TcO_4 ion enters the thyroid gland similar to iodine, although it does not participate any further in thyroid metabolism. Its entry into the gland is essentially unchanged even if the next step of organification is blocked. Hence an accurate measure of trapping function can be obtained even if the patient is on antithyroid drugs.

1. Carotid-to-thyroid transit time:
   Normal 2.5 to 7.5 seconds
   Hyperthyroid 0–2.5 seconds
2. Initial trapping curve:
   Normal plateau at 3 minutes
   Hyperthyroid continuous rise
   Hypothyroid very poor rise
3. 20 minute Technetium uptake (% of injected dose):
   Normal range is 1–2%. The value is higher in hyperthyroidism. In a hyperthyroid patient on anti-thyroid drugs, suppression of uptake indicates that medication may be curtailed or terminated.

Thyroid imaging

Graves' disease: increased; No salivary glands seen
Hypothyroid: No clear image; Salivary glands seen
Thyroiditis: No tracer in thyroid; Salivary glands visualized

The 20 minutes-Tc-image clearly defines the three causes of hyperthyroidism:

Graves' disease: Diffuse uniform increased tracer

Toxic multi-nodular goitre: 'Hot' and 'cold' areas
Toxic nodule: 'Hot' nodule, rest of gland not seen

IV. *Stimulation by exogenous TSH*

   i. To determine if absence of tracer accumulation in one lobe (as seen on scanning), is due to agenesis of a lobe or suppression due to a toxic adenoma.

   ii. To determine before surgery whether the remaining thyroid tissue will be able to resume function after removal of a toxic adenoma.

   iii. To determine if potential for thyroid function exists in a patient taking full replacement dose of thyroxine, to establish or exclude a diagnosis. of thyroprivic hypothyroidism.

V. *Tests for antibodies*

   i. Anti-thyroglobulin antibodies

   ii. Anti-microsomal (thyroid peroxidase) antibodies

   iii. Antibody to a colloid antigen distinct from thyroglobulin

   iv. Antibody to a nuclear component of thyroid cells

Nos. i and ii are commonly carried out. Presence of autoimmune antibodies indicates the possibility of Graves' disease, Hashimoto's disease, or subacute thyroiditis.

In young patients no. i is positive in only about 50 per cent of patients with other evidence of Hashimoto's disease.

In adult patients no. i is positive in 85 per cent and no. ii in 99 per cent.

In Graves' disease no. i is positive in 30 per cent and no. ii in 80 per cent.

A somewhat lower figure is seen in primary hypothyroidism.

Presence of antibodies in ophthalmopathy indicates autoimmune origin rather than an orbital or intracranial tumour.

In women with Graves' disease or Hashimoto's disease, antibodies decrease during pregnancy and increase transiently after delivery, peaking at 3-4 months; this may explain postpartum thyroiditis.

VI. *Tests for thyroglobulin*

Distinct elevation of thyroglobulin (TG) is seen in:

1. Goitre and thyroid hyperfunction (Plummer's disease)

2. Inflammation or physical injury (subacute thyroiditis)

3. Differentiated thyroid cancer

The major clinical value of TG is not for diagnosis but for monitoring the treatment of differentiated thyroid cancer. After removal of the tumour, TG values drop to the normal range and remain so if metastatic disease is not present. Elevation of TG while suppressive thyroxine therapy is being given suggests the presence of residual local cancer or metastatic cancer.

VII. *PBI and BEI*

A high PBI (Protein bound iodine) with normal T_3 and T_4 is suggestive of non-hormonal iodine components (MIT, DIT) seen in dyshormonogenesis, or abnormal thyroglobulin and iodoalbumin as seen in Hashimoto's disease and thyroid malignancy.

VIII. *Fluorescent scanning*

In this technique an exciting radiation beam of photons from an Americium-241 source causes fluorescence in the stable iodine in the, thyroid gland, which is imaged. Benign nodules contain a significant amount of iodine whereas malignant nodules contain less iodine–both are seen as 'cold' nodules on radionuclide scanning. The Hashimoto gland is characteristica1ly found to be devoid of iodine.

IX. *Ultrasonography*

This helps to determine the nature of a 'cold' nodule seen on radionuclide imaging–solid vs cystic. The typical findings of a benign cyst include an echo-free area, sharp backwall, and increased echo behind the cyst. Approximately 20 per cent of single nodules turn out to be benign cysts, which can be aspirated under ultrasonographic guidance.

X. *FNAC*

FNAC (fine needle aspiration cytology) provides the opportunity of morphological confirmation of malignancy and Hashimoto's disease with a

TABLE 54.12 TREATMENT OPTIONS FOR HYPERTHYROIDISM

Patient group	Anti-thyroid drugs	I-131	Surgery
1. Neonatal	+	−	−
2. Juvenile	+	+++	+
3. Young female non-pregnant	+	+++	+
4. Young female pregnant	++++	−	+
5. Male	+	++++	+
6. Elderly	+	++++	−
7. Coexistent nodule	−	−	++++
8. Pressure symptoms & signs	−	−	++++

TABLE 54.13 FACTORS FAVOURING LONG-TERM REMISSION AFTER ANTI-THYROID THERAPY FOR DIFFUSE GOITRE

T3 toxicosis
Small goitre
Decrease in goitre size during therapy
Normal thyroid function tests
Normal serum TSH
Negative tests for Ig of Graves' disease

hazard-free outpatient procedure. It has a reported accuracy of 95 per cent. The problem of sampling error is common to all FNAC procedures, since only 100 cells out of a billion are available for study. No information about invasion of the capsule (indicative of malignancy) is available with FNAC. A positive result for malignancy leads to surgery. A Hashimoto gland should be left alone by the surgeon. If the result is negative or inconclusive, malignancy is not ruled out. Watching the size of the nodule on eltroxin suppressive therapy for three months is a safe policy. In young males, rapidly growing nodules should be excised immediately.

Treatment options in thyrotoxicosis are given in **Table 54.12**. Factors favouring long-term remission after antithyroid therapy for diffuse goitre are listed in **Table 54.13**.

I-131 Treatment for Hyperthyroidism

Radioactive iodine I-131 was first used to treat Graves' disease in 1941 in the USA. The ability to cure a major disorder by a single sip of a medicine represented a landmark in the history of therapeutics. In the subsequent five decades, over a million patients worldwide have received I-131 treatment which today is the most cost-effective option among all therapeutic modalities available. The main problem with I-131 therapy (5-10 mCi dose) is the probable development of hypothyroidism in the subsequent 5-10 years, in about 70 per cent of patients. Hence the physician giving I-131 should be committed to monitor for and treat subsequent hypothyroidism with eltroxin.

Anti-thyroid drugs (mainly neomercazol in India) effectively control the symptoms of Graves' disease in short-term by reducing the formation of thyroxine and lowering the plasma concentration of T_3 and T_4. In Graves' disease the drug has to be given for a minimum period of 6-12 months. On stopping the drug there is a 50 per cent chance of relapse necessitating prolonged continuation of drug therapy. Relapse can be predicated by high levels of TSI (Thyroid stimulating immunoglobulin) which is a stimulating antibody to the TSH receptor. High TSI with subnormal TSH in the presence of normal T3 and T4 in the serum predicts a relapse. This test is not widely available.

The rationale of adding thyroxine to antithyroid drugs is to decrease the release of thyroid antigen by TSH. Improved results have been reported when thyroxine was added to carbimazole.

Anti-thyroid drugs need medical supervision and monitoring for side effects which can occasionally be life-threatening, viz agranulocytosis and hepatitis. In solitary toxic nodules and toxic multinodular goitre, anti-thyroid drugs probably never produce long-term remissions hence for these conditions surgery or I-131 are the therapeutic options.

Surgery is the preferred modality for treating very large glands with pressure symptoms and retrosternal goitre. Further, such goitres may harbour unsuspected cancer hence these are preferably treated by surgery.

The fear of carcinogenesis, mutagenesis and teratogenesis due to I-131 has been proved to be unfounded as shown by 50 years' experience, hence the age restriction on the use of I-131 (previously age 40 and above) was removed in Britain in 1983. Although the general policy is to treat young patients at presentation with a 12-month course of anti-thyroid drugs and to use I-131 for relapse I-131 is found increasingly useful in the initial management of young patients, including children.

I-131 should not be given for Graves' disease in pregnancy. If steps are taken to ensure that the patient is not pregnant at the time of I-131 therapy and she avoids pregnancy for the next 6 months, there is no risk of any harm for a subsequent pregnancy.

I-131 in high doses (100-300 mCi) is the preferred treatment for metastases from well-differentiated thyroid carcinoma, after its surgical removal.

55 Weakness

Patients and physicians may use the words 'weakness', lassitude, fatigue, lethargy, tiredness, asthenia, and listlessness, more or less interchangeably. For diagnosis, it is useful to distinguish between three different entities–weakness, fatigue and tiredness.

Weakness: is a reduction in the strength or force of muscle contraction. The gastrocnemius of a normal person can easily support his body weight hence he can rise on his toes. If a person cannot do this, his gastrocnemius is weak. If he cannot stand up from a squatting position without the support of his hands, his pelvic girdle muscles are weak. If he cannot raise himself from bed in a prone position with the help of his hands then his pectoral girdle muscles are weak.

Table 55.1 gives the causes of generalized weakness, and **Table 55.2** the causes of localized weakness.

Fatigue: is a reduction in the force of muscular contraction with repeated effort. It is a normal phenomenon. If a normal person can rise on his toes one hundred times before fatigue sets in, and another man is able to do this only ten times, the latter is suffering from abnormal fatigue or easy fatiguability. This is revealed in tasks requiring sustained effort (e.g. ironing, shaving, grooming the hair). This typically happens in 'pulseless disease' (Takayashu syndrome), where the arm gets fatigued while bathing.

Tiredness: is the feeling associated with or following sustained physical activity. It is the subjective feeling of lethargy and listlessness. This may bear no close relationship to weakness or fatigue. Thus a person may feel tired constantly and yet be able to rise on his toes a hundred times. Another may be unable to rise on his toes at all and yet does not feel tired.

Demonstrable weakness almost always indicates organic disease. Double vision, drooping of the eyelids, difficulty in swallowing, aspiration of food or liquids during swallowing, are all important objective evidence of true muscle weakness.

On the other hand, complaints of tiredness without demonstrable weakness are most likely due to emotional illness.

Easy fatigue: is more difficult to interpret since it can accompany actual weakness or may accompany a feeling of tiredness.

It is important to ascertain that the patient's complaints are not due to stiffness, or clumsiness, or pain on movement, or difficulty in initiating movement, which he may attribute to 'weakness'.

Causes of Weakness

Weakness, fatigue and pain in the muscles are common accompaniments of derangement of endocrine, cardiac, pulmonary, hepatic, renal, gastrointestinal, or haematological function, essentially mediated through the disturbance of sodium, potassium, calcium, magnesium and phosphorus homeostasis. These are listed in **Table 55.1**. Neuromuscular causes of weakness are listed in **Table 55.2** along with their typical diagnostic features and important disease entities causing them.

Drug-induced myopathies are listed in **Table 55.3**.

Analysis of History Items

The history will usually reveal the site and distribution of weakness–e.g. limited to one or two-fingers, one hand, proximal or distal limb, or one-half of the body or the entire body. The onset and progression of weakness–acute, subacute, slowly progressive, recurrent etc are to be elicited

Acute generalized weakness, developing over the course of less than an hour is usually caused by a metabolic or toxic disorder affecting either the neuromuscular junction or muscles. Botulism and other toxins, aminoglycoside antibiotics and other drugs can produce acute failure of neurotransmission.

Weakness developing over the course of 24 hours may occur in electrolyte, metabolic and toxic disorders and in acute inflammatory myopathies particularly those related to viral and parasitic infections and acute polyneuropathies and paralytic poliomyelitis.

Subacute weakness, developing over days, may indicate poliomyelitis, Guillain-Barre syndrome, porphyria, diphtheria, polymyositis or dermatomyositis. It is also a feature of Addison's disease, and Sheehan's syndrome.

Slowly progressive weakness, involving the proximal muscles, indicates nutritional and alcoholic polyneuropathy, deficiency of vitamins (thiamin, niacin), polymyositis, dermatomyositis or unsuspected endocrinopathy or diabetic proximal mononeuropathy. Proximal muscle weakness is very characteristic of myopathies, but neuropathies such as acute and chronic inflammatory and nutritional polyneuropathy, neuromuscular junction disorder (Lambert-Eaton syndrome) and many anterior horn cell lesions produce predominantly proximal muscle weakness. Hyperparathyroidism, hyperthyroidism and high dose glucocorticoid therapy also cause proximal muscle weakness.

Slowly progressive weakness involving the distal muscles indicates peripheral neuropathy or anterior horn cell lesions or myotonic dystrophy.

Intermittent weakness is a frequent complaint (e.g. potassium loss following diarrhoea or thiazide diuretics) but disorders that cause intermittent or periodic paralysis are not. The challenge is to determine the diagnosis of periodic paralysis by history alone since the physical examination is normal between the attacks.

Primary periodic paralysis is a rare but intriguing disease inherited as an autosomal dominant trait. Symptoms usually begin early in life, usually in adolescence, and rarely commence after age 25.

Attacks typically follow rest or sleep and almost never occur in the midst of vigorous activity. The patient remains alert during the attack.

The hypokalaemic variety is precipitated by meals of high carbohydrate or sodium content. The reflexes are hypoactive. Cardiac arrhythmias or respiratory muscle paralysis may prove fatal.

The hyperkalaemic and normokalaemic varieties are potassium sensitive, and attacks are precipitated by exercise, exposure to cold, pregnancy, or administration of potassium.

Usually patients recover fully after an attack of periodic paralysis. However, permanent weakness may develop after repeated attacks.

Muscle Pain

Muscle pain is common in bone, joint and neuromuscular disease as also in inflammatory and metabolic muscle disease.

The useful questions to ask are:

- Is the pain persistent or intermittent?
- Is it precipitated by exercise or fasting?

Intermittent muscle pain, particularly when precipitated by exercise or fasting indicates a substrate utilization defect such as glycogen or lipid storage myopathy or a muscle enzyme deficiency (e.g. myoadenylate deaminase), or metabolic myopathies.

If fasting precipitates pain, then inquire about associated findings such as dark-coloured urine which may indicate myoglobinuria.

Persistent muscle pain in a patient with normal strength usually indicates a cause other than myopathy.

Physical Examination

Note the muscle bulk (wasting or hypertrophy), fasciculations, and tenderness. Also note the distribution (symmetrical or asymmetrical) of muscle wasting if present.

Without actually touching the patient, it is possible and desirable to quantify the patient's ability to perform tasks required for daily living.

TABLE 55.1 SYSTEMIC CAUSES OF GENERALIZED WEAKNESS

Disease	Features
Endocrinopathies	
Hyperthyroidism	Proximal muscle weakness.
Hypothyroidism	Generalized; calf muscle cramps.
Hyperparathyroidism	Pain due to associated bone disease; characteristic hyperreflexia.
Hypoparathyroidism	Hyporeflexia or areflexia; CPK ↑.
Cushing's syndrome	Severe muscle weakness; wasting.
Adreno-cortical insufficiency	Hypotension; pigmentation.
Panhypopituitarism	Loss of axillary & pubic hair.
Diabetes mellitus	Proximal weakness; neuropathy.
Nutritional	
Vit. D deficiency	Chronic proximal muscle weakness; osteomalacic myopathy.
Vit. C deficiency	Pain due to associated bone disease.
Thiamin deficiency	Heaviness & weakness of legs.
Nicotinic acid deficiency	
Vit. E deficiency	Myopathy.
Protein deficiency	
Anaemia	Weakness & easy fatiguability.
Chronic renal disease	Impaired Vit. D metabolism; anaemia; muscle weakness & fatigue.
Chronic congestive failure	Muscle weakness and wasting 'cardiac cachexia'.
Chronic respiratory failure	Poor chest expansion; chronic cough.
Electrolyte disturbance	
Hyponatraemia	Mainly lassitude.
Hypokalaemia	Muscle weakness, especially lower limbs; very severe or abrupt deficit; total paralysis including respiratory muscles and paralytic ileus; absent tendon reflexes.
Hyperkalaemia	Ascending muscular weakness; flaccid quadruplegia & respiratory paralysis.
Hypercalcaemia	Fatigue, lethargy.
Hypocalcaemia	Muscle spasm.
Hypomagnesaemia	Lethargy & weakness; muscle cramps.

TABLE 55.2 DIAGNOSTIC CLINICAL FEATURES OF NEUROMUSCULAR CAUSES OF WEAKNESS

Location of cause	Clinical features	Typical examples
Psychogenic	Variable weakness; reflexes normal; no wasting; no atrophy of muscle.	Hysteria Compensation neurosis
Pyramidal system	Often unilateral (monoparesis, hemiparesis); more severe distally; clumsiness of finger movement; spasticity, clonus; exaggerated tendon reflexes; extensor plantar response.	Mass lesions Meningioma Tuberculoma Haematoma Syphilitic meningomyelitis Cervical spondylosis Vit. B12 deficiency Myelopathy

(Contd)

TABLE 55.2 (Contd)

Location of cause	Clinical features	Typical examples
Extrapyramidal system	Slowness and difficulty in initiating movement; cog-wheel rigidity; tremors.	Parkinsonism Wilson's disease Manganese poisoning Carbon monoxide poisoning Drug-induced
Anterior horn cell	Asymmetrical limb or bulbar atrophy early & marked; fasciculations; no sensory loss; reflexes variable (depending upon associated UMN lesions).	Spinal muscular atrophy Amyotrophic lateral sclerosis Motor neurone disease
Peripheral nerve (uni-focal or diffuse)	Asymmetrical or symmetrical distal; atrophy moderate; paraesthesia; hypoaesthesia; reflexes decreased out of proportion to weakness.	Diabetic neuropathy Leprosy Carpal tunnel syndrome Mononeuritis multiplex Polyarteritis nodosa Nutritrional neuropathy (thiamin, pyridoxine, B12)
Neuromuscular junction	No atrophy of muscle; No sensory involvement; no fasciculations/cramps; normal reflexes; diurnal variations (Weaker as day progresses).	Myasthenia gravis (extraocular, bulbar) May be associated with: thymoma (CT mass) thyrotoxicosis (increased T_3, T_4) other autoimmune disorders (ANF, RF) Eaton-Lambert syndrome (proximal limb muscles) May indicate hidden cancer (e.g. small cell lung ca.)
Muscle	Symmetrical limb distribution; bulbar in some.\n\nAtrophy slight early, marked later; No sensory involvement. Reflexes diminished in proportion to weakness.	Duchenne's muscular dystrophy Facioscapulo-humeral Limb girdle Periodic paralysis Polymyositis/dermatomyositis Trichinosis Toxoplasmosis Cysticercosis Scleroderma SLE, RA, Mixed connective tissue disorder Sarcoidosis Glycogen storage disease Lipid-carnitine deficiency

TABLE 55.3 DRUG-INDUCED MYOPATHIES

Painless

Without neuropathy	Corticosteroids
With neuropathy	Colchicine
	Chloroquine
	Hydroxy-chloroquine
Myasthenic syndrome	D-penicillamine
	Antibiotics (esp. aminoglycoside)
	Beta blockers (e.g. pindolol, labetalol)

Painful

Polymyositis	D-Penicillamine
	Cimetidine
	Zidovudine
Myopathy	Clofibrate
	Statines
	Cyclosporine
Neuromyopathy	
Eosinophilia-myalgia syndrome	Colchicine + Cyclosporine
	Clofibrate + Statin
Vacuolar myopathy	Colchicine
	Chloroquine
	Amiodarone
	Cyclosporine
	Drugs causing hypokalaemia
Mitochondrial myopathy	Zidovudine
Necrotizing myopathy	Vincristine
	Emetine

- Ask the patient to walk on heels and toes.
- Ask the patient to rise from a chair without the use of his arms.
- Ask the patient to rise from a squatting position.
- Ask the patient to step on to a chair.
- With the patient lying supine, ask him to extend the leg: knee extension lag (inability to fully extend the leg against gravity) indicates quadriceps weakness.
- Ask the patient to sit up from the supine position (trunk muscle weakness).
- Ask the patient to hold his neck when extended beyond the edge of the bed (neck muscles).
- Ask the patient to lift the arms above the head (shoulder girdle muscles).

- Inspect the back for scapular winging as arms are elevated.
- Give your two fingers to the patient's hand to grip them, and note the degree of difficulty in extracting them from his hand.
- Notice blanching of the knuckles when he makes a fist.

Grading of muscle power is useful for future follow-up.

Grade   0 = no movement
1 = trace movement not enough to produce a contraction.
2 = ability to move when gravity is eliminated.
3 = ability to move against gravity but not against resistance.
4 = ability to oppose gravity plus resistance.
5 = normal.

If one has limited time for testing muscle strength the assessment of function as described earlier is likely to be of greater value than formal muscle testing.

Investigations

History and physical examination will lead to a diagnosis in a majority of patients whose presenting symptom is weakness and is most probably due to a neuro-muscular disease. Failure to arrive at a diagnostic impression before routine and sophisticated tests often leads to diagnostic inaccuracy and confusion. Few of the biochemical, histologic and electrophysiological studies used to evaluate patients with neuromuscular disease are pathognomonic since nerve and muscle can respond to disease processes only in a limited number of ways.

The laboratory assessment of a case of unexplained weakness is given below:

Hb and ESR
Total and differential WBC count
BUN, Creatinine
Electrolytes
    Na, K, Ca, Mg, P
Liver function tests-SGOT, SGPT, Alk.
    Phosp
CPK MB and MM.
T3 T4, TSH.
Cortisol and ACTH

Urine for myoglobin (+ test for blood in the urine in absence of RBCs).

CPK MM isoenzyme predominates in the skeletal muscle.

In long-standing necrotizing muscle disease and in athletes, CPK MB also rises.

The clinical diagnosis of corticosteroid-induced myopathy can be difficult if the drug is given to treat an inflammatory myopathy. The presence of normal CPK, no myopathic changes on EMG, and a type II muscle fibre atrophy on biopsy (see below) are helpful in making the diagnosis.

A single dose alternate day regime of corticosteroid therapy has the greatest muscle-sparing effect.

EMG

Normal resting skeletal muscle is electrically silent.

- Spontaneous resting activity = denervation
  Also seen in polymyositis but not in other myopathies.
- Single fibre EMG : Increased 'jitter' = myasthenia gravis.
- Motor Unit Potential (MUP) at mild effort.
  High amplitude, long duration polyphasic potentials = MND.
  Low amplitude, brief duration potentials = acute polymyositis.
- Recruitment pattern at maximum effort.
  Incomplete recruitment pattern = earliest feature of neurogenic lesion.
  Complete recruitment = myopathic lesion
- Nerve conduction studies Evoked motor response (EMR) < velocity = demyelinating neuropathies.

Muscle biopsy

Distinguishes between neurogenic and myopathic disease.

Helps in recognizing specific muscle disorders:
    Congenital myopathies,
    Muscular dystrophies,
    Specific metabolic defects by histochemical or biochemical techniques.

Criteria for diagnosis of drug-induced myopathy

1. Lack of pre-existing muscle weakness
2. Lack of alternative cause for myopathy
3. A time interval between onset of treatment and myopathy
4. Complete or partial improvement after drug withdrawal
5. Rechallenge-not advisable because of the risk of serious relapse

Management of Myasthenic Crisis

A major complication of myasthenia gravis is respiratory failure which may lead to respiratory arrest in a few minutes if not treated promptly with ventilatory support and pharmacological intervention (plasma exchanges and I.V. immunoglobulin).

2 mg Edrophonium (tensilon) in 1 ml solution is administered IV. If it improves the weakness myasthenic crisis is confirmed. If the weakness is increased, then cholenergic crisis (cc) resulting from over medication with anti-cholinesterase drugs (like pyridostigmine) is postulated, hence the subsequent 8 mg additional dose should not be given, which may be fatal in CC.

Most normal persons maintain a steady weight because their food intake is matched to their energy expenditure, by the coordinated activity of the 'feeding' and 'satiety' centres in the hypothalamus. This mechanism works efficiently over months or years so that one is not required to consciously watch the calories. If the food intake continues to be the same as in youth, but the energy expenditure gradually becomes less, there is imperceptible gain in weight particularly in the waistline.

A general practitioner would be rendering a great service to his patients if he weighs them regularly and measures their abdominal and hip girths (normally the abdominal girth at the umbilicus should be at least 2 inches less than the hip girth). When they are equal it represents 2-3 kilograms of excess fat deposition at the waistline, which should be taken, among other things, as a risk factor for disease.

Weight record to be comparable, should be on the same machine, with the same clothes and at the same time of the day, preferably in the morning before breakfast.

Weight Gain

Gradual gain In weight is due to obesity or myxoedema.

Sudden gain in weight over 3-4 days is due to fluid retention (and *not* fat which takes time to accumulate). Similarly, sudden weight loss over 4-7 days is mainly due to fluid loss (and *not* fat loss which takes time to be decreased), but this rapid weight loss impresses many gullible people undergoing crash programmes of weight reduction.

Weight record is particularly important during pregnancy. Weight gain is predictable at a certain rate; excessive gain is a warning for pre-eclampsia. Keeping a record of the height and weight in infants and growing children is also an important service. Failure to gain weight in children is as serious as spontaneous weight loss in adults.

Weight Loss

Spontaneous weight loss (i.e. not due to deliberate dieting) in an adult is always a serious symptom which needs thorough investigation. Mechanisms of weight loss include lack of food availability, anorexia leading to diminished food intake, obstruction to the passage of food, or repeated vomiting, malabsorption of nutrients, accelerated catabolism, and loss of calories in the urine and stools. Infection and malignancy produce weight loss through many mechanisms including anorexia, excessive catabolism mediated by lymphokines and cytokines such as tumour necrosis factor, and Interleukin-6. Severe mental depression causes weight loss through poor appetite and poor intake of food.

Table 56.1 lists the causes of weight loss with the underlying mechanisms, and diagnostic clues.

One useful clinical approach is to consider (a) weight loss in spite of a good appetite and intake of food, and (b) weight loss with poor appetite.

(a) *Weight loss in spite of good appetite and good intake of food*

Common	Rare
Diabetes mellitus	Pheochromocytoma
Thyrotoxicosis	Leukaemia
Malabsorption	Lymphoma
Worm load	(excessive metabolism)
(in children)	

TABLE 56.1 CAUSES OF WEIGHT LOSS

Disease	Mechanism	Diagnostic clues
I. *Oesophagus*		
Stricture	Obstruction to the passage of food	Dysphagia.
Malignancy		Endoscopy.
II. *Stomach*		
Pyloric obstruction	Vomiting	History of ulcer pain.
secondary to peptic ulcer		Endoscopy.
Carcinoma	Anorexia	
III. *Intestines*		
Sprue	Malabsorption	Bulky fatty stools
Parasities	Competition for nutrients	Stools for ova
Inflammatory bowel disease	Loss of protein from gut	(See Chapter 30).
Tuberculous enteritis	Malabsorption and loss of protein	Barium studies.
Cancer colon	Cytokines	Stools for occult blood.
IV. *Liver*		
Acute and chronic hepatitis	Anorexia	Jaundice.
Alcoholic liver disease	Loss of protein in ascitic fluid	Ascites.
Hepatoma		
Amoebic liver abscess		
V. *Pancreas*		
Chronic pancreatitis	Deficient exocrine secretion	CT abdomen.
Carcinoma pancreas	Deficient bile action	
VI. *Endocrine*		
Diabetes mellitus	Gluconeogenesis from protein and fat	Urine sugar and blood sugar.
Thyrotoxicosis	Excessive metabolism	Tremors, tachycardia.
Pheochromocytoma	Excessive metabolism	Hypertension, tremors.
Addison's disease	Anorexia due to	Pigmentation.
	cortisol deficiency	Hypotension.
		Loss of axillary and pubic hair.
Panhypopituitarism		
VII. *Renal*		
Chronic renal failure	Anorexia	BUN, Creatinine high.
		Anaemia. urine albumin.
VIII. *Infection*		
Tuberculosis	Excessive catabolism	Thorough search for hidden infection.
AIDS	Anorexia, diarrhoea	CT, gallium scanning.
Bacterial endocarditis	Lymphokines and cytokines	HIV testing.
IX. *Malignancy*		
Leukaemia, lymphoma	Excessive metabolism	Lymphadenopathy.
		Hepatosplenomegaly.
		Other features: CBC.
X. *Retroperitoneal fibrosis*	Anorexia; involvement of duodenum, small intestine, colon; renal failure	Abdominal pain, anorexia, fatigue, malaise, raised ESR, IVP: medial displacement of ureters.
XI. *Psychiatric illness*		
Anorexia nervosa	Anorexia	Other features of depression.
Depressive illness		

NOTE: See also **Table 58.I** in Chapter 58 on Medical Oncology, for GI tumour syndromes causing weight loss.

(b) *Weight loss with poor appetite and diminished intake of food*

Common	Rare
Hidden infection	Anorexia Nervosa
Hidden malignancy	Addison's disease
Renal failure	Panhypopituitarism
Depression	

The tricky situations are:

'Silent thyroiditis' with transient thyrotoxicosis: no thyromegaly, but *tenderness over gland.*

'Apathetic thyrotoxicosis': no tremors or eye signs.

'Occult steatorrhoea': Normal appearance of stools, but faecal fat > 6 g.

Hidden infection:

HIV: not detected unless specially tested for.

Tuberculosis: extrapulmonary (hepatic, renal, spine etc).

Amoebic abscess without palpable tender liver.

Hidden malignancy:

This is the most common cause of weight loss in the absence of major signs and symptoms.

Hidden renal failure:

Weight loss due to anorexia is the earliest manifestation of chronic renal failure. There is nothing in the symptoms and signs to suggest kidney disease hence it is very important to *routinely examine the urine* for specific gravity, albumin and RBC, and the blood for BUN and creatinine in every patient of anorexia and weight loss.

Women's Health

Introduction

The United Nation Decade of Women (1975-1985) highlighted women's socio-economic plight in the declaration that women do two-third of the world's work, earn only 10% of its income and own 1% of its property.

Women in India suffer a triple jeopardy economic, caste/religion and gender. Apart from the consequences of poverty, irregularity and exploitation suffered by both men & women. Contain suffering are unique to Indian women.

1. Gender bias against girls even before birth, and abortion selectively of female fetuses.

2. Infanticide of girl infant, tragically motivated by the desire to spare her future misery if she lives upto adult life.

3. Poor mother gives less time to breast-feed the female child. Nutritious food (milk, eggs etc.) are preferentially given to the male child.

   Medical care especially if it costs money is preferentially given to the male child. Not surprisingly, upto the age of 5 years female mortality exceeds that of males by 20%.

4. Female literacy is much less than males in India. In the 4 BIMARU states 75% women cannot read or write, 75% of girls aged 6-14 are school drop-outs.

5. Although child marriage is a legal offence, a large number of marriages in BIMARU states take place when the girl is under 15. More than 15 million girls aged 15-19 delivery every year, with high maternal mortality. Over 200,000 deaths occurs due to unsafe abortions conducted by unqualified persons under non-sterile conditions.

6. One mother dies during delivery every six minutes in India. Twenty percent deaths are due to severe iron deficiency, anaemia which is totally preventable.

7. As a result of maternal malnutrition, 20 million Indian children are born every year with a low birth weight (< 2.5 kg) and insulin resistance, which will make them patients of hypertension, atherosclerosis and diabetes when they grow up to adult life.

8. Sexual offences (rape & sexual harassment) on women occurs on a scale which is difficult to quantify since few women dare to prosecute the offenders. The victim may be 4 months old, 4 years old or 80 years old.

Gender-based differences in disease

Sex-based differences in disease are those related to biological and physiological factors (chromosomes, gonads, and hormones), whereas gender-based differences are those related to socio-cultural, behavioral and psychological factors, affecting the natural history of a disease and the prognosis, treatment response and outcome in the management of disease. This applies to neurological, gastrointestinal, cardiovascular and thyroid conditions.

Gender-based differences are seen in paediatric population are often inherent in the embryology of the fetus and sex-determination factors that influence development of male & female anatomy.

Endometriosis

Endometriosis is a common gynecological disorder estimated to affects 176 million women and girls worldwide. Endometriosis affects 10-15% of all women of reproductive age, 20%-50% of all women with infertility and 25%-70% of women and adolescents with chronic pelvic pain or pelvic pain and dysmenorrheal (Goa et al 2006).

26 million Indian women between the ages of 18-35 years suffer from endometriosis. Endometriosis is a considerable burden in terms of both direct and indirect healthcare costs, leads to significant loss of productivity, reduces quality of life and causes impact on physical and mental health (Simoens et al 2007; Nnoaham et al 2011).

Endometriosis is defined as the presence of functional endometrial glands and stroma in ectopic locations outside the uterine cavity - ovaries, pelvic peritoneum uterosacral ligaments, but may affect any part of the body.

The signs and symptoms of endometriosis are often non-specific as they are also observed in other chronic pain disorders such as irritable bowel syndrome and pelvic inflammatory disease (May et al 2011).

Presently, the gold standard for diagnosis of endometriosis is direct visualization on laparoscopy or laparotomy, ideally with histological confirmation. However, laparoscopy is an expensive, invasive procedure requiring general anesthesia, surgical skills and associated with potential complications. Certain pathological conditions like splenosis, endosalpingiosis, mesothelial hyperplasia, hemosiderin deposition, hemangiomas, adrenal rests etc. may be confused visually with endometriotic implants.

There is an urgent need to develop non-invasive biomarkers for early diagnosis, prognosis and to monitor the treatment of endometriosis.

Autoimmunity has been shown to be responsible for endometriosis in a significant number of cases.

Endometriosis is associated with a decreased pregnancy rate after IVF treatment.

Several investigators reported presence of anti-endometrial antibodies (AEA) in women with endometriosis.

The sensitivity of anti-PDIK1L - autoAb was comparatively better than CA125.

CA125 are usually increased in many physiological and pathological conditions like arrival of menstrual period, pregnancy, inflammation of the abdominal cavity, intimal arteritis, breast cancer, liver cancer, lung cancer. etc. The sensitivity is only about 10%-40% in diagnosis of endometriosis.

ELISA based on the biomarkers (peptides of TPM3, SLP2 and TMOD3) for detection of endometriosis.

Tropomyosin 3, Stomatin like protein 2 and Tropomodulin 3 for non-invasive diagnosis of endometriosis and to analyze and correlate the reactivity against these peptides.

Osteoporosis

After age 30, bone density continues to fall in both sexes, with accelerated loss in women after menopause - bone resorption exceeding bone formation. This effect is reduced by estrogen replacement therapy, yet only 4%-6% of women are diagnosed and treated. An estimated 80% are neither diagnosed nor treated, 16% are diagnosed but not treated.

Three fractures occur as a result of fall from a standing height or less – vertebral fracture, femoral head and distal radius (Colles' fracture).

The life time risk of fracture in women over age 50 is 50%, higher than the risk of breast cancer (12%) morbidity and mortality of hip fractures is high with death in > 30% within 6 months.

WHO Fracture Risk Assessment. Tool (FRAX) provides physicians with a way to determine the 10 year risk of osteoporotic fractures and effectively choose candidates for therapy. A number of potent skeletal anti resorptive and anabolic drug have become available to treat osteoporosis, hence the importance of routine bone densitometry in elderly population.

Ischaemic Heart Disease (IHD) in Women

IHD is a leading cause of death in women with higher mortality compared to age-matched men. Microvascular dysfunction with normal epicardial coronary arteries (Syndrome X) is more common in women. Myocardial perfusion and function list with Nuclear medicine SPECT and Rubidium - PET (with regional coronary flow reserve measurement) should be more frequently utilized so as not to miss a preventable and treatable condition.

Hypertension in Pregnancy

Chronic hypertension : Known history of HT pre-pregnancy ≥ 140/90. Normal fall of blood pressure commencing in the first Trimester, may mask pre-existing hypertension.

Gestational Hypertension : Occurring in second half of pregnancy in a previously normotensive woman without significant proteinuria.

Pre-eclampsia usually occurs after 20 weeks of 7gestation (HT, proteinuria > 0.3g /24 hrs).

Eclampsia occurrence of grand mal convulsion on top of pre-eclampsia. 75 mg aspirin daily from 12 weeks until delivery is recommended for women with high risk for pre-eclampsia.

Diabetes and Pregnancy

Diabetes in pregnancy is becoming a major health concern for the mother and fetus. Diabetes before pregnancy [Pre-Gestational Diabetes Mellitus (PGDM)], and hyperglycemia developing for the first time in pregnancy is defined as Gestational Diabetes Mellitus (GDM).

The incidence of congenital fetal anomalies is higher in poorly controlled diabetes. First generation sulfonylureas (tollntamide, chlorpro pcmide) were formed to be associated with congenital malformations in animal studies. On the other hand there studies have shown no association between oral antidiabetic agents and congenital malformations (Towner et al Diabetes Care 1995, 18, 1446-51).

Langer O et al Am J. Obgy 1999, 180, 538.

Ekpebegh C et al Diab Med 2007, 24, 253-58.

Current guidelines recommend use of insulin in women with PGDM, with the use of oral metformin for GDM (Rowan J et al NEJM 2008, 358, 2002-15). At present Meglitenides Gliptins and S6L2 inhibitors cannot be advocated in pregnancy.

During breast feeding, metformin can be continued while other oral hypoglycimic agents should be avoided. This topic is particularly important in India and poorly resourced countries where the price and availability of insulin injections may be important factors.

Pre-Natal Screening

Pre-Natal screening aids in assesing health of the unborn child, provides information on developmental abnormalities to the clinician.

Increasing maternal age increases the risk of a neuploidy - increase or decrease in chromosomal number.

Multiple miscarriages may be caused by chromosomal abnormalities.

Family histroy of genetic disorders (monogenic or polygenic) is also an indicator for need of prenatal testing.

Ethnic groups with high risk of genetic abnormalities (e.g. sickle cell and thalassemia) being common among the Sindhi community) deserve prenatal testing for determining health of the fetus.

Ultrasonography is generally recommended during the 18th - 20th week of gestation. It can performed on the abdomen or Trans-vaginally. Nuchal Translucency thickness (NT) determined by ultrasound alongwith results of other biochemical tests help accurate diagnosis.

Biomarker in maternal amniotic fluid (20ml) such as AFP, HCG, UE_3, in hibin a help detection of aneuploidres such as Trisomy 21, 18, 13, Turners syndrome.

Chronic villus sampling (CVS) helps in diagnosis of single gene disorders and information about factal chromosomal statues.

Precutaneous Umbilical Blood Sampling (PUBS)

Under ultrasound guidance blood is collected from umbilical vein - Diagnosis of haematological disorders, toxoplasma infection, aneuploidy chromosomal instabilities and in utero blood transfusion is possible.

Common Breast – Concerns

Palpable breast mass : Although majority of breast lumps are benign, there is significant anxiety in the patients mind about malignancy which should be addressed by the clinician.

A detailed history to assess the location and duration of the breast lump, changes in size over time, and with the menstrual cycle and overlying skin changes, family history of breast or ovarian cancer, age at menarche at first parity (prior benign breast biopsies including hyperplasia etc.).

The clinical breast examination involves inspection of the breasts in both upright and supine positions for signs of asymmetry, overlying skin & nipple rash, erythema or peau d'orange.

Palpation is performed to assess discrete or dominant mass, and palpation of axillay and supraclavicular areas for lymphadenopathy.

Mammography in women 30 years and older is done to confirm presence of breast mass or areas of asymmetric density or presence of pleomorphic calcifications associated with breast cancer.

In women with dense breast the sensitivity of mammography is reduced, hence the next step is *targeted ultrasound* to determine if the mass is solid or cystic. Benign cysts are thin-walled structure with clear fluid. They can be aspirated with a fine needle if they are causing pain. Complex cysts are thick-walled or have echogenic contains which should be biopsied. Solid masses should be biopsied.

MRI of the breast has high sensitivity (> 95%) but lower specificity.

Newer technologies such as molecular imaging and tomosynthesis are being utilized.

Nipple Discharge can be physiological or pathological. Physiological discharge is usually thick, white, cream or greenish colour, noted on manual pressing of the nipple. Pathological discharge is usually spontaneous, due to intraductal papilloma duct ectasia or periductual mastitis, but may also represent malignancy.

Milky nipple (Galactoria) can be related to hyper-prolactinemia hypothyroidisim, oral contraceptives, metoclopramide, cimetidine phenothiazine etc.

Breast Pain (mastalgia) may or may not be related to the menstrual cycle. Cyclic mastalgia mostly occurs in the pre-menstrual phase and resolves after menstruation. Non-Cyclic mastalgia may be a marker

of mastitis, hematoma from trauma fibrocystic disease.

Gynecologic Oncologic Imaging with PET/CT

Cervical cancer is typically very FDG avid and hence FDG PET/CT is most valuable for initial staging radiation therapy planning and detection of recurrence.

For ovarian cancer, in the setting of rising CA 125 level FDG PET/CT detects recurrence and evaluating response to therapy.

Some of the most common findings relate to cyclical changes that occur as part of the menstrual cycle in pre-menopausal women Mucinous toumours and low-volume or peritoneal carcinomatosis are causes of false - positive FDG/ PET/ CT studies.

Cervical Cancer is the third most common neoplasus in women worldwide (after breast, ovaries) Risk factors include Human Papilloma Virus (HPV), multiple sexual partners.

FDG PET/CT detects both cervical cancer (FDG avid).

Testing for circulatory tumor cells (CTCs) is an important adjunct to imaging. Use of specific fluorescent mAbs and magnetic nanoparticle based separation (immunomagnetic assay) help identification of rare tumor cells in blood and body fluids, in metastatic breast, colorectal lung, prostate, lung and epithelial cancers.

$\geq$ 5 CTCs and imaging findings predict shorter overall survival. Rising CTC levels occur before imaging to detect metastases.

Chemoprevention of Cancer

Cancer is a multi-step process extending over 10-30 years. Angelina Jolie underwent bilateral preventive mastectomy because of strong family history of cancer and BRCA 1 and BRCA2 +. It is not known if she also had mutation of p53 (Cancer - preventing gene). Starting chemoprevention with dietary phytochemicals at age 10 and continuing throughout life is a workable strategy to prevent or ever reverse the multi-step process (Surh 2004).

SECTION FOUR

SPECIAL TOPICS

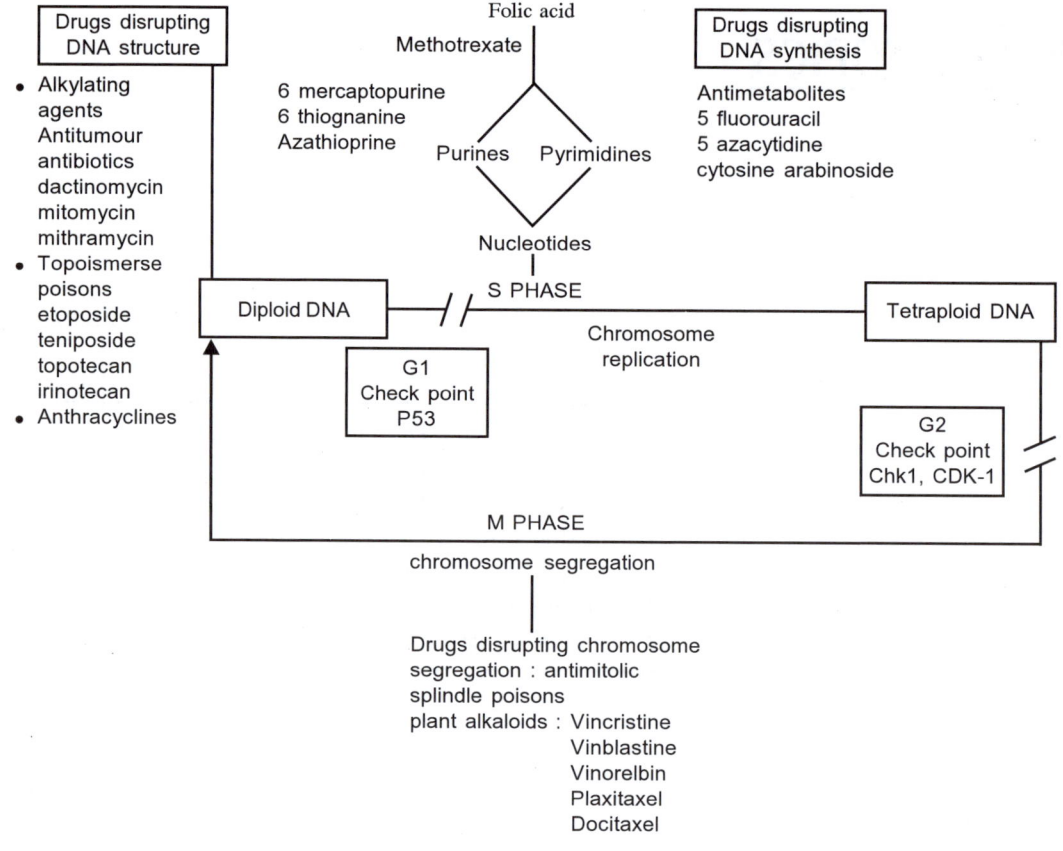

Fig. 58.1:   Sites of drug action in cancer cell cycle :
Phase-specific agents act on S phase (antimetabolites) and M phase (spindle poisons).
Phase non-specific agents act throughout the cycle but cause arrest of cell cycle
progression at G1 and G2 check points.

Comment:

Conventional chemotherapy of cancer cannot be curative since it targets cancer cells as well as host normal cells.

New approaches aim at targets uniquely expressed by cancer clls, or over-expressed by cancer cells compared to normal cells - specific monoclonal antibiodies, or aptamers which can be delivered specifically to cancer cells via new devices such as liposomes, dendramers etc.

eg. CD20 on B cells - Rituximab
Her-2 on Breast Ca Trastuzumab
RGD peptide anti-integrin mAb
VEGF Bevacizumab

Cancer Biology

Growing knowledge about the attributes of the cancer cell as distinct from normal cells opens new ways for blocking cell signalling pathways that regulate cell proliferation and differentiation and apoptosis, with dietary phytochemicals.

Cancer cells differ from normal cells in the following nine attributes:

1. *Deregulated cell proliferation*:
   a) Loss of negative regulators (suppressor oncogenes- P53, Rb etc.) and lack of normal check-point responses.
   b) Increase in positive regulators - Ras, Myc, etc.
   c) Increased membrane transport activity pgp, ABCG2 (BCRP) glucose transporters, aminoacid transporters, Na+K+ ATPase etc.

2. *Failure to differentiate*: Retain properties of stem cells - Bmi-1, Notch wnt and sonic Hedgehog (SHH) pathways are stem cell regulators.

3. *Loss of normal apoptosis pathways*
   a) Mutation or inactivation of p 53
   b) Increased expression of BCl2.

4. *Genomic instability*: defects in DNA repair pathways. Micro satellite instability, chromosomal instability.

5. *Loss of replicative senescence*: Active telomerase gene expression and unlimited supply of telomers- contrast normal depletion of telomers after 25-30 doublings).

6. *Increased angiogenesis* (a) Increased expression of VEGF, FGF, IL-8, proangiogenic factors. (b) loss of negative regulators-endostatin, tumstatin, thrombospondin.

7. Invasion:
   a) Loss of cell- cell contact through gap junctions Cadherins.
   b) Increased production of matrix metalloproteinases (MMPs).

8. Metastases: Expression of integrins for spread to lymph nodes or distant sites.

9. Evasion of normal immune Surveillance:
   a) Down-regulation of MHC class I and II expression to evade recognition and destruction by Cytotoxic T cells.
   b) Induction of T cell tolerance.

Recent emphasis is on cancer stem cells (CSCs) which are resistant to current therapeutic approaches hence the cause of recurrence / relapse and ultimate death. CSCs have been identified in several solid tumors including brain, breast, ovary, colon, pancreas, prostate, melanoma & multiple myeloma. Identification of cancer stem cells markers (eg. Lin (-) CD44(+) CD24 (+ low) ESA (+) for breast, CSCs, CD34+ / CD38- for leukaemia. CSCs will provide new targets for effective therapy as well as prevention, such as Hedgehog inhibitors, HH antagonists, Notch 1 antagonists and wtn antagonists. Salinomycin selectively reduces breast CSCs in mice by more than 100 fold relative to paclitaxel, a commonly used chemotherapeutic agent. The role of dietary phyto-chemicals for these CSC targets needs to be investigated afresh. Sonic Hedgehog (SHH) blockers such as cyclopamine, and DMAPT (parthenoloid derivative) are suitable candidates for CSC elimination.

Oncology is the study of tumours. Neoplasia means abnormal new growth, which may be benign or malignant. Although the term 'benign' implies that the tumour is harmless, poses no threat to normal health and life, and so should be left alone, it is not always so. A benign tumour, located strategically may produce serious consequences (e.g. a benign cyst in the 3rd or 4th ventricle causing obstructive hydrocephalus). Benign adenomas that secrete powerful hormones (e.g. insulinoma, pheochromocytoma) can produce serious and life-threatening consequences; hence the need to recognize them, and cure the patient by removing them. For this reason these tumours get emphasis far out of proportion to their prevalence in the population.

Cancer is the term used to describe a wide variety of malignant diseases. It is necessary for all doctors to be aware of the protean clinical manifestations of various cancers which are summarized in **Tables 58.1, 58.2 and 58.3.**

Importance of Team work

Coordination between surgeon, radio therapist and chemotherapist is essential, because the sequence of treatment is critical to success, which is different from the standard surgery first approach. Although surgery is the most effective means of treating cancer, curing 40% of the cases, in some settings e.g. bulky testicular cancer or stage III breast cancer surgery is not the first treatment modality employed–chemotherapy and/or radiation therapy are used to reduce the size of the tumour and control clinically undetected metastatic disease followed by surgery to remove residual masses.

Traditionally, oncology has been the domain of surgeons and radiotherapists. But with the development of cytotoxic drugs and hormone therapy, physicians have now a greater involvement in the overall management of malignancy.

Although cancer chemotherapy is given by experts in the domain, all doctors should be aware of what drugs are currently used, what to expect from chemotherapy, and what are the complications of chemotherapy. These are summarized in **Fig. 58.1** and **Tables 58.4** and **58.5.**

Recognition of paraneoplastic syndromes (although they are relatively rare) is important for the following reasons:

1. They may *precede* the clinical presentation of the primary malignancy, thereby facilitating early detection.

2. They may *mimic metastatic disease* and thus confuse grading, prognosis and management decisions.

3. They may also serve as *tumour markers* to monitor therapy and recurrence **Table 58.6.**

The hope of clinicians is to be able to detect cancer at an early (if possible pre-cancerous) stage where surgical excision offers the prospect of cure. Patient education and participation (e.g. self-examination of the breast and routine Papanicolaou smears in females, stools for occult blood in middle-aged males) are all efforts directed towards the hope of early detection.

Modalities of Giving Chemotherapy

Chemotherapy is administered by several routes:

A. *Oral route:* To minimize nausea and vomiting drugs are best given at bedtime, except cyclophosphamide which is given early in the day since hydration and frequent urination are desired to avoid haemorrhagic cystitis.

Table 58.1 CLINICAL PRESENTATIONS OF MALIGNANT DISEASES

	Examples
A. *Mass lesion itself*	Painless swelling in breast (carcinoma). Painless swelling in muscle (sarcoma). Lymph node enlargement (lymphoma). Spleen enlargement (lymphoma).
B. *Secondary effects of mass lesion (organ-related)*	Tumour in the brain: headache, vomiting, visual disturbance, papilloedema—due to raised intracranial pressure, convulsions–focal neurologic deficits. Tumour in spinal cord vicinity: Spinal cord compression, meningeal carcinomatosis (leukaemia, lymphoma). Bronchogenic carcinoma: partial/complete airway obstruction, superior vena cava obstruction, mediastinal structure compression. Distal colon: Alterations in bowel habits. Cancer head of pancreas: jaundice. Cancer oesophagus: dysphagia.
C. *Haemorrhage from eroded structures* (a) epithelial surface	Haemoptysis: bronchogenic ca or adenoma. Haematemesis: gastric ca. Bleeding per rectum: colonic ca. Haematuria: renal and bladder ca.
(b) serous surface	Malignant pleural effusion, pericardial effusion, peritoneal effusion.
D. *Pain (not common at presentation)* (a) due to nerve compression	Brachial plexus: ca. bronchus / ca. breast Sacral plexus: ca. rectum / ca. cervix Paraspinal nerve: ca. pancreas
(b) distension/distortion of organs	Hepatoma, hepatic metastases: distension of liver capsule. Bone pain from primary or secondary vertebrae, ribs.
E. *Cachexia (due to various mechanisms)*	Rare in breast and CNS tumours (except glioblastoma); uncommon in leukaemia, lymphoma; common in ca. of gastrointestinal tract, lung ovary, testes.
(a) Difficult passage of food	Ca oesophagus.
(b) Anorexia, vomiting	Ca stomach.

(Contd)

TABLE 58.1 (Contd)

	Examples
(c) Reduced exocrine function	Ca pancreas.
(d) Malabsorption-obstructed biliary flow	Ca pancreas, gallbladder.
(e) Secretory diarrhoea	Gastrinoma VIPoma.
(f) Cytokines	Tumour necrosis factor.

F. *Bone marrow suppression*
   (a) Bone marrow replacement by primary or secondary tumour
   (b) Bone marrow fibrosis
   (c) Bone marrow injury
   (d) Nutritional deficiency
   (e) Interference with normal control of erythropoiesis

G. *Hypercalcaemia*
   (a) Due to extensive bony metastases   Ca breast, prostate, lung.
   (b) Due to PTH-like peptide
   (c) Due to bone-resorbing cytokines   Interleukin-I,
                                      Tumour necrosis factor,
                                      Lymphotoxin.

H. *Paraneoplstic syndromes*
   (a) Due to hormones and hormone precursors produced by cancers (**Table 58.2**)
   (b) Nervous system   Cerebellar syndrome
                                      cerebellar cortical degeneration.
                                  Myoclonic encephalopathy.
                                  Subacute sensory neuropathy.
                                  Visual paraneoplastic syndrome.
                                  Limbic and bulbar encephalitis.
                                  Multifocal leucoencephalopathy.
                                  Skeletal muscle syndromes
                                      polymyositis, dermatomyositis,
                                      carcinomatous neuromyopathy.
                                  Myaesthenic syndromes
                                  e.g. Eaton-Lambert.

I. *Miscellaneous syndromes*   Anorexia (TNF or catechin) produced by macrophages.
                                  Fever.
                                  Glomerular kidney disease.
                                  Digital clubbing-pulmonary osteoarthropathy.
                                  Haematological syndrome i.e.
                                      idiopathic thrombocytopenic purpura.

TABLE 58.2 ECTOPIC PRODUCTION OF HORMONES AND HORMONE PRECURSORS BY CANCERS

A. *Hormones and hormone precursors*
Pro-opiomelanocortin and related peptides
Corticotrophin-releasing hormone
Chorionic gonadotrophin and its alpha & beta subunits
Vasopressin
Growth factors e.g. transforming growth factor B, epidermal growth factor, insulin-line growth factor II
Parathyroid hormone-like protein
Erythrophiloprotein
Eosinophiloprotein
Growth hormone
Gastrin
Prolactin
Gastrin-releasing peptide (and bombesin)
Secretin
Glucagon
Calcitonin
Renin
Vasoactive intestinal peptide
Somatostatin
Hypophosphataemia-producing factor
Oestrone and oestradiol

B. *Enzyme production*
e.g. alkaline phosphatase, thymidine kinase

C. *Foetal protein production*
e.g. alpha foeto-protein, CEA

B. *IV route:* Extreme care is needed to avoid extravasation (which can cause serious local tissue injury) and venous thrombosis. For patients with poor peripheral venous access, in-dwelling central venous catheters with subdermal ports, or ports external to the skin are available.

C. *Intrathecal route:* This is needed for the treatment of meningeal involvement. To achieve high levels in the ventricles and cisterns (not always possible by usual lumbar puncture), neurosurgical placement of an intraventricular reservoir in the lateral ventricle is more satisfactory.

D. *Intra-arterial route:* This has been used primarily for patients with hepatoma or hepatic metastases from colon cancer. An implantable pump is used to deliver the drug via a hepatic arterial route.

E. *Intra-cavitary route:* Intrapleural, intraperitoneal or bladder instillation are also used to deliver chemotherapy locally.

Complications of Chemotherapy

These are listed in **Table 58.5**. Two complications deserve special mention, along with their management.

Tumour lysis syndrome: is often seen with treatment of rapidly progressive, chemotherapyresponsive, bulky tumours (e.g. Burkitt's lymphoma). It is associated with hyperuricaemia, hyperphosphataemia and hypocalcaemia. Vigorous hydration and allopurinol minimize the risk of acute renal failure caused by Uric acid nephropathy.

Hypercalcaemia: Acute management consists of the following:

(a) Volume expansion with IV 0.9 per cent saline infusion at the rate of 300-500 ml/hour until intravascular volume has been restored.

(b) Forced saline diuresis (sodium inhibits renal tubular reabsorption of calcium) along with frusemide 20-40 mg IV to prevent volume overload.
0.45 per cent saline and 0.9 per cent saline are alternately infused at rates of 300-500 ml/hour to maintain adequate diuresis.

(c) Hydrocortisone 5 mg/kg IV every 8 hours followed by a maintenance dose of prednisolone 40-80 mg PO qid is given in hypercalcaemia due to lymphoma, leukaemia and multiple myeloma.

(d) Synthetic salmon calcitonin may temporarily lower the serum calcium by 1-3 mg/dl. This expensive drug should be used only if (a) and (b) above have proved ineffective. The usual starting dose is 4 IU/kg SC or IM over 12-24 hr, maximum dose 8 IU/kg IM 6 hrly.

TABLE 58.3 CLINICAL FEATURES OF GI TUMOUR SYNDROMES

Tumour syndrome	Clinical features	Diagnosis
1. Glucagonoma (patient age 40)	Necrolytic migratory erythema Mild diabetes long history Diarrhoea Venous thrombosis Liver metastases.	Increased glucagon after IV tolbutamide. CT: pancreatic mass.
2. Somatostatinoma	Dyspepsia, gallstones Steatorrhoea Hypochlorhydria Diabetes.	Hyperglycaemia with ketonaemia. Stool bulky 400-800 g/d; stool fat 1-30 g/d. CT: pancreatic mass.
3. P Poma	Secretory diarrhoea.	None known.
4. Gastrinoma	Severe peptic ulcer disease Secretory diarrhoea, which stops on H$_2$ receptor antagonist tr.	Increased serum gastrin after IV secretin. High gastric acid secretion.
5. VIPoma 'pancreatic cholera'	Large volume secretory diarrhoea, hypokalaemia, hypochlorhydria (gastrin inhibitor). Metabolic acidosis Occ. co secretion of 5, 3 & hetodermin.	Stool pH < 8 on fasting (chronic bicarbonate secretion). Increased plasma PHM.
6. Calcitoninoma	Diarrhoea.	Secretory diarrhoea while fasting, osmotic component while eating.
7. GHRHoma	Acromegaly (long history).	Normal sella. CT/MRI no mass. GH release by exogenous GHRH blunted.
8. Neurotensinoma	Oesophageal reflux (one case).	None known.

NOTE: Some tumours have been diagnosed only during investigation of weight loss. Tumour localization is done by CT/MRI/PET or US. Periodic repeating imaging tests are essential to assess response to treatment and recurrence.

(e) Plicamycin (formerly called mithramycin), a potent toxin to osteoclasts, inhibits boneresorption. 25 µg/kg is given IV over 4-6 hours. Circulating calcium levels begin to fall within 12 hours, and the effect lasts 3-7 days, after which the dose may be repeated. Thrombocytopenia, azotaemia and hepatotoxicity limit the long-term usefulness of the drug.

In hypercalcaemic patients in whom volume expansion is precluded by the presence of renal or cardiac failure, dialysis with calcium-free dialysate is effective.

Relief of Pain

Effective antineoplastic therapy itself may relieve pain, but often it requires additional measures.

Local pain may be symptomatically relieved by radiotherapy or by nerve block, cordotomy, or commisurotomy.

General pain needs systemic analgesics. The opium group of drugs may be given for severe pain without undue concern for addiction.

Severe bone pain requiring frequent narcotic analgesics can be palliated by radioactive strontium–Sr 89 or radioactive phosphorus–P 32. This can be done on an outpatient basis.

TABLE 58.4 CURABILITY OF CANCERS WITH CHEMOTHERAPY

A. *Advanced cancers with possible cure*

Acute lymphoid leukemia
Acute myeloid leukemia
Germ cell neoplasms
    Embryonal carcinoma
    Terato carcinoma
    Seminoma
    Chorio carcinoma
Gestational trophoblastic neoplasia
Paediatric neoplasms
    Ewing's sarcoma
    Embryonal rhabdomyo carcinoma
    Neuroblastoma
    Neuroepithelioma
    Wilm's Tumour
Small cell lung cancer
Ovarian cancer

B. *Advanced cancers possible cure with chemotherapy & radiation*

Breast Ca.
Ca uterine cervix
Squamous carcinoma
    Head & neck, anus
Carcinoma
Small cell lung carcinoma
Non-small cell lung carcinoma.

C. *Cancers possibly cured with high dose chemotherapy with stem cell support*

Chronic myeloid leukemia
Multiple myeloma
Relapsed leukemias and lymphomas

D. *Useful palliation but not cure*

Bladder carcinoma
Breast carcinoma
Endometrial carcinoma
Hairy cell leukemia
Gastric carcinoma
Colorectal carcinoma

E. *Poorly responsive in advanced stages*

Biliary tract neoplasms
Carcinoma of vulva
Hepatocellular carcinoma
Melanoma
    Prostate carcinoma
    Renal carcinoma
    Pancreatitic Ca

TABLE 58.5 COMPLICATIONS OF CANCER CHEMOTHERAPY

1. Nausea, vomiting, diarrhoea
2. Extravasation of drug : sloughing
3. Tumour lysis syndrome
4. Hyperuricaemia
5. Stomatitis-mouth ulcers
6. Bone marrow suppression
7. Cardiotoxicity e.g. adriamycin
8. Pulmonary fibrosis e.g. bleomycin
9. Renal toxicity e.g. cisplatin
10. Neuropathy e.g. vincristine
11. Alopecia e.g. cyclophosphamide
12. Development of a second malignancy e.g. alkylating agent: acute leukaemia

Emotional support:
Patients who receive emotional support from their families have shown a longer life span for the same grade and stage of malignancy compared to those patients who did not get it. Depression also depresses the immune surveilance.

Anticancer drugs of the future

Currently used anti-cancer drugs focus principally on the proximate biochemistry of nucleic acids and mitotic spindle structure or function. Drugs of the future may seek to replace lost function of tumour suppressor genes (such as p. 53); counter the action of activated oncogenes; influence the capacity of cells to die (induce apoptosis); prevent chromosomal end replication (telomerase inhibition); induce differentiation of cells with exit from the cell cycle (retinoic acid); actually infect cells with viruses designed to replicate in the milieu of cancer cells but not in normal cells; use immunological strategies (nanobodies) to target molecules expressed on the surface of cancer cells but not on normal cells; and to prevent angiogenesis. Some successful examples are listed in **Table 58.7.**

TABLE 58.6 TUMOUR MARKERS

Tumour markers	Cancer	Non-cancer conditions
Alfa-feto protein (AFP)	Hepatocellular Ca gonadal germ cell Ca	Cirrhosis, hepatitis
Carcinoembryonic antigen (CEA)	Colon, pancreas, lung breast, ovary	Pancreatitis Hepatitis, Inflamm Bowel Dis. Smoking
Calcitonin	Medullary Ca thyroid	–
Catecholamines	Pheochromocytoma	Panic attacks
CA 125	Ovarian Ca, lymphomas	menustruation, pregnancy
CA 19.9	Colon, pancreas, breast	pancreatitis, ulcerative colitis
CD 30	Hodgkins' D Lymphoma	–
CD25	Hairy cell leukemic Adult T cell leukemia/ lyphoma	–
HCG (Human Chorionic Gonadotropin)	Gestational trophoplastic disease, gonadal gern cell tumour	Preganancy
Lactate Dehydrogenase	Lymphoma, Ewing's sarcoma	Hepatitis Haemolysis
Neuron-specific enolase	Small cell lung cancer neuroblastoma	–
Proatate specific antigen (PSA)	Prostate cancer	Prostatitis BPH, infection
Prostate acid phosphatase	prostate cancer	ditto

TABLE 58.7 MOLECULAR TARGETS FOR CANCER THERAPY

Imatinib mesylate (Gleevec, also known as STI-571) Gefitinib (Iressa, also known as ZD1839)	Targets the epidermal growth factor receptor (EGFR) tyrosine kinase and is approved in the U.S. for non small cell lung cancer is approved for chronic myelogenous leukemia, gastrointestinal stromal tumor and some other types of cancer. Early clinical trials indicate that imatinib may be effective in treatment of dermatofibrosarcoma protuberans.
Erlotinib (marketed as Tarceva) Erlotinib	Inhibits epidermal growth factor receptor[6], and works through a similar mechanism as gefitinib. Erlotinib has been shown to increase survival in metastatic non small cell lung cancer when used as second line therapy. Because of this finding, erlotinib has replaced gefitinib in this setting.
Sorafenib (Nexavar)[7]	Renal cell carcinoma, hepatocellular carcinoma, and radioactive iodine resistant advanced thyroid carcinoma.
Sunitinib (Sutent)	Renal cell carcinoma (RCC) and imatinib-resistant gastrointestinal stromal tumor (GIST).
Dasatinib (Srycel)	Chronic myelogenous leukemia (CML) and Philadelphia chromosome-positive acute lymphoblastic leukemia (Ph+ ALL).

(Contd)

TABLE 58.7 (Contd)

Lapatinib (Tykerb)	Orally active drug for breast cancer and whose tumors overexpress HER2
Nilotinib (Tasigna)	Imatinib-resistant chronic myelogenous leukemia
Bortezomib (Velcade)	Apoptosis-inducing proteasome inhibitor drug treat multiple myeloma that has not responded to other treatments.
Tofacitinib	Janus kinase inhibitors
Crizotinib	ALK inhibitors
Obatoclax Navitoclax and Gossypol	Bcl-2 inhibitors
Iniparib, Olaparib	PARP inhibitors
Pperifosine	PI3K inhibitors
Apatinib	VEGF Receptor 2 inhibitor which has shown encouraging anti-tumor activity in a broad range of malignancies in clinical trials[10]. Apatinib is currently in clinical development for metastatic gastric carcinoma, metastatic breast cancer and advanced hepatocellular carcinoma[11].
AN-152, (AEZS-108) doxorubicin linked to [D-Lys(6)]- LHRH	Phase II results for ovarian cancer[12].
Braf inhibitors (vemurafenib, dabrafenib, LGX818)	Metastatic melanoma that harbors BRAF V600E mutation
MEK inhibitors (trametinib, MEK162)	Are used in experiments, often in combination with BRAF inhibitors to treat melanoma
e.g. PD-0332991, LEE011 in clinical trials	CDK inhibitors
Hsp90 inhibitors, some in clinical trials	
Salinomycin	Demonstrated potency in killing cancer stem cells in both laboratory-created and naturally occurring breast tumors in mice.
Vintafolide	Small molecule drug conjugate consisting of a small molecule targeting the folate receptor. It is currently in clinical trials for platinum-resistant ovarian cancer (PROCEED trial) and a Phase 2b study (TARGET trial) in non-small-cell lung carcinoma (NSCLC)[13].
Temsirolimus (Torisel) Everolimus (Afinitor) Vemurafenib (Zelboraf) Trametinib (Mekinist) Dabrafenib (Tafinlar)	Serine/threonine kinase inhibitors
Rituximab (marketed as MabThera or Rituxan)	Targets CD20 found on B cells. It is used in non Hodgkin lymphoma
Trastuzumab (Herceptin)	Targets the Her2/neu (also known as ErbB2) receptor expressed in some types of breast cancer

(Contd)

TABLE 58.7 (Contd)

Alemtuzumab	
Cetuximab (marketed as Erbitux) and Panitumumab	Target the epidermal growth factor receptor (EGFR). They are used in the treatment of colon cancer and non-small cell lung cancer
Bevacizumab (marketed as Avastin)	Targets circulating VEGF ligand. It is approved for use in the treatment of colon cancer, breast cancer, non-small cell lung cancer, and is investigational in the treatment of sarcoma. Its use for the treatment of brain tumors has been recommended[14].
Ipilimumab (Yervoy)	Anti CTLA-4 Used in melanoma, NSCLC, SCLC, Bladder Ca hormone refractory Ca prostate.

Chemoprevention of Cancer

Young John Surh (Nature review Oct. 2003 Vol. 3 pg. 768-780) has published an excellent review on cancer chempoprevention with dietary phytochemicals. **Fig. 58.2** depicts eleven chemopreventive phytochemical with their dietary sources- Turmeric (curcumin), chilli pepper (capsaicin) Ginger (6-gingerol), green tea (epigallocatechin- 3 gallate) soyabeans (genistein), tomatos (lycopene), grapes (resveratrol), Honey (Caffeic acid phenethyl ester) Garlic (diallyl sulphane). Not shown in the figure are pinebark and grape seed (procyanidin-GSPE) and red wine.

TABLE **58.8** DESCRIBES THE MODE OF ACTION OF DIETARY
PHYTOCHEMICALS AT THE MOLECULAR LEVEL

1.	Curcumin	Inhibits TNFα induced COX2 gene transcription and NFKB & AP1 activation; anti-proliferative, pro-apoptotic and anti-metastatic activities via suppression of B Catenin.
2.	Capsaisin	Blockade of IKbα degradation and NFKB Translocation into nucleus; induces apoptosis by activation of CJUN. NH2 terminal kinase (JNK) and p 38.
3.	Gingerol	Inhibits EGF-induced AP.1 activation and neoplastic transformation.
4.	EGCG: Epigallocatechin 3 Gallate	Blocks activation of AP1 & NFKB, inhibits PI3K. AKT-NFKB and HER2/NEU receptor tyrosine phosphorylation; inhibits VEGF, β catenin expression. G0/G1 phase arrest and apoptosis.
5.	Genistein	Inhibits AP1, cFOS and ERK activity, inhibits AKT mediated NFKB activation.
6.	Resveratrol	Inhibits PMA-induced COX-2, PKC and AP1, MMP-9 NFKB; induces apoptosis via activation of p53 via ErK and p. 38 Down-regulates β catenin.
7.	Procyanidin:	Naturally occurring polyphenolic bioflavonoid in grape-seed & pine bark; powerful antioxidant.
8.	Caffeic acid phenethylester (CAPE)	Disrupts the NRF2-KEAP1 complex. Decrease β Catenin expression; suppress NFKB activation.
9.	Diallyl sulphide	Prevents mutagenesis by suppressing ROS.
10.	Indole 3 Carbinol	Decreases β catenin, inhibits adhesion, migration and invasion of cancer cells.
11.	Sulphoraphane:	Directly interacts with KEPA1; stimulates nuclear translocation of NRF2 which subsequently activates ARE for expression of many anti-oxidant or detoxification enzymes.
12.	Lycopene	Anti-oxidant-suppresses ROS.

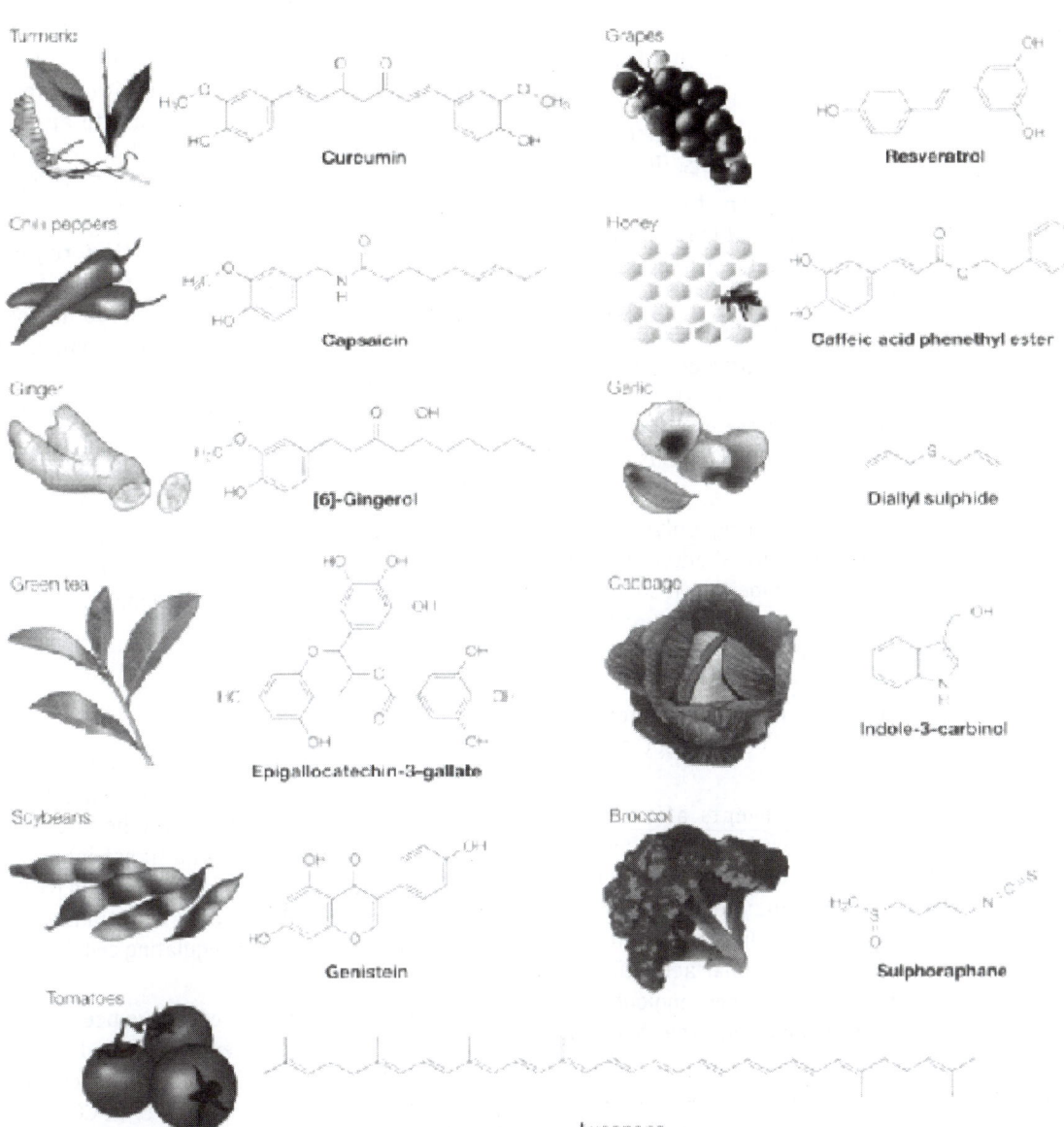

Turmeric

Curcumin

Chili peppers

Capsaicin

Ginger

[6]-Gingerol

Green tea

Epigallocatechin-3-gallate

Soybeans

Genistein

Tomatoes

Lycopene

Grapes

Resveratrol

Honey

Caffeic acid phenethyl ester

Garlic

Diallyl sulphide

Cabbage

Indole-3-carbinol

Broccoli

Sulphoraphane

Fig 58.2

Mechanisms of Chemoprevention:

Carcinogenesis is a multi-step process- initiation, promotion, progression.

Lee Wattenberg proposed a classification of chemopreventive agents into two main categories : blocking agents and suppressing agents. (Ref. 4).

Blocking agents prevent carcinogens from reaching the target sites, from undergoing metabolic activation or interaction with crucial cellular molecules such as DNA, RNA or protein.

Suppressing agents, on the other hand, inhibit the malignant transformation of initiated cells in either the promotion or progression stage. This categorization is an outcome of the combination of several distinct sets of intracellular effects, rather than a single biological response.

Procyanidin, a naturally occurring polyphenolic bioflavonoid, has anti-viral, anti-bacterial anti-inflammator and antiallergic properties; it suppreses endothelin-1 and stimulates production of anti-oxidant enzymes inside the cell. Its anti-oxidant capability is 20 times more powerful than Vit. C and 50 times more than Vit. E.. It enhances the effects of Vit. C and strengthens the connective tissue around capillaries.

The cellular and molecular events affected or regulated by these chemopreventive phytochemicals include carcinogen activation/detoxification by xenobiotic metabolizing enzymes, cell cycle progression, cell proliferation, differentiation and apoptosis; expression and functional activation of oncogenes or tumor-suppressor genes, angiogenesis and metastasis, and hormonal and growth factor activity.

Abnormal or improper activation or silencing of the mitogen-activated protein kinase (MAPK) pathway or its down-stream transcriptional factors can result in uncontrolled cell growth leading to malignant transformation. Some phytochemicals "switch on" or "turn off" the specific signalling molecules, depending on the nature of the signalling cascade they target, preventing abnormal cell proliferation and growth.

Other cell-signaling kinases other than MAPK are protein kinase C (PKC) and phosphatidyl inosital-3

kinase (PI3K). These upstream kinases activate a distinct set of transcription factors including NFKB and AP-1 which act independently or co-ordinately to regulate target gene expression. Aberrant activation of NFKB stimulates proliferation and prevents apoptosis in malignant cells. Many dietary phytochemicals suppresses constitutive NFKB and AP1.

NRF2 is a transcription factor that regulates expression of many antioxidant or detoxification enzymes. NRF2 null mice develop large number of tumors due to failure of combating oxidative stress and carcinogen detoxification.

The Kelch-like ECH associated protein (KEAP-1) is a cytoplasmic repressor of NRF2, that inhibits its ability to translocate to the nucleus. Curcumin and CAPE disrupt the NRF2- KEAP1 complex leading to increased NRF2 binding to ARE. Phytochemicals that activate NRF include EGCG, sulphoraphane, which activation ARE for expression of many anti-oxidant and detoxification enzymes.

β Catenin signalling

β catenin is a multifunctional protein, a component of cell-cell adhesion machinery. It binds with the cytosolic tail of E cadherin and connects actin filaments through β catenin to form the cytoskeleton. β catenin can also function as a transcription factor and nuclear translocation of β. Catenin and β Catenin - TCF/LEF complex is associated with transcriptional activation of various genes regulating cellular growth processes.

Several dietary phytochemicals have been shown to down-regulate the β catenin mediated signalling pathway as a part of their molecular mechanism of chemoprevention. Curcumin, CAPE, EGCG, indole-3 carbinol, resveratrol.

The recent report of Anjelina Jolie undergoing Prophylactic Bilateral Mastectomy in view of strong family history of breast cancer and BRCA I & II positivity raises important conceptual issues and brings into prominence the approach of chemoprevention.

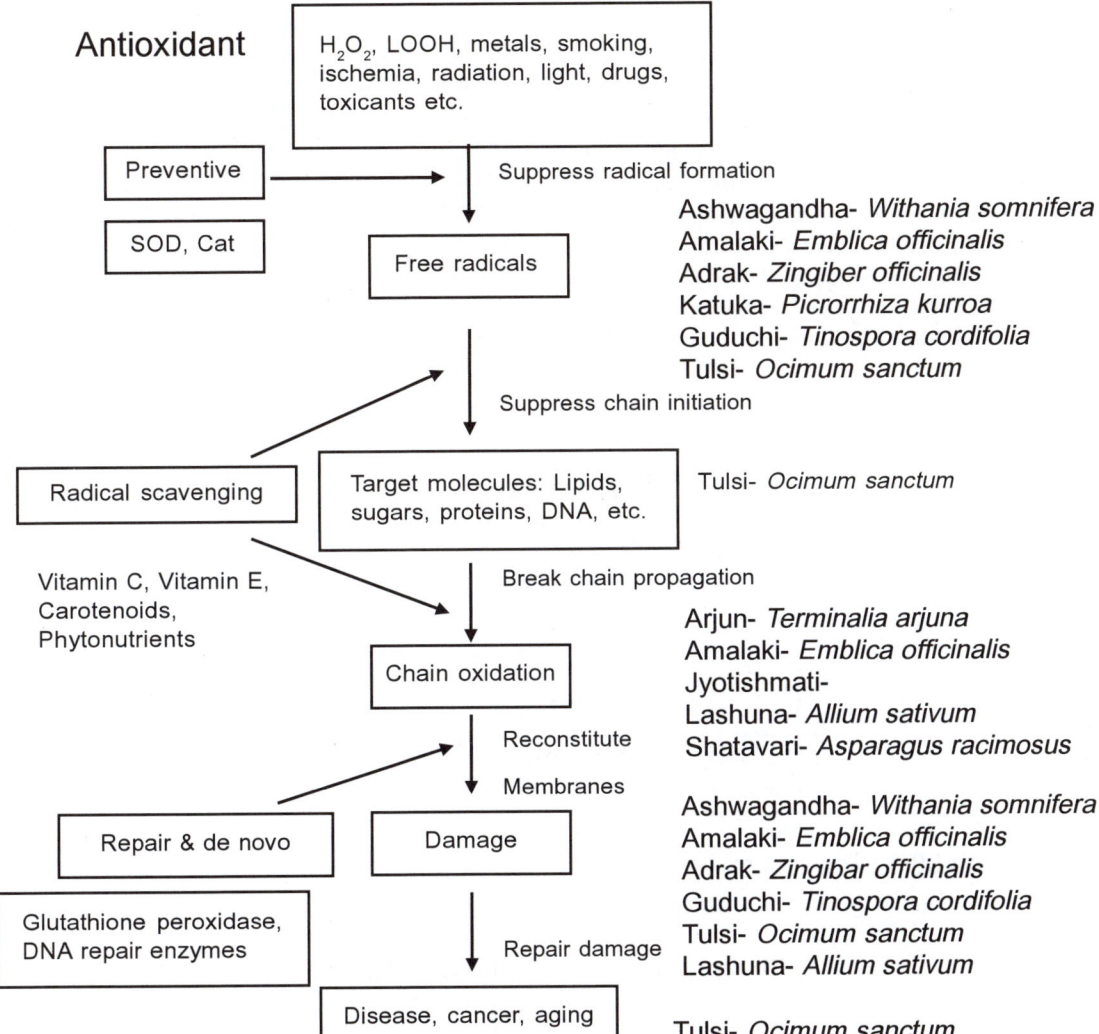

Antioxidant

	H₂O₂, LOOH, metals, smoking, ischemia, radiation, light, drugs, toxicants etc.	

Preventive — → Suppress radical formation

SOD, Cat

Free radicals

Ashwagandha- *Withania somnifera*
Amalaki- *Emblica officinalis*
Adrak- *Zingiber officinalis*
Katuka- *Picrorrhiza kurroa*
Guduchi- *Tinospora cordifolia*
Tulsi- *Ocimum sanctum*

Suppress chain initiation

Radical scavenging

Target molecules: Lipids, sugars, proteins, DNA, etc.

Tulsi- *Ocimum sanctum*

Vitamin C, Vitamin E, Carotenoids, Phytonutrients

Break chain propagation

Chain oxidation

Arjun- *Terminalia arjuna*
Amalaki- *Emblica officinalis*
Jyotishmati-
Lashuna- *Allium sativum*
Shatavari- *Asparagus racimosus*

Reconstitute

Membranes

Repair & de novo

Damage

Ashwagandha- *Withania somnifera*
Amalaki- *Emblica officinalis*
Adrak- *Zingibar officinalis*
Guduchi- *Tinospora cordifolia*
Tulsi- *Ocimum sanctum*
Lashuna- *Allium sativum*

Glutathione peroxidase, DNA repair enzymes

Repair damage

Disease, cancer, aging

Tulsi- *Ocimum sanctum*

Level of Antioxidant Action
Non-enzymatic, enzymatic and ancillary enzymes &
Defense systems in vivo against oxidative damage

Fig. 58.3: Ayurvedic herbal drugs with antioxidant activity at various levels
Reference: Devasagaum TPA, Lele RD et al JAPI, 2004, 52, 794–803

Antisense oligonucleotides

Radiolabeled antisense oligonuclides (RASONs) have been designed for specific mRNAs (e.g. C myc, Erb B2, telomerase) expressed in breast cancer cells. Such sequences of 15 - 25 nucleotides can traverse the membrane of living cells and bind to specific mRNAs (in vitro hybridization) and provide an image of the cancer in vivo. T he specificity of the "Molecular Velcro" for target cells is excellent and provides therapy to kill the cells by using ? emitters or Auger electrons - "Molecular Surgery". T hus by selecting appropriate antisense oligonucleotide sequence it is possible to inhibit the expression of virtually any gene in cells without attacking any other cellular components. Although the word "gene silencing" was not used for this activity it was precisely that, with the, potential for therapy - prevention of production of harmful proteins by virus - infected cells, bacteria - infected cells, tumor cells or genetically transformed cells.16-18 T he oligonucleotide drug Vitravene, the first of such drugs to be approved by FDA in USA, is used to treat cytomegalovirus retinitis in AIDS patients. Antisense oligonuclides have been developed to block the c-myc proto-oncogene m RNA which codes for substances that cause atheroma in blood vessels. Table I lists the currently tested antisense agents and their mRNA targets.

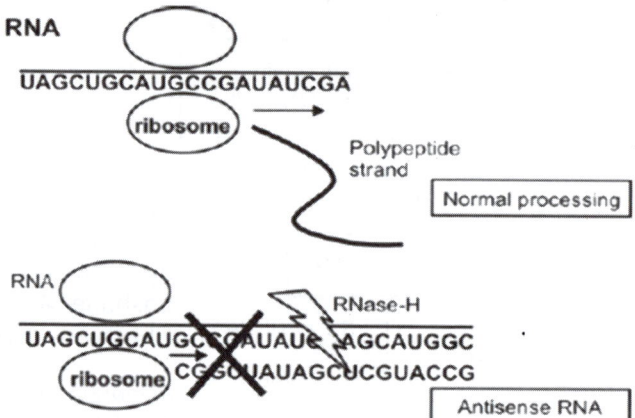

Fig 58.4 : The schematic representation of antisense oligonuclides that inhibit transcription of mRNA

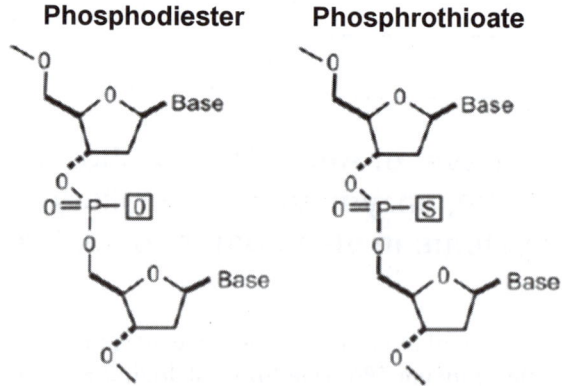

Fig 58.5 : Creation of phosphorothioate backbone

TABLE 58.9. ASON for cancer therapy

Cancer			
	-	OGX–011	Clusterin (survival protein in Cancer cell in response to therapy)
	-	LY2181308	Survivin over expressed in cancer cell only
	-	LY2275796	Eukaryote initiation factor 4E (eIF4E) critical switch for cancer progression
	-	O6X427	Heat shock protein HSP 27 cell Survival protein.
	-	Wickstrom's ASON	C-myc in Burkitt's lymphoma
	-	Genasense (G3139)	BCl2 over expressed in all cancer cells.
	-	Affinitak ISIS13521	Protein kinase C (PKC)
	-	AP12009	TGF β 2
	-	AP11014	TGF β 1
	-	Le raf AON (ISIS 5132)	C-raf 1
	-	ISIS2503	H-ras
	-	GEM 231	Protein Kinase A (PKA)
	-	GEM 240	MDM2
	-	IGF–IR ASON	Insulin- like growth
	-	ALT 1103	factor (IGF)
	-	MG 98	DNA methyl transferase
	-	GTI 2040	Ribonucleotide reductase
	-	Ki 67 AON	Ki-67

TABLE 58.10. Neuroendocrine tumors

Neuroendocrine tumors: Site of origin	
foregut	Respiratory tract, oesophagus, thymus, lung, stomach, duodenum and pancreas (insulinoma, Glucagonoma, VIPoma, pancreatic polypeptidoma)
midgut	Small bowel, appendix, ascending colon
hindgut	Transverse and descending colon, rectum
Histological grade:	G1 (Ki67 index < 2) G2 (Ki67 index 3-20) G3 (Ki67 index > 20) (neuroendocrine carcinoma) All express Somatostatin Receptor (SSTR) subtypes 1-5 in varying densities which can be imaged with 68Ga-DOTANOC PET-CT

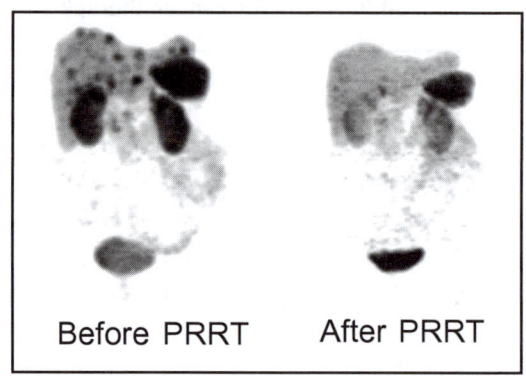

Fig 58.6

Peptide receptor radionuclide therapy (PRRT) With lutetium-177 dotatate

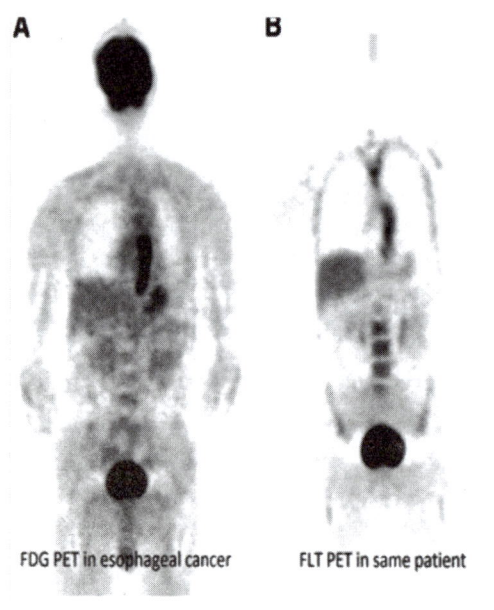

Fig 58.7

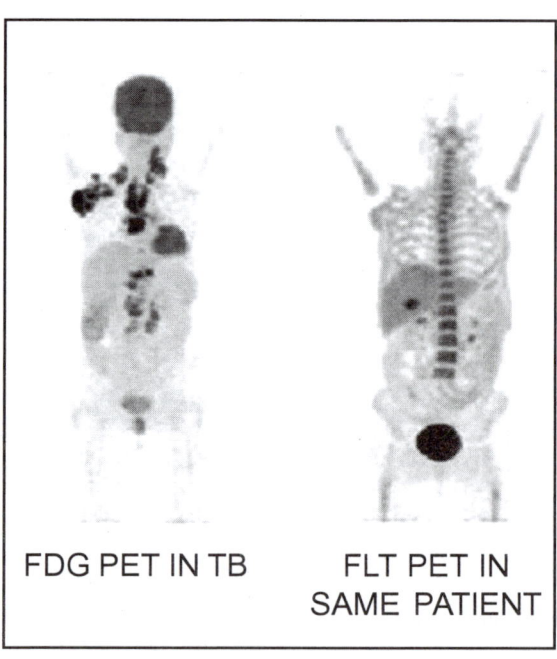

Fig 58.8

59 Multisystem/Multi-organ Diseases

In describing clinical manifestations of diseases, it is convenient to approach them organ-wise or system-wise, such as those associated with the heart, lungs, kidneys, liver, pancreas, gastrointestinal tract, brain etc.

But there are several diseases (or more correctly, disease mechanisms) which affect multiple systems/multiple organs simultaneously or sequentially. Hence it is worth recapitulating these disorders and considering the mechanisms by which they become multisystem/multi-organ diseases and the diagnostic features of each one of these diseases which can help in their clinical recognition.

A good clinician makes use of this knowledge for several practical ends including diagnosis, prognosis and management plan which ensure optimal patient care, and the anticipation and prevention of complications if possible.

In the beginning of the twentieth century William Osler had said, 'Know syphilis and you will know the entire medicine'. This was to emphasize the multisystem/multi-organ involvement in syphilis. Hence syphilis entered the differential diagnosis of every clinical syndrome which could be produced, among other diseases, by syphilis, and blood for VDRL became a routine test.

With the decline in the prevalence of syphilis and an increase in the prevalence of diabetes mellitus, another disease which affects multiple systems and organs, it could well be said, 'Know diabetes mellitus and you will know the entire medicine'. Since the diabetic may present to the doctor for the first time with any of the so-called 'complications' of diabetes, the alert clinician always includes a blood sugar (or glycosylated Hb) and urine sugar as routine tests in every patient who presents with any syndrome that can result from diabetes (retinopathy, neuropathy,

nephropathy, dermopathy etc). In today's context HIV infection has taken the place that syphilis held at the beginning of this century, hence the full clinical spectrum of HIV infection is described at the end of this chapter.

In developing countries tuberculosis is an important multisystem/multi-organ disease (**Fig. 59.1**). It should be considered in *any* age group or any socio-economic stratum of society. This has become all the more important in the context of HIV infection.

To illustrate the importance of recognizing a disease with multisystem/multi-organ involvement, the clinical features of polyarteritis nodosa (PAN) in one hundred patients (ultimately proved by muscle biopsy and angiography) are given in **Table 59.1**. The patient may present to different specialists or

Table 59.1 CLINICAL FEATURES OF POLYARTERITIS NODOSA (PAN) IN 100 PATIENTS

(In order of occurrence)

Manifestations		Laboratory features	
Renal	65%	High ESR	89%
Hypertension	58%	Leucocytosis	78%
Fever	49%	Anaemia	66%
Pulmonary	42%	Thrombocytosis	58%
Skin rash	41%	Rheumatoid factor	37%
Arthralgia/arthritis	40%	HBs Ag +	26%
Peripheral neuropathy	40%	Cryoglobulinaemia	25%
Myalgia	33%	Hypocomplemen-	
Cardiac	30%	taemia	21%
CNS	26%	Thrombocytopenia	18%
Hepatomegaly	22%	Eosinophilia	5%
Intestinal perforation	11%		

doctors at different times with 'arthralgia', or 'asthma' or 'haematuria' or jaundice' or 'hypertension', without the doctors appreciating the common underlying pathology, viz vasculitis of medium-sized vessels in different organs. Hence an experienced clinician will always bear in mind the presenting manifestations arousing suspicion of PAN (**Table 59.2** and **Fig. 59.2**).

Table 59.3 and **Figs. 59.1, 59.2, 59.3** and **59.4** show the various categories of diseases which can present as multisystem/multi-organ syndromes (infection, metabolic, immune-mediated, autoimmune, malignant, haematological and undetermined aetiologies). It is worth remembering that the symptomatology of depression and anxiety is also

TABLE 59.2 PRESENTING MANIFESTATIONS AROUSING SUSPICION OF PAN

1. A non-specific subacute or chronic febrile illness with loss of weight and leucocytosis.
2. An atypical abdominal illness which may simulate a condition requiring laparotomy.
3. A primary renal disease frequently thought to be acute or subacute glomerulonephritis.
4. Polyneuropathy, sometimes in combination with myositis.
5. Bronchial asthma or focal pulmonary infiltrates suggesting infection.
6. Myocardial infarction or coronary insufficiency especially in association with any of the above.
7. Unexplained severe hypertension.

TABLE 59.3 MULTISYSTEM/MULTI-ORGAN DISEASES

Disease entity	Mechanisms
I. Infections	
(a) Septicaemia	Disseminated intravascular clotting
(b) Specific infections:	
Tuberculosis ⎫ Fungal infections ⎭	Granuloma formation; arteritis
Brucellosis	Granuloma formation
Syphilis	Endarteritis obliterans; gumma
Lyme Disease	Endarteritis
Malaria (falciparum)	Blockage of capillaries by parasitized RBCs
Viral infections	Vasculitis (e.g. Varicella gangrenosa)
II. Cardiovascular	
Bacterial endocarditis ⎫ Atrial myxoma ⎭	Emboli in multiple organs
III. Unclassified	
Sarcoidosis	Granuloma formation (behaviour similar to tuberculosis) Hypercalcaemia
IV. Metabolic & Endocrine Disorders	
i. Diabetes mellitus	Free radical-induced tissue damage Glycosylation of structural proteins Capillary basement membrane thickening: microangiopathy Atherosclerosis: macroangiopathy
ii. Multiple endocrine neoplasia Types I & II	Hyperplasia/adenoma accompanied by excessive autonomous hormone secretion
iii. Renal failure	Acidosis, anaemia, anorexia, potassium and phosphate retention, secondary hyperparathyroidism
iv. Acute intermittent porphyria	Unknown mechanism: demyelination of nerves
v. Amyloidosis	Deposition of amyloid in vessels, in multiple organs.

(Contd)

TABLE 59.3 (Contd)

Disease entity	Mechanisms
V. *Haematological diseases*	
Sickle cell disease	Obliteration of capillaries by deformed red blood cells
Agranulocytosis	Superadded infection
Paroxysmal nocturnal haemoglobinuria	Haemolytic anaemia; vascular thrombosis
Polycythaemia vera	Thrombosis of veins in different organs
Thrombocytopenia	Bleeding in various organs
Bleeding disorders	Bleeding in various organs
Hyperviscocity syndromes	Platelet dysfunction leading to bleeding in different organs
VI. *Malignant diseases*	
Solid tumours	Direct pressure of lesion on surrounding structures
Leukaemia	Erosion of nearby blood vessels & serous sacs
Hodgkin's disease	Paraneoplastic syndromes due to ectopic hormone production
Plasmacytoma	Complications of chemotherapy
VII. *Immunological injury*	
Serum sickness, anaphylaxis & angio-oedema	Release of histamine immune-complex deposition in various organs (kidney, synovium, blood vessels)
VIII. *Autoimmune diseases*	
Organ-specific:	Both hyperfunction and hypofunction can occur
Autoimmune	depending upon the stimulating effect (e.g. Graves' disease)
Polyglandular syndromes	or blocking effect (e.g. Hashimoto's disease)
(Table 59.4)	
Non-organ specific:	Immune complexes
SLE	Vasculitis: different-sized vessels
Polyarteritis nodosa	T-cell-mediated toxicity
Polymyalgic rheumatism & giant cell arteritis	Antibody mediated toxicity
Rheumatoid arthritis	Hyperviscosity
IX. *Immunosuppressed states*	
Congenital defects ⎱	Superadded infection by opportunistic organisms
Acquired defects ⎰	
AIDS	Apoptosis & death of cells infected with HIV
X. *Drug toxicity and hypersensitivity*	Multiple mechanisms (**See Chapter 59**, **Fig. 59.1**)
XI. *Depression and anxiety*	Symptoms related to all systems: e.g. headache, dizziness, insomnia, weakness, fatigue, anorexia, nausea, vomiting, diarrhoea, chest pain, shortness of breath, palpitations, abdominal pain, back pain, joint pains, amenorrhoea, impotence, but not matched by physical findings

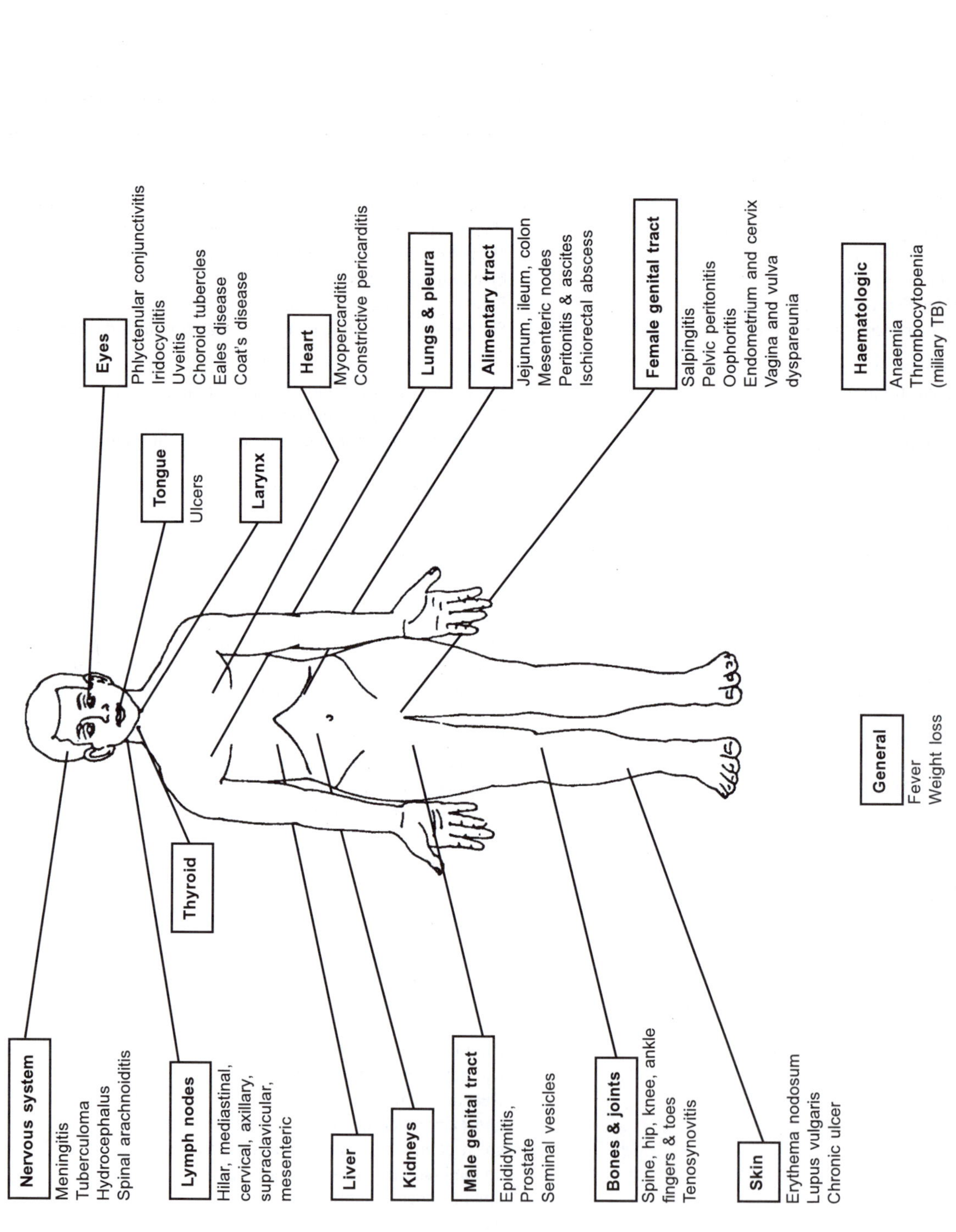

Eyes
Phlyctenular conjunctivitis
Iridocyclitis
Uveitis
Choroid tubercles
Eales disease
Coat's disease

Tongue
Ulcers

Larynx

Heart
Myopercarditis
Constrictive pericarditis

Lungs & pleura

Alimentary tract
Jejunum, ileum, colon
Mesenteric nodes
Peritonitis & ascites
Ischiorectal abscess

Female genital tract
Salpingitis
Pelvic peritonitis
Oophoritis
Endometrium and cervix
Vagina and vulva
dyspareunia

Haematologic
Anaemia
Thrombocytopenia
(miliary TB)

Nervous system
Meningitis
Tuberculoma
Hydrocephalus
Spinal arachnoiditis

Lymph nodes
Hilar, mediastinal,
cervical, axillary,
supraclavicular,
mesenteric

Thyroid

Liver

Kidneys

Male genital tract
Epididymitis,
Prostate
Seminal vesicles

Bones & joints
Spine, hip, knee, ankle
fingers & toes
Tenosynovitis

Skin
Erythema nodosum
Lupus vulgaris
Chronic ulcer

General
Fever
Weight loss

Fig. 59.1: Tuberculosis as a multi-organ disease

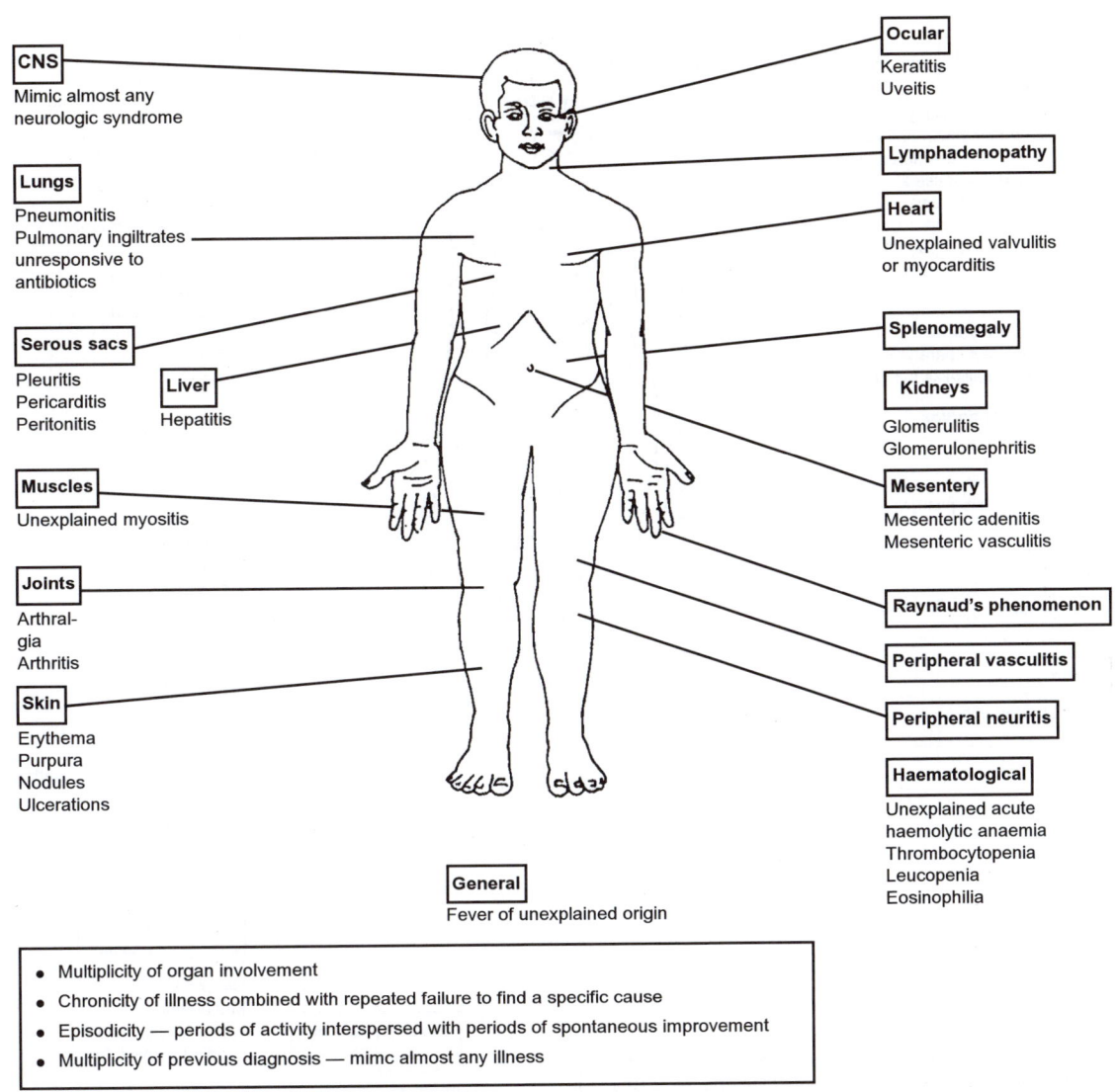

CNS
Mimic almost any
neurologic syndrome

Lungs
Pneumonitis
Pulmonary ingiltrates
unresponsive to
antibiotics

Serous sacs
Pleuritis
Pericarditis   **Liver**
Peritonitis   Hepatitis

Muscles
Unexplained myositis

Joints
Arthral-
gia
Arthritis

Skin
Erythema
Purpura
Nodules
Ulcerations

Ocular
Keratitis
Uveitis

Lymphadenopathy

Heart
Unexplained valvulitis
or myocarditis

Splenomegaly

Kidneys
Glomerulitis
Glomerulonephritis

Mesentery
Mesenteric adenitis
Mesenteric vasculitis

Raynaud's phenomenon

Peripheral vasculitis

Peripheral neuritis

Haematological
Unexplained acute
haemolytic anaemia
Thrombocytopenia
Leucopenia
Eosinophilia

General
Fever of unexplained origin

- Multiplicity of organ involvement
- Chronicity of illness combined with repeated failure to find a specific cause
- Episodicity — periods of activity interspersed with periods of spontaneous improvement
- Multiplicity of previous diagnosis — mimc almost any illness

Fig. 59.2: SLE as a multi-organ disease

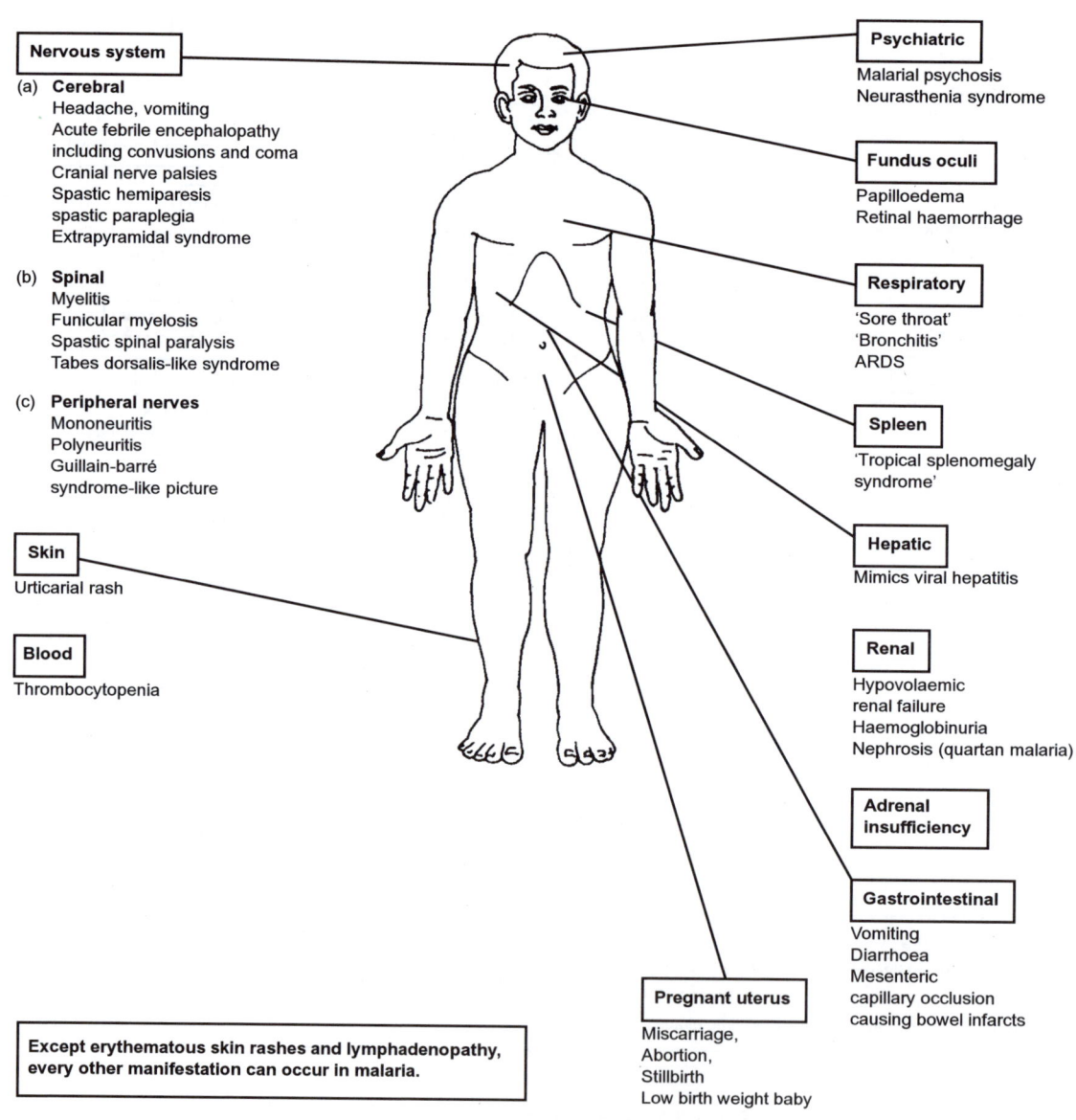

Nervous system

(a) **Cerebral**
Headache, vomiting
Acute febrile encephalopathy
including convusions and coma
Cranial nerve palsies
Spastic hemiparesis
spastic paraplegia
Extrapyramidal syndrome

(b) **Spinal**
Myelitis
Funicular myelosis
Spastic spinal paralysis
Tabes dorsalis-like syndrome

(c) **Peripheral nerves**
Mononeuritis
Polyneuritis
Guillain-barré
syndrome-like picture

Skin
Urticarial rash

Blood
Thrombocytopenia

Psychiatric
Malarial psychosis
Neurasthenia syndrome

Fundus oculi
Papilloedema
Retinal haemorrhage

Respiratory
'Sore throat'
'Bronchitis'
ARDS

Spleen
'Tropical splenomegaly
syndrome'

Hepatic
Mimics viral hepatitis

Renal
Hypovolaemic
renal failure
Haemoglobinuria
Nephrosis (quartan malaria)

**Adrenal
insufficiency**

Gastrointestinal
Vomiting
Diarrhoea
Mesenteric
capillary occlusion
causing bowel infarcts

Pregnant uterus
Miscarriage,
Abortion,
Stillbirth
Low birth weight baby

Except erythematous skin rashes and lymphadenopathy,
every other manifestation can occur in malaria.

Fig. 59.3: Malaria as a multi-system disease

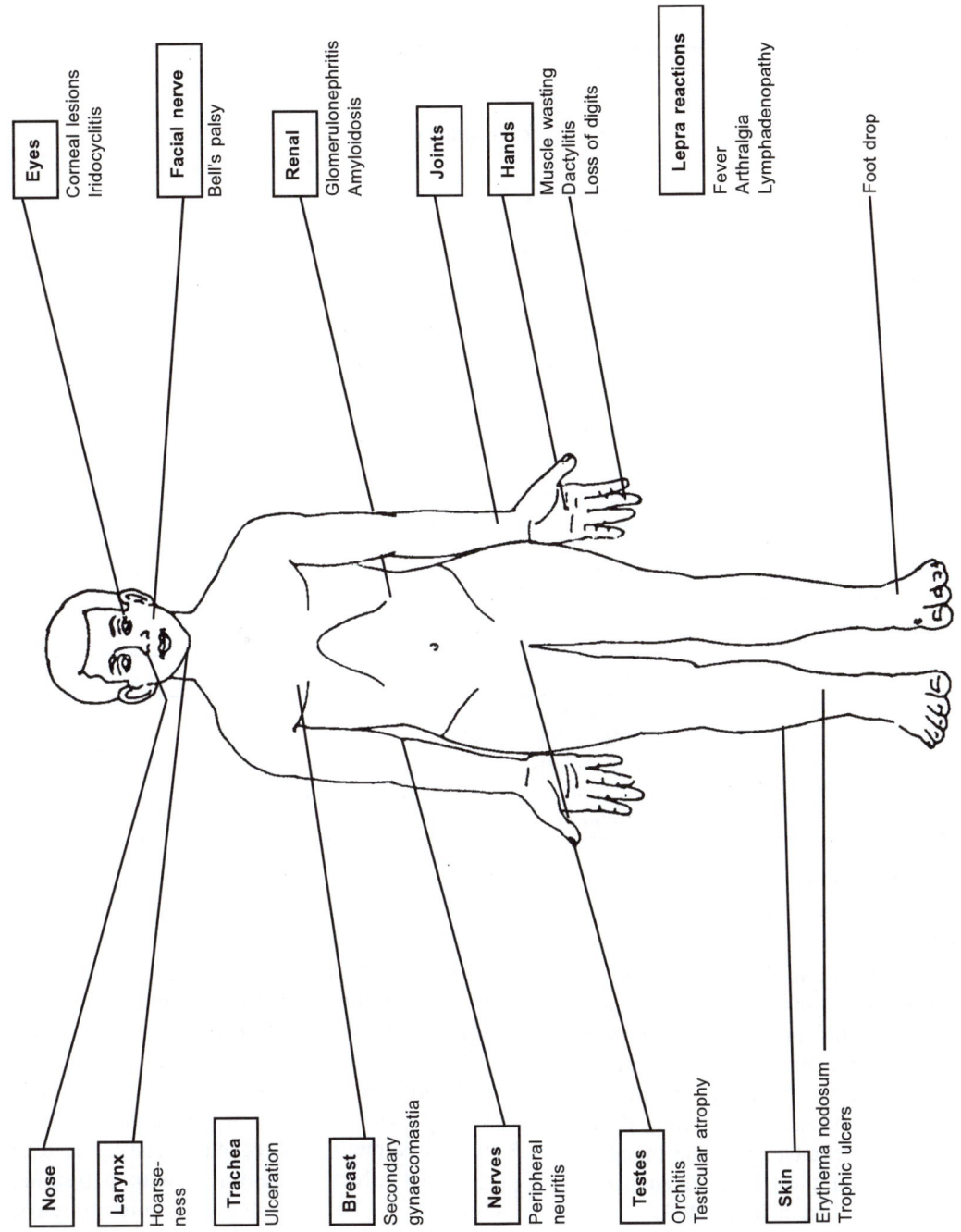

Eyes
Corneal lesions
Iridocyclitis

Facial nerve
Bell's palsy

Renal
Glomerulonephritis
Amyloidosis

Joints

Hands
Muscle wasting
Dactylitis
Loss of digits

Lepra reactions
Fever
Arthralgia
Lymphadenopathy

Foot drop

Nose

Larynx
Hoarse-
ness

Trachea
Ulceration

Breast
Secondary
gynaecomastia

Nerves
Peripheral
neuritis

Testes
Orchitis
Testicular atrophy

Skin
Erythema nodosum
Trophic ulcers

Fig. 59.4: Leprosy as a multi-organ disease

TABLE 59.4 AUTOIMMUNE POLYGLANDULAR SYNDROMES

Component disorders of Type I & Type II syndromes

Type I	Type II
Adrenal insufficiency	Adrenal insufficiency
Mucocutaneous candidiasis	
Hypoparathyroidism	Geriatric hypoparathyroidism
Chronic active hepatitis	
Graves' disease	Graves' disease
Hypothyroidism	Hypothyroidism
Pernicious anaemia	
IDDM	IDDM
Vitiligo	Vitiligo
Malabsorption syndrome ? secondary to hypocalcaemia	Coeliac disease
Alopecia	Alopecia
Hypophysitis	Hypophysitis
Primary hypogonadism	Primary hypogonadism Myasthenia gravis Parkinson's disease
Keratoconjunctivitis	Serositis

Contrasting features of Type I & Type II syndromes

Type I	Type II
Only siblings affected	Multiple generations affected
No HLA-DR association	HLA DR3/DR4 association
Mucocutaneous candidiasis	No candidiasis
Destructive hypoparathyroidism	Rare hyoparathyroidism (antibody mediated)
IDDM more than 4%	IDDM 50%

multisystem/multiorgan-only there are no positive physical findings to match the symptoms. Drug toxicity also involves multiple systems or organs.

The autoimmune polyglandular syndromes are described in **Table 59.4**. It may be noted that both hyperfunction and hypofunction can occur in these syndromes. Failure to recognize pernicious anaemia as part of the syndrome (antibodies to gastric intrinsic factor) may lead to unnecessary suffering of the patient from a totally treatable condition (monthly injection of Vit. B12 100 µg IM). Multiple endocrine neoplasia (MEN) is described in **Table 59.5**.

Although these tumours (APUDomas) are rare, they are worth remembering because they can now be easily diagnosed and treated. Most of these tumours express somatostatin receptors on their surface, and thereby lend themselves to detection by imaging with radiolabelled octreotide (a somatostatin analogue). Thus carcinoid tumours, pituitary secreting GH, TSH, ACTH, prolactin, pancreatic endocrine tumours such as gastrinoma, insulinoma, VIPoma, glucagonoma etc can be detected in an easy, non-invasive manner. Apart from the detection of the tumour site for surgical treatment, this technique can be used to predict the effect of treatment with octreotide (sandostatin). For instance carcinoid tumours, gastrinomas and acromegaly patients have been successfully managed with octreotide.

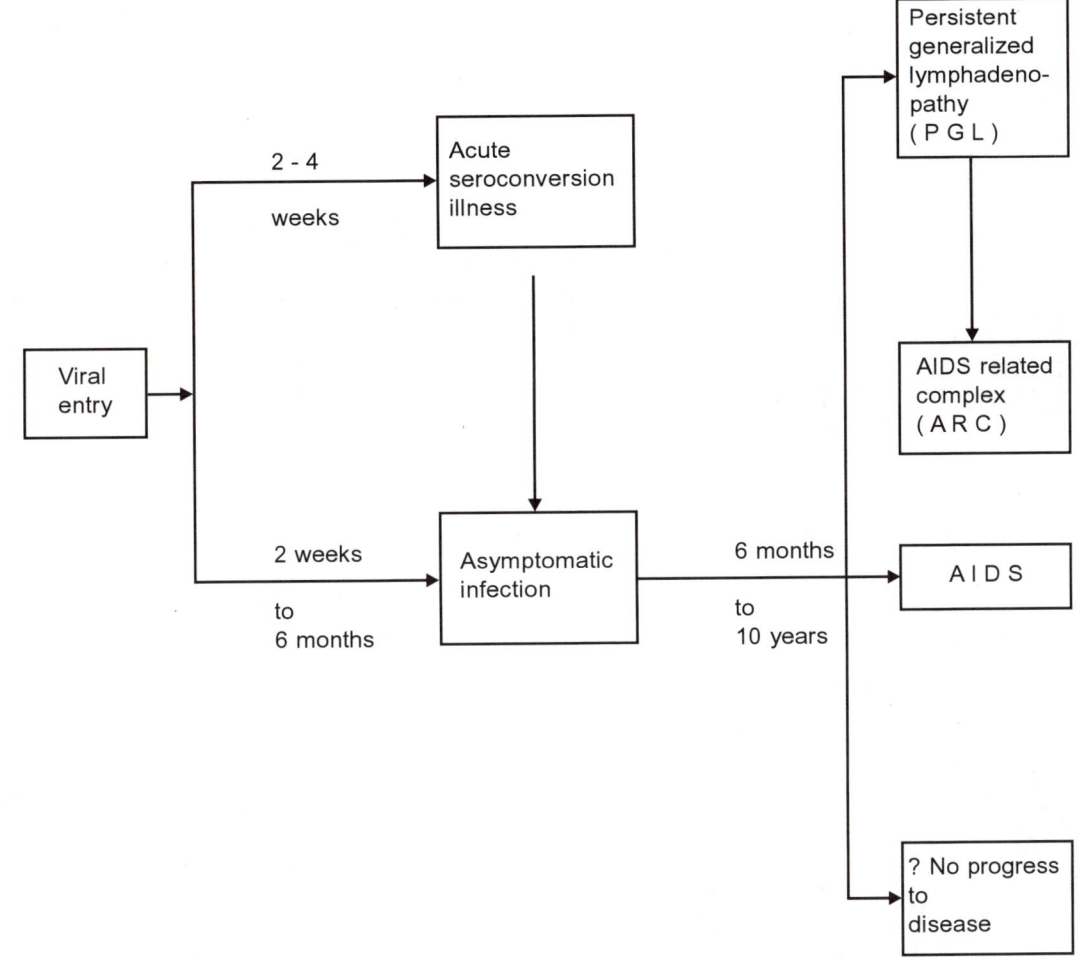

Fig. 59.5: The progression of HIV infection

Clinical Manifestations of HIV Infection

The clinical manifestations of HIV infection form a wide spectrum ranging from asymptomatic Infection to fatal AIDS (**Figs. 59.5** and **59.6**).

I. *Acute infection*

    An acute seroconversion illness occurs in some HIV infected persons within 2-6 weeks of viral entry. Features of this illness include fever, maculopapular rash mainly on the trunk and limbs, malaise, myalgia, arthralgia, lymphadenopathy, anorexia, sore throat, diarrhoea, etc. The illness is self-limiting and lasts between 1 and 3 weeks. In a few cases acute-

onset reversible encephalitis and meningitis have also been noticed.

The seroconversion illness mimics many viral illnesses (infectious mononucleosis, rubella, Epstein-Barr virus, and toxoplasmosis.

II. *Asymptomatic infection*

    Whether or not a well-defined seroconversion illness is experienced, all HIV infected persons experience an asymptomatic period ranging from months. to years. A small number of persons have stopped at this stage, the rest progressing to further stages with increasing immunodeficiency, usually within 2-3 years.

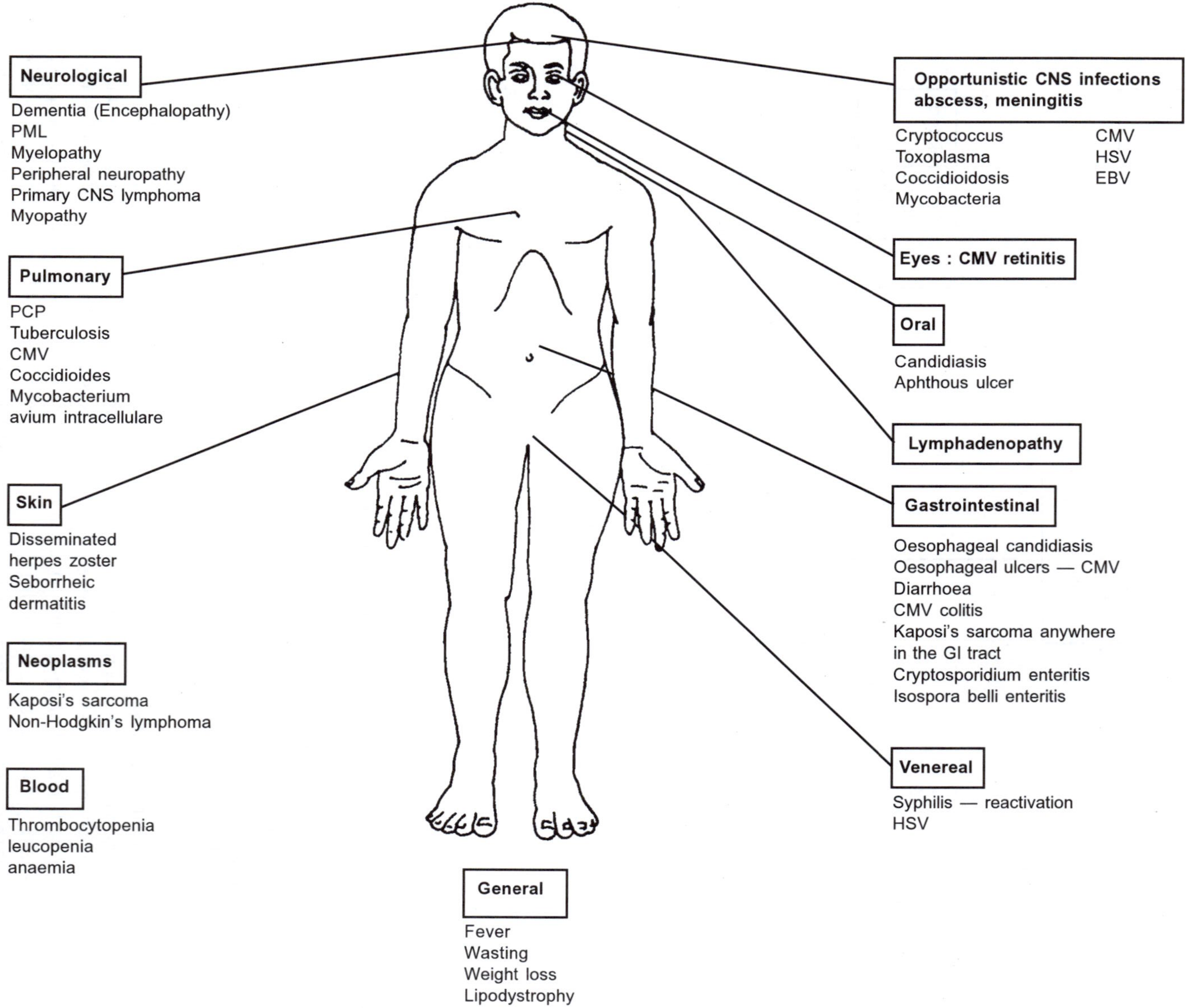

Opportunistic CNS infections abscess, meningitis

Cryptococcus   CMV
Toxoplasma   HSV
Coccidioidosis   EBV
Mycobacteria

Eyes : CMV retinitis

Oral

Candidiasis
Aphthous ulcer

Lymphadenopathy

Gastrointestinal

Oesophageal candidiasis
Oesophageal ulcers — CMV
Diarrhoea
CMV colitis
Kaposi's sarcoma anywhere
in the GI tract
Cryptosporidium enteritis
Isospora belli enteritis

Venereal

Syphilis — reactivation
HSV

General

Fever
Wasting
Weight loss
Lipodystrophy

Neurological

Dementia (Encephalopathy)
PML
Myelopathy
Peripheral neuropathy
Primary CNS lymphoma
Myopathy

Pulmonary

PCP
Tuberculosis
CMV
Coccidioides
Mycobacterium
avium intracellulare

Skin

Disseminated
herpes zoster
Seborrheic
dermatitis

Neoplasms

Kaposi's sarcoma
Non-Hodgkin's lymphoma

Blood

Thrombocytopenia
leucopenia
anaemia

Fig. 59.6: HIV infection as a multi-organ disease

TABLE 59.5 MULTIPLE ENDOCRINE NEOPLASIA (MEN)

Autosomal dominant pattern of inheritance

MEN 1

Gene on chromosome 11 Deletion of a regulatory gene	Familial association. Parathyroid hyperplasia– tends to recur following surgery. Pancreatic islet cells hyperplasia gastrin, insulin, glucagon, PP. Pituitary hyperplasia prolactin, GH, ACTH. Carcinoid tumour less common. Lipomas in some.

MEN 2 A

Gene on chromosome 10	Medullary Ca. Thyroid: bilateral multicentric. Pheochromocytoma: unilateral or bilateral. Parathyroid hyperplasia less common.

MEN 2 B

	Medullary Ca. Thyroid. Pheochromocytoma. Multiple mucosal neurinomas: distal tongue, lips, sub-conjunctival, entire GI tract. Colonic polyps can occur.

- Overlap syndromes can occur.
- Histological progression from hyperplasia → adenoma → carcinoma in some.
- Embryonic derivation from neuro-ectoderm—cells have some neurone-like properties
  APUD (Amine precursor uptake and decarboxylation)
  APUDomas may arise from the pituitary, thyroid, autonomic nervous system (paraganglioma, neuroblastoma, pheochromo cytoma), lung, gastrointestinal tract, or pancreas.

III. *Persistent generalized lymphadenopathy (PGL)*

This group includes patients who have palpable lymph nodes more than 1 cm in diameter at two or more extrainguinal sites lasting for three or more months, without any apparent explanation for the same. The lymph nodes, commonly seen in the cervical and axillary regions, are nonmatted. Splenomegaly may also be present.

As the disease progresses there may be a regression in the lymph node size. Malaise, fatigue, fever and night sweats may accompany the lymphadenopathy, resembling tuberculosis.

IV. *AIDS-related complex (ARC)*
ARC is characterized by two or more of the constitutional signs and symptoms listed below, lasting for three months or more in the absence of additional diagnostic features of AIDS.
- Lymphadenopathy
- Fever, night sweats, fatigue
- Weight loss without apparent explanation
- Persistent diarrhoea without apparent cause
- Oral cavity : thrush, aphthous ulcers etc.
  (Table 59.6)
- Skin manifestations **(Table 59.6)**
- Thrombocytopenia

V. *Neurological disease*
(1) Neurological involvement can occur independent of the manifestations of immunodeficiency, since the brain cells have receptors for the irus and infected cells undergo death by apoptosis. (2) Neurological manifestations may also be secondary to a variety of opportunistic infections (CMV, herpes simplex, EB virus, papovavirus, cryptococcus, candida, toxoplasma, mycobacteria). (3) They may be due to primary CNS lymphoma or Kaposi's sarcoma. A wide spectrum of neurological manifestations can result:
- AIDS dementia
- Primary lymphoma of CNS
- Progressive multifocal leucoencephalopathy
- Aseptic meningitis
- Cerebral abscess
- Myelopathy
- Peripheral neuropathy

VI. Pulmonary manifestations Pneumocystis carinii pneumonia (PCP) is the most common opportunistic lung infection in developed countries. Mycobacterial infections are more common in developing countries. M. tuberculosis infection in AIDS shows different clinical features (absence of granuloma formulation, resistance

TABLE 59.6 OPPORTUNISTIC INFECTIONS IN HIV PATIENTS

I.   *Viral:*
  CMV   Upper & lower respiratory tract, oesophagitis, gastritis, enterocolitis, chorioretinitis, necrotizing adrenalitis, bone marrow suppression.
  HSV   Large persistent ulcers, oesophagitis, pulmonary disease.
  Varicella   Typical dermatomal lesions or disseminated recurrent disease,
  zoster   meningoencephalitis, cranial neuritis.
  EBV   Clinical manifestations unclear.
  JC   Papovavirus associated with progressive multifocal leucodystrophy (PML), altered mental status, visual loss, weakness and abnormal gait.

II. *Bacterial:*
  Non-typhoid salmonella Esp. S. typhimurium: invasive disease that recurs or persists despite appropriate antibiotic tr.
  Syphilis   Reactivation of previously treated disease, active disease with negative serology, asymptomatic neurosyphilis & relapse after standard tr.
  Bacterial pneumonias   S. pneumoniae, H. influenzae, group B Streptococcus.

III. *Mycobacterial:*
  Mycobacterium   Increasing frequency esp, in IV drug abuse, atypical radiographic patterns,
  tuberculosis   apical cavitary disease rare, extrapulmonary disease. Prophylaxis with INAH recommended for all.
  M. avium   One of the most frequent opportunistic infections.
  intracellulare   Generalized infection or gastrointestinal disease.

IV. *Fungal:*
  Candidiasis   Persistent oral, oesophageal, vaginal infection, dissemination e.g., IV catheters used.
  Cryptococcus   Most common cause of fungal CNS disease in AIDS.
  neofonnans   Symptoms may be mild hence high index of suspicion to perform LP.
  Histoplasma   May cause disseminated disease & septicaemia;
  capsulatum   relapses common on amphotericin B tr.
  Coccidioides   Extensive pulmonary disease with extrapulmonary spread. Meningitis requires
  immitis   intra-cisternal or intra-ventricular amphotericin.

V.   *Protozoal:*
  Pneumocystis   Most common opportunistic infection in AIDS, leading cause of mortality;
  carinii pneumonia   otitis and cutaneous lesions also described.
  (PCP)   Prophylaxis TMP/SMZ 160 mg/800 mg/day or pentamidine aerosols 200 mg/ each month recommended for all patients with CD_4 cell count less than 200.
  Toxoplasma   Multiple CNS lesions: encephalopathy, focal neurologic findings,
  gondii   choreoretinitis. Sulfadiazine 25 mg/kg 6 hrly plus pyrimethamine 75 mg on day 1, 50 mg on day 2 and 25 mg/ d thereafter result in improvement. Indetinite therapy is needed to prevent relapse.
  Cryptosporidium and   Enteric infection; no effective treatment;
  Isospora belli   TMP/SMZ 160 mg /800 mg PO qid for 10 days, then bid for 3 weeks for Isospora belli.

(Contd)

TABLE 59.6 (Contd)

VI.	Neoplasms associated with AIDS:	Non-Hodgkin's lymphoma. Primary CNS lymphoma. Kaposi's sarcoma: skin & mucosa anywhere in the body.
VII.	Gastrointestinal manifestations:	Oesophageal candidiasis. Oesophageal ulcers due to CMV. Diarrhoea. Kaposi's sarcoma anywhere in the GI tract. CMV colitis which may mimic ulcerative colitis.
VIII.	Skin manifestations:	Seborrhoeic dermatitis. Folliculitis. Psoriasis. Molluscum contagiosum—warts. Kaposi's sarcoma. Herpes zoster-multiple sites.

to chemotherapy). HIV infection may reactivate dormant tuberculosis anywhere in the body.

Treatment of HIV/AIDS

The discovery of a diagnosis of HIV infection is a devastating event, hence the paramount need for pre-test and post test counseling and active medical as well as emotional support in which experienced social workers play a vital role. Combination of 3 anti-retroviral drugs is the cornerstone of management. The least expensive is the combination of Lamivudine (RTI) 150 mg b. d., Stavudine (RTI) 30 mg b. d., Nevirapine (NNRTI) 200 mg b. d. Given the complexity of this field, especially treatment of concurrent tuberculosis, and the drug —drug interactions, decisions regarding choice of drugs are best made in consultation with experts. Compliance is an important part of ensuring maximal effect of therapy. The simpler the regimen the easier it is for the patient to be compliant.

Fig. 59.7 and Table 59.7.

Emphasis on prevention

Education counseling and behaviour modification are the cornerstones of HIV prevention strategy. The practice of "safe sex" by use of latex condoms, avoidance of sharing needles among intravenous drug users (IDU) by providing sterile needles; mandatory HIV testing of blood donors by blood banks, and treatment of an HIV infected mother with ART during pregnancy and the newborn during the first week following birth are proven strategies, which should be rigorously implemented.

Prophylaxis against tuberculosis with INAH for 12 months in HIV positive patients with a positive P skin test, is recommended.

Candida is treated with ketoconazole.

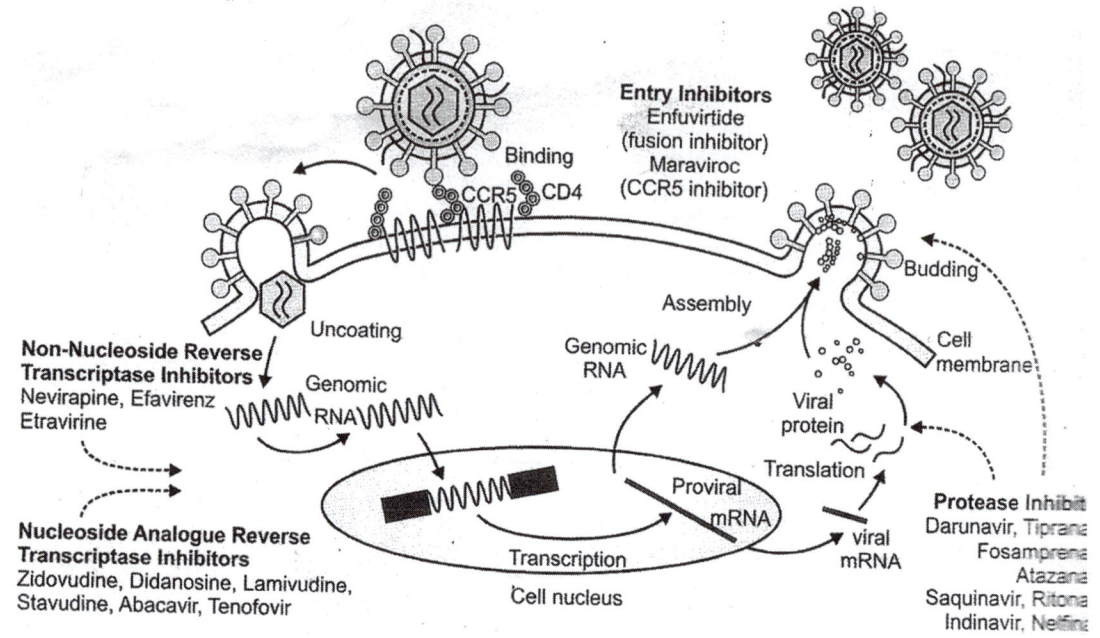

Fig. 59.7. Target sites of drugs for HIV.

TABLE 59.7 CLASSES OF ANTIRETROVIRAL DRUGS**

Nucleoside and Nucleotide Reverse Transcriptase Inhibitors (NRTIs/NtRTIs)	Non-Nucleoside Reverse Transcriptase Inhibitors (NNRTIs)	Protease Inhibitors (PIs)	Entry Inhibitors	Integrase Inhibitors
NRTIs	Nevirapine* (NVP)	Atazanavir* (ATV)	Fusion inhibitor	Raltegravir
Abacavir* (ABC)	Efavirenz* (EFV)	Darunavir* (DRV)	Enfuvirtide* (T20)	
Didanosine* (ddI)	Etravirine (ETV)	Fosamprenavir* (fAMP)	Entry blocker	
Emtricitabine* (FTC)		Indinavir (IDV)	Maraviroc	
Lamivudine* (3TC)		Lopinavir / Ritonavir*		
Stavudine*'' (d4T)		(LPV)		
Zidovudine* (AZT)		Nelfinavir* (NLF)		
NtRTI		Ritonavir* (RTV)		
Tenofovir disoproxil		Saquinavir (SQV)		
fumarate (TDF)		Tipranavir* (TPR)		

*   Approved for use in children

**   Three drugs–zalcitabine, amprenavir and delavirdine–are no longer manufactured, and do not appear in this table.

60 Stem Cell Therapy

Introduction

Stem cells are cells which have the potential to divide indefinitely and are required to renew worn-out tissues throughout life. These are immortal cells (unlike normal cells with a definite life span with programmed cell death-apoptosis). Stem cells have the ability to self-replicate for indefinite periods of time, and can differentiate into different cell types in response to specific signals. In dermatology it has cosmetic applications to improve the skin, treatment of burn injuries and scars.

Totipotent cells are found only in early embryos, which can differentiate into any of the over 200 cell types in the body. Pluripotent cells are found in the fetus (Obtained from Medical Termination of Pregnancy and it is legal in India). The placenta and umbilical cord are a rich source of multipotent stem cells. Menstrual blood is also a source of multipotent cells.

Apart from pluripotent embryonic stem cells, which can differentiate into an endoderm-gastrointestinal (GI) tract, liver, lungs, mesoderm-hematopoietic and mesodermal/ectoderm-skin and Central Nervous System, **(Fig. 60.1)**, there are resident stem cells in adults in all tissues which are capable of generating the cell type of the tissue in which they reside. The skin and mucosa and the endometrium are constantly renewing systems due to resident stem cells.

Lipo-aspirate from liposuction provides a rich source of MSCs and EPCs.

A new discovery is the presence of resident mesenchymal stem cells (MSCs) in the liver, kidneys, skeletal and cardiac muscle, endothelial progenitor cells (EPCs), dental, retinal, cerebral neurons specially hippocampus, and peripheral nervous system. The scope of stem cell therapy is depicted in Fig. 60.2.

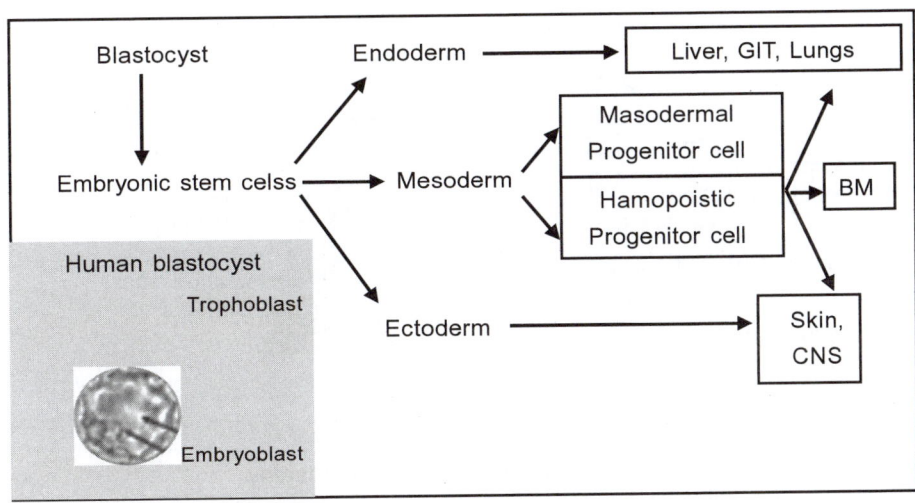

Fig. 60.1 : Embryonic Stem Cells

A further attribute of resident stem cells is their plasticity-capability of giving rise to a cell type of completely different tissue. For example, skin cells can be transformed into neurons. This approach will bypass the need of embryonic or fetal stem cells and play a major potential role in the treatment of neurodegenerative disorders.

In vitro, in vivo animal and human studies have shown a wide range of potential applications of MSCs in regenerative medicine. MSCs migrate to sites of tissue injury in response to local signal, with critical phenotypic changes and intense paracrine activity that contributes to reparative process. Allogenic MSCs have unique immunomodulatory properties. MSCs have been shown to pass through the blood-brain barrier and migrate throughout the forebrain and cerebellum without disrupting the host brain architecture. Allogenic MSC in mice with experimental autoimmune encephalomyelitis led to a significant decrease in score over time and cells expressing nerve growth factor and BDNF.

At present there are a significant number of clinical trials exploring the use of MSCs for treatment of various diseases including myocardial infarction and stroke and diabetes. MSCs have regenerative capacity to suppress autoimmunity which causes 90 human autoimmune disorders, in multiple sclerosis, type 1 diabetes, Crohn's disease etc. Allogenic and Autologous MSCs and EPCs have the ability to restore myocardial myogenesis and angiogenesis with improvement in cardiac function.

Pancreatic Islet β cells are destroyed by autoimmune mechanism in type 1 diabetes mellitus. Adult human MSCs have restored islet β cell and disappearance of β cell specific T cells .

MSCs have the capacity to improve diabetic nephropathy by reconstituting necrotic segments of diabetic kidneys.

Cartilage defects of knee can be repaired with autologous MSCs.

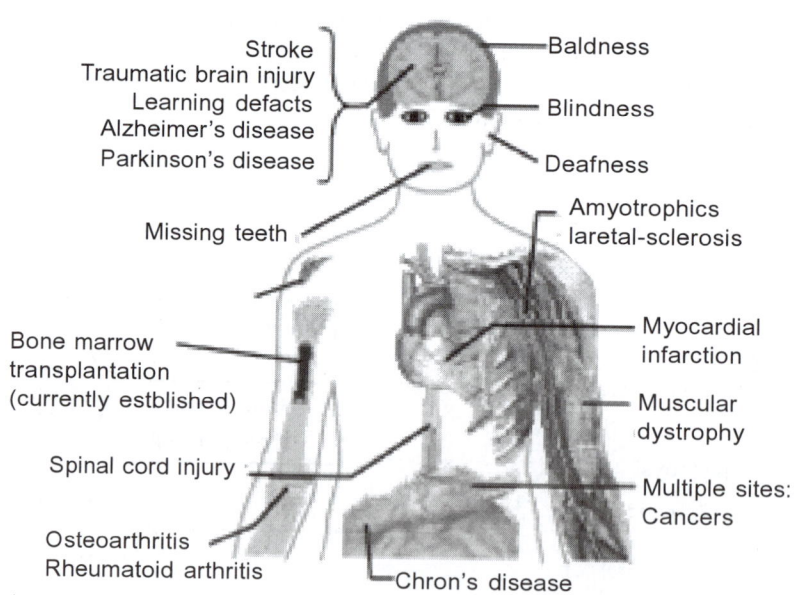

Fig. 60.2 : Scope of Stem Cell Therapy

Stem Cell Therapy

Autologous MSCs have a clear advantage of avoidance of undesirable immune reactions. Their procurement requires bone marrow aspiration, which may not be suitable in elderly patients with poor nutritional condition. The limited number of available autologous MSCs represents a major obstacle.

Allogenic MSCs need a Good Manufacturing Practice Facility and extensive preclinical evaluation prior to their application.

Stem cell therapy for intractable skin disease

Bone marrow provides fibroblast-like cells in the dermis and keratinocytes in the epidermis. Both embryonic and postnatal transplantation of bone marrow cells in mouse models of Epidermolysis bullosa (EB), a heritable blistering skin disease due to a genetic mutation of cutaneous basement membrane components, promote skin wound healing and correct the intrinsic basement membrane defect. The source of epithelial progenitor cells in bone marrow was the nonhematopoietic, platelet derived growth factor receptor α (PDGFRα) positive mesenchymal stem cell (MSC) population.

Prospective cell-based therapies for EB have been discussed by Uitto. Heritable forms of EB are characterized by chronic, lifelong blistering and erosions at the cutaneous basement membrane zone.

Wong et al demonstrated the feasibility of direct intradermal injection of allogeneic fibroblasts in the lesional skin of patients with recessive dystrophic EB, with improvement in skin fragility. It is considered more difficult to restore structural proteins than restore secretory enzymes. EB is caused by defects in Keratinocyte structural proteins (Collagen 17). Both hemopoietic and MSCs from bone marrow have the potential to produce Col 17. Furthermore, human cord blood has CD34+ cells and can also differentiate into keratinocytes and express human skin component protein.

Wound Healing

The nonhematopoietic component of bone marrow includes multipotent MSCs capable of differentiating into fat, bone muscle, cartilage, and endothelium.

Human MSCs are characterized by a profile CD29+ CD44+ CD105+ CD166+ CD34- CD45-. Autologous

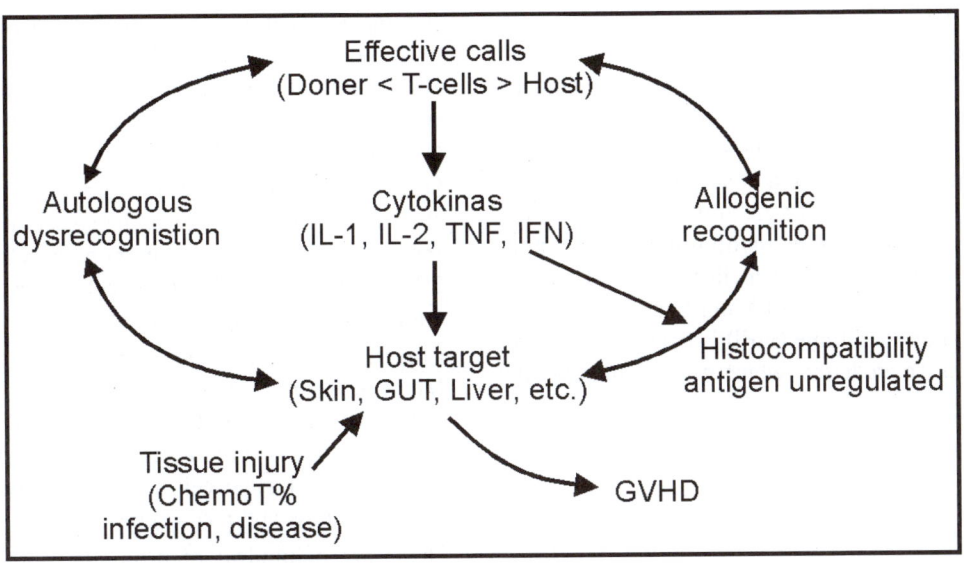

Fig. 60.3 :

bone marrow-derived cultured MSCs have been delivered into a fibrin polymer spray system with a double barrel syringe, into patients with acute wounds from skin cancer surgery, and in patients with chronic, long-standing, nonhealing lower limb wounds. 6 Cells were grown in vitro under conditions favouring the multiplication of MSCs. The cultured autologous MSCs were applied up to four times to wounds. Both fibrinogen (containing the MSCs) and thrombin were diluted to optimally deliver a polymerized gel that immediately adhered to the wound without run-off and yet allowing the MSCs to remain viable and migrate from the gel. Sequential adjacent sections biopsy specimens showed elongated spindle cells, which immunostained for MSC markers.

Generation of new elastic fibers was evident by both special stains and antibodies to human elastin and stimulated closure of full thickness wounds. Tracking of green fluorescent protein (GFP) showed GFP in blood vessels.

Graft Versus Host Disease

Dermatologic manifestations of graft versus host disease (GVHD) have been reviewed by Scheinfeld et al. 7 MSCs can be used for the treatment of therapy-resistant GVHD. Factors involved in GVHD are shown in **Fig. 60.3**.

Dermatologic manifestations are an important aspect of (GVHD), and dermatologists are crucial members of the treatment team. Acute GVHD occurs within the first 100 days of transplantation, with the triad of dermatitis, enteritis, and hepatitis. Chronic GVHD develops after 100 days and consists of an autoimmune syndrome involving the skin and multiple organs. Evidence of liver and/or GI tract GVHD without skin involvement is rare. A skin manifestation of chrome GVHD is lichen planus-like eruption or scleroderma, which present therapeutic challenges.

Staging and scoring system for skin involvement in acute GVHD is as follows:

Stage 1 involvement of < 25% of body surface

Stage 2 involvement of 25%-50% of body surface

Stage 3 involvement of 50%-100% (erythroderma)

Stage 4 vesicles and bullae.

MSCs have been used for the treatment of therapy-resistant GVHD.

Somatic Cell Nuclear Transfer (SCNT)

Human embryonic stem cells (hES) are a promising source for transplantation to replace diseased or damage tissue, but their differentiated progeny expresses human leukocyte antigens (HLA) that will probably cause graft rejection. Taylor et al (Lancet 2005, 366, 2019-25) have estimated that a bank of 150 consecutive blood group compatible donors, 100 consecutive blood group donors provided a full match at HLA-A, HLA-B, and HLA DR match for approximately 85%.

A new technique involving reprogramming of adult skin cells to induce pluripotent stem cells (iPS) has become feasible. (Yuj et al Science 2007, 318, 1917-20). Amazing things like bone re-growth, formation of teeth, retinal repair, cure of deafness, skin replacement have been demonstrated in animal models of iP5. Four factors (OCT4, SOX2, NANO6 and LIN28) are sufficient to reprogram human somatic cells to luripotent stem cells exhibiting the essential characteristics of embryonic stem cells.

SCNT is an approach to create autologous pluripotent stem cell lines, to enable patient-specific stem cell therapy without the risk of immune rejection. During SCNT, patient-specific donor cell is fused into an enucleated donor oocyte to produce blastocyst.

Chris Mason, Director of London Regenerative Medicine Network in United Kingdom has estimated that more than 323,000 patients worldwide have received cell-based therapies, and has predicted that the market for stem cell and regenerative therapy will rival drugs and medical devices.

There are a handful of products in the market, including a synthetic skin.

61

Making Effective Therapy Safer: Personalized Therapy

Introduction

The public perception worldwide about modern medicine is that just as it has the immense potential to give benefits, it has immense potential to do harm. The Institute of Medicine (IOM) in USA, in a 1999 report entitled "To Err is Human" estimated that about 100,000 deaths occurred annually in USA alone due to adverse effects of therapy. The cost of adverse drug reactions (ADRs) related to morbidity and mortality in USA alone ranges between $ 3-130 billion.

Some times rare but important ADRs are not detected in randomized controlled drug trials prior to FDA's drug approval (e.g. troglitazone's hepatotoxicity or viovax's adverse effect on CAD), hence physicians need to be cautious in the prescription of new drugs and to be alert and vigilant about the appearance of previously unrecognized ADRs. The publication of a newly recognized adverse effect can in a very short time stimulate many similar reports of ADRs which had previously gone unnoticed. The Internet now makes available a wide range of information about ADRs almost instantaneously, at any time, at any part of the world. Patients themselves are increasingly accessing the internet for information hence the doctors must ensure that they know at least as much as the patients do!

It is important to realise that a major motivation of public recourse to alternative therapies is the fear of adverse reactions to modern drugs and the public perception about the safety of alternative therapies. In their quest for safety more and more people are likely to seek safe but ineffective therapy which is no better than placebo. This will result in two undesirable social consequences: (1) wasteful expenditure on ineffective alternative therapy (2) Genuine deprivation of effective therapy provided by modern medicine.

Most ADRs are preventable hence the utmost concern of practitioners of modern medicine is to make effective therapy safer for the individual patient.

During hospitalization patients receive as many as 10 different drugs. The sicker the patient, the more drugs he receives, with a corresponding increase in the likelihood of ADRs. The elderly patients as a group have a greater burden of disease, and hence receive a greater number of medications, hence a greater frequency of ADRs in them, which can be very subtle hence the clinician must be alert to the possibility that their symptoms and signs reflect an ADR.

The ADR often present diagnostic problems because they can involve every organ and system of the body and are frequently mistaken for signs of the underlying disease. For example drugs can cause toxic effects which can mimic almost every naturally occuring liver disease in humans. About 2 per cent of all causes of jaundice in hospitalized patients are drug-induced. About a quarter of fulminant hepatic failure are drug-induced.

Drug history should be an integral component of a patient's history. It is a sobering thought for all doctors that about 10-20 per cent of hospitalized patients, and 2-5 per cent of outpatients develop adverse effects while taking medications. This frequency varies greatly, depending upon the drugs administered, the patient population treated, and the definition of adverse effects. A small group of frequently administered drugs accounts for the majority of adverse drug reactions. Since these drugs produce most of the problems, familiarity with their adverse effects is important (**Tables 61.1, 61.2**).

I. Some adverse effects are *predictable* since they are produced by the *intended pharmacological actions* of the drugs, and are *dose-dependent*. Common examples are:

TABLE 61.1 ADVERSE EFFECTS OF COMMONLY USED DRUGS

Drugs	Adverse effect	Drugs	Adverse effect
Penicillins and cephalosporins	Hypersensitivity reactions, Neutropenia, Interstitial nephritis, Pseudomembranous colitis, Coagulation abnormalities.	Frusemide	Hypovolaemia, Hypokalaemia, Hyponatraemia, Hyperuricaemia, Hyperglycaemia, Ototoxicity.
Aminoglycoside antibiotics	Nephrotoxicity, Autotoxicity, Neuromuscular paralysis.	Thiazides	Hypokalaemia, Hyperuricaemia, Hypercalcaemia, Hyperglycaemia, Thrombocytopenia, Pancreatitis, Pulmonary oedema.
Tetracyclines	Nausea, Metallic taste, Photosensitivity, Pseudomembranous colitis, Vertigo (doxycycline), Candida superinfection.		
Trimethoprim/ sulphamethoxazole (TMP/SMZ)	Skin rash, Nausea, Diarrhoea, Neutropenia, Thrombocytopenia.	Insulin	Hypoglycaemia, Allergic reactions, Lipoatrophy.
Aspifin	Nausea, Epigastric discomfort, Gastritis, Ulcers, Tinnitus, Prolonged bleeding time.	Prednisolone	Osteoporosis, Proximal muscle weakness, Skin atrophy, Vascular fragility, Adrenal suppression, Hyperglycaemia, Hyperlipidaemia, Centripetal obesity, Hirsutism, Pancreatitis, Cataract, Glaucoma, Psychosis, Depression of cell-mediated immunity.
NSAIDs	Nausea, Epigastric discomfort, Gastritis, Diarrhoea, Headache, Interstitial nephritis, Oedema, Hepatitis, Neutropenia, Thrombocytopenia.		
Acetaminophen	Skin rash, Leucopenia, Hepatic necrosis, Renal papillary necrosis.	Propranolol	Bronchospasm, Congestive heart failure, Bradycardia, Fatigue, Depression, Vivid dreams, Impotence.
Digoxin	Anorexia, Nausea, Vomiting, Yellow-green vision, Gynaecomastia, Cardiac arrhythmias Bradycardia.		
Warfarin	Anorexia, Nausea, Haematuria, Haemorrhage, Haemorrhagic necrosis of breast, skin or toes.	Captopril	Hyperkalaemia, Eczema, Fixed drug eruption, Photodermatitis, Urticaria, Taste disturbance Agranulocytosis, Nephrotic syndrome, Troublesome cough.

(Contd)

TABLE **61.1** (Contd)

Drugs	Adverse effects
Tricyclic antidepressants	Fatigue, Somnolence, Orthostatic hypotension, Dry mouth Glaucoma, Blurred vision Headache, Seizures, Constipation, Urine retention, Delayed ejaculation, Parkinsonism, Tardive dyskinesia, Arrhythmias, Congestive cardiac failure.
Oral contraceptives	Hyperglycaemia, Nausea, Headache, Breast tenderness, Weight gain, Thromboembolism, Stroke, Cholelithiasis Secondary amenorrhoea, Hypertension, Myopathy.

Hypoglycaemia: caused by overdose of insulin or sulfonylurea.

Hypotension: caused by overdose of antihypertensive drugs.

Sodium and water depletion: caused by overdose of diuretics.

Altered drug pharmacokinetics are a frequent cause of dose-dependent adverse effects. For example, when the clearance of a drug is reduced (due to hepatic or renal dysfunction), excessive drug concentration at the receptor sites occurs, causing exaggerated pharmacologic effects.

II. Adverse effects caused by unintended actions of the drug may be categorized into those due to

1. Physical and chemical properties of the drug or its excipients, usually caused by decomposition of the drug, or effects of excipients commonly used for stabilization or solubilization.

2. Direct cytotoxic effect of the drug or its metabolites that covalently bind to tissue macro molecules.

e.g. hepatotoxicity caused by isoniazid.

3. Induction of an abnormal immune response. This occurs by one of three mechanisms:

i. The drug binds to proteins or cells and directly induces an antibody response, e.g. quinidine-induced thrombocytopenia.

ii. The drug alters tissue and induces an autoimmune response directed against the altered tissue, e.g. alphamethyl dopa causes haemolytic anaemia (Coomb's positive), which disappears on stopping the drug.

iii. The drug induces production of antibodies that are cross-reactive with other proteins or tissues, e.g. penicillin.

4. Drug reaction due to heritable enzyme defects. e.g.

(a) Succinylcholine: prolonged neuromuscular blockade due to deficiency of pseudocholinesterase.

(b) Sulphonamides or primaquine: haemolytic anaemia due to glucose-6-phosphate dehydrogenase deficiency.

Time Frame of Adverse Drug Effects

1. Most adverse drug reactions occur soon after administration.

2. Many effects are seen after a month or more e.g. INAH hepatitis.

3. Many effects may occur after several months, e.g. chloroquine.

4. Some may take years (mutagenesis or teratogenesis).

5. Some may be seen in the next generation e.g. stilboesterol given to mothers causes vaginal tumours in offspring.

The evidence of teratogenesis is strong for anti-cancer drugs, some hormones (androgens, oestrogens, corticosteroids) warfarin, phenytoin, inhaled anaesthetics, phenothiazines, tricyclic antidepressants, tobacco, and alcohol. Antineoplastic agents like cyclophosphamide have been linked to the development of chromosomal damage and subsequent malignancy.

TABLE 61.2 DRUG-DRUG INTERACTIONS (illustrative examples)

Drug	Interactor	Effects
Oral hypoglycaemics		
Chlorpropamide Glybenclamide	(1) Antacids (aluminium & magnesium hydroxide)	Increased absorption: *Increased* hypoglycaemic
Metformin Gliclazide Glipizide	(2) Rifampicin Phenytoin Carbamazepine Phenobarbitone	Enzyme induction Increased metabolism: *Reduced* hypoglycaemic effect.
	(3) Chloramphemicol Cotrimoxazole Fluconazole Phenylbutazone Cimetidine	Enzyme inhibition: *Increased* hypoglycaemic effect.
	(4) Expectorants (ammonium chloride) Allopurinol	Decreased renal excretion: *Increased* hypoglycaemic effect.
	(5) Beta blockers Thiazides ACE inhibitors	Delayed recovery from hypoglycaemia.
	(6) Corticosteroids Oral contraceptives	Increased blood sugar.
Anticoagulants		
Coumarins	(1) Aspirin & NSAIDs	Increased bleeding.
	(2) Barbiturates	Reduced anticoagulation.
	(3) Carbamazepine	
	(4) Chloramphenicol	Increased bleeding.
	(5) Cimetidine	
	(6) Eltroxine	
Antidepressants		
Amitriptyline Amoxapine Desipramine Doxepin	(1) Enzyme inducers Barbiturates Carbamazepine Phenytoin (Cytochrome P450 system)	Reduced antidepressant effect. Exacerbation of affective disorders. Need to increase dose of antidepressant.
Imapramine Maprotiline Nortryptyline Trimipramine	(2) Enzyme inhibitors Cimetidine Diltiazem Fluoxetine Neuroleptics Propoxyphene Quinidine Verapamil	Increased antidepressant effect and toxicity. Dose of antidepressant should be reduced. Ranitidine may replace cimetidine.

Pregnancy and Drugs

Since most drugs cross the placenta, foetal drug concentrations are directly related to maternal plasma levels. During the first trimester of pregnancy, when organogenesis is taking place, the risk of drug-induced defects is the greatest, but exposure any time during pregnancy may delay or distort normal development. Hence extreme conservatism in prescribing drugs to pregnant women is essential.

Patients at Risk

Certain patients may be at greater risk for developing adverse reactions to drugs.

Advanced age: Lower glomerular filtration as compared to young patients, reduces drug clearance for the same dose.

Hepatic and renal disease: Alteration of drug pharmacokinetics.

Inherited enzyme defects: e.g. G-6-PD deficiency.

Alcohol: can increase toxicity of benzodiazepines, phenothiazines, and phenytoin.

Drug–drug Interactions (Table 61.2)

A drug-drug interaction is defined as an alteration in the action of a drug resulting from the prior, concurrent, or subsequent administration or discontinuation of another drug. The net result of the interaction may be *enhancement* of action (toxicity), *reduction* in the effect of a drug, a *new action*, or no significant change in the effect.

While the list of drug interactions is large, only a small number of drug interactions are clinically relevant. Knowledge of drug interactions enables the doctor to prevent or minimize either toxicity or reduced therapeutic response, by choosing alternative drugs, or by adjusting the dose or the time of administration of different drugs. During hospital stay a patient may receive on an average 3-8 medicines at a time. In general practice a patient may be taking several drugs concurrently prescribed by either the same doctor or by different doctors, or drugs from different alternative systems of medicine, or self-administered drugs.

Hence it is very essential to understand the basic mechanisms of drug interactions.

1. Pharmaceutical incompatibility

Drug interaction which occurs in a syringe ora bottle when some drugs are mixed together is termed pharmaceutical incompatibility. This can occur with or without a visible change in the solution, and the net result is the loss of efficacy. The intravenous administration of incompatible drug mixtures may result in a serious, even fatal, outcome. Examples of pharmaceutical incompatibility are:

> Thiopentone + succinyl choline: Precipitation.
> Penicillin + gentamicin/heparin/phenytoin:
> Neutralization.
> Heparin + hydrocortisone/lignocaine:
> Neutralization.
> Protein Hydrolysate + tetracycline: Protein
> binding.

2. Pharmacokinetic phase

Drugs may interact during their absorption, distribution, metabolism, or excretion.

i. *Absorption:* Antacids interfere with the absorption of tetracyclines, isoniazid and digoxin. By increasing the pH in the stomach, antacids decrease absorption of aspirin and fluoroquinolones.

These interactions can be minimized or avoided by administering the interacting drugs 23 hours apart.

ii. *Distribution:* A number of acidic drugs are reversibly bound to plasma proteins. The pharmacological action of a drug is due to the free circulating (unbound) drug. Competitive displacement of a highly bound (over 90 per cent) drug by another drug administered subsequently with a higher binding affinity, will lead to an increase in the free drug concentration of one drug. These interactions become clinically important only if the metabolic or excretion processes are not functioning normally.

Examples of drugs with high binding to plasma proteins are:

NSAIDs: ibuprofen, phenylbutazone, etc.

Antibiotics: cloxacillin, dicloxacillin, ketoconazole.

Psychotropic drugs: amitriptyline, chlorfrmazine, diazepam.

Cardiac drugs: amiodarone, digitalis, felodipine.

iii. *Metabolism:*

(a) *Enzyme induction:* Drugs that induce hepatic metabolic enzymes (cytochrome P450) can increase the metabolism of a drug leading to *gradual loss of effect*, thus necessitating an increase in the dosage of the parent drug. If the inducing drug is discontinued, the effect of the parent drug may result in toxicity unless the dose of the parent drug is also reduced. For instance, a patient stabilized on an oral anticoagulant drug while also on phenylbutazone therapy, will develop haemorrhage on stopping phenylbutazone, unless the dose of anticoagulant is titrated downwards. Some potent metabolic enzyme-inducing drugs are listed in **Table 61.2**.

(b) *Enzyme inhibition:* Drugs that inhibit hepatic metabolic enzymes cause an *increase* in the blood levels of the parent drug and resultant *toxicity*. These effects develop quickly, unlike enzyme induction which develops slowly over 2-3 weeks, and also wash out quickly. For example, isoniazid given along with oral hypoglycaemic agents, *enhances* the hypoglycaemic effects. Important drugs in this category are: allopurinol, chloramphenicol, ciprofloxacin, cimetidine, cotromoxazole, indomethacin, isoniazid, metrolidazole, paracetamol, phenylbutazone, sulphonyureas and sulphonamides.

iv. Renal excretion: Some drugs are actively secreted by the proximal tubules. This is a nonspecific and saturable process. Drug interaction can occur by competition between two drugs for the secretory process. For instance, probenecid decreases penicillin and methotrexate excretion.

Many drugs are passively diffused back into the distal tubules. Weak acid drugs, because of poor ionization in acid urine, are better absorbed in acid urine. The reverse happens in alkaline urine. Alkaline urine increases the excretion of barbiturates, lithium salts, salicylates and sulphonarnides, while it decreases the excretion of amphetamine, procainamide, quinidine and antidepressants.

3. *Pharmacodynamic phase*

Pharmacodynamic drug interactions occur quite commonly in clinical practice and are used to advantage, e.g. theophylline and terbutalin in bronchial asthma; diuretics and beta-blockers in hypertension. Combined use may also produce additive toxicity, e.g. increased ototoxicity with combined use of gentamicin and frusemide.

Medication Error

This is an avoidable cause of adverse drug reactions. Errors can be made by several persons including the prescribing doctor, nursing staff, pharmacist, and the patient or his relatives. Each one of them has a responsibility to take every possible precaution to prevent errors.

i. Prescribe the *correct* medicine.

ii. Write the generic name *legibly* so that there is no scope for misinterpretation. Avoid abbreviations; drugs may have similar names e.g. acetohexamide and acetazolamide. Drugs may be packaged in similar containers and the tablets may look alike.

iii. Indicate clearly the correct *dose, frequency* and *route*. An effective method of preventing dose error is to place a zero before a decimal point e.g. 0.1 mg instead of 0.1 mg. Do not confuse mg, mmol and mEq.

iv. Encourage the patient to read the drug information literature and caution him about possible side effects. Warn him to *stop the drug* immediately if he experiences any untoward effects, and to *report* to the prescribing doctor immediately for further instructions.

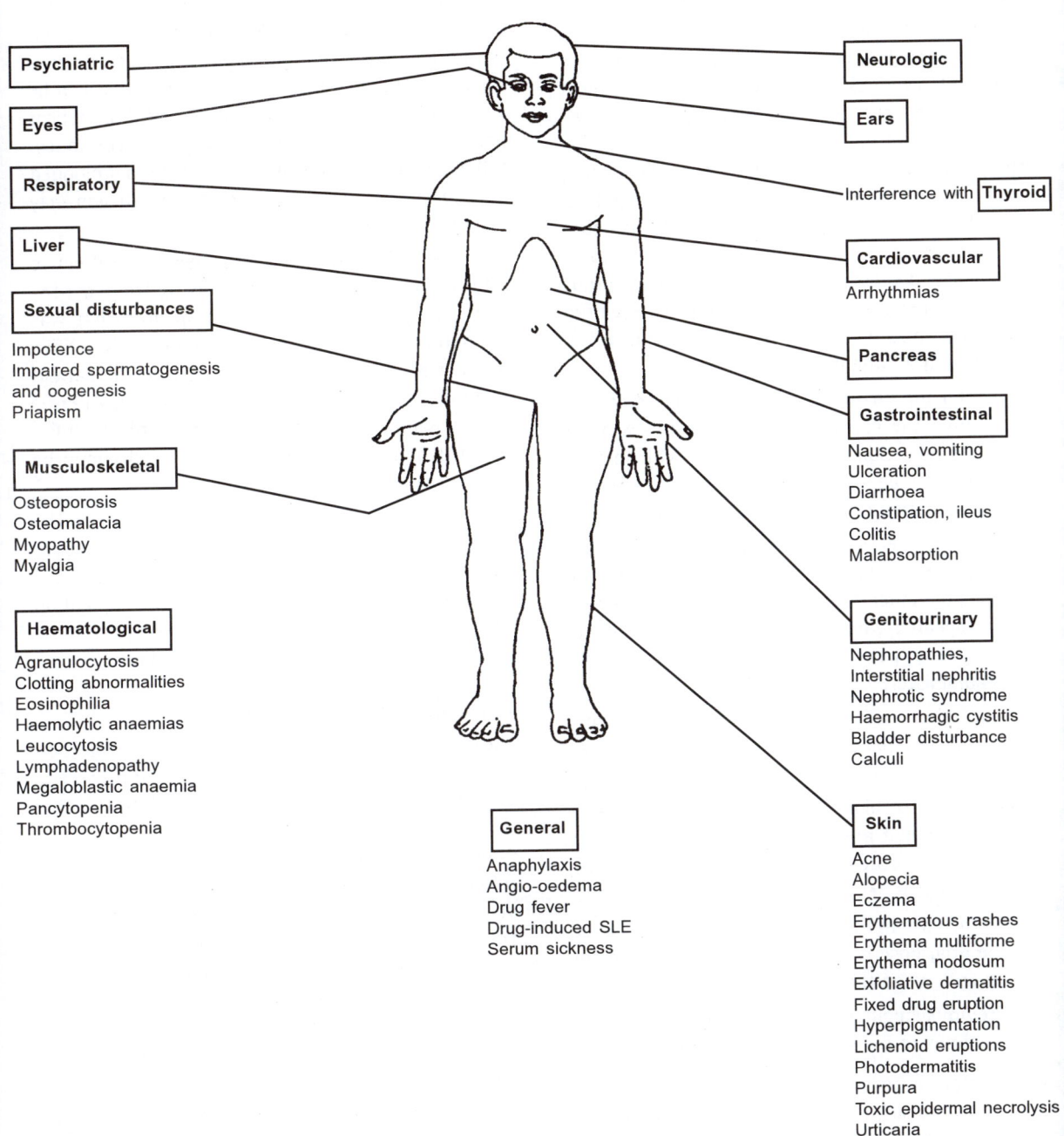

Psychiatric

Eyes

Respiratory

Liver

Sexual disturbances
Impotence
Impaired spermatogenesis
and oogenesis
Priapism

Musculoskeletal
Osteoporosis
Osteomalacia
Myopathy
Myalgia

Haematological
Agranulocytosis
Clotting abnormalities
Eosinophilia
Haemolytic anaemias
Leucocytosis
Lymphadenopathy
Megaloblastic anaemia
Pancytopenia
Thrombocytopenia

General
Anaphylaxis
Angio-oedema
Drug fever
Drug-induced SLE
Serum sickness

Neurologic

Ears

Interference with **Thyroid**

Cardiovascular
Arrhythmias

Pancreas

Gastrointestinal
Nausea, vomiting
Ulceration
Diarrhoea
Constipation, ileus
Colitis
Malabsorption

Genitourinary
Nephropathies,
Interstitial nephritis
Nephrotic syndrome
Haemorrhagic cystitis
Bladder disturbance
Calculi

Skin
Acne
Alopecia
Eczema
Erythematous rashes
Erythema multiforme
Erythema nodosum
Exfoliative dermatitis
Fixed drug eruption
Hyperpigmentation
Lichenoid eruptions
Photodermatitis
Purpura
Toxic epidermal necrolysis
Urticaria

Fig. 61.1: Adverse Drug Reactions

Establishing a Diagnosis of Adverse Drug Reaction (ADR)

A broad spectrum of diseases is produced by adverse drug reactions (**Fig. 61.1**). Drugs causing them have been listed in various chapters of this book. The most common manifestations are skin rash, pruritus, fever, nausea, vomiting, diarrhoea, dizziness, and headache. Other important and relatively frequent adverse drug effects include bone marrow suppression, hepatitis, nephrotoxicity, arrhythmias and a variety of neuro psychiatric symptoms including hallucinations, somnolence, depression, and confusion. Since drugs can induce such a variety of conditions, adverse drug reactions should always be considered when investigating a patient's complaints.

Suspecting the possibility of ADR is one thing and establishing the cause-effect relationship is quite another thing. Some useful criteria will help to establish the diagnosis of an adverse drug reaction as an explanation of the patient's problem.

1. Temporal relationship, establishing that the suspected drug was administered before the reaction under investigation began, the reaction disappeared when the drug was discontinued, and reappeared when the drug was readministered.

2. Published literature which conclusively establishes that the drug produces the suspected reaction.

3. Detection of blood or tissue concentrations of the drug that are known to be toxic e.g. blood levels of digoxin, cyclosporine, dilantin, aminoglycosides etc.

4. An increase in the severity of the reaction when the drug dose is increased or a decrease in the severity when the dose is decreased.

5. Previous occurrence of the same or similar reactions to the same or similar drugs.

Drug history is to be elicited thoroughly from the patient with a suspected adverse drug reaction. The patient should be questioned about all drugs he has recently taken or is currently taking. A thorough probe is necessary since the patient may not recall or may overlook a course of therapy he considered inconsequential.

The management of ADR should be systematic and tailored to the severity of the reaction. When a patient is taking multiple drugs and a severe reaction occurs, all drugs that are thought to be likely culprits should be stopped, as well as all others that can be discontinued safely. Fortunately, most ADRs disappear promptly when the offending drug is discontinued. If the reaction is severe and the drug has a prolonged duration of action, dialysis or haemoperfusion may be required to remove the drug.

After the ADR has subsided, what next? If no effective alternative therapy is available to treat a life-threatening disease, each essential drug that was discontinued should be readministered one at a time, in order of importance, while observing the patient carefully for recurrence of the reaction. Allergic reactions may often be lessened by antihistaminics or corticosteroids. Dose-dependent ADRs may be reduced by lowering the dose.

Although most ADRs are recognized during the development of a new drug, post-marketing surveillance is constantly required to identify unusual reactions, drug interactions and patient population at increased risk. Eternal vigilance is the price to be paid for the privilege of practising medicine.

Uniqueness of each individual

The greatest impact of the Human Genome Project on clinical medicine is the appreciation of the extraordinary molecular and biochemical individuality of each patient. Gene polymorphism occurs in 1 in 1000 DNA base pairs in the human genome. This is reflected in the diversity of the gene products - structural proteins, enzymes, channel proteins, transporters and binding proteins, receptors and post-receptor signaling cascades. Polymorphism can occur not only in the protein-coding sequences but also in the up-stream promoter sequences - such polymorphism can influence the activities of several enzyme-mediated processes.

The most common gene polymorphism is single nucleotide polymorphism (SNP). There are over 3 million SNPs in the entire human genome, out of which 60,000 are in the exons or coding regions of DNA (cSNPs) which help in the hunt for genes of clinical interest. There are, on an average 4-8 SNPs in every gene either in the exons or in the nearby exon-intron boundaries in the upstream regulatory regions. Gene of interest can be pin pointed using SNPs. At the molecular level mutations in gene, leading to altered gene products or altered regulation of gene expression provide an understanding of disease. It follows logically that understanding disease at the molecular level will lead to therapy at the molecular level. New technologies such as complimentary DNA (cDNA) microarrays now available will facilitate analysis of individual variations in the whole genome and the expression profile of all genes in all types of cells and tissues, for understanding our basic genetic makeup and how variations in our genetic instructions, in response to environmental influences cause disease. Every individual is a product of the interaction of his genes and the environment throughout a lifetime. How nutrition influences gene expression is the subject of Nutrigenomics.

Table 61.3 gives examples of genetic determinants of response to drugs.

As important as predicting the efficacy of a drug is predicting and thus preventing adverse drug reactions. Pharmacogenomics now provides the opportunity of analyzing the drug metabolizing enzymes (super family of cytochrome P450 CYP1, CYP2 and CYP3) Approximately 50 percent of the elimination of commonly used drugs is accounted for by the P450 enzymes taken together. Clinicians are dealing with a polymodal population- some having an extensive while others having a poor ability to metabolise the same drug. No wonder that the effectiveness of most major drugs falls in a range of 20-60 per cent of patients!

Determination of an individual patients' genotype will be particularly important in treatment with anti-psychotic drugs. For example the drug remoxipride has to occupy 70-85% of the dopamine D2 receptors in the brain to be effective. To achieve this end point some patients need only 50 mg/day while others may need more than 1 g/day. Optimal drug dosage for the individual patient can be determined from information about receptor occupancy (by using radiolabelled receptor ligands and external detector probes). This approach will prospectively identify responders and non-responders, thereby making the treatment of mental illness far more effective than at present.

Guidelines for prescribers

1. Prescribers should use only a limited number of drugs with which they are thoroughly familiar, and have confidence about their beneficial effects far out weighing risks.

2. Prescribers should use the smallest dose necessary to produce the desirable effect.

3. The number of drugs and doses per day should be minimised to three or less. Once a day medications are likely to have the largest patient compliance.

4. Every prescriber should determine what drugs a patient has been taking, at least during the preceding 30 days, before prescribing any medication. The prescriber may be unaware of the drugs his patient is receiving from other care-gives (including alternative therapies) which may result in duplicative, additive, synergistic or counter active interactions.

5. Prescriber should be particularly wary when adding or stopping specific drugs that are especially liable to provoke interactions and adverse reactions (See Table 61.2 for examples).

In future drug therapy will be individualised to suit the genotype of the individual as adjudged by the DNA microchip. Drugs will be prescribed only to those in whom a high probability of efficacy without significant adverse events is predicted. This approach will drastically change the design of future clinical drug trials, and will ensure that effective therapy is safe for the individual patient.

Computerized physician order entry (CPOE) and Computerized Prescriptions

Medication is an important therapeutic tool in care of the sick. However the entire medication process – from the determination of the patients' need for a drug, through the physician's decision to prescribe the drug, the actual hand-written prescription, its communication to the pharmacy, dispensing by the

TABLE 61.3 EXAMPLES OF GENETIC DETERMINANTS OF RESPONSES TO DRUGS

Polymorphism of drug-metabolizing enzymes	Mechanism	Consequences
TPMT (Thiopurine S-methyl transferase)	[Inactivation of azathioprine and 6 mercaptopurine] = full activity enzyme EM:extensive metabolism deficient activity enzyme PM : poor metabolism	PM phenotype patients show Excessive bone marrow toxicity with "usual" dose EM phenotype patients show undertreatment with "usual" dose of azathioprine.
NAT-2 (n-acetyl transferase)	acetylation of isoniazid, hydralazine, sulfonamides, procainamide etc. "slow", "rapid" and "intermediate" acetylators	slow acetylators likely to produce INAH neuropathy
Cytochrome P450 monooxygenases	isoforms with different substrate specificities multiple pathways EM (extensive metabolizers) PM (poor metabolizers) IM (intermediate metabolizers)	Range of activity can vary ten-fold between individuals on same dose. eg. chlorpromazine
CYP2D6	metabolic pathway for antiarrhythmic drugs, β blockers, tricyclic antidepressants, neuroleptic drugs, selective serotonin reuptake inhibitors	PM phenotypes show exaggerated drug effect on same dose of β blockers can be identified by test drug debrisoquine
CYP2C19	catalyzes omeprazole Proguanil, diazepam and etalopram	EM genotype patients show only 29%, cure rate for eradicating H. Pylori vs 100% cure rate in PM genotype for same dose 20 mg omeprazole
CYP2C9	Metabolism of warfarin and phenytoin, Loss of catalytic function in PM phenotype causes bleeding even with low warfarin dose.	100-200 fold difference in clearance of mephentoin between EM & PM phenotype Increased toxicity in PM phenotype.
Genes coding ion Channel proteins	mutant genes, remain subclinical until challenged by drugs such as quinidine which prolong action potentials.	prolonged QT and polymorphic VTachycardia

Making Effective Therapy Safer: Personalized Therapy

pharmacist and the eventual administration of the medication to the patient, and the patient's compliance with instructions – is extremely complex. Many providers are involved in the process and opportunities for errors abound.

Prescription errors often occur because the prescriber does not have immediate access to relevant information relating to the patient's condition (especially hepatic and renal function) and the drug (especially toxicity profile and drug-drug interactions). With the deluge of new drugs in the market, the physicians' memory can no longer serve as a bridge between advancing knowledge and clinical practice involving tremendous individual patient variables. There are several key areas in which computerized prescriptions will transform the care process and treatment outcomes.

The computerized prescription system design has 3 components :

1. Drug Database and drug dictionary

2. Patient data base including age, sex, weight, drug allergies, genetic data eg. G6PD deficiency, diagnosis, relevant laboratory results (esp. liver and kidney function)

3. Scientific drug information reference and guidelines such as treatment protocols for particular conditions.

For instance if a clinician diagnoses a patient with gonorrhoea, the system will help him with the recommended updated guideline (eg. CDC-STD Rx). The patient database will direct him to the already known allergies (e.g. penicillin) which helps him to select an alternative drug such as doxycycline recommended by the system.

The laboratory data can interact with the pharmacy data : examples : the most recent digoxin and serum potassium levels before renewing a prescription for digoxin; or to question the propriety of a vancomycin prescription for a patient who has no blood culture, or one positive for a methicillin–sensitive organism. Adjustment of drug dosage in elderly patients with impaired renal function (even if serum creatinine may be in the normal range) is incorporated in the computer program for prescribing drugs eliminated by the kidneys. Computerized prescription eliminates dosing mistake which are the most common and preventable type of medication error. Dose calculations and automated checks on drug toxicity (e.g. fatal agranulocytosis during cancer chemotherapy) and adding time dimensions including out-patient scheduling ensure safety. Barcoded medication administration (BCMA) eliminates transcription errors. Patient instructions are given in the form of clear legible statements in his own language regarding how to take the medicine (with meals– cimetidine, corticosteroids; on a full stomach– aspirin, NSAIDS; on an empty stomach–one hour before meals or 2hours after meals for most antibiotics); not to take antacids and antibiotics together etc. Simple as these instructions are, it is amazing how many patients have never been told about them. The patient is also alerted about possible adverse reactions which should be reported immediately (bleeding on anticoagulants, hypoglycemia on insulin or sulphonylureas). Just as pilots and ground engineers are expected to check a list of potential problems before taking an aeroplane back into the sky, the computer check list, completed by a patient while waiting in the clinic (or on-line on phone from home) enables a clinician to check for any drug problem before renewing a prescription.

By combining drug indication data (automatically recorded when the prescription is written) with adverse effect data, usage patterns and the reasons for discontinuing therapy (problem resolved/failure to achieve desired result/adverse reaction/availability of a more effective alternative), a valuable data base is created for post-marketing surveillance of newly introduced drugs, which has eluded the FDA for decades viz-**pharmacovigilence**.

Personalized Medicine

A key goal of 21st Century medicine is to develop personalized therapy tailored to an individual patients' biology (genotype and phenotype), so also personalized preventive care In future medicines will be prescribed only to those patients in whom a high probability of efficacy without significant side effects & adverse events is predicted. This approach will change the design of fulltime clinical trials.

Affymetrix in Santa Clara California, has developed a tiny chip that can analyze 1000 to 20000 SNPs to probe 6817 genes in 15 minutes. Drug companies have an enlightened self-interest in making this chip available and affordable to all patients since it will decrease their liability for damages through adverse drug reactions (ADRs). The cost of ADR-related morbidity and mortality in USA alone ranges between $30-130 million. The entire medical community and the general public should be interested in the availability of an affordable chip as soon as possible.

Metabolic Phenotyping in Health and Disease

Analyzing metabolites (small molecules < 1 KDa) in body fluids such as plasma, urine and saliva using various spectroscopic methods provides information on the metabolic phenotype of individuals and populations, information that can be applied to personalized and public health care.

The metabolic phenotype (metabotype) is the product of genetic and environmental influences (diet, lifestyle, gut microbial activity). Xenobiotics, such as plastieizers, food preservatives, pesticides and plant secondary metabolities (caffeine flavonoids, phytoestrogens) also contribute to metabotype variations as does gut microbiome activity through the production of co-metabolites.

The Human Metabolome Database contains 41,500 entries including water-soluble and lipid soluble metabolites, 5680 genes and protein sequences and 440 human metabolic and disease pathways.

Insulin Resistance syndrome/Cardiovascular dysmetabolic syndrome (IRS/CDS) is of great importance to the Indian population; in which endothelial dysfunction coupled with insulin resistance give rise to a constellation of syndromes: visceral obesity, hypertension, type 2 diabetes mellitus and coronary artery disease. The putative multiple genes and their polymorphisms can now be studied in individual patients as well as their healthy siblings and offsprings, taking advantage of the SNPs that are present in the coding regions as well as in the upstream regulatory regions, and which can be detected by DNA chips. Considering that Hypertension, type 2 diabetes and coronary artery disease have attained epidemic proportions in India prevention becomes supremely important. The childhood origins of atherosclerosis are now very well recognized. In future genetic profile analysis of a sample of blood from a child will give indication of his/her susceptibility to these diseases. Lifestyle modification (diet, exercise, anti-oxidants, stress control) can begin early in life. This is really practice of preventive medicine at its best.

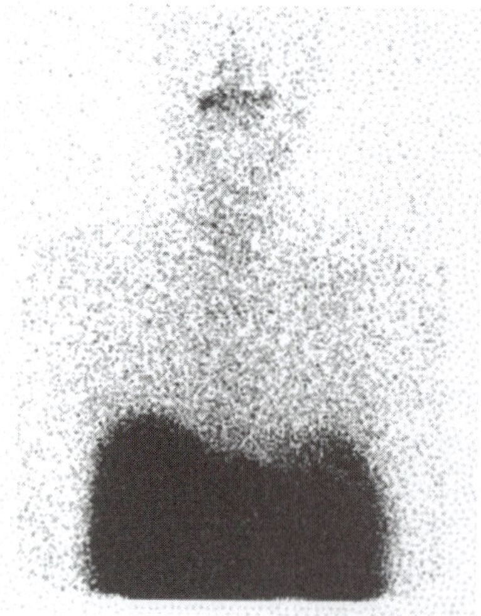

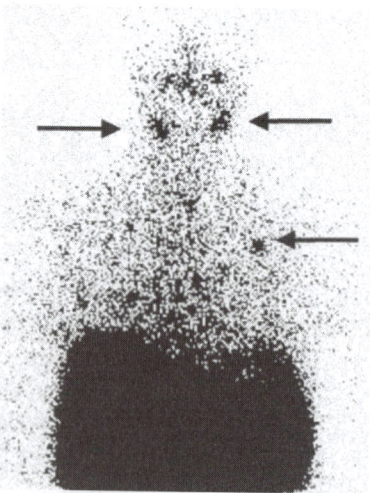

Fig. 61.2 Before Treatment
Annexin apoptosis imaging before
chemotherapy in Lymphoma

Fig. 61.3 After Treatment
After chemotherapy showing apoptosis in
lymph nodes predictive of success

Ancient Indian Insights

"Ayurveda" (Science of Life) represents experiential wisdom of over 5000 years. A unique feature of Ayurveda is its emphasis on the promotion of positive health, physical, mental, social and spiritual.

"The wise man should control the impulses of greed, grief, fear, anger, vanity, impudence, jelousy, malice and excessive attachment".

"He alone can remain healthy - who takes proper, diet, exercise and recreation, who controls his sexual pleasures, who is just, generous, truthful and forgiving and who can get along with his kins".

Importance of Diet- "Ahar"

Charak Samhita discusses "wholesome" and "unwholesome" food. "The use of a wholesome diet is the only factor that promotes the healthy growth of humans; and the factor that makes for disease is the indulgence in unwholesome diet". "That class of food which helps the harmonised body elements to retain their state of equilibrium, and the discordant body elements to gain equilibrium, is the wholesome one; and the unwholesome one to be that which acts in the opposite manner".

Regarding Energy requirements, Charak States: "Even light, easily digested and nutritious food should not be taken in excess of bodily requirements, or after the appetite has been satisfied. Food difficult to digest should not be taken habitually. Even if used, the quantity should not exceed a fraction of a full meal". "An excess or surfeit of food is markedly harmful unless the gastric fire is increased by hard exercise".

Shushruta, who described Diabetes (Madhumeha) for the first time in the history of medicine advised the corpulent diabetic to indulge in vigorous physical exercise (such as walking 20 "yojanas" or physical effort (digging a well). At the same time Shushruta exorted the thin diabetic not to exert too much.

Ayurveda describes 3 kinds of "ahar" or diet – "satwik", "rajasik" and "tamasik": The "Rishis" took "Satwik ahar" consisting of kanda, moola, phala" (vegetables and fruits) and lived for hundred years. In today's parlence, this represents a 1300 caloric diet (which causes the least oxidative stress), high fibre, low fat, low sodium, high potassium & minerals and plenty of antioxidants (**Fig. 62.1**). Excessive oxidative stress is central in most human disorders including ageing process as shown by increased levels of F2 Isoprostanes in peripheral blood and urine and increased F4 neuroprostanes in the cerebrospinal fluid (CSF).

Osmotin, a recently discovered plant analog of mammalian adiponectin, is abundant in fruits & vegetable and acts through adiponectin receptors (Narsimhan et al 2005). Adiponectin and osmotin act via Adipo R1 receptors in muscles and Adipo R2 receptors in liver and act as insulin sensilizers and regulators of energy homeostasis via AMPK activation (Wolf G 2003). Part of the beneficial effects of fruits and vegetables is due to their osmotin content, which remains stable in the digestive tract.

Kashyap Samhita (which deals with paediatrics) stresses the importance of breast milk as essential promoter of growth and development and tonic for all tissues. "If the mother does not have enough breast milk, it is better to employ a "Dhatri" (wet nurse) as no other milk can compete with human milk". Ayurveda also gives details of the qualities of Cow's milk, also milk from buffaloes, goats, sheep, camels, horses and elephants. The insight about mother's milk is fully vindicated today in terms of its ideal content of essential fatty acid (EPA/DHA) and their effects on the composition of the cell membrane (as discussed in the next section).

Diet and Inflammation

Prof. PC Calder (2002) has given an excellent review of inflammation in health and disease. He has

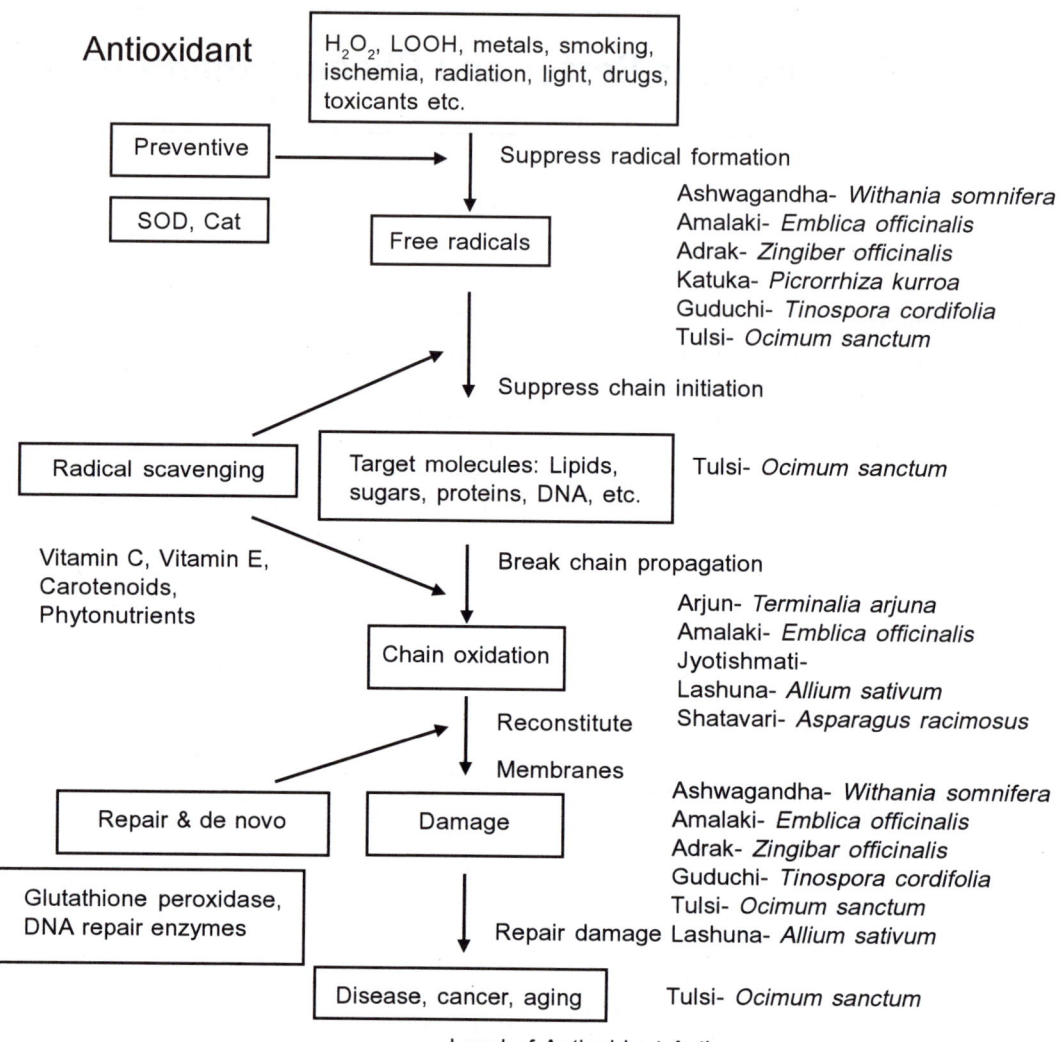

Fig. 62.1: Depicts the Ayurvedic anti-oxidants according to the various levels at which they act (Devasgayam et at. 2004)

emphasized the important role of dietary essential fatty acid omega 3 PUFA, EPA and DHA, in the suppression of pro-inflammatory cytokines and production of anti-inflammatory lipoxins, resolvins and protectins in the resolution of inflammatory response **(Fig. 62.2)**. This is crucial in many disease states including inflammatory disorders (such as arthritis), atherosclerosis, asthma and cancer.

Zinc, selenium, Vit. A, Vit. C, Vit. E, folic acid Vit., B6 and Vit. B12 are important nutrients whose deficiency affects susceptibility to infection and host immune response. The role of Vit. D. in relation to immune competence has only recently been discovered. Dendritic cells and macrophages have receptors for Vit. D. Deficiency of Vit. D and Vit. D receptor polymorphism increase susceptibility to tuberculosis (Wilkinson 2000). There is a two-way interaction between nutrients and human genes (Roche HM

2004). How genetic variation influences response to nutrients and how nutrients influence gene expression, transcription and metabolism are the subject of Nutrigenomics. The effect of maternal malnutritional on suppression of foetal insulin receptor substrate – Phosphoinositide 3-Kinase (IRS-PI3K), AKT pathway is well known as the basis of Metabolic Syndrome and insulin resistance with consequent hyperuinsulinemia.

Diet and Chemoprevention of cancer

Diet contains several non-nutritional phytochemicals whose active principles have been identified: Haldi (Curcumin), red chilli peper (capsaicin), ginger (gingerol), green tea (epigallocatechin), honey (caffeic acid) garlic (diallylsulphide), cabbage (indol-3-carbinol) broccoli (sulpharaphane), carrot (β-carotene), grapes (resveratrol), grape seeds, pine bark (procyanadine), tomatoes (lycopenes). Their mode of action at the moleuclar level is described in on Page 362. Non-nutrient dietary phytochemicals exert their substantial anti-mutagenic and anti-carcinogenic properties by blocking cell signalling pathway that regulate cell proliferation and differentiation - such as the family of mitogen- activated protein kinases (MAPKs), NFKB-API, NRF2 as well as β-catenin a component of cell-cell adhesion machinery. Carcinogenesis is a multi-step

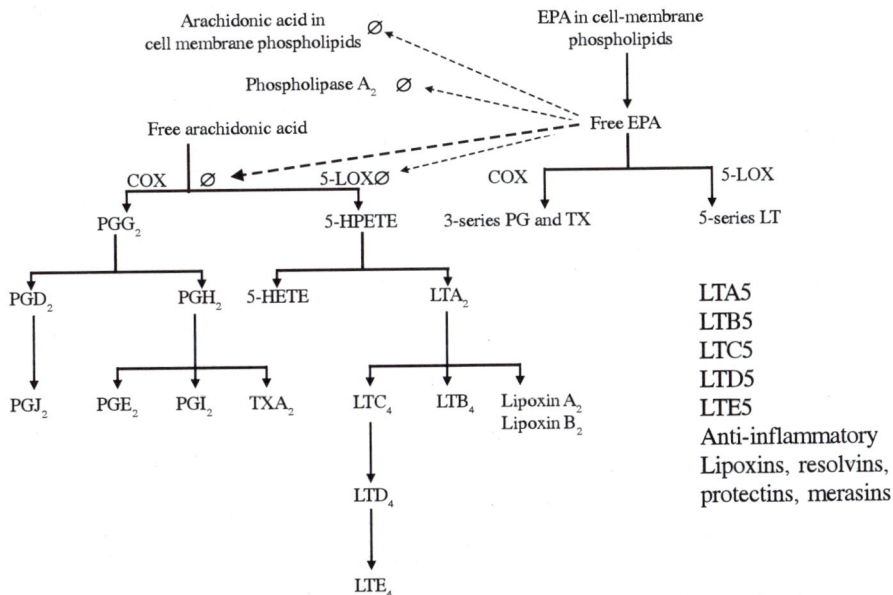

Fig. 62.2: Beneficial effects of EPA/ DHA in cells membrane phospholipids

process, the initiation of which can be blocked or suppressed by dietary phytochemicals. They can also halt or retard the progression of pre-cancerous cells into malignant cells (Surh YH 2004). How dietary phytochemicals can modify gene expression or transcriptional gene silencing is the subject of nutrigenomics and epigenetics.

Importance of Exercise

Charak states "Physical exercise increases the body's strength and firmness. It should be practised regularly in the right measure. Lightness, capacity for work, firmness, tolerance to hardship, subsidence of humoral discordance and stimulation of gastric fire accrue from exercise". "Fatigue, exhaustion, wasting thirst, asthma, cough, fever & vomiting result form over-exercise".

"A person who is habituated to pampering his belly even when a previous meal has not been thoroughly digested; who is addicted to a habit of sleeping in the day or leading a sedentary life, who is averse to taking any sort of physical exercise, will suffer from excessive stoutness. He is likely to be afflicted by many diseases that invariably terminate in death, due to obstruction of internal channels due to deposition of fat. Hence all things and conditions which foster the growth of abnormal fat should be carefully avoided".

"The excessive corpulence is caused by over eating, lack of exercise, lack of mental exertion and by inherited tendency". "The corpulent person is afflicted with eight disabilities viz. dimunition of lifespan, lack of agility, debility, difficulty in sex act, fetor, distressing sweats, excessive appetite and excessive thirst".

Prevention of stress

The World Health organization (WHO) has determined that about 80% of illness is behaviorally related. People are often harrased, worried, anxious, afraid and seek help and reassurance. Their complaints are physical: headache, back ache, weakness, tiredness, palpitations, breathing difficulty, poor appetite, poor sleep etc. but they originate in mental stress.

Folklore language is full of expressions which show the appreciation of the impact of the mind on bodily functions. We "see red" with rage or become "blind with rage", we are struck "dumb with horror", we experience "heartache" or "heart break", fear makes one's heart come up into one's mouth" or "sink into one's boots"; fear may make one's flesh creep" or make one "limp as a rag" or "go weak at the knees" it makes our mouth dry or cause the teeth to chatter". Disgust makes one sick, we cannot "stomach or swallow a situation". Anxiety produces "a load on the chest". Relief is expressed as "getting something off one's chest. Certainly there is nothing new in the recognition of body - mind unity in medicine.

Ischaemia induced by mental stress

John Hunter, the famous British surgeon who had angina pectoris, was well aware of the effect of anger when he said, "my life is in the hands of any rascal who chooses to provoke me". Effects of anger on left ventricular ejection fraction (LVEF) have been well documented. Sudden cardiac death has been triggered by an earth quake.

More often, mental stress induces silent ischemia as first demonstrated by Deanfield in 1984 and several other studies. Mental stress-induced ischaemia has been reproduced in the laboratory and has been compared with ambulatory ischaemia during daily life along with haemodynamic features.

It is important to note that mental stress can induce silent ischaemia more frequently than physical exercise in the same patient. Laboratory protocols involving mental stress (arithmetic problems, speaking assignments) have been used along with continuous monitoring of LVEF by ambulatory vest. The prognostic value of mental stress testing in coronary artery disease (CAD) has been established. Mental stress can induce adverse cardiac events in stable angina patients. FMD studies have shown significant reduction (47%) in forearm blood flow during mental stress, and significant improvement (15%) during laughter.

A study of men in depressive mood (4-12 score on the 13 point Welsh depression subscale) has shown 46% higher hsCRP, 16% higher IL-6 and 10% higher (ICAM-1) expression compared to controls.

How to improve endothelial function?

Dean Ornish set up a study in 1977 to explore the effect of diet and lifestyle modification on the reversal of coronary atherosclerosis, using the techniques of quantitative coronary arteriography and quantitative myocardial blood flow using N-13 ammonia positron emission tomography (PET) imaging. The findings were published in JAMA (1983), Circulation (1989), Lancet (1990), JAMA (1995) and JAMA (1998). It became obvious that modification of cardiovascular risk factors that contribute to endothelial dysfunction improve patient outcome disproportionately to the regression in the anatomic atherosclerotic lesions. Patients with "mild" coronary artery lesions can have severe endothelial dysfunction. Long term follow-up showed more cardiac events in such patients. Myocardial ischaemia can occur during exercise in patients without significant epicardial vessel stenosis, due to endothelial dysfunction. Recent insights into vascular biology help us to understand how the benefit occurs in relation to endothelial dysfunction.

Newer Insights

Modern research in neuro-science have revealed many new insights into our complex mental processes and their regulation by an intricate network of electrical and chemical circuits – neuro transmitters (both excitatory and inhibitory) connect the brain, the neuro-endocrine and the immune system (psycho-neuroendocrinology and psychoneuroimmunology).

Cannabinoid CB2 receptors are expressed or cells on the peripheral immune system and are coupled to inhibition of adenylyl cyclase, suggesting a potential anti-inflammatory role. Mental depression also depresses the immune system. Functional brain imaging with PET and MRI have revealed characteristic changes in blood flow, metabolism and neurochemical activity in anxiety, depression, obsessive-compulsive neurosis, schizophrenia and manic-depressive psychosis. A unique Fludeoxyglucose (FDG)-PET study of glucose metabolism of the brain (Lele et al. 1989) has shown that the ancient Indian practice of meditation causes a generalised hypometabolism in the brain – the reverse happens in stress. The GABA, encephalin-endorphin – dynophrin and endocannabinoid system become activated during stress. Cannabiniod CB1 receptors are found in high abundance in the brain, especially basal ganglia, cerebellum, hippocampus and cerebral cortex. Considerably lower expression is found in peripheral tissues including lungs, testes, uterus and vascular tissue. Following agonist binding CB1, receptors cause inhibition of adenylcyclase, inhibition of the N and Q type voltage operated calcium channels and stimulation of inwardly rectifying and A type K^+ channnles. Signaling by endocannabinoid system represents a mechanism by which neurons can communicate backwards across synapses to modulate their inputs. The endocannabinoids reduce pain and anxiety, cause sedation or slowing down, increase appetite and promote food intake.

The lipid anandamide (arachidonyl – ethanolamide) exemplifies cannabinoids in the brain, analogus to the endogenous opiate receptor agonists. Their physiological role is increasingly appreciated, as Natural Healers of the body.

Functional brain studies of pain perception have shown that when a peripheral pain stimulus is applied, the contralateral thalamus gets activated and relays the pain sensation to the cingulate cortex, which also become activated. Studies during hypnosis have shown that while the thalamus continues to be activated, the cirgulate cortex is not, hence there is no awareness of pain – possibly due to activation of the cannabinoid system.

Burn out syndrome

Herbert Freudenberger, a New York psychoanalyst coined the term "burnout syndrome" in the early 1970's to describe a state of mental and physical exhaustion caused by one's professional life and its chronic stresses. In response to mounting task loads, the wretch piles on the hours at work, pulling late nights at the office, ignoring exercise, skipping meals or eating unhealthful fast food on the run, cancells personal commitments to family and friends. Sooner or later the work efficiency declines, with poor concentration, fewer creative ideas, self-dissatisfaction and lagging self-esteem and anxiety about failure, and depression. Some may seek solace in alcohol or pills. Some even attempt suicide.

The anti-stress measures that are required are as simple as they are effective. They include eating wholesome food at regular meal time, exercising regularly and getting enough sleep, spending time with family and friends and developing a hobby or a pleasurable activity like listening to music or relaxation techniques including Yoga and meditation ("Yoga" literally means equilibrium).

Unfortunately commercial pressures world-wide have distorted the scientific practice of medicine. Dean Ornish has said in his book "Reversing Heart Disease" says "The insurance company will pay at least $ 30,000 for a CABG, at least $ 7500 for a balloon angioplasty, but only $ 150 if a doctor spends the same amount of time and effort educating a heart patient about nutrition, exercise, stress-coping and, life style management. If someone spends the same amount of time and effort teaching a well person how to remain healthy, the insurance company will pay nothing at all. It is nor surprising that doctors spend time doing what is reimbursed".

To educate and motivate the general public to adopt a healthy life-style including diet (caloric restricted diet with 400 g fruits & vegetables and essential fatty acids and avoidance of transfats), regular physical exercise, avoidance of tobacco and alcohol use and stress management, takes time and persistent effort **(Tables 62.1 & 62.2)**. To educate and motivate the patient to implement the advice takes at least 10 minutes per visit, while it takes only 10 seconds to write a drug prescription. There is a very powerful drug lobby but no lobby to promote nutrition exercise and stress control. The medical community should be reminded that the word "doctor" is derived from "docere"- to teach.

TABLE 62.1 Describes the full scope of prevention, including primary and secondary prevention patient can adopt

The Wide Spectrum of Patient Care

Scope of primary prevention

Advice and guidance for the following:

Nutrition: calories, proteins, minerals (iron, iodine, calcium), vitamin A and D, essential fatty acids, green leafy vegetables and fruits.

Mother and Child care: Family planning advice.

Immunization against major infectious diseases.

Abstinence from tobacco, alcohol and narcotic drugs.

Regular physical exercise and weight control.

Safe sex (use of condoms) for avoidance of HIV.

Safety measures in home, workplace, roads, beaches to prevent accidents and environmental pollution. Use of safety belts for cars and helmets for motorcyclists and scotterists.

Scope of secondary prevention

Penicillin prophylaxis to prevent rheumatic valvular disease.

Control of hypertension to prevent its complications.

Control of diabetes mellitus to prevent its complications.

Aspirin in TIA (transient ischemic attacks) to prevent strokes.

Anticoagulant and thrombolytic therapy in acute myocardial infarction and ischemic strokes to prevent further damage to myocardium and brain.

Revascularization and angioplasty: heart, kidney and peripheral vessels.

Scope of curative measures

Infections: antimicrobial therapy, immunoglobulins and antivenins.

Replacement of deficient nutrients and hormones; correction of excess nutrients and hormones;

Surgical removal of tumors, foreign bodies and obstructions; organ transplants, prostheses, implants; plastic and reconstructive surgery, restoration of severed limbs.

Desensitization of allergic patients.

Desensitization of phobic patients.

Gene therapy (futuristic).

Scope of supportive measures

Restoration of circulating volume: blood, plasma, volume expanders, saline.

Restoration of electrolytes and acid-base equilibrium.

Maintenance of ventilation and circulation.

Measures to reduce cerebral edema.

Hemodialysis and peritoneal dialysis; hemoperfusion.

Plasmapheresis.

Immunomodulators, immunosuppressants and immunostimulants.

Scope of symptomatic measures

Pain relief: analgesics, anti-spasmodic, antacids, antianginal drugs etc.

Sedative and hypnotics.

Anxiety reducing drugs.

Anti-depressants.

Anti-convulsants.

Anti-tussive and bronchodilators.

Diuretics for edema.

Laxatives for constipation.

Antiemetic drugs.

Antiallergic and anti-inflammatory drugs.

Rehabilitation

Medical rehabilitation

Vocational rehabilitation.

Social rehabilitation.

Psychological rehabilitation.

TABLE 62.2 Promotive and preventive care and health education provided by FP

Pregnancy
  Weight, Hb, DP, Urine examination for albumin and sugar

Prenatal care
  Supplement of iron, folic acid, calcium, Vit. D

Post partum
  Family planning, IUCD
  Encourage breast-feeding 6-12 months
  Emergency contraception

Newborn
  Neonatal hypothyroidism screen (TSH)
  Neonatal jaundice (Rh, viral hepatitis, HIV)
  Immunization

Childhood
  Height-weight charts to monitor growth
  Records of milestones: Detection of mental retardation
  Dental care: Caries, orthodontic conditions
  Check for refractive errors: Squint
  Check for hearing defects

Adolescence
  Sex education: Awareness about STD and HIV
  Avoidance of teenage pregnancy
  Health-related behavior: Alcohol, drugs, smoking
  Prevention of vehicular accidents
  Emotional support: Broken families

Adult life
Training for parenthood and family planning
Family dysfunction: Marital and sexual problems
Guidance on health-related behavior exercise, weight control, alcohol, tobacco smoking
Coping with stress:
  Relaxation techniques
  Early detection of high BP, diabetes
  Hypercholesterolemia, and hyperlipidemia
  Early detection of ischemic heart disease in high-risk groups

Middle age
  Females: Prevention of osteoporosis
  Self-examination of breasts
  Papanicolaoi smears
  Males: Rectal examination for prostate
  Stools for occult blood
  Annual blood test PSA
  Both sexes: "Empty nest syndrome"
  Joint families: closing generation gap

Old age:
  Coping with progressive
  incapacity of old age:
  Loneliness
  Memory loss
  Falls and fractures

63 | Mobile Smart Phones: Revolution in Healthcare

The recent wide spread availability of mobile phones has made a tremendous impact on health care, by engaging all stake-holders - patients and their relatives, nursing and para-medical health workers, general public doctors and medical institutions. 70% of India's 1.23 billion population is rural and today there are more mobiles than latrines in rural India. This is an opportunity for improving rural health care through mobile information technology which is now available and affordable. Mobile real-time data acquisition is now possible for application in preventive medicine.

The advantages of mobile technology are many- information at point-of-care; direct communication between patient and care-giver; clinical help at crisis time and direct access to medical & drug databases. Physicians can share PDA/Smart phone findings with their patients.

For the practicing doctor, mobile smart phone helps also in secretarial work - appointment scheduling and charges; two way communication with patients; patient data base making payment on-line by HCP gateway - keep track on important health days declared by WHO; etc.

All smart phones have high end cameras, email schedulers, fast web browsers, scanner, visiting card reader, remote watch CCTV, medical photography and medical records. There are thousands of medical applications available on internet, both free and paid.

Information at point of care

With Internet	Without Internet
Medscape	Epocrates
Skyscape	Micromedex
UMMS	Medscape Web MD
NEJM this week	Qxmedical calculations
Black Berry medical resources	Human Anatomy

Most common platforms used by smart phones are the Android, Apple iOS, Research in Motion (RIM) Black Berry, Symbian, Samsungs, Bada.

Smart phones provide current clinical information and decision support at the point of care. Medical calculators simplify the bedside use of medical equations, scores stratification, risk prediction and prevention models, Smart phones assist in physical examination with photography of physical findings.

Radiology and USG

Handheld ultrasound Doppler uses commercial USB ultrasound probes with Microsoft windows smart phones. Images can be sent to a centralized service for review.

Radiology investigations' interpretation can be made by friendly software Radiopaedia.

Google glass

Google Glass is a type of *wearable technology* with an *optical head-mounted display* (OHMD). It was developed by *Google* with the mission of producing a mass-market *ubiquitous computer*. Google Glass displays information in a *smartphone*-like hands-free format Wearers communicate with the Internet via *natural language* voice commands, headtilt, touch or change of gaze.

Similar gadgets are available from Optinvent-France. Ora X features a front-facing 1080p 5MP camera, a 9-axis motion sensor, wireless connectivity with Bluetooth, Wi-Fi and GPS as well as a trackpad for tactile interactions with the device, the eyewear, powered by a dual-core chip, can support complex applications can well and even has an augmented reality mode. Variety of Healthcare applications exists:

Medopad and Google Glass being used in a hospital to review the medical records, check live patient

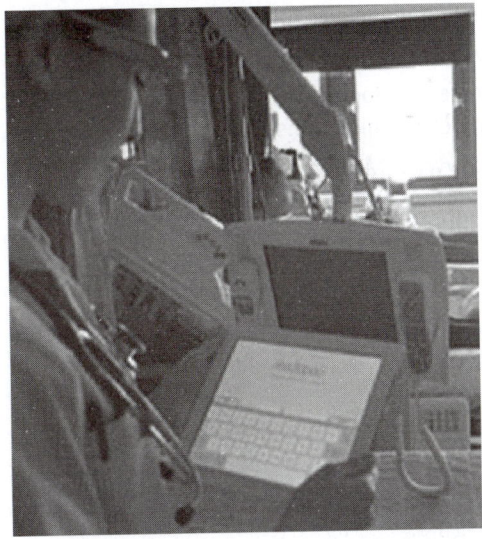

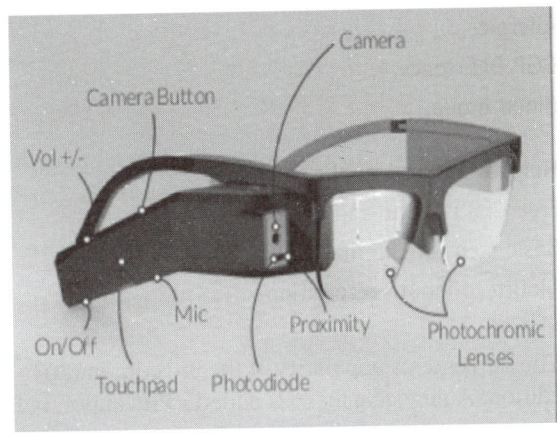

vitals, collaborate by sharing what they are viewing in surgery with up to 5 other doctors, and record video or take pictures at point of care.

Dr. Chrono, has developed a new application for the device a "wearable health record". It has a great potential in health education for medical community as well as well as masses. Sharing technical expertise with others.

The *Phillips accenture Google Glass* allows surgeons to simultaneously monitor a patient's vital signs while performing surgery, accessing a near real-time feed of vital signs in Google Glass, it also helps in calling up images and other patient data by clinicians from anywhere in the hospital, accessing a pre-surgery safety checklist, giving clinicians the ability to view the patient in the recovery room after surgery, conducting live, first-person point-of-view video conferences with other surgeons or medical personnel and recording surgeries from a first-person point-of-view for training purposes.

Unlimited & unexplored possibilities exist in health & fitness & need to be explored for the use of such a helpful electronic device.

Mobile Phone based microscopy

Light microscopy - smears sent for analysis at main centre QBC fluorescent microscope.

Cell Scope - Compact high resolution handheld microscope on site disease diagnosis via data-transmission on smears to main centres.

Smart Phone Scans for oral cancer detection – Oscan

A mouth positioner, a circuit board and two rows of fluorescent light emitting diodes - attached to any smart phones built in camera - a quick swipe to take high resolution panoramic image of a person's entire month cavity, by the devices blue fluorescent light, malignant lesions are seen as dark sports. Images can be sent to oral surgeons for diagnosis and plan biopsies at site of lesion.

For dermatological diagnosis Visual DX-Visual clinical Decision support System idoc24 is useful.

NETRA

Near Eye tool for Refractive Errors assessment preventive blindness screening.

Mobile Diabetes Monitoring - Blood sugar.

Patient with chest pain - ECG analysis in emergency OCM and medical alerts.

Mobile phone pulse oximeter, i stethoscope.

Help to patients

Symptom checker for emergency medicine: Direct contact with health provider shows patient his cardiovascular risk age, gender, BP, total cholesterol, HDL, Smoking and Diabetes. Encourage patient for lifestyle modification and to quit smoking.

Diet prescription and exercise to lose weight.

Information about drugs and procedures - poisoning and drug overdose.

Allergies,

GGP Deficiency,

Blood group.

Help to general public

Free CPR i phone applications.

Basic steps in external cardiac message.

Mouth to mouth respiration.

Heimlich maneuver for choking.

How to get noticed in Emergency.

Register in Google Maps so that people can locate you, getting directions to go to nearest hospital.

Ref: www: iMedical Apps.com

www: mobilehealthnews.com

www: peakvision.org

www.thecommunityguide.org/tobacco/mobilephone.html

The tremendous popularity of the 3rd edition (2015) which is all sold out has prompted me to trying out a 4th edition. A new chapter (62) added - Prevention is Better and Cheaper than Cure, includig a

Table 1 describing the full scope of prevention including primary and secondary prevention and the scope of curative measures, supportive measures and symptomatic measures.

Table 2 describes promotive and preventive care and health education provided by the family physician.

The last chapter 63 Mobile Smart Phones Revolution in health care have an added new section initiative for mother and child healthcare.

In India 60% pregnant women are devoid of healthcare facilities. In 2014 Aditya Kulkarni, working in science for society developed a Care Mother Kit for estimation of Hb, urine proteins, weight, fetal heart sounds - total nine parameters giving results in a few minutes. He developed an AP through which patients reports are communicated to the doctor almost instantaneously enabling timely medical care. In 2015 this was tested in Aurangabad and Govandi near Mumbai with great success. This has now reached 9 states through 15 institutions, benefiting 30,000 pregnant women. It is hoped to reach 1.5 lakh pregnant women by 2020. In July 2018 Aditya Kulkarni was felicitated by Queen Elizabeth of England at the Buckingham Palace, for this achievement. Care nx.

Cellscope-Skin to micro

- Transforms it into a compact, high-resolution, handheld microscope .
- On-site disease diagnosis
- Wireless transmission

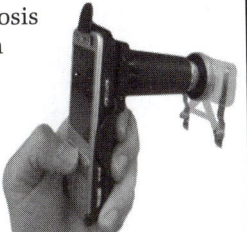

Using QBC-Fluoroscent Microscopy

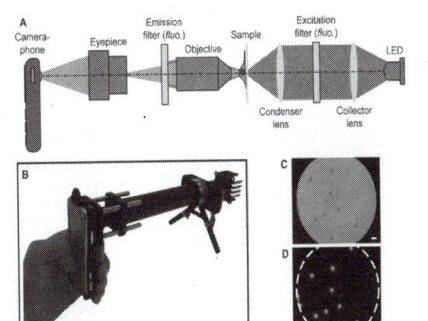

Smears analyzed at the main center

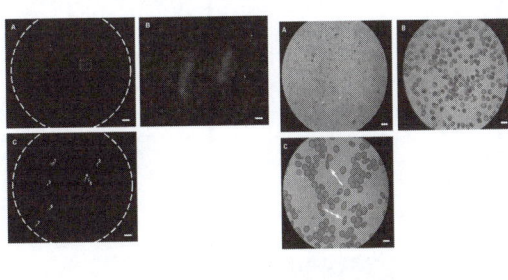

NETRA (Near-Eye Tool for Refractive Assesment

- looks@ lens attached to the phone
- creating an eye prescription.
- Colour blindness test
- Mass screening

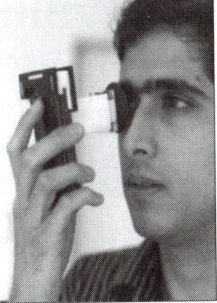

Smartphone scans for oral cancer detection - O scan

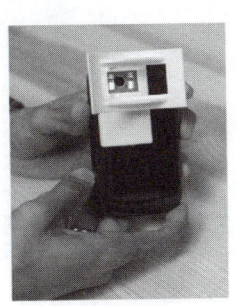 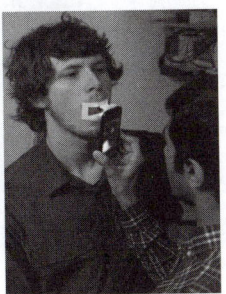

Boon for staff- residents- Nurse

- Keeping primary data-can be entered by self.
- BODY MASS INDEX.-surface area
- Reminder-allergies-deficiencies-G-6-PD.
- Own set of contradictions-interactions.
- Dictation software apps.-speech –to Text
- Epidemiological data-Indian evidence

Mobile phone Pulse oximeter, Instant Heart Rate-Android App.

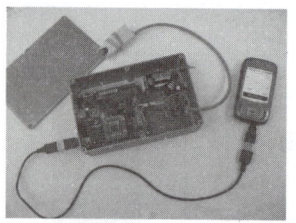 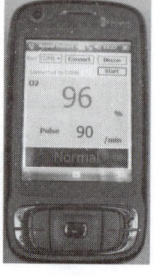

i-stethoscope

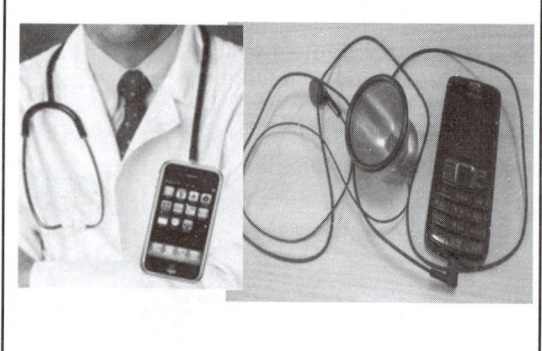

Mobile Diabetes Monitoring

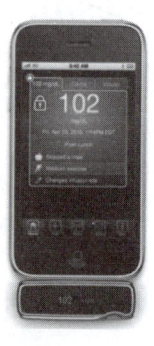 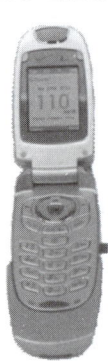

ECG Analysis-Emergency

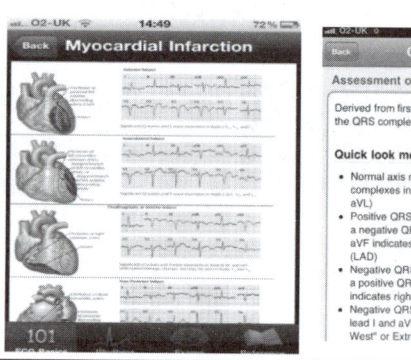

AirStrip Cardiology,

- Emergency Medical Systems,

- Emergency Department and Cardiology teams – especially when transporting potential AMI-

  STEMI patients."

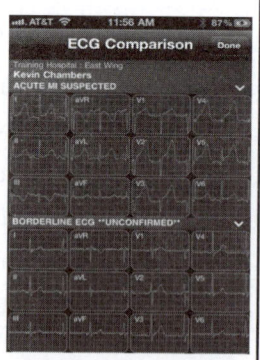

Superb Image collections

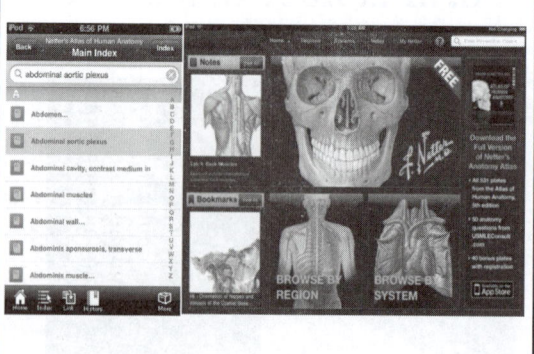

Virtual dissection - 3 D concepts

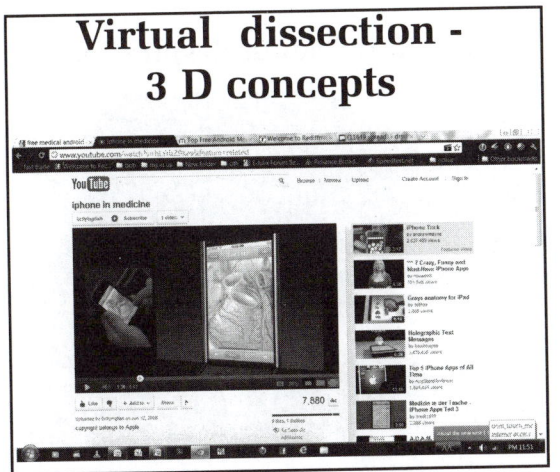

NEJM this week

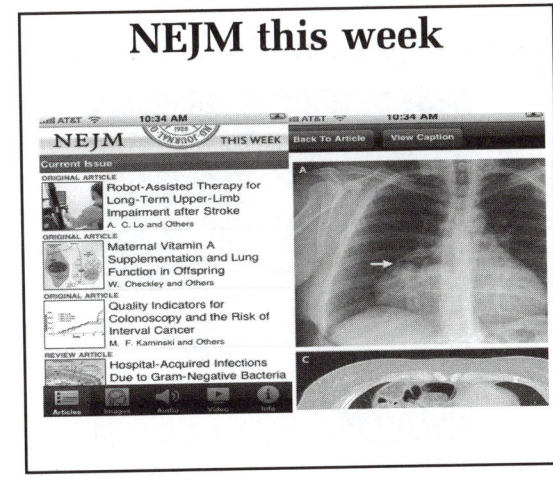

New face of any conference

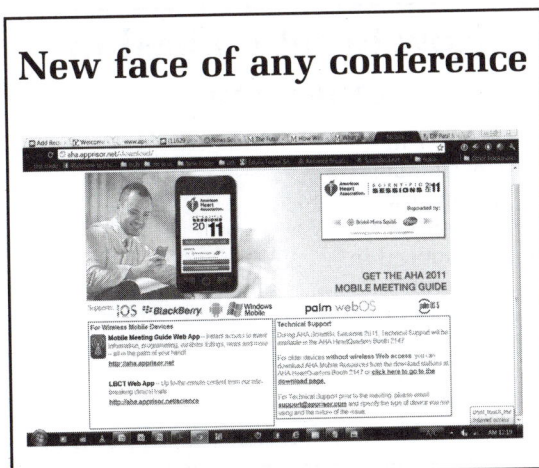

What mMEDICINE does

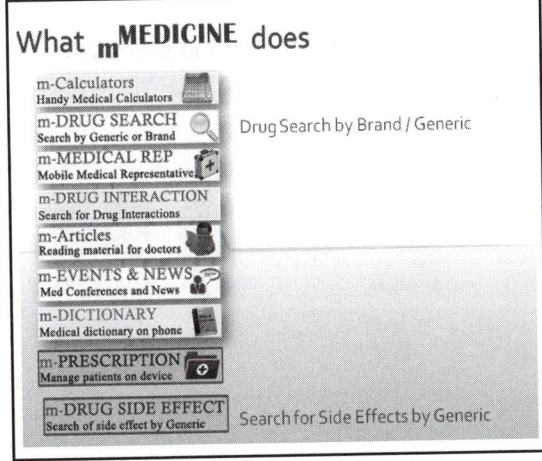

- m-Calculators — Handy Medical Calculators
- m-DRUG SEARCH — Search by Generic or Brand — Drug Search by Brand / Generic
- m-MEDICAL REP — Mobile Medical Representative
- m-DRUG INTERACTION — Search for Drug Interactions
- m-Articles — Reading material for doctors
- m-EVENTS & NEWS — Med Conferences and News
- m-DICTIONARY — Medical dictionary on phone
- m-PRESCRIPTION — Manage patients on device
- m-DRUG SIDE EFFECT — Search of side effect by Generic — Search for Side Effects by Generic

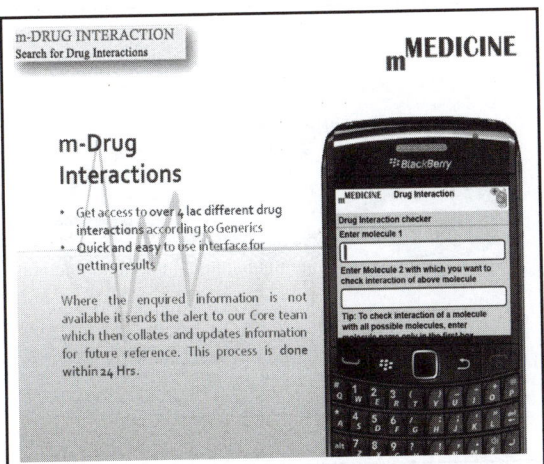

Free CPR iPhone Application

- **CPR & Choking**
- **By Stone Meadow Development LLC**
- They are convinced that teaching these life saving techniques to as many people as possible will save lives.

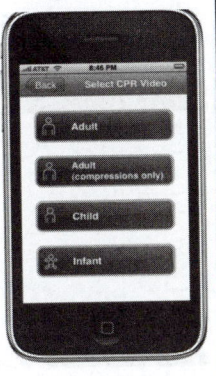

Basic steps-External compressions

Mouth to Mouth Respiration

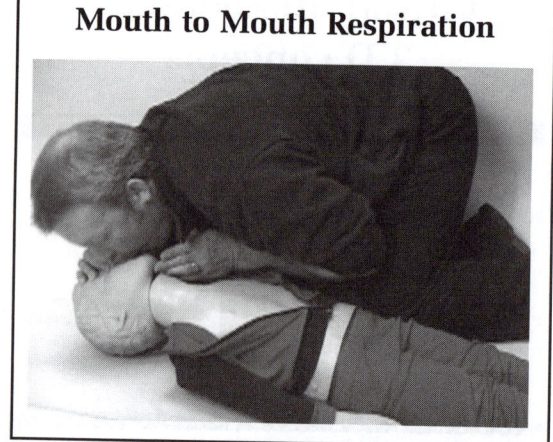

Heimlich maneuver

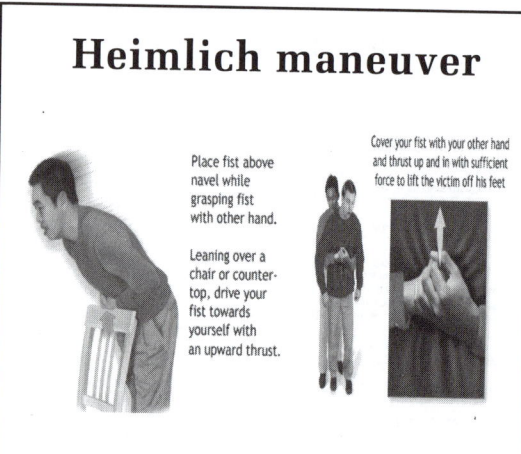

Place fist above navel while grasping fist with other hand.

Leaning over a chair or counter-top, drive your fist towards yourself with an upward thrust.

Cover your fist with your other hand and thrust up and in with sufficient force to lift the victim off his feet

How to get noticed in Emergency.

- Register in Google Maps
- Having own website.
- Get noticed in different searches of medical database Or doctors list.
- People can locate you-

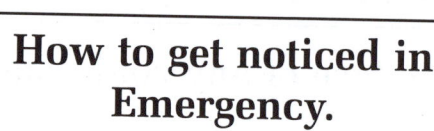

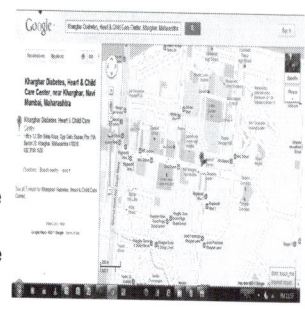

Getting Directions from Nearby.

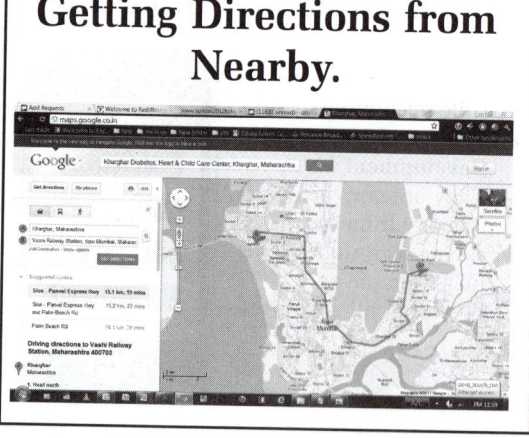

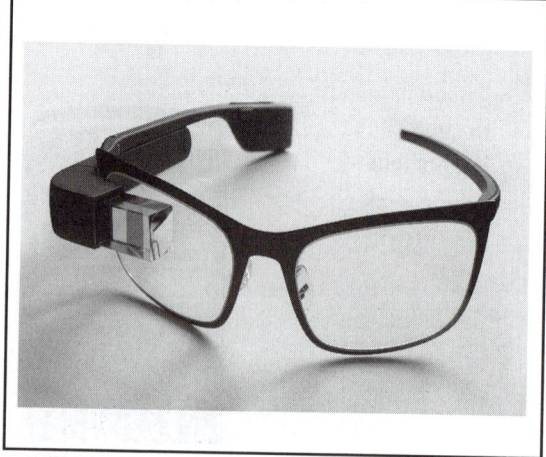

INDEX